W9-AUF-963

BENJAMIN F. MILLER, M.D.
University of Pennsylvania Medical School

JOHN J. BURT, Ed.D.
Division of Physical Education, Health
Education and Recreation
University of Toledo

W. B. SAUNDERS COMPANY · Philadelphia &

GOOD HEALTH

PERSONAL AND COMMUNITY

London

SECOND EDITION

W. B. Saunders Company:

West Washington Square
Philadelphia, Pa. 19105

12 Dyott Street
London W.C.1

Reprinted November, 1966, September, 1967, February, 1968 and May, 1968

Good Health

Press of W. B. Saunders Company. Library of Congress catalog card number 66-12325.

To
JUDITH W. MILLER
and
to
PEARL and JOHNNY BURT

This edition of Good Health: Personal and Community *appears under changed authorship owing to the untimely death of Zelma Miller, Ph.D., who collaborated in the writing of the First Edition. The new coauthor, Dr. John Burt, is Associate Professor of Physical Education and Health at the University of Toledo, Toledo, Ohio. His special field of knowledge in human physiology, applied programs, and educational organization has been blended with the medical science areas for which I retain responsibility. Our association has been rewarding in personal and professional results.*

BENJAMIN F. MILLER

PREFACE

From the moment of publication of the First Edition of *Good Health*, we have queried teachers and students on preference of content and method of presentation. Their suggestions have proved most helpful to us in preparing this revision. The reader will note that federal legislation, changing public health patterns, and modified religious attitudes on many socioeconomic problems have also influenced content. The chapters on degenerative and organic diseases have received special attention, as have sections on marriage and family planning, sex education, tobacco, alcohol and drugs, personal medical care programs, and mental health.

Many new illustrations, including an eight-page folio of anatomical drawings, have been added to the text. The authors wish to thank Simon and Schuster, and Golden Press for materials borrowed from *The Complete Medical Guide* and *The Modern Medical Encyclopedia*. We are grateful to Dr. Edward B. Rosenberg for his editorial help in preparation of the manuscript. Our thanks also to W. B. Saunders Company and their employees, who have given generously of time and resources to speed this endeavor.

Benjamin F. Miller
John J. Burt

ACKNOWLEDGMENTS

The authors and publisher gratefully acknowledge the help of those who have granted use of photographs and illustrations for this book. Credits appear in the legends of many illustrations throughout the book. Additional credits are given alphabetically below. Pages on which illustrations appear follow the name of the person or company granting permission for use of this material.

Abbott Laboratories, North Chicago, Illinois, 193
American Cancer Society, Inc., New York, New York, 244
American Heart Association, New York, New York, 232, 233, 238
Bergman Associates, Brooklyn, New York, 220, 390, 391
Department of Health, New York, New York, 200, 444 (right), 455, 457
Harry F. Dowling and Tom Jones: *That the Patient May Know*, Philadelphia, W. B. Saunders Co., 126, 140, 439
Fairchild Aerial Surveys, New York, New York, 469
Philip Gendreau, New York, New York, 306
General Electric, Milwaukee, Wisconsin, 249, 297, 476
Gesell Institute, New Haven, Connecticut, 123
Ormond Gigli, New York, New York, 307
John Henderson: *Emergency Medical Guide,* New York, McGraw-Hill Book Company, 38
Illuminating Engineering Society, New York, New York, 416
National Association for Mental Health, New York, New York, 83
National Institute for Mental Health, Bethesda, Maryland, 75, 231
National Tuberculosis Association, New York, New York, 171
Stephenson Corporation, Shrewsbury, New Jersey, 266
Suzanne Szasz, New York, New York, 152, 153, 154, 386
Taylor Instrument Company, Rochester, New York, 30
United Cerebral Palsy Association, New York, New York, 212, 213
United States Department of Health, Education and Welfare, 444 (left), 468
Western Publishing Company, 73, 89, 123, 166, 205, 269, 282, 299, 317, 414, 419
Wide World Photos, New York, New York, 268
Elizabeth Wilcox, Riverdale, New York, 301, 302

CONTENTS

SECTION ONE

INTRODUCTION

1

HEALTH EDUCATION

The aim of health education is to help people to achieve health by their own actions and efforts. Health education begins therefore with the interest of people in improving their conditions of living, and aims at developing a sense of responsibility for their own health betterment as individuals, and as members of families, communities, or governments.

WORLD HEALTH ORGANIZATION TECHNICAL REPORT, SERIES NO. 89, 1954

College years are perhaps the most challenging and exciting ones in our lives. It is during these years that we leap forward from girlhood or boyhood into adulthood. Indeed, some of you will be married, some even parents, by the time you graduate. For many of you college will mark the last rung on a long ladder of formal education.

When you reach graduation day, will you be a fully realized, mature graduate? Will you have become the person you truly wanted to become? Will the impressions, the general knowledge, and the special skills you have acquired be worth the time, work, and worry you had to expend? The answers to these important questions depend on you—and how fully, wisely, and advantageously you use your college years. Thomas Edison said that he never invented anything by accident but only through careful planning and hard work. So it is with becoming educated; it does not happen by accident or without hard work.

It is an important task to decide what one wants from college; moreover, it is a decision that you and you alone can make. In the course of making this important decision, however, it is helpful to discuss the problem with your friends, teachers, and parents.

Having decided on the goal of your college years, you should then plan your courses carefully. Much of your future happiness will depend on the adequacy of cultural and professional knowledge gained in the college classroom. In addition to formal classwork, you should devote yourself to the problems of good social adjustments; of rewarding relationships with your contemporaries, teachers, and parents; and of thoughts about approaching marriage and parenthood.

To a large extent, success in all these important areas depends on good physical and emotional health and also on the confidence that comes from understanding how to use and to protect the precious possessions of your body and mind.

HEALTH SCIENCE AS A PART OF THE COLLEGE CURRICULUM

Many colleges and universities are currently requiring students to take a group of courses considered to be valuable, irrespective of the individual's chosen field of study.

Health science is included in these required subjects because the state of your health is basic to your ability to perform well in classes and throughout life. No one denies the importance of good health, and if there were some way to obtain a guarantee of lifelong good health, we would all be willing to pay a handsome price for it.

The real question, therefore, is not the importance of health but rather how a course in health science can aid you in maintaining good health. Such a course can help you to achieve a long, healthy life; it cannot guarantee it. The authors of this text and the instructor in your course believe that if the knowledge gained from a study of health science is put to use in daily living, the chances for attaining optimal—even superb—good health will be greatly increased. It is for this reason that a course in personal and community health is included in the general curriculum and the authors have undertaken to write this text.

Understanding the Human Body. The human body is a unique and remarkable possession, but we are provided with "only one to a customer."

Two hundred and six bones provide the basic structure on which over 600 muscles enable you to make every conceivable type of movement and gesture. Within this framework are supported the organs that carry out miracles of chemistry and physics needed for the coordination of activity and conscious thought. The human heart does a pumping job that has never been duplicated. Without ever shutting down for repairs it works away, pumping in a lifetime 60 million pounds of blood.

The kidneys, responsible for purifying the blood of waste chemicals, do this by means of 2 million tiny filter units. Each unit works so perfectly that our most expert engineers have been able to approach with only a crude approximation the selectiveness and sensitiveness of the kidney. Yet these 2 million elaborate microfilter units can fit into the space of your two fists.

The liver works so silently that we are unaware of its function. Yet it carries out more than 500 different chemical operations vitally needed for proper functioning of our bodies.

Certainly no less remarkable is the human brain. With some 15 billion nerve units, it produces memory imprints in ways still to be understood and not yet duplicated by even the greatest chemists and physicists. It is a marvelously effective machine, operating through chemical and electrical systems to control thought, memory, sensory responses, movement, heart rate, respiration, and dozens of other important physiological activities.

We are indeed, as the Bible tells us, "fearfully and wonderfully made."

As far as is known, our brains exemplify the highest level of evolutionary development. We are capable of an almost infinite range of creativity and artistry. Truly magnificent advances in science, mathematics, medicine, and every other intellectual area have been made in our time, and these advances continue. It is conceivable that within our lifetime many of the activities and aberrations of the human mind will no longer be a mystery, but will be explained in relatively simple chemical and physical terms.

Perhaps the most remarkable feature of our bodies and minds is the degree to which they are intertwined. The flesh and the spirit powerfully influence each other. The amazing manner of our response to sensory perception and our ability to conceive and carry out complex activities reflects the intricate interplay of nerve, muscle, and mental control in our daily activities.

A general description of the body and how it works is essential to the study of health science. Therefore, basic material on anatomy and physiology is presented in Chapter 2 as an aid to understanding normal development, as well as abnormal function and structure.

Understanding Disease. Many persons know virtually none of the elementary facts about illness, although this information might some day represent the difference between life and death to them. Some real life cases will serve to sharpen this point.

For a number of weeks a young boy, whose name was Freddy, had complained to his parents of feeling out of sorts. He was slowly and steadily losing weight and also appeared to be losing his strength. He spoke frequently of how thirsty he was much of the time.

His parents were not really alarmed until they noticed one afternoon that he was unusually drowsy, almost stuporous. At that time, unfortunately several weeks too late, they telephoned the doctor. It was his busy season—flu, sore throats, and a measles epidemic—and they had difficulty locating him. By the time the doctor heard the story and made the diagnosis of diabetes, the child was unconscious.

Freddy was rushed to one of our best medical centers. Doctors stayed with him continuously through the night injecting insulin and administering other necessary medicines. But the boy died.

Freddy could have been saved, for today we can treat diabetes successfully, almost routinely, with insulin. Even the serious complications of acidosis and coma can be overcome if recognized early. The parents meant well, but they were ignorant of basic health science.

People often assume that the doctor takes full responsibility for their health. They consult him when they get sick and pay him for treatment and cure. But from the doctor's side of the fence a different situation is seen. Often the physician is consulted only when the illness has become dangerously far advanced. For example, Freddy's parents were unaware of the approaching tragedy during all those weeks when diabetes, untreated, was progressing toward its inevitable end. Other parents, more sensitive to medical problems, might have recognized, weeks earlier, the danger signals of excessive thirst and weight loss. The problem is one of education.

Fortunately, most potentially fatal diseases signal their onset with obvious symptoms. When a fever of 105 degrees and a violent chill strike, you know you need medical attention. And whether your symptoms result from pneumonia, meningitis, or malaria, your doctor can usually cure you if you heed the warnings.

But many serious medical conditions develop silently, without obvious warning. A woman with cancer of the uterus may suffer no illness or pain until the growth has progressed to such an extent that it may cost her life. However, it is possible to prevent serious damage from this and other insidious diseases by learning to watch for specific danger signals. Indeed, the American Cancer Society estimates that 90,000 lives could be saved annually by early detection of cancer. After you have read this book, you should know when to call the doctor and why.

A knowledge of disease is also a weapon against fear and concern. For example, a young college graduate, whose name was Janet, became emotionally upset when a friend told her that "awful things could happen to your baby if you become pregnant." Janet knew that she was Rh-negative, but that was about all she knew concerning the topic.[1] A short explanation from her physician set her mind at ease.

Ignorance of health science, as noted in Janet's case, is often a cause of real concern. An education that doesn't eliminate such basic ignorance is not complete.

Understanding Marriage and Family Living. The college years are very convenient for selecting a marriage partner. In fact, three of five Americans are married before the age of 24 years. According to the Population Reference Bureau, more girls in the United States marry at 18 than at any other age, and more men at 21. Twenty-five per cent of all 1964 college graduates were married by the time they graduated. It is likely, therefore, that you will find your mate during college and get married either before or within a short time after graduation.

---

[1]Complications in pregnancy sometimes develop when the mother builds up antibodies against the red blood cells of the developing embryo. However, modern medical science can now effectively handle these cases. A more complete discussion is found on page 154.

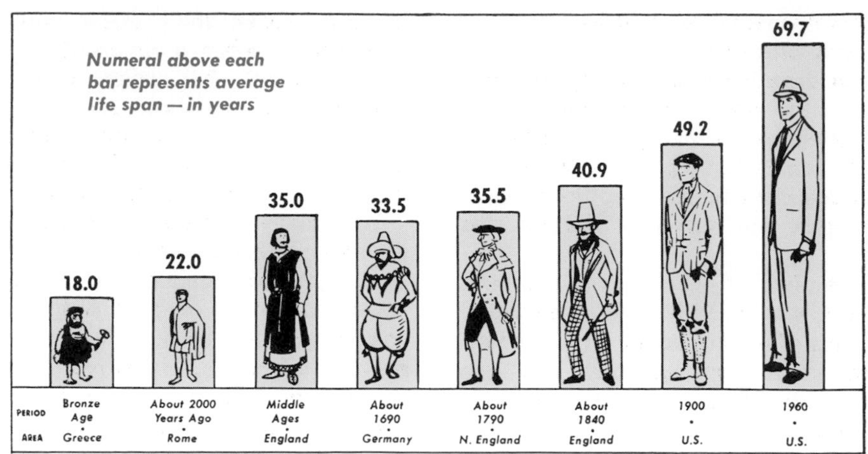

Figure 1–1. Knowledge has helped to nearly quadruple man's life-span. (Adapted from *New Medical Materia.*)

Although courtship is a time of fun and excitement, engagement and marriage should receive the most serious consideration. It is said that the average American devotes more caution to the selection of an automobile than to a marriage partner. This is attested to by the fact that the partners in one of three marriages today turn out to be mismatched. Perhaps this is because there are more objective criteria by which to select an automobile! Nevertheless, there are many basic factors to be considered in selecting a mate. These factors are discussed in Chapter 9.

In addition to selection of a husband or wife, there is much to be learned about family living—for example, pregnancy, child birth, infant care, and birth control. The college student should study all these areas carefully.

Understanding Doctors and Medicines. To obtain the best medical care for yourself and your family requires at least an elementary knowledge of doctors and their professional training. Unlicensed quacks, pretenders, and racketeers collect nearly a billion dollars each year from people who are in trouble. Frequently, their methods and machines for treating the sick are so subtle that even highly educated people are deluded by them. A discussion of the various types of doctors and their training is included in this book along with information to help you select a personal physician, intelligently purchase and use medicines prescribed by your doctor, and deal with personal problems of daily emotional stress, personal appearance, and physical safety.

SECTION TWO

THE HUMAN BODY AT WORK AND REST

2

UNDERSTANDING THE HUMAN BODY

Our total health is the summation of smooth functioning and integration of the individual parts of the body. If the mind is free from excess nervous tension, and all the vital organ systems are working at maximum efficiency, we possess the mental and physical basis for joyful, successful living.

Understanding how the body functions helps us maintain this prized state of optimum health and performance.

THE BRAIN AND THE CENTRAL NERVOUS SYSTEM

The brain is the master organ of our bodies. With it we carry out functions possible only to human beings: complex thought, creative work in the arts and sciences, and the control of speech. This remarkable organ contains 10 to 15 billion nerve units which permit the storage of millions of memory images and all the other learning that we accumulate. In addition to the memory cells, the brain has a huge number of connections, through its wide network of nerves, which control the more than 600 muscles in our bodies. The *afferent* nerves bring messages to the brain, and the *efferent* nerves carry the brain's directives to the tissues.

When we use the word "brain," we frequently imply the entire *central nervous system.* This comprises many areas in addition to the "gray matter" through which we think, remember, and carry on the functions of the conscious mind. Automatic centers in the brain control the rate and intensity of breathing, and the pumping of the heart. Certain areas react specifically to hunger, thirst, sex impulses and other primal urges.

The many brain relay stations receive the input of the sensory organs, decode the messages and translate them into appro-

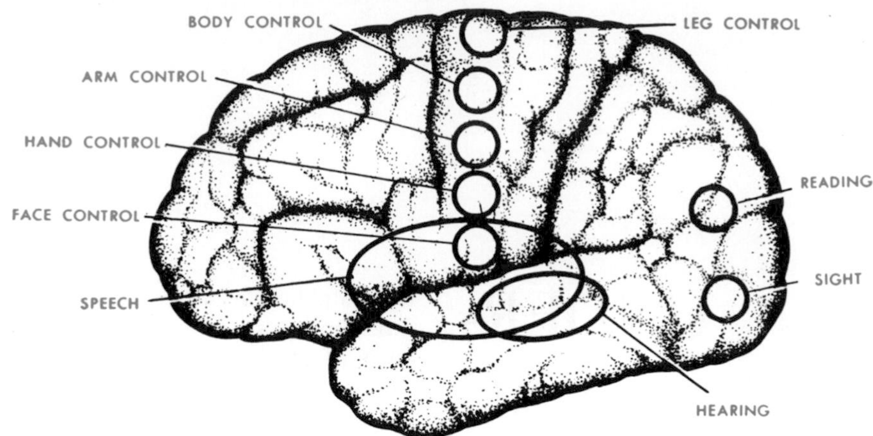

Figure 2–1. Control zones of the cerebral cortex. Nerve cells that control physical and mental activities are located in specific centers or zones of the cerebral cortex, the largest part of the human brain. The left side of the cerebral cortex with its control zones is diagrammed here. If the normal flow of blood to one of these zones is stopped, the activity controlled by the zone will be impaired. (From the pamphlet *Strokes,* American Heart Assoc.)

priate responses, such as memory storage, the recognition of sights and sounds, and immediate motor activities.

The nerves which motivate muscles are under the control of the conscious mind. In addition, there is a large section of the central nervous system which is *autonomic,* i.e., not under our conscious control. These nerve fibers carry messages to many organs and tissues, such as the heart, the sweat glands, the digestive glands, and the intestines, regulating them at their optimum point of activity.

Protection of the Brain

It is not surprising that nature had to evolve a system of defenses to guard this amazing three pound structure against injuries. The bony skull protects the brain. The scalp is the tough wrapping outside the skull that can take up blows. A tough membrane inside protects the brain. Also, the brain has an additional protective device against blows and falls: it is encased in fluid and "floats" in liquid which helps absorb traumatic shocks.

But nature can provide protection for the brain only within definite limits. She apparently never anticipated the automobile and other modern devices that can deal terrific blows.

We can help nature by protecting our brains against severe trauma. To do this we should know the hazards of boxing, football, diving, and other sports, and act to avoid skull injuries. Employ recognized safeguards learned from your athletic coach. Using safety measures does not make you a "sissy." It stamps you as a resourceful, rather than a reckless, human being. Automobile drivers should remember the terrible consequences of brain injuries when indulging in reckless speeding or other hazards. Workers must learn the physical as well as the chemical hazards on the job to prevent brain and nerve injuries.

You can help your brain operate at maximum efficiency by providing enough sleep to rest and revitalize it. And your general health and disposition will be better if you don't overstimulate the brain with too many "pep pills," too much caffeine from coffee, cola drinks, or tea; and if you don't depress it with too frequent use of alcohol, or sedatives such as the barbiturates and bromides.

You don't need special "brain foods" and tonics to keep your brain in good condition. Any well balanced diet provides all the vitamins and nourishment it needs. Fish is no better for the brain than any other protein food.

Can the effects of aging on the brain be prevented? Some of this is due to hardening of the arteries and can be prevented or diminished by maintaining a normal weight and blood pressure and taking other precautions (Chapters 18 and 26).

Headaches, dizziness, fainting, impaired

memory and other brain symptoms can be caused by conditions in and around the brain: for example, sinus trouble or a tumor. However, these symptoms could also be the result of poisons, because damaged kidneys are not removing toxic materials from the blood. In other words, any continual, unusual brain symptom calls for a complete medical checkup.

Always be on the optimistic side about your brain and its future. Think of Michelangelo, producing some of the greatest art of all times when he was more than 80; of Toscanini at 87, directing a hundred-piece symphony orchestra without referring to any musical score; and the many other people we meet in everyday life, who continue to have active, useful brains long beyond the traditional "three score and ten years."

Intellect and Memory

The brain is the only organ that can store everything we learn, all our impressions and memories. Damage to certain areas of the brain at birth can produce mental retardation. If the brain is seriously injured in later life, or affected by a tumor, this can cause loss of learned acts and impairment of the intellect and of memory.

One of the most fascinating problems in brain research is to discover how we store the images and memories of past experiences. Certain areas of the brain seem to be uniquely concerned with memory, according to investigations at the Montreal Neurological Institute of McGill University.

It has been known for some time that when the portion of the brain concerned in speech is stimulated electrically, the patient cannot speak and he behaves as though the area had been destroyed. If the patient's brain is stimulated in the area controlling vision, he experiences strange sensations—"dancing lights" and "colored balls whirling."

The brain also contains "memory centers," and stimulation of these centers with a tiny electric needle produces specific memories.

This was discovered during an attempt to locate the area of the brain responsible for epileptic seizures. The patient was a woman, under local anesthesia. When the surgeon stimulated a particular point on her brain electrically, she remarked that she was seeing herself give birth to her baby girl, more than 20 years before.

In another surgical exploration, stimulation of the brain at a specific area made the patient remark, "I hear music!" A nearby area was touched, evoking a memory of fear. When the original area was again contacted, the patient heard music, and this time she described an orchestra playing a song, which she proceeded to sing in its entirety—"Marching Along Together."

It is believed that memories are stored over a large area of the brain, and that brain cells accomplish this feat by undergoing subtle, relatively permanent changes—the equivalent of "grooving" on a phonograph record.

Consciousness

The capacity for consciousness, for "MEness" and awareness, resides in the brain, mediated by its numerous neuron pathways. But the precise mechanisms which make consciousness possible are still not understood.

In a highly personal manner, Homer Smith, physiologist at New York University Medical School, has speculated about this fascinating problem:

> . . . It is clear that my consciousness resides not in any particular atoms because the atoms that are part of me today, tomorrow will be gone from me to be replaced by others—there is scarcely one that is 'mine' for more than just a few weeks at most—but rather in their unique and transient patterns of activity.
>
> The bald facts are that, for matter to know itself in ME, ten billion neurons in my brain, and many, many times that number of functional connections are required to give me the past, the present, and the future all too inaccurately divined future that contrive this moment. Five hundred million years of vertebrate evolution have been required to produce that brain, composed of a dozen-odd sort of atoms; and, given an adequate internal environment, it can know itself in self-awareness for at most some three- or fourscore years.
>
> How all this comes about in the transient interplay of atoms and molecules, no one can answer, but this does not mean that the answer is unattainable. Science advances so rapidly that it would be rash to place a limit on its possibilities.[1]

---

[1]Smith, H. W.: *From Fish to Philosopher,* Little, Brown & Co., Boston, 1953.

What Electroencephalograms Reveal

The nervous system actually resembles a huge electrical network, in which the brain acts as the central control panel for the nervous connections to and from tissues and organs. The nerve cells themselves can be compared to batteries, and the nerve fibers—which transmit the messages—to electrical wires. Apparently the impulses carried by the nerves are electrical in nature, and this activity can be determined by the machine called the *electroencephalograph,* which picks up these electrical discharges.

Electroencephalograms are made by placing wires at various points on the scalp, and recording the electrical wave patterns or impulses which the brain emits. Much like one's fingerprints, the electroencephalogram, called the EEG, remains remarkably constant throughout adult life. The fetus and the infant show very little electrical activity, and only one rather slow rhythm. After about three months, more definite rhythms manifest themselves in the EEG. Three-year-old children possess EEG's which resemble those of adults, but the truly adult pattern emerges only at about the age of 10 or 11.

Surprisingly little difference can be found between the EEG curves of stupid and very brilliant individuals. The important difference observed is a greater minute-to-minute variation in the records of brilliant and temperamental people; dull individuals generally show unchanging records. The EEG usually changes so little with age that the record of a man of 80 looks essentially the same as that of a young adult.

The EEG's of persons suffering from various types of mental disorder are not marked by any particularly distinguishing characteristics, which has been disappointing to physicians in this field. However, these brain waves do help diagnose some abnormal conditions such as epilepsy, tumors, infections and hemorrhages in the brain.

Brain Injuries and Skull Fractures

Head injuries occur quite frequently. They may range from relatively minor bruises and cuts of the scalp to serious injuries accompanied by loss of consciousness. *Concussion* is the term used when head injury causes a jarring of the brain, usually followed by a period of unconsciousness. In most cases, recovery is spontaneous and requires no special treatment other than rest. But anyone who suffers a concussion should be watched for a few days. Increased drowsiness or development of weakness of the limbs suggests that there may be hemorrhage within the skull.

Contusion is usually less serious than concussion, and means a bruise. The terms subdural or extradural hematoma are sometimes used in connection with brain

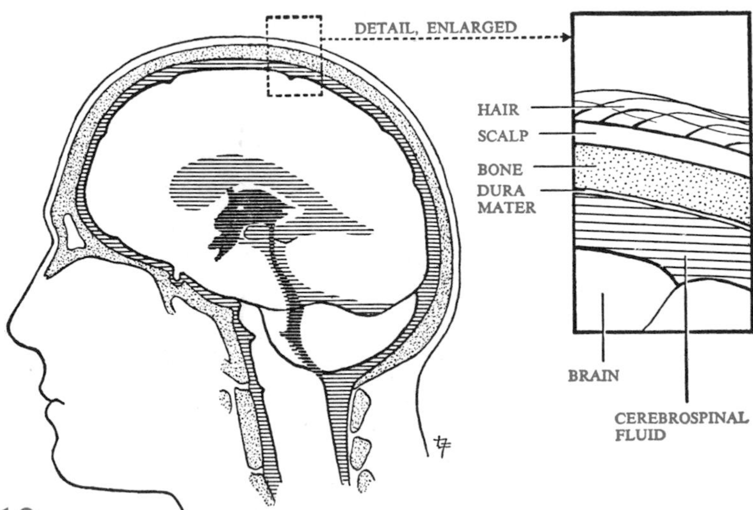

Figure 2–2. How the brain is protected. Note the number of outer coverings that provide excellent protection for the brain, and the fluid that helps absorb shocks.

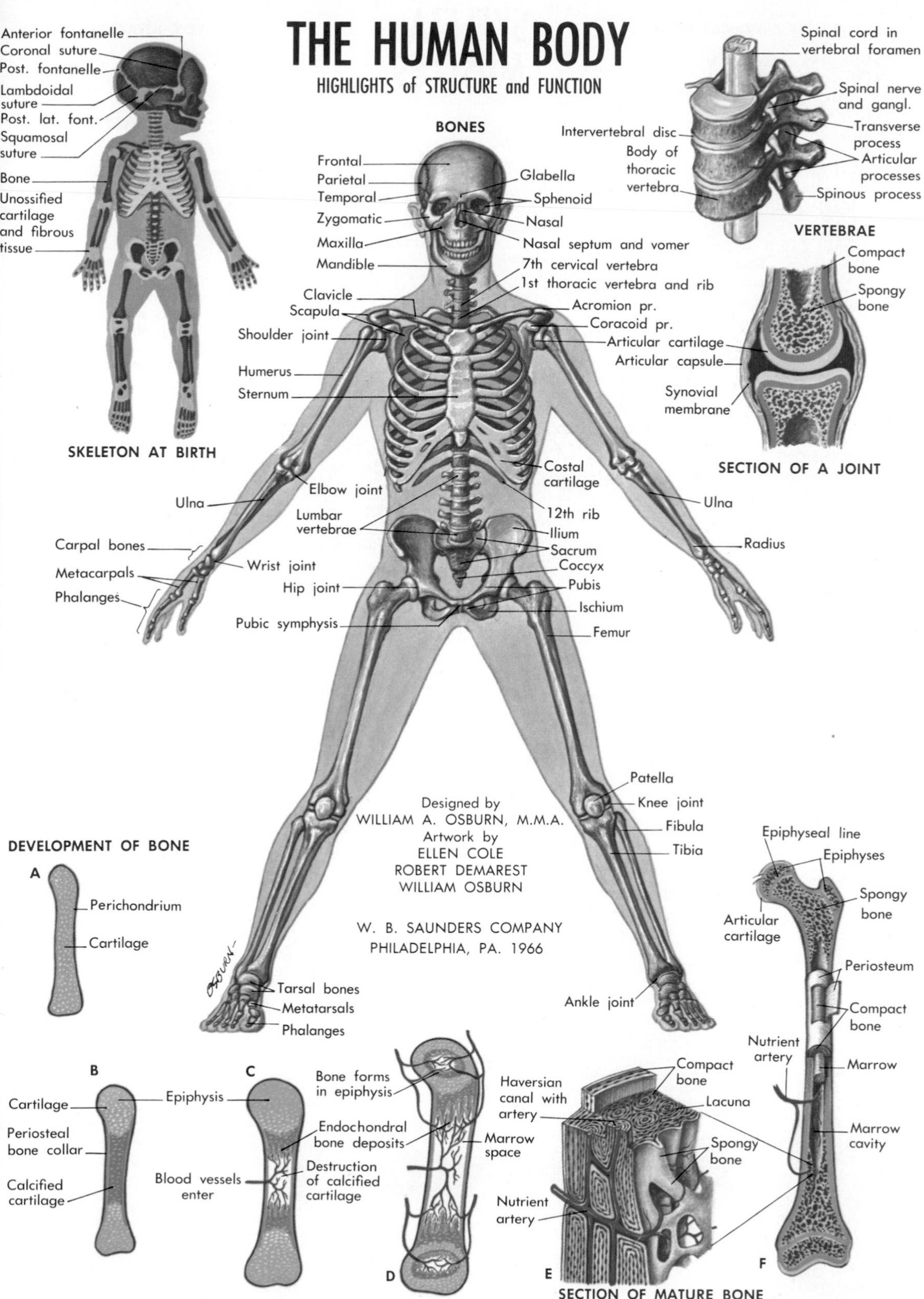
THE HUMAN BODY
HIGHLIGHTS of STRUCTURE and FUNCTION
BONES
Frontal
Parietal
Temporal
Zygomatic
Maxilla
Mandible
Glabella
Sphenoid
Nasal
Nasal septum and vomer
7th cervical vertebra
1st thoracic vertebra and rib
Clavicle
Scapula
Shoulder joint
Acromion pr.
Coracoid pr.
Humerus
Sternum
Costal cartilage
Elbow joint
Ulna
12th rib
Lumbar vertebrae
Ilium
Sacrum
Coccyx
Carpal bones
Metacarpals
Phalanges
Wrist joint
Hip joint
Pubis
Ischium
Pubic symphysis
Femur
Ulna
Radius
Patella
Knee joint
Fibula
Tibia
Tarsal bones
Metatarsals
Phalanges
Ankle joint
Anterior fontanelle
Coronal suture
Post. fontanelle
Lambdoidal suture
Post. lat. font.
Squamosal suture
Bone
Unossified cartilage and fibrous tissue
SKELETON AT BIRTH
Spinal cord in vertebral foramen
Spinal nerve and gangl.
Intervertebral disc
Transverse process
Body of thoracic vertebra
Articular processes
Spinous process
VERTEBRAE
Compact bone
Spongy bone
Articular cartilage
Articular capsule
Synovial membrane
SECTION OF A JOINT
Designed by
WILLIAM A. OSBURN, M.M.A.
Artwork by
ELLEN COLE
ROBERT DEMAREST
WILLIAM OSBURN
W. B. SAUNDERS COMPANY
PHILADELPHIA, PA. 1966
DEVELOPMENT OF BONE
A
Perichondrium
Cartilage
B
Cartilage
Periosteal bone collar
Calcified cartilage
Epiphysis
C
Blood vessels enter
Endochondral bone deposits
Destruction of calcified cartilage
Bone forms in epiphysis
Marrow space
D
Haversian canal with artery
Compact bone
Lacuna
Spongy bone
Nutrient artery
E
SECTION OF MATURE BONE
Epiphyseal line
Epiphyses
Spongy bone
Articular cartilage
Periosteum
Compact bone
Nutrient artery
Marrow
Marrow cavity
F

Plate I

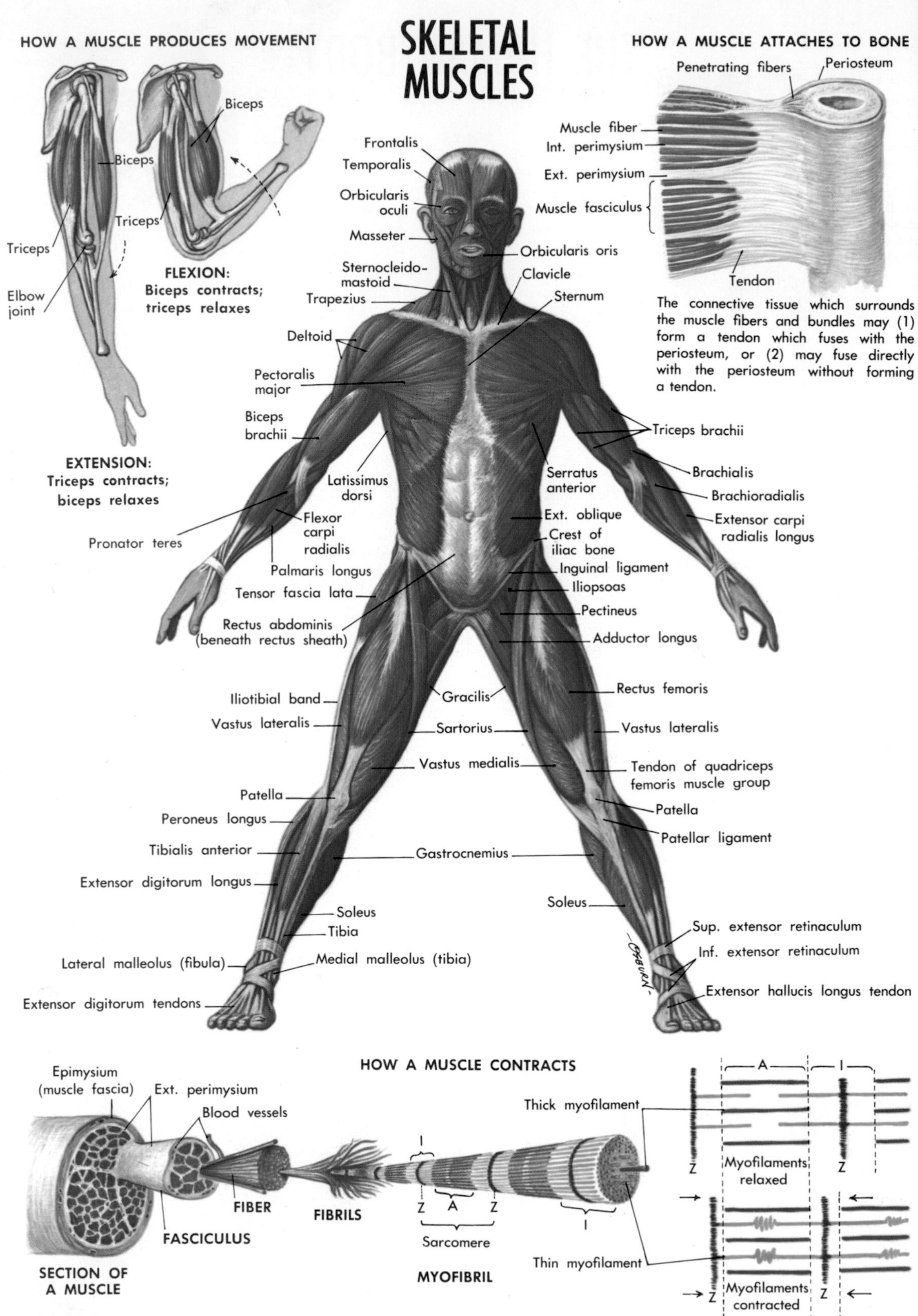
SKELETAL MUSCLES
HOW A MUSCLE PRODUCES MOVEMENT
Biceps
Biceps
Triceps
Triceps
Elbow joint
FLEXION: Biceps contracts; triceps relaxes
EXTENSION: Triceps contracts; biceps relaxes
HOW A MUSCLE ATTACHES TO BONE
Penetrating fibers
Periosteum
Muscle fiber
Int. perimysium
Ext. perimysium
Muscle fasciculus
Tendon
The connective tissue which surrounds the muscle fibers and bundles may (1) form a tendon which fuses with the periosteum, or (2) may fuse directly with the periosteum without forming a tendon.
Frontalis
Temporalis
Orbicularis oculi
Masseter
Orbicularis oris
Sternocleido-mastoid
Clavicle
Trapezius
Sternum
Deltoid
Pectoralis major
Biceps brachii
Triceps brachii
Brachialis
Latissimus dorsi
Serratus anterior
Brachioradialis
Flexor carpi radialis
Ext. oblique
Extensor carpi radialis longus
Pronator teres
Crest of iliac bone
Palmaris longus
Inguinal ligament
Tensor fascia lata
Iliopsoas
Pectineus
Rectus abdominis (beneath rectus sheath)
Adductor longus
Iliotibial band
Gracilis
Rectus femoris
Vastus lateralis
Sartorius
Vastus lateralis
Vastus medialis
Tendon of quadriceps femoris muscle group
Patella
Patella
Peroneus longus
Patellar ligament
Tibialis anterior
Gastrocnemius
Extensor digitorum longus
Soleus
Soleus
Tibia
Sup. extensor retinaculum
Lateral malleolus (fibula)
Medial malleolus (tibia)
Inf. extensor retinaculum
Extensor digitorum tendons
Extensor hallucis longus tendon
HOW A MUSCLE CONTRACTS
Epimysium (muscle fascia)
Ext. perimysium
Blood vessels
FIBER
FIBRILS
FASCICULUS
SECTION OF A MUSCLE
I
Z
A
Z
Sarcomere
I
MYOFIBRIL
Thick myofilament
Thin myofilament
A
I
Z
Myofilaments relaxed
Z
Z
Myofilaments contracted
Z

Plate II

THE ORGANS OF DIGESTION

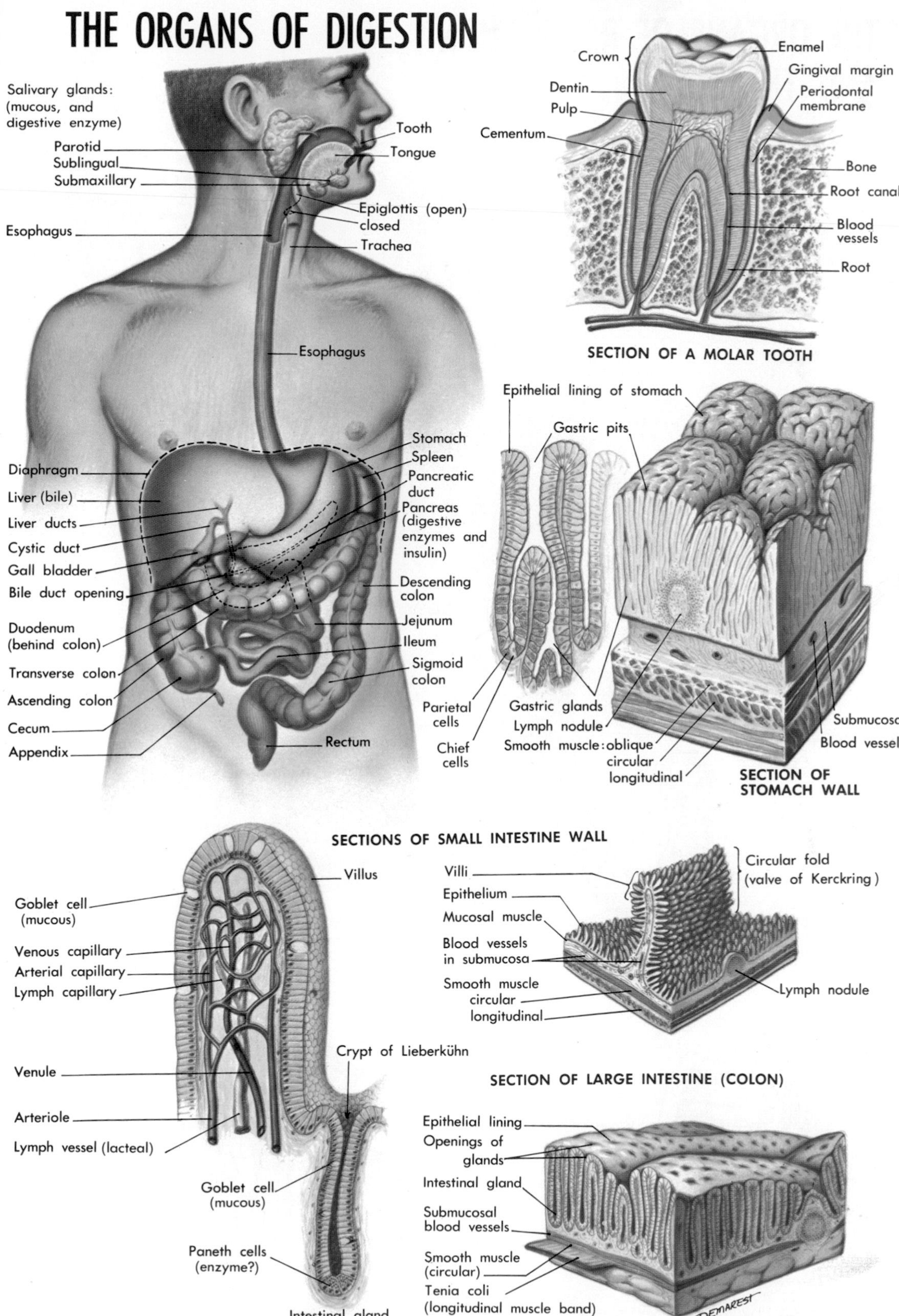

Plate III

THE ORGANS OF RESPIRATION AND THE HEART

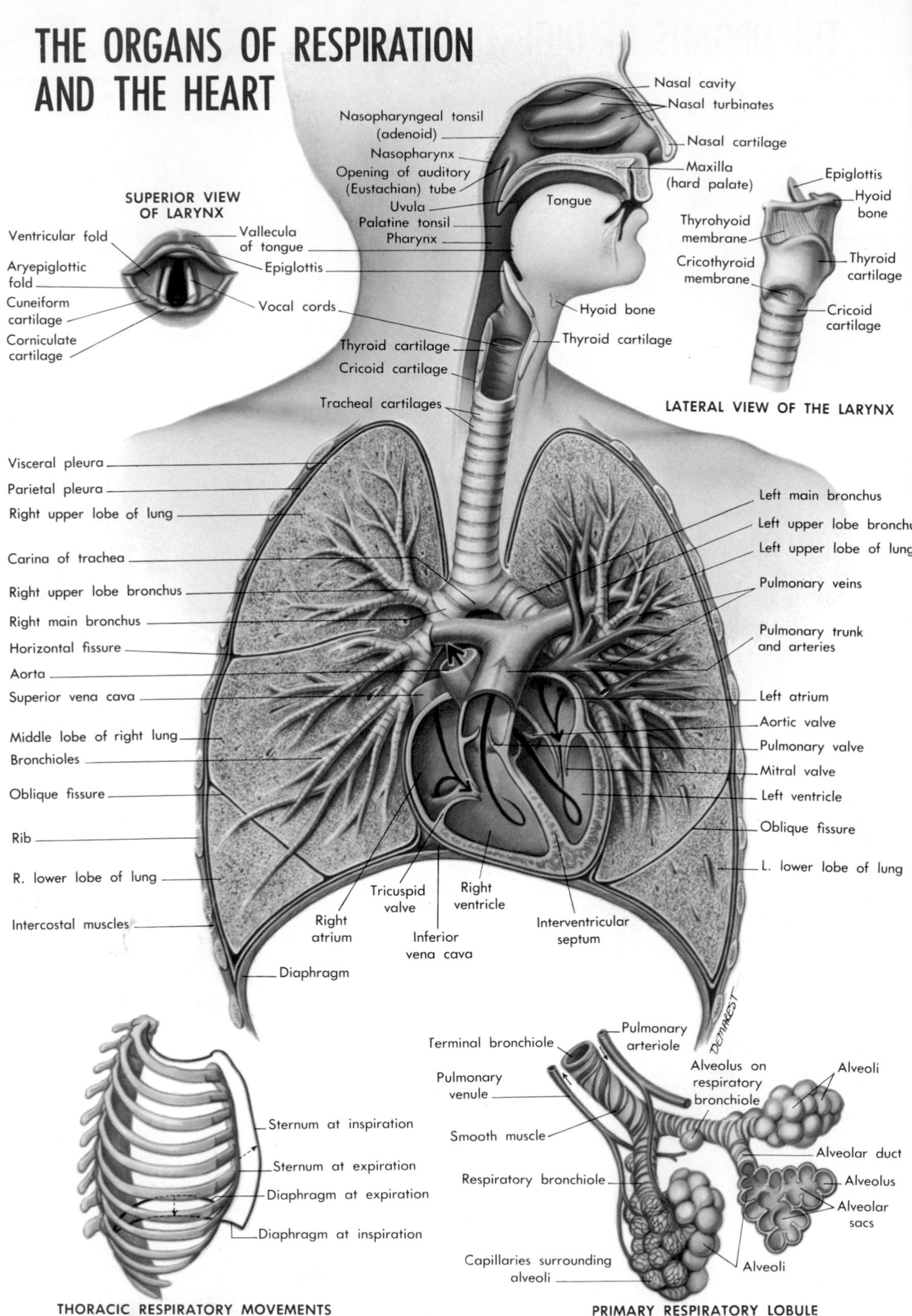

Plate IV

THE MAJOR BLOOD VESSELS

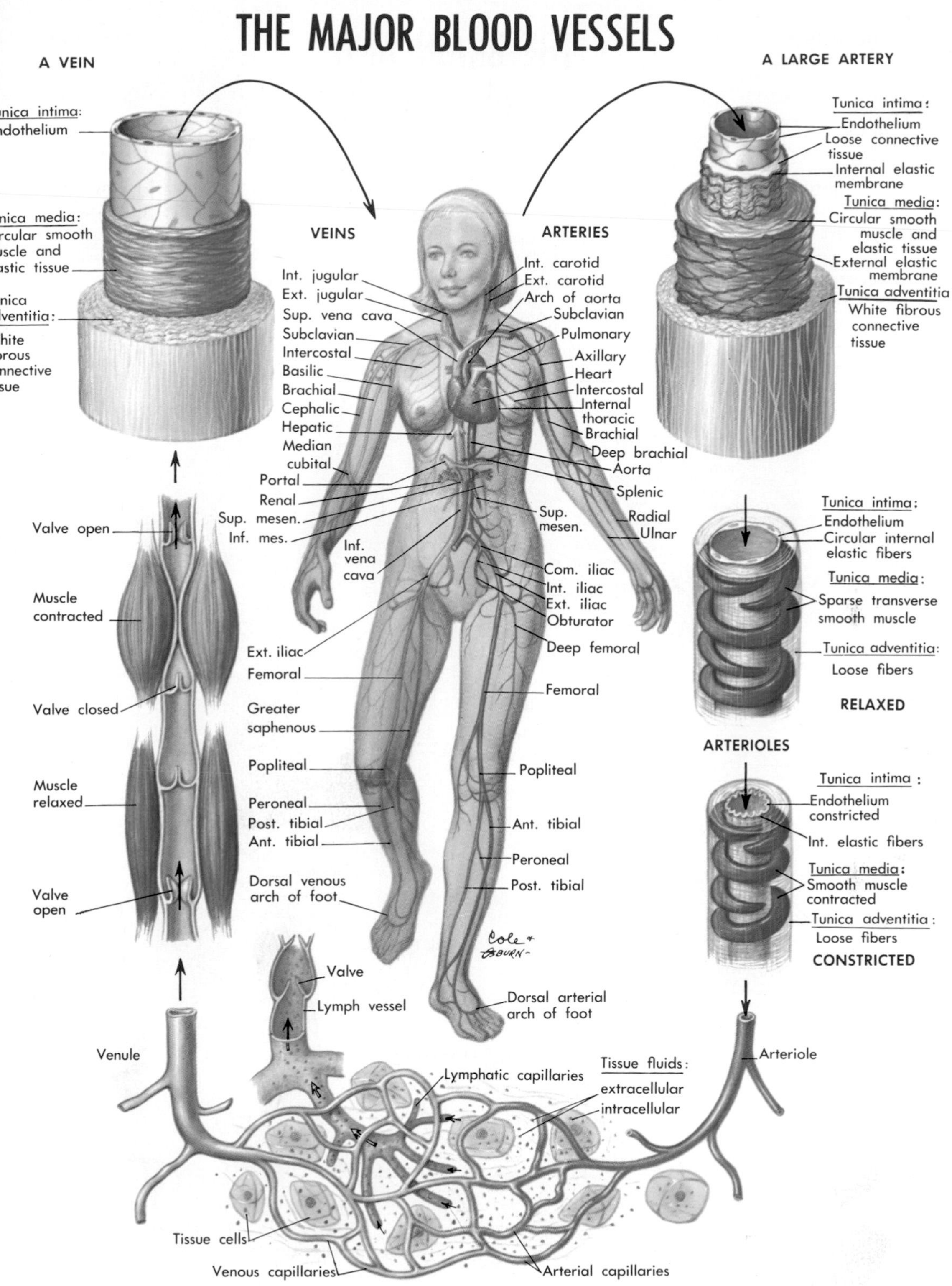

Plate V

THE BRAIN AND SPINAL NERVES

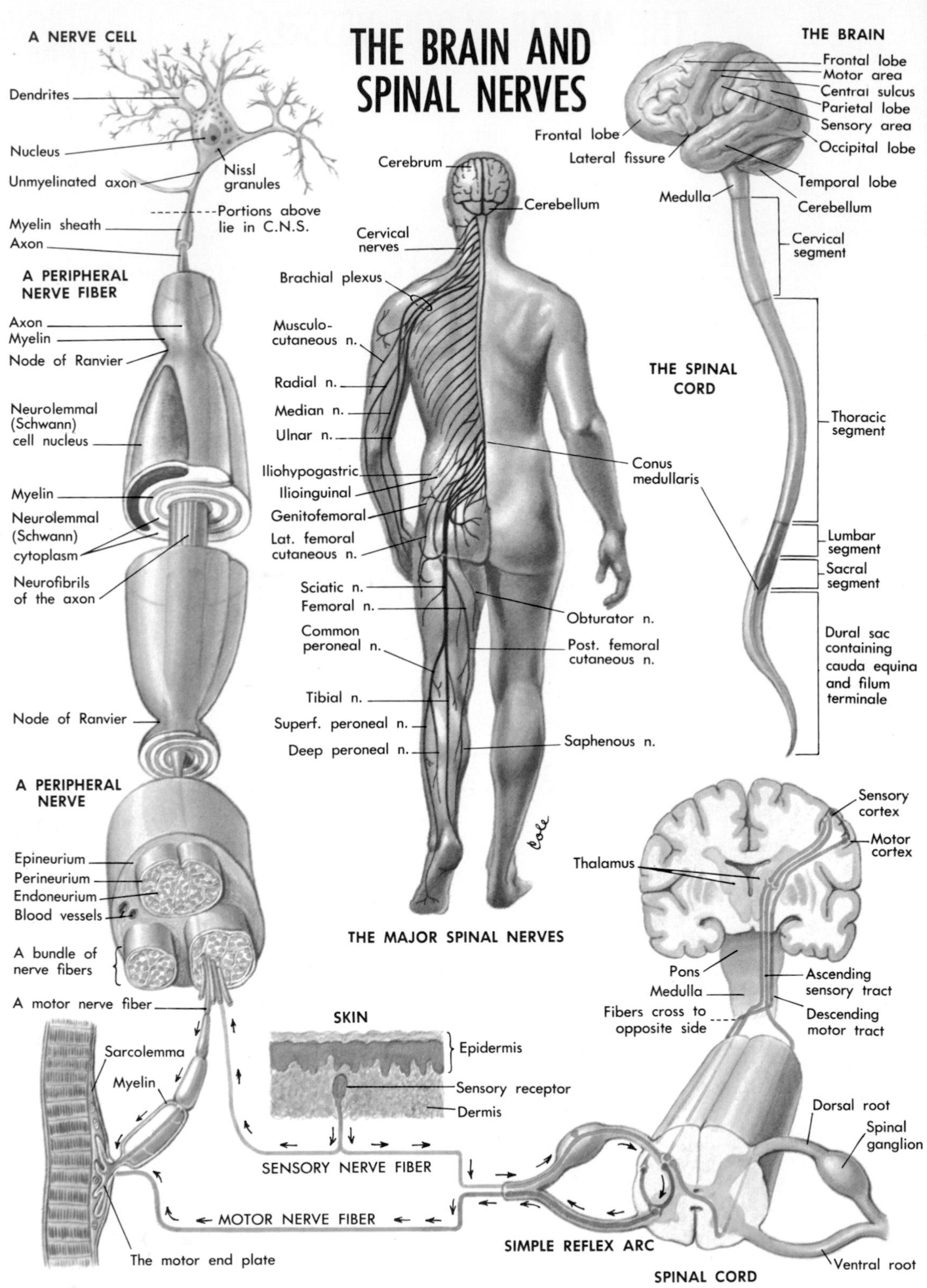

Plate VI

ORGANS OF SPECIAL SENSE AND THE PARANASAL SINUSES

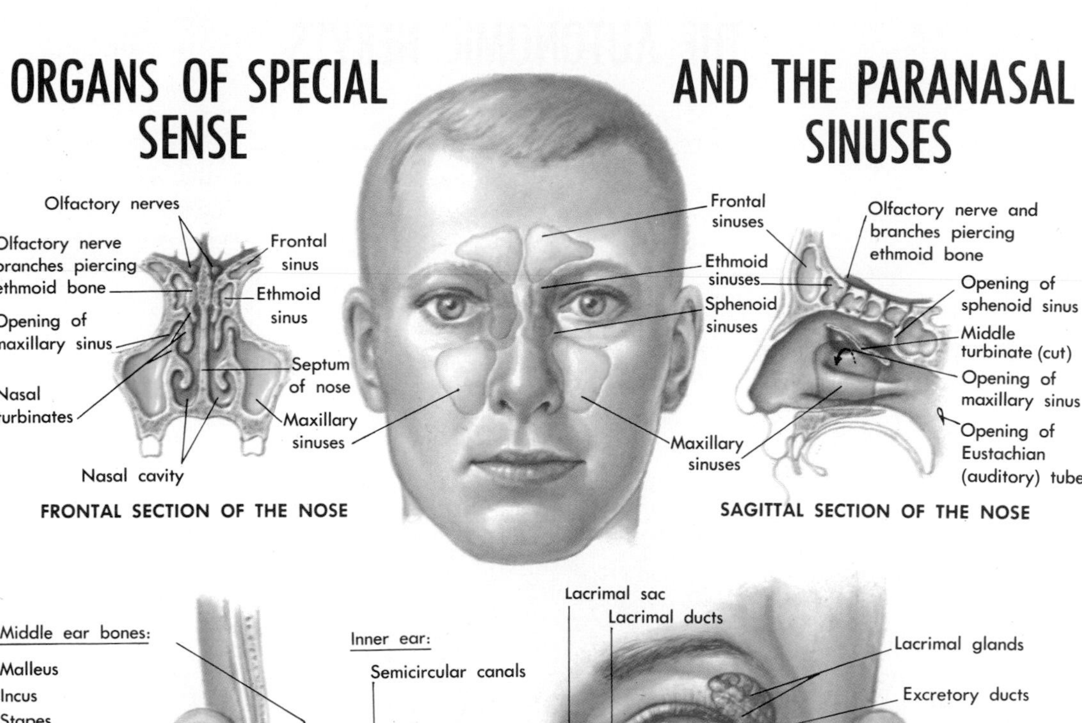

FRONTAL SECTION OF THE NOSE

SAGITTAL SECTION OF THE NOSE

THE ORGAN OF HEARING

THE LACRIMAL APPARATUS AND THE EYE

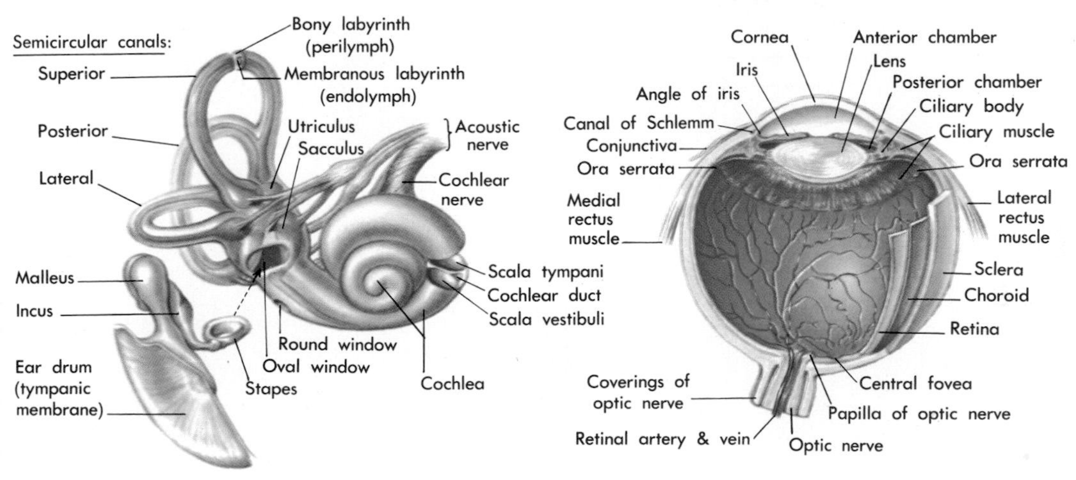

THE MIDDLE EAR AND INNER EAR

HORIZONTAL SECTION OF THE EYE

Plate VII

THE AUTONOMIC NERVES

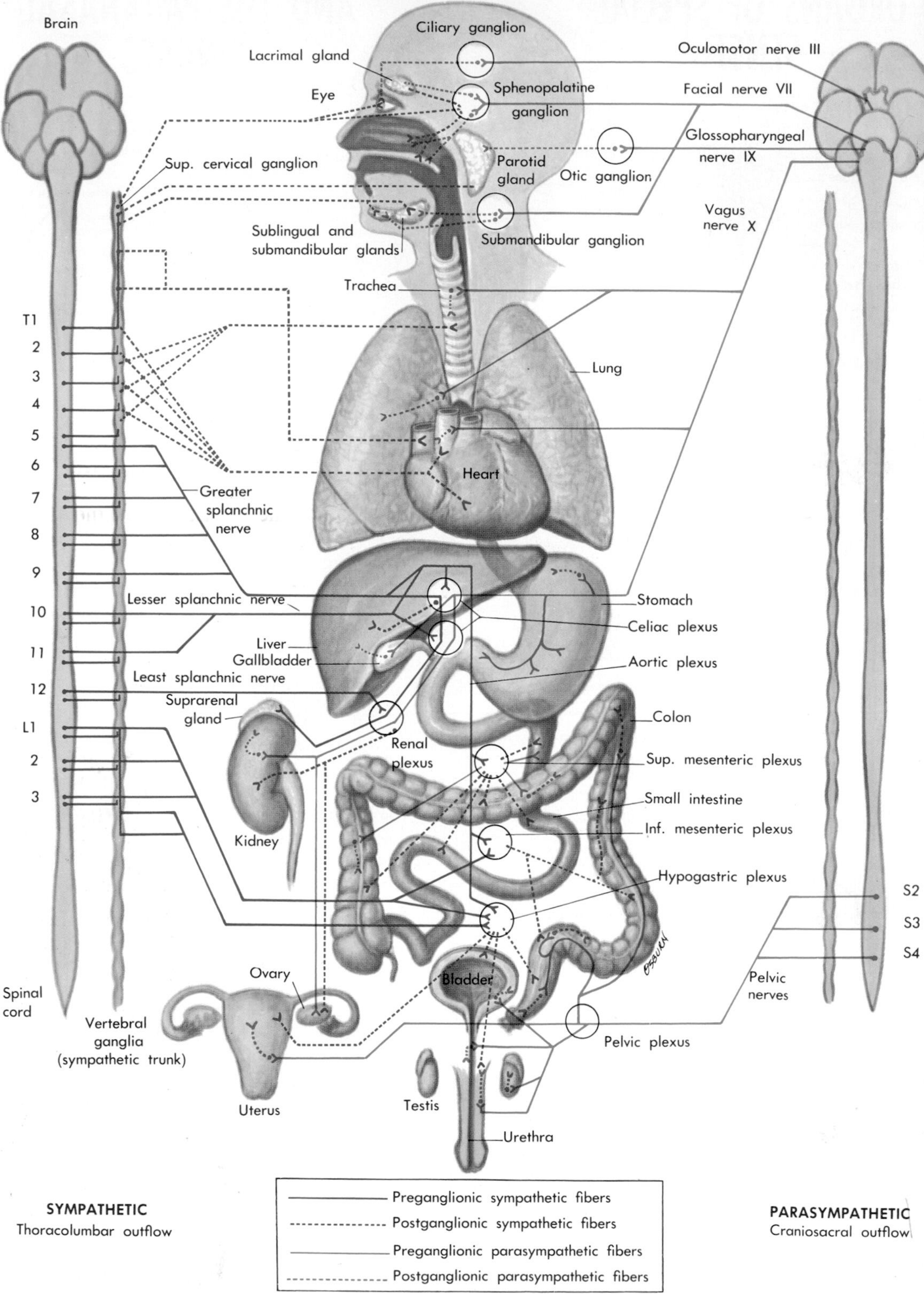

Plate VIII

injuries. These mean bleeding either underneath or above the *dura*, which is the brain covering (Fig. 2–2). Many boxers suffer repeated concussions and contusions, and their punch-drunk state is the final result.

Fractures of the skull, the bony covering of the brain, can frequently be surprisingly uncomplicated by symptoms, and cause no damage. However, healing may take a long time. You may have heard of simple versus compound fracture of the skull. Simple fractures involve a break in the bone of the skull, and they may vary from a slight fracture line to a very extensive cracking. As long as no fragments of bone penetrate the brain, they are usually uncomplicated. A compound fracture is one in which the damage is extensive enough to expose or tear the brain substance, and can be dangerous because of the possibility of direct damage to brain tissue or subsequent bacterial infection.

RESPIRATION AND CIRCULATION

The circulation of the blood can be compared to the transportation system of a large city. The individual cells of the body are the people in the city to whom the blood brings food, oxygen and all other necessities. It also trucks away the waste products. If this transportation system fails, the cells cannot survive. Death of the body results.

Food is digested in the intestinal tract to breakdown products which the body cells can use. These are absorbed from the intestines and transported by the blood to all the tissues. In the same way, cells receive their full supply of hormones, which are also secreted into the blood.

Blood is also essential for the transport of oxygen to tissues and of waste gases away from them. In the lungs continuous oxygenation of the blood and discharge of carbon dioxide and other waste gases occur.

This would be a useless system without a very efficient pump to send the blood on its various routes around the body. We possess just such a pump in the heart and its auxiliary valves, which are discussed in Chapter 18.

Lungs and Respiration

The two lungs, which, like the heart, are completely encased by the ribs of the *thorax* (chest cavity), lie on each side of the heart. They act like bellows, sucking in air through the trachea when the chest cavity gets bigger, and expelling it when the cavity contracts. The *diaphragm* and other muscles expand the chest during respiration. This process goes on at the rate of about 12 to 16 times a minute, increasing in speed when the body is active and more oxygen is needed. It is an automatic process, although we can deliberately take in a breath and keep from expelling it for a while. It is possible to work these "bellows" by artificial respiration or with an iron lung, if they can't function by themselves.

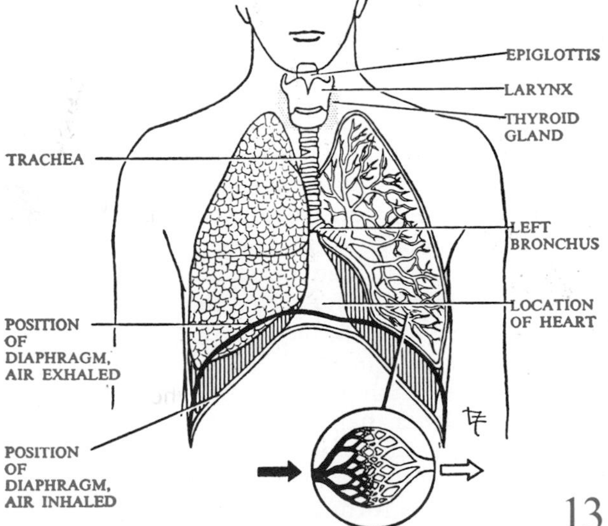

Figure 2–3. The lungs. **Left,** Outer surface of the lung. **Right,** Internal structure of the lung. **Inset,** Network of blood vessels in a microscopic section of the lung, showing (in black) the blood before picking up oxygen, and (in white) the blood containing oxygen.

The air goes to the lungs via the *trachea* (windpipe), which divides into smaller tubes called the *bronchi.* The lungs are subdivided into lobes. Hence, *broncho-pneumonia* means infection of the bronchial tubes, and *lobar pneumonia* refers to infection of one of the large portions of the lungs. Asthma is properly called *bronchial asthma* because it affects the air tubes.

Fortunately, the lungs have a tremendous reserve capacity. It is possible to live comfortably even if one lung has been completely destroyed or removed. But there must be a definite amount of healthy lung tissue in order to breathe adequately. If too much of it becomes infected or destroyed, the patient eventually succumbs because of lack of oxygen. In severe infections of the lungs, such as pneumonia and tuberculosis, the sick person faces an additional danger from the toxins, or poisons, of the bacteria causing these diseases.

The Heart and Circulation

The heart is a muscular, pear shaped organ, slightly bigger than your fist, and it is composed of four chambers, separated by valves. Enclosed by a protecting sac (the *pericardium*), it is located in the left front portion of the chest. Actually, the heart is a four-chambered pump, sending blood to all parts of the body through the *arteries* which divide and subdivide, eventually forming the tiny *capillary* vessels. These, in turn, merge with *veins* that carry the blood back to the heart.

Your heart beats automatically at the rate of 70 to 80 times a minute, or about 40,000,000 times a year, every year of your life. Its pace increases when the body is active, decreases when it is at rest. Most people can't consciously influence its speed. If your heart beats at a slower rate, that doesn't mean there is anything wrong with it. In fact, a well trained athlete may have a heart rate of 30 to 40 beats a minute. Your heart may also beat somewhat faster than 80 times a minute and still be perfectly normal.

Because the heart is such an essential organ, it is fortunate that it is an extremely tough one. Protected by the tough and resilient ribs, the heart is rarely damaged by a blow. Although you may have heard that it is "delicate," the heart has been handled by surgeons who have successfully sewn up wounds in it, and have even repaired the valves and corrected malformations.

Care of the Heart. The great enemies of the heart are: *coronary artery disease* (hardening of the arteries); *high blood pressure* (hypertension); *rheumatic fever* (*not* rheumatism, which does not affect the heart); *congenital heart disease; nephritis* (Bright's disease); *diabetes;* and *syphilis.* These include the *cardiovascular-renal* diseases, so called because they involve the circulatory system and the kidneys, as well as the heart.

The human body has often been compared to an automobile: the *brain* would be the steering wheel; the *heart,* the motor; the *kidneys,* the exhaust pipes; and the *glands,* the accelerators and brakes. E. Hunter Wilson has pointed out that "there are only two major differences between the human body and a car. One is that the body is a more intricate mechanism. The other is that most people take better care of their automobiles than they do of themselves." *This applies particularly to the heart.* You're usually very careful of what you put into your car, and choose the best oil for smooth running, the best gas for the most mileage, and you check the battery water regularly. Very few people employ as much care in choosing their diets and general hygiene habits to obtain maximum "mileage" and performance from their hearts.

Loading a car excessively makes the motor overwork and overheat. Overloading the human body—putting on excess weight—causes an even greater strain on the heart. *Overweight is one of the greatest preventable causes of heart disease in the world today.* In addition, it increases the tendency to high blood pressure and diabetes, both of which are harmful to the heart. Mortality rates are 80 per cent higher in obese persons 20 to 29 years old than in persons of the same age group whose weights are normal. And about 20 per cent of Americans are overweight.

You don't race your car motor exces-

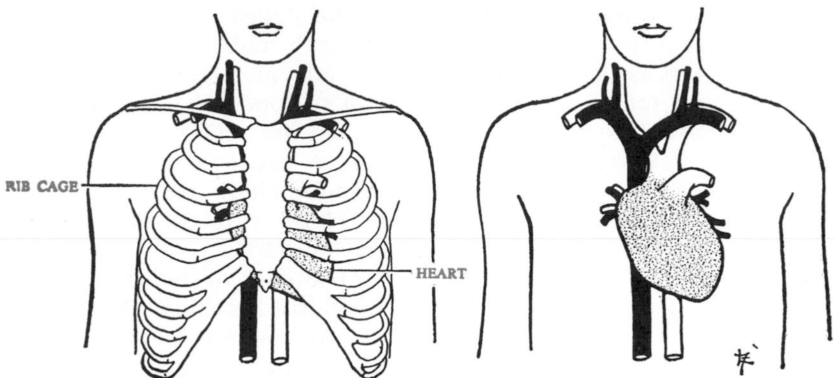

Figure 2-4. Location of the heart. **Left,** The protective bony structure. **Right,** The blood vessels from the body (in black) and to the body (in white).

sively, nor deliberately take it over rough roads, nor run it at high speed all the time. Why not give your heart similar care? Far too many people strain their hearts and increase their blood pressure by working too hard and not getting enough rest.

When a car gets older, one doesn't expect the same performance as when it was young. The human heart, too, should get some extra consideration when it becomes older. Above all, the thousand mile checkup and lubrication you give your car should be extended to your heart, in the form of a regular, periodic medical checkup, especially when you reach the age at which you are prone to heart disease. (Heart diseases, a major cause of death today, are discussed in Chapter 18.)

Cardiac Surgery. Without a doubt, one of the most thrilling chapters of medical science is found in the remarkable advances in cardiac surgery within the past ten years. Today, because of specialized surgical methods, doctors are able to rehabilitate thousands of patients who would previously have died or have lived as chronic invalids. There are now operations for such heart conditions as certain types of damaged valves and for birth deformities such as patent ductus arteriosus, coarctation of the aorta, and the defects which give rise to "blue babies." Techniques have been perfected to empty the heart of blood completely during surgery and to connect the patient's circulation to an "artificial heart" while the surgeon repairs the damaged heart.

As an indication of their gratitude because, like Lazarus, they "have risen from the dead," a group of heart surgery patients who were operated on at the Peter Bent Brigham Hospital in Boston have formed a national organization called *Mended*

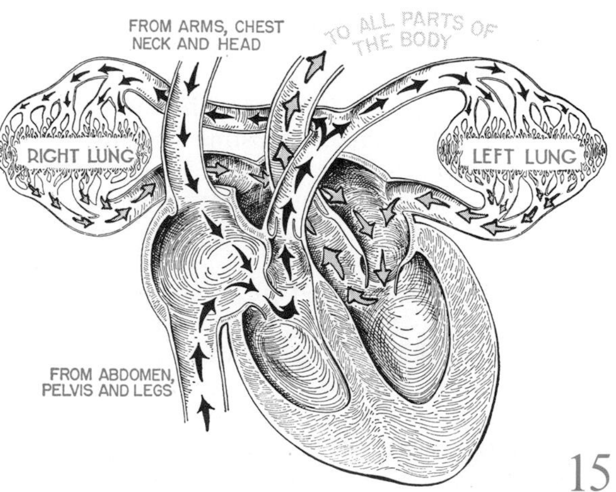

Figure 2–5. Course of blood through the heart. The blood flows from the body (black arrows) into the right side of the heart. From there (black arrows) it goes to the lungs, it returns (grey arrows) to the left side of the heart, and is sent through the body (grey arrows). (From Dowling and Jones: *That the Patient May Know.*)

Hearts, Incorporated. Active membership is limited to individuals who have undergone heart surgery, and associate membership to friends and relatives of heart surgery patients who wish to participate in the program. They visit, write to, encourage and help in whatever ways they can, other people undergoing or preparing for heart surgery.

Ingestion, Digestion and Excretion

By a remarkable and economical process, the human body is able to digest food to forms it can use for energy or for building and replenishing the body's tissues and organs. The human body is a very efficient factory, carrying out extremely complicated chemical reactions under very mild conditions. The secret is that the living cell produces efficient chemical catalysts, called *enzymes,* which perform a multitude of reactions, normally requiring conditions of very high temperature, acidity or pressure. The foods the body wants are then absorbed from the intestines, and distributed to the tissues by the blood stream or the lymph circulation. The residue is excreted through the kidneys, in the form of urine, or by way of the large bowel, as feces.

STOMACH, INTESTINES AND COLON

The *stomach,* which is located in the abdominal cavity, resembles a bag, approximately a foot long and six inches wide. The narrow small intestines are about twenty feet long, and the *colon,* or large intestine, is about five feet long. The *esophagus* is the tube which connects the throat to the stomach. The stomach ends and the small intestine begins at the *duodenum.* This structure is very important because the main ducts from the *pancreas, liver,* and *gallbladder* discharge juices and bile into it.

Food is churned up, acted upon by juices, and digested in the stomach and intestines, the residue being eliminated through the *rectum* and *anus.* Actually, the mouth itself, in which the food is chewed and mixed with saliva, is a part of the *digestive,* or *gastrointestinal, system.*

The delicate and sensitive lining of the stomach and intestines synthesizes juices and enzymes for the digestion and absorption of food. The stomach and intestines, which are controlled by a network of nerves, are constantly in motion, pushing the food along. It takes about 24 hours for the food you eat to move through the digestive tract.

Disorders of the gastrointestinal system are fairly common. Almost everyone has had some degree of difficulty in this area at one time or another.

These disorders can be functional. Because of the extensive nerve connections in the digestive system, fear, anger, and other nervous upsets may set off attacks of nausea, cramps, or diarrhea. This is probably the origin of the expression, "You give me a bellyache!" Organic diseases such as ulcer and cancer can also affect these organs, as do contagious diseases, such as typhoid fever and virus infections, as well as food poisoning, constipation, dyspepsia, allergies—and a list almost as long as the digestive tract itself.

You can protect your digestive system by taking precautions against infectious diseases by being sensible about the food you eat and the way you eat it, by avoiding poisonous and irritating substances (including excessive amounts of alcohol), and by maintaining "peace of mind" in order to prevent "nervous stomach" and other psychosomatic digestive diseases.

Perhaps even more important, you can guard the health of your stomach and intestines by *letting them alone.* Don't take enemas to "clean out the colon and get rid of germs." Nature intended the germs to be there, and a great many people would have better digestions if they had never heard the term *autointoxication.* The words *acid stomach, alkaline stomach,* and *heartburn* are equally meaningless. You cannot "cure" these nonexistent diseases by taking stomach "sweeteners," or "aids" to digestion. In fact, these medications can do real harm.

It is unfortunate that there are so many "simple remedies" for indigestion on the market, because it is by no means a simple disease. In fact, it isn't a disease at all, but a condition or group of symptoms which can be caused by any number of

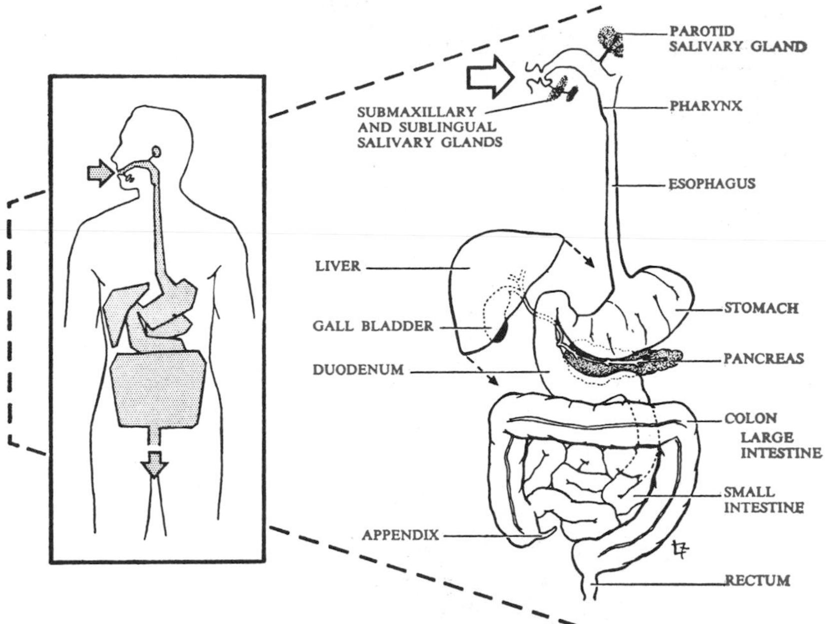

Figure 2–6. The gastrointestinal (digestive) tract. **Left,** Shaded areas indicate the location of the organs associated with digestion. **Right,** As food passes through the mouth, stomach, and small and large intestines, it is worked upon by juices manufactured in these and other organs (such as the liver and pancreas). The food is then absorbed, mainly through the intestinal walls. The residue is excreted through the rectum.

diseases, from migraine headaches to heart disease, gallbladder trouble, the onset of the flu—or simply to the fact that you bolted your dinner when you were tense and tired.

Even a skilled physician may find it a long and difficult task to determine the cause, and hence the treatment, of indigestion. He may require a complete set of x-rays after the patient takes a drink containing barium, which is opaque to x-rays; or he may have to examine the stomach with a prism-equipped instrument called a *gastroscope*. These tests are well worth while. Almost every disturbance of the gastrointestinal system which makes itself known by the symptoms of indigestion can be helped if it is identified in time.

On the other hand, a disease can progress to a serious, even fatal, stage while the patient is "treating" his indigestion—for example, taking cathartics for indigestion which happened to be caused by appendicitis. Let the doctor decide whether or not you should take any medicine, except for an occasional *mildly upset stomach.*

LIVER AND GALLBLADDER

If you place your left hand over the lowermost ribs on the right side of your chest, it will cover the liver, which is one of the largest organs in the body. It has many functions, and is involved in the processes of digestion, nutrition, and the development of the red blood cells. It also produces *bile,* which flows out through a channel into the small intestine and helps detoxify harmful substances in the blood.

There is only one *liver* in our bodies and it is an absolutely indispensable organ. Complete removal or destruction will be followed by death in a very short time. Fortunately, nature has given us a tremendous amount of reserve liver tissue. It has been estimated that more than 80 per cent of the liver cells can be damaged or destroyed before symptoms of liver insufficiency will appear. Another saving feature is the liver's great capacity for regeneration and rebuilding itself after disease has injured the cells, or even destroyed large numbers of them.

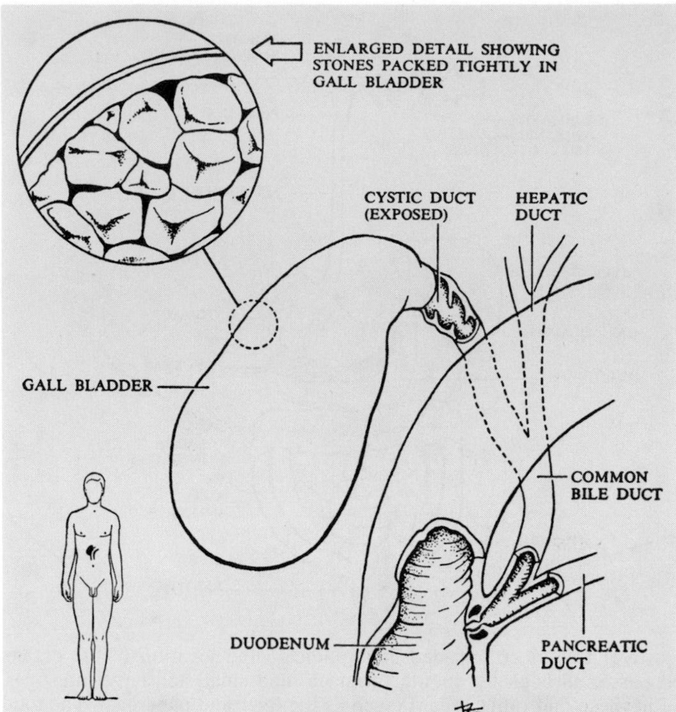

Figure 2–7. The gallbladder.

The liver in a healthy body does *not* need to be "stimulated" by medicines such as those which claim to "increase the flow of bile." However, there are ways to prevent damage to your liver. Protect it from the harm which can result from excessive drinking of alcoholic beverages, and from poisons such as *carbon tetrachloride* to which you may be exposed at work or while engaged in hobbies that require solvents. Obesity also damages the liver. A good, balanced diet and normal weight prevents this.

Damage to the liver, such as that caused by a virus infection, can manifest itself by the appearance of jaundice. This causes a yellowing of the skin and, particularly, of the whites of the eyes.

The gallbladder is a "side pocket" in the channel through which the bile flows from the liver into the intestine. It acts as a storage place for the bile, which is important in digestion, especially the digestion of fats. Infection may cause an acute or chronic inflammation of the gallbladder. Gallstones sometimes cause a great deal of pain, or they may block the flow of bile, causing jaundice and infection in the liver and gallbladder. Fortunately, the gallbladder can be surgically removed. The body can get along without it.

KIDNEYS

The kidneys are two organs located deep in the abdomen at about the level of the lowest ("floating") ribs. By means of more than two million tiny, separate filters, they filter out and remove from the blood, the urea and other useless material. They excrete these substances in the urine. The kidneys also regulate the volume of fluid in the body. When you drink a large amount of fluid, the kidneys excrete the excess, but in hot weather, when extra fluid is lost via sweat, the kidneys excrete smaller amounts of urine.

Your kidneys do *not* need to be "flushed" or "stimulated" by useless patent medicines. Trouble in the kidneys can cause pain in the lower back, and this symptom, together with changes in the urine, should always be reported to a doctor. However, contrary to the claims made for certain "kidney medicines," they can't cure *chronic pain in the back,* which is *seldom* caused by kidney trouble.

Some of the causes of kidney stones (renal calculi) are beyond our control, but preventing or curing infections helps to keep them from forming. An adequate flow of urine also helps prevent the formation of stones. The output should amount to at least a quart or more a day. When the urine becomes highly concentrated because of hot weather or because of excessive sweating at work, there is an increased tendency toward the formation of stones and the occurrence of infections. These conditions too can be avoided by drinking sufficient water.

A floating (or movable) kidney is usually not serious, although it may cause discomfort.

URINARY BLADDER

The urinary bladder and the tubes leading to and from it form, together with the kidneys, the *urinary system.* The tubes called the *ureters* carry waste products from the kidneys to the bladder. After a sufficient quantity has collected there, it is eliminated by urination through the tube called the *urethra.* The external opening of the urethra is called the *meatus.*

Infections and inflammations are fairly common, especially in the bladder. (*Cystitis* is the name for infections of the bladder.) They usually yield to treatment with antibiotic or other medicines, which *must* be given under the supervision of a doctor. Infections can be the cause of incontinence—the inability to control urination. Incontinence is natural in young children, because they have not yet developed

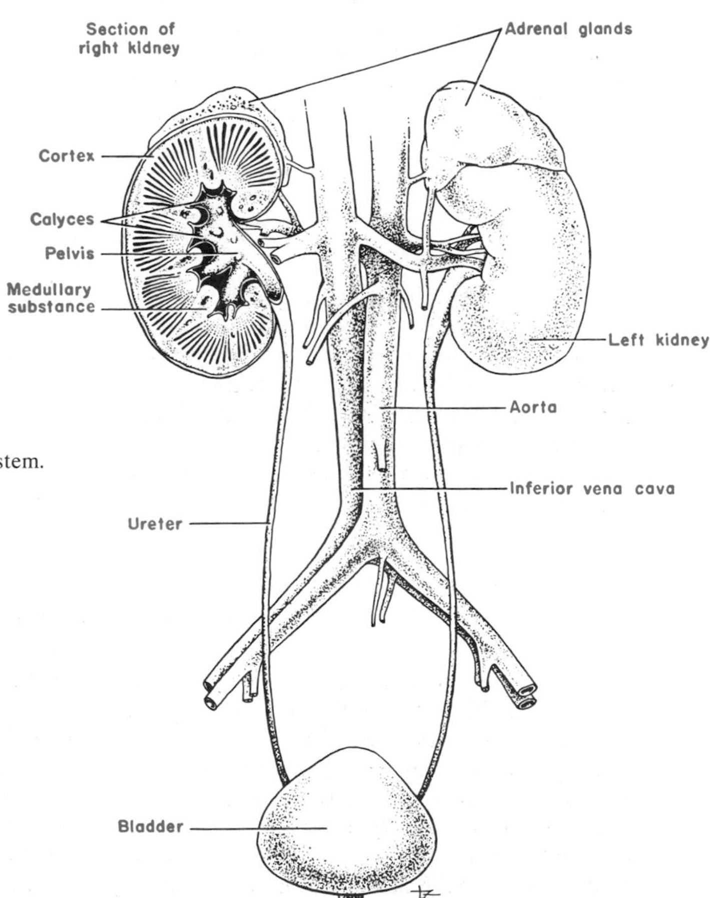

Figure 2–8. The human urinary system. (From Ville: *Biology*, 3rd Ed.)

adequate control. In older children, however, bedwetting is frequently due to emotional tension, although it can have a physical cause. Always consult a doctor if you experience *frequent, difficult, or painful urination.* It may result from an easily cured inflammation. However, it can also be caused by a disease, such as diabetes, a urethral stricture, or enlargement of the prostate gland. Stones can also form in the urinary bladder. Never take any home remedies to "dissolve" them. If necessary, stones can be removed by a surgeon.

SPLEEN

This pulpy organ is tucked away under the ribs in the upper lefthand corner of the abdomen. Its chief function is to produce certain blood cells and to store blood. Internal abdominal bleeding following an accident may come from a broken or ruptured spleen. Fortunately, the body can get along without the spleen and it can be removed surgically if injury or disease affect it.

PANCREAS

The pancreas lies high up in the abdomen, situated deep behind the stomach. In animals, the pancreas is called the sweetbread. It produces important digestive juices which flow into the small intestine. Equally important are its *islets of Langerhans,* which produce insulin. A lack of insulin causes *diabetes.*

BODY STRUCTURE AND MOVEMENT: THE SKELETOMUSCULAR SYSTEM

A human being is almost continuously in movement. His legs shift, the arms move, the head nods, the eyes blink. As he sits quietly reading, his eyes travel across the page, and fingers tilt the book to catch the light or bring the type nearer. Even in deepest sleep, when he thinks himself motionless, the human being is often in motion.

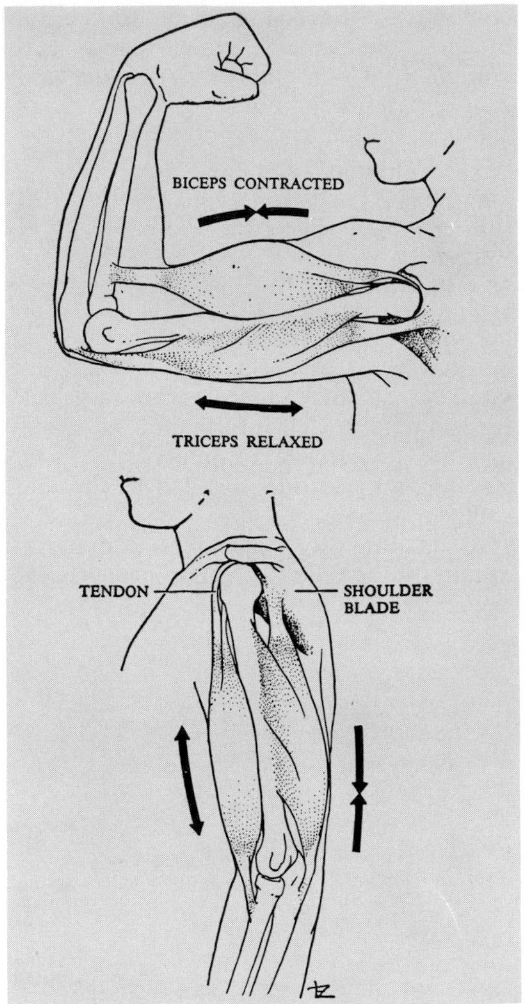

Figure 2–9. Voluntary muscular action.

Muscles: Generators of Motion

It is muscle tissue which makes this motion possible. The muscle is a collection of threadlike fibers, surrounded by a protective sheath, each fiber consisting of special tissue cells which are able to contract, and shrink in length. When a muscle is stimulated, its afferent nerve transmits a message to the brain. The efferent nerve from the brain carries the directive back to the muscle, telling it what to do. The muscle then contracts, changes its form, liberates its stored-up energy, and thus generates motion.

There are over 600 *voluntary* muscles in the human body. These give us the power to carry out an enormous variety of movements, and it is these muscles which move the bones. The muscles of movement are called voluntary, skeletal, striped, or striated muscles. These synonyms refer to muscles such as the biceps, the powerful one in the front of your upper arm, which lifts the forearm. You can feel the strong tendon in the elbow where the biceps muscle is attached to the bone.

The voluntary muscles are quick-acting, and are controlled by the conscious part of our brains. There is another group of muscles in the body which carries on activities over which we have little or no control. They propel the food along the intestines; they contract the heart; they control the pupil of the eye. These are the *involuntary muscles*.

Muscles remain in good condition only when they are exercised properly. Healthy muscles are important to a sense of well-being, and to good posture, graceful walking, and other movements. Also, strong muscles protect the bones, joints, and contents of the abdomen against injury.

Because the muscles are composed chiefly of protein, a good diet containing protein is essential for the maintenance of muscular structure.

Almost everyone has experienced a "Charley horse." This results from too violent use of a muscle or group of muscles before they have been properly trained, for example, starting summer sports or football practice.

The muscles "protest" against this unaccustomed work by soreness, stiffness and pain. The "charley horse" will clear up by resting the sore muscle. Warm baths and aspirin will also help relieve the pain. *Muscle twitchings* result from various causes, usually minor ones like temporary fatigue, overwork of a group of muscles, nervousness or insomnia. If muscle twitches become frequent or painful, or if they involve the face, producing unpleasant grimaces, then you should discuss them without delay with your doctor. The same is true of *muscle cramps,* especially the ones that sometimes wake people from their sleep because of intense pain in the calf of the leg or other areas.

In a *strain,* the muscle stretches and becomes quite painful. You can get a strain by taking a wrong step and stretching the muscle that supports the ankle, for example. Treatment consists of rest for the injured part, application of heat, and light massage.

A *sprain* occurs when a ligament connecting bone or supporting a joint is torn. In this case the pain is severe, and if the ankle is injured, you cannot walk at all, or only with great difficulty. The injured part swells, and there is pain and discoloration of the skin, which becomes red or reddish blue.

Bones

The bones form the basic framework or chassis of the human body. There are 206 bones in the body. Some of these, such as the skull, which encloses the brain, the eyes and the inner ear, have chiefly a protective function. Others are mainly supporting structures, such as the vertebral column with its 24 individual bones. This encases the vital spinal cord, and also helps support the back. Other bones are concerned chiefly with movements, for example, those of the fingers. The various types of bones are shown in Figure 2–10.

Bones contain a hard, stony chemical structure which gives them the tremendous strength required of them. Yet they are so marvelously constructed that they are resilient and light enough to permit the wonderful feats of strength and agility of which the human being is capable. The basic chemical of bones is calcium phosphate, found so plentifully in milk. That is why milk is so essential to growing infants and children, as well as to the pregnant and nursing mother. Vitamins, especially vitamin D, are also required in the proper manufacture of the bones.

The bones have another quite different function in addition to protection, support and movement. They are vital elements in the manufacture of the blood cells. The *bone marrow* carries on this important work. After the red and white blood cells

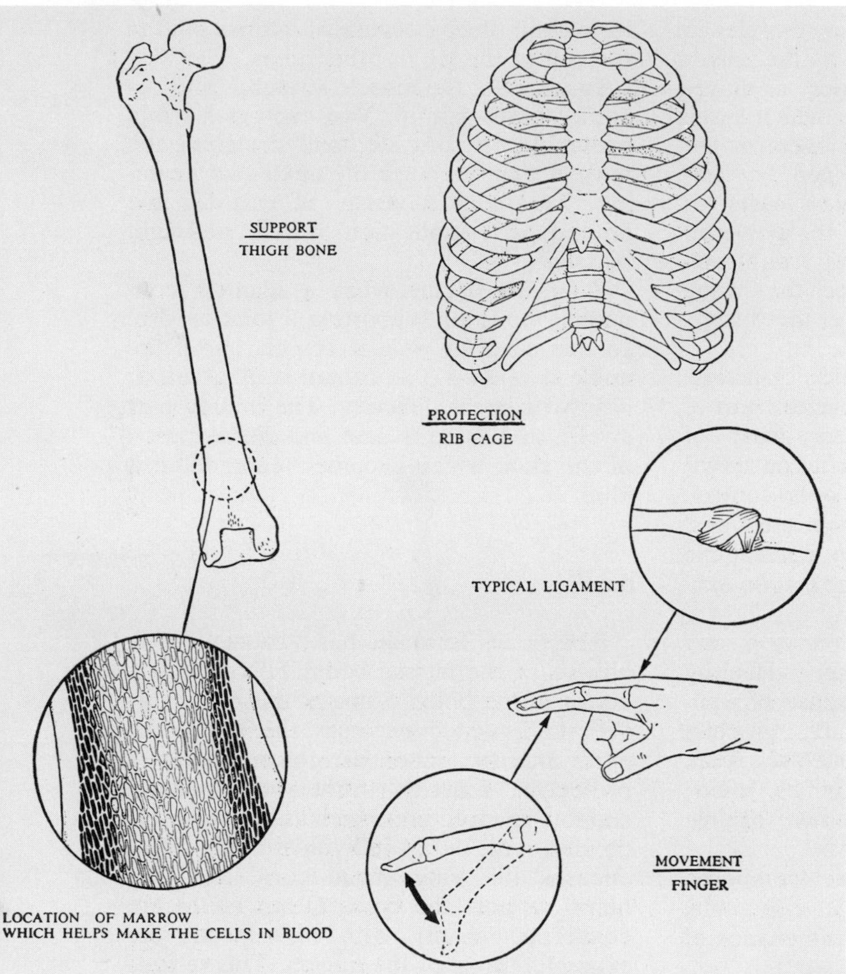

Figure 2–10. Main types of bones.

are manufactured in the marrow of the various bones, these cells enter the blood to carry out their special functions.

The bone marrow requires nutrient foods and vitamins different from those needed by the hard, outer, calcified part of the bones. The red blood cells must have iron and proteins to build hemoglobin, their important oxygen-carrying pigment. Other vitamins, such as folic acid and B_{12}, are also required to nourish bone marrow.

A *dislocation* is a bone out of place at the joint. *Congenital dislocations* are present at birth in a small percentage of children. Hip dislocations, found more frequently in female than male children, may not be evident until the child starts to walk. Then it will be noticed that the gait is not symmetrical. It is extremely important to diagnose this condition before the child does much walking with the weakened hip joint. At this time, proper treatment can cure the condition without surgical operation. If the condition is neglected, even for a year or two, orthopedic surgery will be needed to reconstruct the hip joint. A neglected dislocated hip joint can wear out so badly in later life that major reconstructive surgery will be required to prevent total incapacitation.

Dislocations can also result from injury or strain. Shoulder, finger and jaw dislocations are the more common types. Frequently, manipulation of the bones will restore them to their normal positions.

Clubfoot is another congenital condition which seriously affects the foot. It can be corrected by early treatment, sometimes requiring only strapping or casts. Serious cases need expert orthopedic surgery.

Frozen shoulder is a very disabling

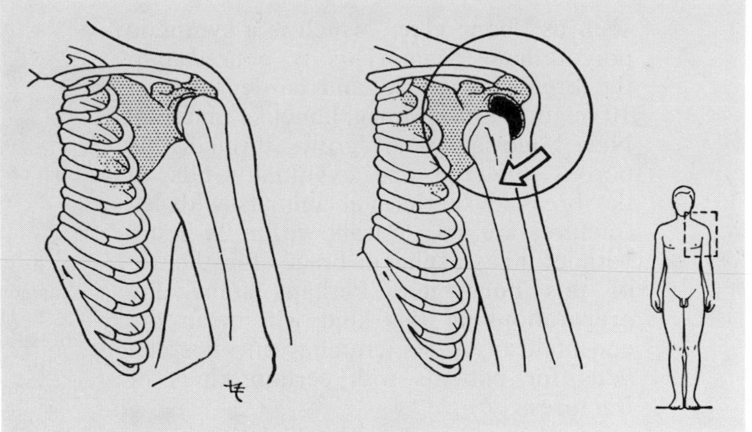

Figure 2–11. Dislocation of the shoulder. **Left,** Normal shoulder The shaded area indicates the scapula (shoulder blade). **Right,** Dislocation. The end of the humerus (upper arm bone) has completely separated from its socket (darkened area) and moved forward in the direction of the arrow.

limitation of motion of the important shoulder joint which sometimes develops after bursitis. It usually results from bands of adhesions around the joint, but can also be due to other causes. If exercises, rest, and medicines don't help, then a doctor who has had experience in the technique may be able to free the adhesions by manipulation of the shoulder. This is done under anesthesia, and must be performed expertly to avoid tearing or breaking important structures in and around the joint.

A bone fracture means a broken bone. When no break in the skin occurs, it is called a *simple* fracture. If the broken bone pierces the skin and is exposed, it is a *compound* fracture.

Fractures usually cause only temporary disability. However, if the bone does not heal properly, there may be disability for life. Fractures in elderly people tend to knit poorly, and may need special attention. Also, in the growing child, fractures must be set correctly so that there is no interference with growth.

There is a tremendous difference in fractures and in the time and skill required to treat them. A noncomplicated fracture usually requires only a plaster cast which can be applied by the family doctor, and heals over in several weeks. However, a double break of the forearm, for example, presents a serious problem. A specialist in orthopedic surgery may have to insert a metal pin in one bone and fasten a plate on the other. It is well worth the effort involved as it will result in a strong, normal arm. Fractures of the long bones, especially of the thigh, usually require special apparatus, and cannot be treated successfully by casts.

Tremendous advances have been made in the field of orthopedic surgery in recent years. Perhaps part of this has been sparked by serious war wounds and automobile injuries! Many new materials have come into use to speed up healing of fractures,

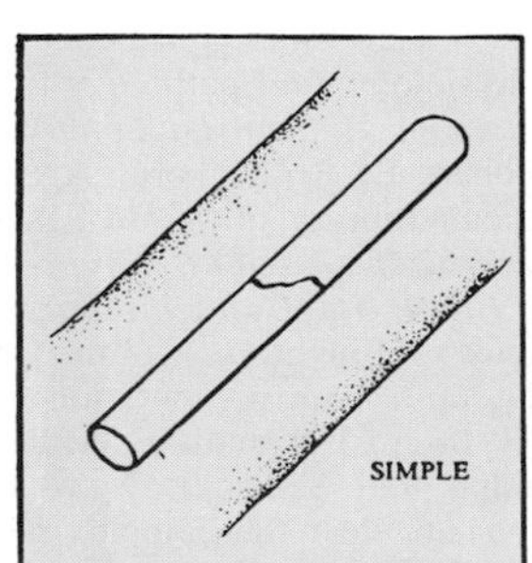

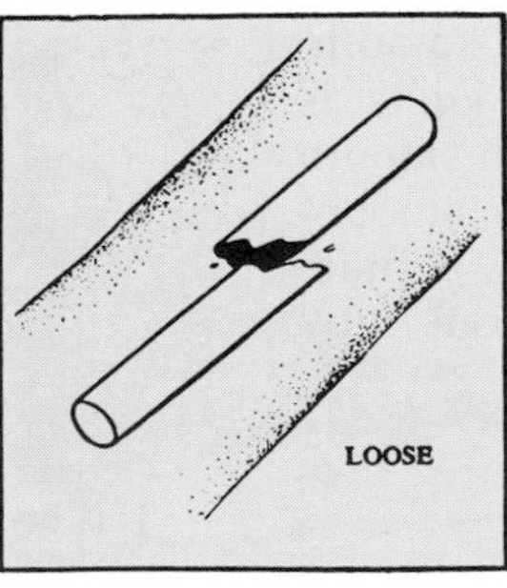

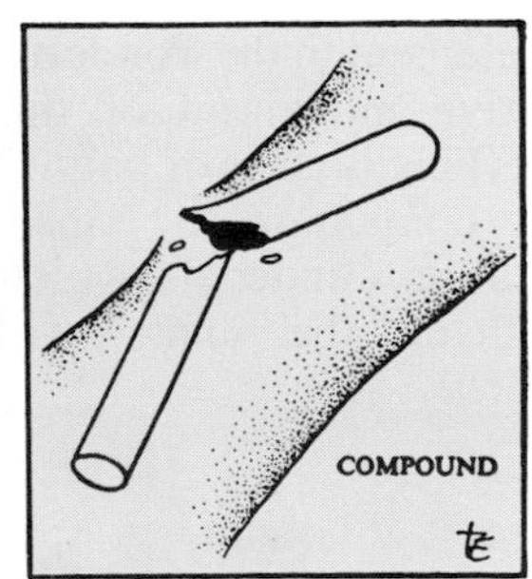

Figure 2–12. Main types of fractures. **Left,** The bone is broken, but the ends have not separated. **Center,** The ends of the broken bone have separated to some extent. **Right,** The end of the broken bone penetrates through the skin.

such as "bone glue," which is a synthetic polyurethane foam. This is poured into the break in a bone, and hardens within 10 minutes into a strong, bonelike material. New bone apparently grows through this porous material and eventually fills in the break. Experimental animals with leg fractures are able to walk within 24 hours without a cast, splint or brace after the use of this bone glue. Perhaps some day preparations of this kind will mean the end of heavy casts, crutches and hospital beds for patients with certain kinds of fractures.

Another new material which has been used in bone grafts is a white, porous substance called *anorganic bone*. This is made from bovine bone, by extracting all the organic material, and can be shaped with a scalpel to fit the contours of a bone defect before it is implanted.

Joints, Ligaments and Bursae

The joints and ligaments connect the bones to each other. The joints provide the smooth, gliding surfaces at the ends of the bones so that movements can be carried out easily and painlessly. For the ends of the bones concerned in body movements, nature provides a special material, called *cartilage*. This has unusual resiliency and smoothness so that fingers, arms and legs can move thousands of times daily without our being conscious of their activities.

To bind bones together, or to strengthen joints, the body uses a special type of tough binding cord called *tendons*. These are attached to the bones so well that only exceptional pulls or twists will tear a ligament away from the bone.

A final element in the wonderful, smooth, and effective movement of the joints is the *bursa*. This is a sac or bag with smooth surfaces, containing a small amount of lubricating material which permits movement of the joints without any friction.

Questions

1. Why is the brain called the master organ of our bodies?
2. How is the human brain protected?
3. What is an electroencephalograph and what does it measure?
4. Trace the passage of air from mouth to lungs. What happens when a piece of food goes down "the wrong way" and causes a coughing spell?
5. What is the special function of the arteries and of the veins and how do they interconnect?
6. What are some of the great enemies of the heart?
7. Trace the course of blood through the heart.
8. Why do you think "nervous stomach" is such a common ailment?
9. How do the liver and gallbladder participate in digestion?
10. What is the difference between a tendon, a joint, and a bursa?
11. What is the function of the bones? Of the bone marrow?

Topics for Discussion

What the college student should know about his body.

Mechanics of breathing and exchange of respiratory gases.

The process of memory.

Artificial kidney.

Brain injuries and skull fractures.

Reading Suggestions

Function of the Human Body, Arthur C. Guyton. 2nd Ed., W. B. Saunders Co., Philadelphia, 1964. A well written, college-level textbook of human physiology.

Human Anatomy and Physiology, Barry G. King and Mary Jane Showers. 5th Ed., W. B. Saunders Co., Philadelphia, 1963. A college-level text describing the human body and how it works.

The Physics and Chemistry of Life, A Scientific American Book. Simon and Schuster, New York, 1955. An excellent book for the student of science.

The Wonderful Human Machine, adapted from Today's Health and published by American Medical Association, Chicago, 1961. A well written and well illustrated account of how the human body works.

That The Patient May Know, Harry F. Dowling and Tom Jones. W. B. Saunders Co., Philadelphia, 1959. An atlas used by the physician in explaining anatomy, physiology, and pathology to the patient.

The New American Medical Dictionary and Health Manual, Robert E. Rothenberg. A Signet Book, New American Library of World Literature, Inc., New York, 1962 (paperback).

The Human Brain: Its Capacities and Functions, Isaac Asimov. Houghton Mifflin Co., Boston, 1964. Clear, up-to-date presentation of the topic.

Man and His Body, Benjamin F. Miller and Ruth Goode. Simon and Schuster, New York, 1960. This book makes clear the complex mechanism of the human body.

Structure and Function in Man, Stanley W. Jacob and Clarice A. Francone. W. B. Saunders Co., Philadelphia, 1965. Excellently illustrated text for students of the allied medical sciences.

3

PHYSICAL FITNESS IN THE MODERN WORLD

A Caution to Everybody

Consider the auk;
Becoming extinct because he forgot to fly,
and could only walk,
Consider man, who may well become extinct
Because he forgot how to walk and learned
how to fly before he thinked.

OGDEN NASH
(Private Dining Room and Other Verses)

Man's long journey up and out of the caves and jungles into a modern "push-button" society is a tribute to our magnificent advances in science and technology. These advances have created golden potentialities for the human race, and many thoughtful individuals taking advantage of the relief from routine and dull tasks have more nearly approached the good life than any generation since the ancient Greeks. But for others, the conveniences of modern living have resulted in an all-embracing philosophy of mental and physical take-it-easy-ism—a trend that years ago helped lead to the decay and death of the all-powerful Roman Empire.

Today, this philosophy is responsible for a decrease of physical fitness in an ever-increasing portion of the American population. That this trend cannot continue without detrimental effects on the health of our nation is attested to by the statements of many physicians.

Drs. Hans Kraus and Wilhelm Raab warn us, in a book entitled *Hypokinetic Disease,* that those individuals in our society who do not exercise are more likely to suffer from coronary heart disease, diabetes, duodenal ulcer and low back pain than active persons who do exercise. In addition, sedentary people, as a statistical class, can expect higher blood pressure, more neuromuscular tension, more body fat, higher resting pulse rates, less adaptability to stress, less strength, and less flexibility.[1]

Dr. Paul Dudley White, Boston cardiologist and physician to former President Eisenhower, tells the American public that "proper exercise is as essential to

[1]Kraus, H., and Raab, W.: *Hypokinetic Disease: Role of Inactivity in Production of Disease,* Charles C Thomas, Springfield, Ill., 1961.

good health as eating and sleeping."[2] Dr. Wilhelm Raab, University of Vermont College of Medicine, in describing a pathological condition that he aptly calls "loafer's heart," writes:[3] "Since antiquity, physically lazy, overfed persons of the social upper crust have been popularly known as candidates for ailments of at least partially cardiac origin—shortness of breath, palpitations, chest pain and 'heart attack.'"

Dr. Irvine Page, Director of Research at the Cleveland Clinic, notes that[4] "exercise seems to have several mechanisms by which it reduces the tendency to develop arteriosclerosis [hardening of the arteries]."

Dr. Edward Bortz, a past president of the American Medical Association, states:[5] "It would appear that exercise strengthens the adaptive mechanism of the body. In a physically fit person, there appears to be a better adrenal reserve with an increased amount of steroids available to counter prolonged tension."

The American Medical Association states:[6]

> The successful use of physical activity in the medical management of patients indicates the beneficial effects of exercise in preventing or delaying organic disease and degeneration . . . obesity, muscle atrophy, cardiovascular inefficiency, joint stiffness, and impairment of various metabolic functions are possible effects of prolonged inactivity.

In view of the possible effects of physical inactivity on the health and welfare of our nation, and perhaps because exercise was credited with ameliorating his own heart condition, former President Dwight D. Eisenhower created, in 1956, the American Council on Youth Fitness. Shortly thereafter, 29 governors created councils in their states to lead the attack on "soft living," "loafer's heart," and hypokinetic diseases in general.

[2]White, P. D.: Man's best medicine, in *New York Times Magazine,* June 23, 1957.

[3]Raab, W.: Loafer's heart. *Archives of Internal Medicine, 101*:194, 1958.

[4]*Report to the Nation,* American Heart Association, 1959.

[5]Bortz, E. L.: Exercise, Fitness and Aging, in *Exercise and Fitness,* a collection of papers presented at a Colloquium on Exercise and Fitness, The Athletic Institute, Chicago, 1959.

[6]Joint Committee of American Medical Association and American Association for Health, Physical Education and Recreation: Exercise and fitness, Journal of the American Medical Association, *188*:433, 1964.

John F. Kennedy, who succeeded Dwight D. Eisenhower as president, was an even stronger advocate of physical fitness. In a press release prior to taking office, he proposed a four point program to combat "soft living":

> 1. Establish a White House Committee on Health and Fitness to formulate and carry out a program to improve the physical condition of the nation.
> 2. Make physical fitness of our youth the direct responsibility of HEW (Health, Education and Welfare).
> 3. Invite the governor of each state to attend an annual national youth fitness congress.
> 4. Proclaim through all departments of the government that the promotion of sports participation and physical fitness is a basic and continuing policy of the United States.

COLLEGE PHYSICAL EDUCATION

Physical education is an important part of your college curriculum, and you should take advantage of the opportunity to develop skills that you can use throughout life. It is axiomatic that people do most what they can do well; therefore, it is likely that you will enjoy physical activity in later life if you set the stage in your college years by becoming skilled in some selected sport or recreational program.

In selecting your physical education courses, try to take those that have carry-over value. With all due respect to youth fitness, it is during middle and later years of life in which exercise needs more emphasis.[7] Tennis, handball, squash, badminton, swimming, and golf are good examples of carry-over sports.

Also, it is important that you enjoy whatever activities you finally select as a means of maintaining fitness. For instance, although a program of calisthenics can play an important role in maintaining fitness, the tendency is to discard such a program after a short period of use. But if you derive pleasure from the activity, it is probable that you will continue it as a regular routine.

Today, sports skills are only a part of the physical education program. The

[7]It is interesting to note that during John F. Kennedy's administration the President's Council on Youth Fitness changed its name; now it is known as the President's Council on Physical Fitness.

modern physical educator, aware that intelligent persons are easy to lead but difficult to drive, draws from the various scientific disciplines to help you understand the benefits of fitness as well as the various methods of obtaining it. Whether you maintain a reasonable level of fitness throughout life, of course, is entirely up to you; before deciding, you should be aware of evidence for the health benefits of exercise.

THE BENEFITS OF EXERCISE

Physical Fitness and Cardiovascular Health

The normal heart, pumping more than 4000 quarts of blood daily, is one of the most efficient organs of the human body. In fact, it is even more efficient than our best made machines. For example, the heart converts 50 per cent of its fuel into energy, whereas the automobile is only 25 per cent efficient. This "perpetual" pump works night and day for over 70 years without stopping to rest. Indeed, while the rest of our body sleeps each night, the heart accomplishes a work load roughly equivalent to carrying a 30 pound pack to the top of the 102-story Empire State Building.

It is a sobering fact, however, that when you neglect your fitness, this wonderful pump begins to lose some of its efficiency. For example, subjects undergoing three weeks of bed rest experience an acceleration in the resting heart rate; this indicates that the heart, after a period of bodily inactivity, must work harder to pump the same amount of blood. Conversely, it has been amply demonstrated that the resting heart rate can be lowered with training. Jim Beatty, the famous miler, has a heart rate 50 per cent slower than the average person. Also, it is not unusual for highly trained persons to have a rate of 30 to 40 heart beats a minute, as compared with the average 72 for male college students. Also, it is a familiar observation that wild animals have a lower heart rate than domestic animals—for example, the tame rabbit has a heart rate of approximately 200 beats a minute, whereas the wild hare has a rate of around 64 beats a minute.

That the trained heart works more

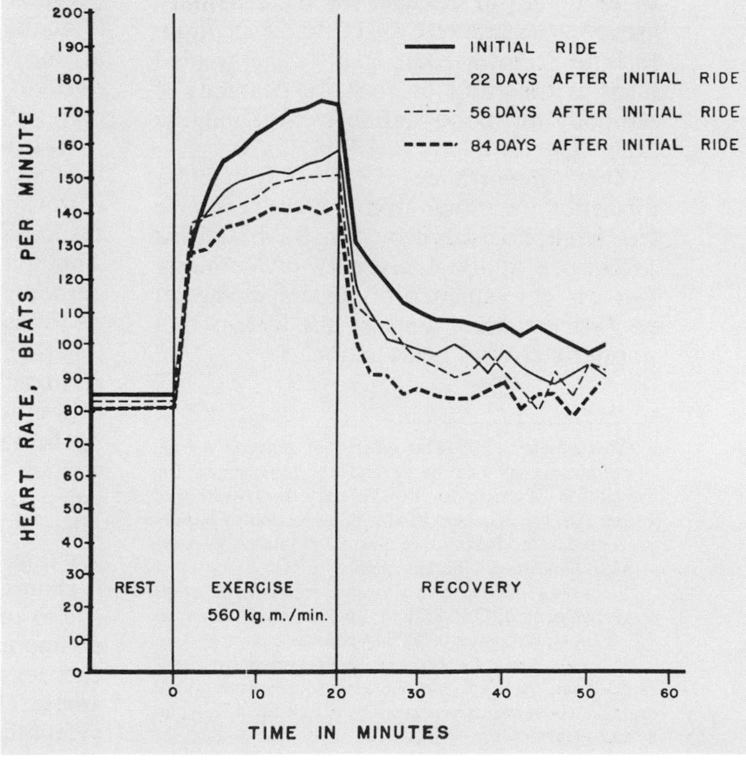

Figure 3–1. Effect of training on heart rate for a standard amount of exercise: pedaling a bicycle ergometer for 20 minutes with a work load of 560 kg. m./min. Training was achieved by riding the bicycle four days a week with the same work load. (From Brouha, L.: In *Science and Medicine of Exercise and Sports*, Johnson, W. R., ed. New York, Harper & Brothers, 1960.)

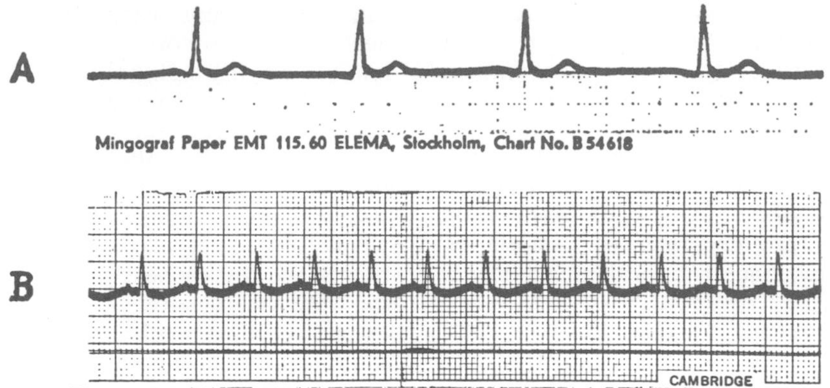

Figure 3–2. Electrocardiograms of (*A*) an 87 year old extremely physically active alpinist (heart rate, 48) and (*B*) a 69 year old spinster who had spent 30 years voluntarily in bed (heart rate, 140). (From Kraus, H. and Raab, W.: Hypokinetic Disease, Charles C Thomas, Springfield, 1961.)

efficiently is a matter of simple physics. Dr. Harald Mellerowicz, a West Berlin cardiologist, has computed the workload of trained and untrained hearts when the body is at rest.[8] For sedentary office workers, this amounted to a daily workload of 10,000 to 15,000 kilogram meters; whereas for 107 well trained sportsmen the daily workload was only 5000 to 10,000 kilogram meters.[9] Subsequently, the oxygen consumption of the heart was estimated to be 25 to 40 cc./min. for the sedentary group as compared to 15 to 25 cc./min. for the trained sportsmen.[10] The trained heart is thus able to meet the demands of the body for blood with less effort and less fuel.

The importance of cardiovascular efficiency resulting from regular exercise has been elucidated by Dr. Raab and his associates at the University of Vermont. But for convenience of understanding let us first examine some of the factors that normally control heart action.

Regulation of Heart Action. The heart is regulated by the autonomic nervous system. This involuntary control system is divided into two parts—the parasympathetic division and the sympathetic division. The parasympathetic division, in turn, is composed of nerves that have their origin in the cranium and in the sacral, or lower, portion of the spinal cord (Fig. 3-3). For this reason, it is sometimes called the craniosacral division of the autonomic nervous system. The sympathetic division is made up of nerves that have their origin in the thoracic and lumbar, or middle, portions of the spinal cord; it is sometimes referred to as the thoracolumbar division.

In general, the parasympathetic division is concerned with the conservation and restoration of energy; therefore, its responsibility is to slow down the heart. The sympathetic division is primarily concerned with the expenditure of energy; its job is to speed up heart action. Working together these nervous components are responsible for the exceptional efficiency of the heart—that is, they interact to speed up heart action when the body requires a greater blood delivery and to slow it down when the requirements have been met. In other words, they prevent the heart from wasting energy by working too hard when it should slow down.

Yet under certain conditions, one of the components of the autonomic nervous system tends to dominate the other. For example, habitual lack of exercise causes sympathetic dominance, which is charac-

[8]Mellerowicz, H.: The effects of training on O_2 consumption of the heart and its importance for prevention of coronary insufficiency, in *Health and Fitness in the Modern World,* A collection of papers presented at the Institute of Normal Human Anatomy, Athletic Institute, Chicago, 1961.

[9]Scientists use the term *kilogram meters* to describe work performed. One kilogram meter is equivalent to 7.233 foot-pounds or 0.002344 calorie.

[10]These values for oxygen consumption were derived from the fact that the hearts of warmblooded animals consume approximately 3 to 4 cc. of oxygen per kilogram meter of work.

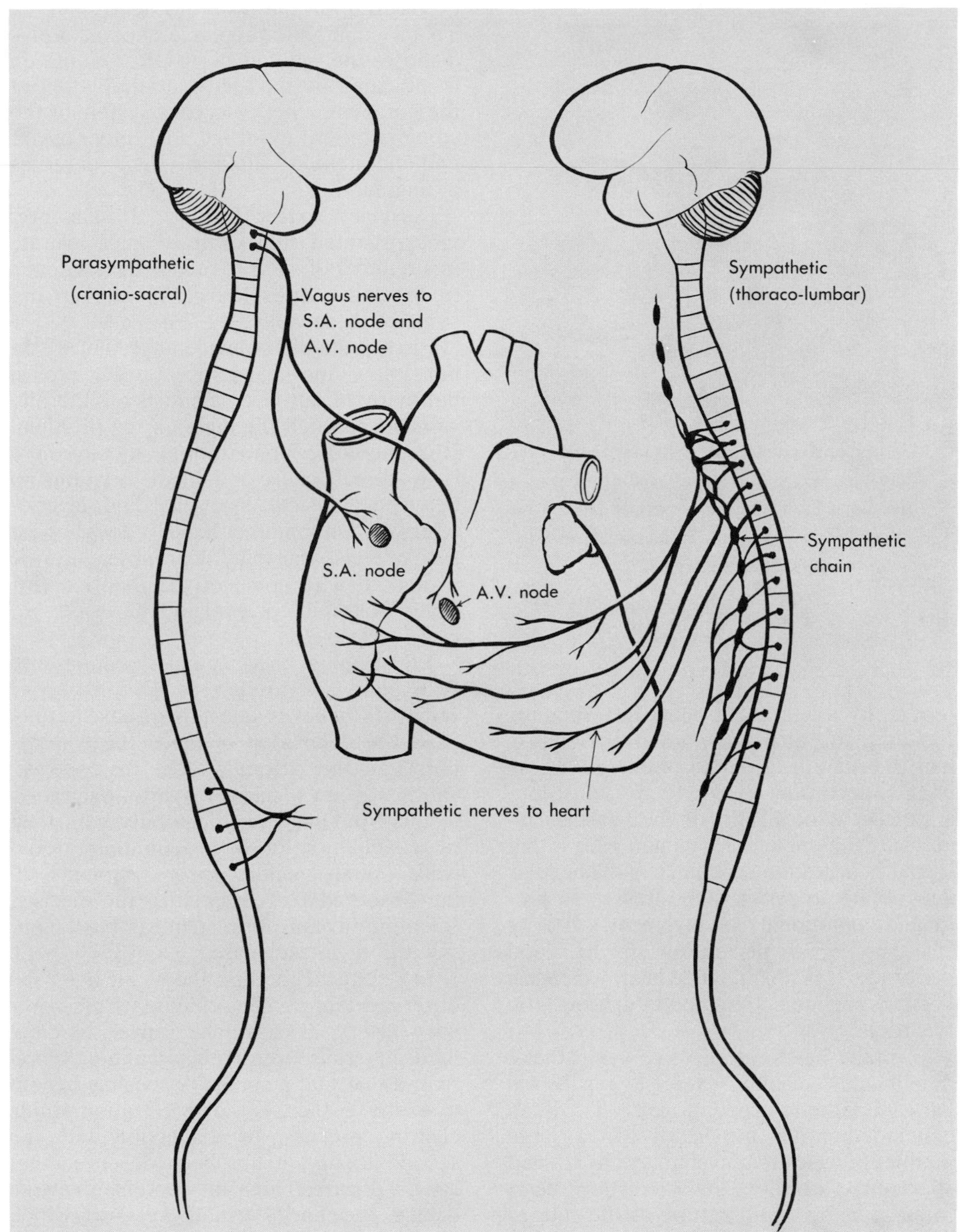

Figure 3–3. Regulation of heart action by the autonomic nervous system. (Redrawn from King and Showers, Human Anatomy and Physiology. 5th Ed. Philadelphia, W. B. Saunders, 1963.)

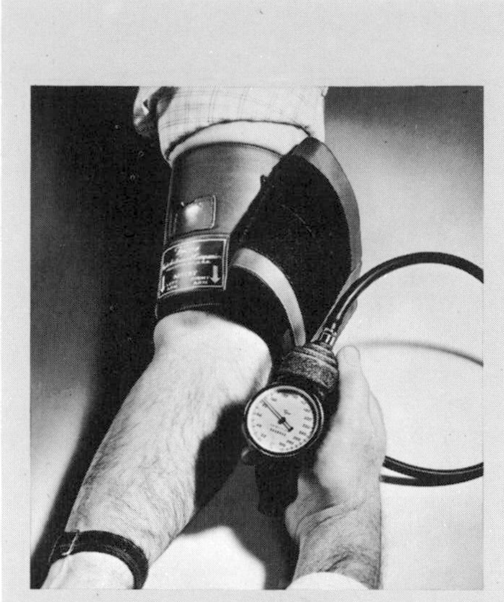

Sphygmomanometer, the instrument used to measure blood pressure, used here on the upper arm. Because normal blood pressure can vary widely, only a doctor can tell if changes indicate illness.

terized by a heart that beats fast, requires too long to return to normal after stress and is generally wasteful of energy. These effects, according to Dr. Raab,[3] constitute a threat to the health of the heart by increasing its metabolic vulnerability—that is, the heart of the sedentary individual has less ability to resist such stresses as prolonged emotional involvement, arteriosclerosis or hypertension (high blood pressure). It is a vulnerable heart which has been designated the "loafer's heart" by Dr. Raab.

Whereas inactivity leads to sympathetic dominance, regular exercise results in parasympathetic preponderance. Dr. Raab concluded after the study of a large number of cases that systematically trained sportsmen display lower resting heart rates, a more rapid return of the rate to normal after stress and a generally more efficient heart—the antithesis of "loafer's heart."

The clinical value of parasympathetic dominance has been demonstrated by Dr. Raab and his associates while working with patients suffering from angina pectoris. This condition, which is characterized by sharp pains in the chest, results from a lack of oxygen to the working heart muscle. That sympathetic preponderance may predispose the individual to this condition is indicated by the fact that stimulation of the parasympathetic nervous system or the administration of drugs that block sympathetic activity diminish the symptoms of angina.

Coronary Artery Disease. It was previously noted that exercise may operate in a number of ways to reduce the tendency to develop arteriosclerosis. What, then, are some of these ways?

First, it should be made clear that we do not know the cause of arteriosclerosis, but many of our best scientists are literally working through the night on the problem. It is, therefore, premature to say that there is a direct cause-and-effect relationship between physical inactivity and arteriosclerosis. On the other hand, it does appear that exercise can play a prophylactic role in accord with some of the theories currently offered to explain the onset of arteriosclerosis.

Two popular theories have been offered to explain arteriosclerosis. One group of scientists believes that this disease results from the deposition of lipids (fatty materials) in the arterial wall. In contrast, another group suggests that arteriosclerosis results from the deposition of fibrin (formed by coagulation of blood) on the arterial walls. While neither theory explains all the observed facts related to the disease, scientific investigation supports basic considerations in each case.

In regard to the first theory, it has been observed that persons suffering from coronary artery disease take longer to clear lipid materials from their circulating blood than do normal persons. A possible benefit of exercise, then, is the acceleration of this clearing process. In connection with the second theory, it has been observed that after a meal of high fat content, exercise delays the fibrin-forming system (which may otherwise be accelerated by the fat), and exercise at the same time activates a system that destroys fibrin. Thus, exercise may play a role in both theories of the mechanism currently offered to explain the etiology of arteriosclerosis. This condition and its relationship to exercise are

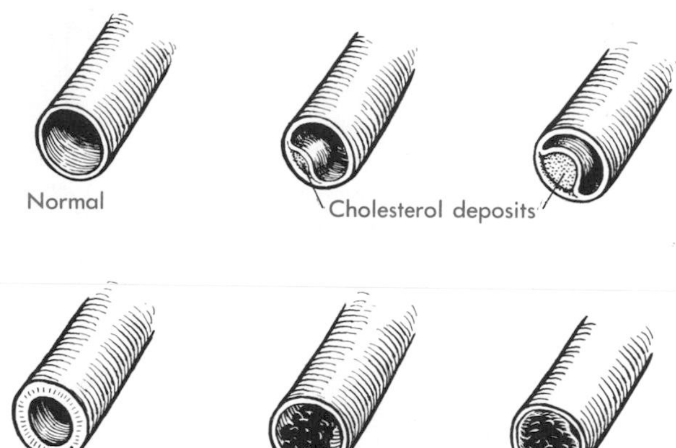

Figure 3–4. Arteriosclerosis.

discussed in Chapter 18, pages 235–236.

An additional benefit of exercise in the problem of heart disease has been reported by Dr. Richard Eckstein of Western Reserve University.[11] This study was designed to determine the effects of exercise on dogs whose coronary arteries had been surgically constricted to approximate the condition of arteriosclerosis. A group of 45 dogs was exercised four times daily for several weeks, while a control group was confined to cages.

At the end of the training period, the amount of blood able to reach the damaged portion of the heart by routes other than the primary route (which had been surgically constricted) was measured. These alternate routes by which blood can frequently reach a damaged area of the heart are referred to clinically as the collateral coronary circulation (Fig. 3–5).

When compared, the dogs in the exercise group were found to have significantly more collateral coronary circulation than the caged group. In fact, complete occlusion of the primary blood supply had little effect on the trained dogs; their new blood supply was functionally adequate.

On the basis of this study, Dr. Eckstein concluded that "since the onset of coronary disease is not recognizable, it would probably be advisable to encourage middleaged human beings who are without symptoms to exercise." It seems equally important to extend these recommendations to younger age groups since the autopsy reports of men (average age, 22 years) killed during the Korean War revealed that 77 per cent had lipid deposits in their arteries.[12] These findings have been substantiated by the autopsy reports of 222 young air force personnel.[13] Moreover, in 1959, 25 children under 5 years of age died of arteriosclerotic heart disease.

Because of the increasing incidence of heart disease, which annually claims 849,000 persons in the United States alone, an International Conference on Preventive Cardiology was held in 1964. A major topic of consideration at this conference was the prophylactic effects of exercise for heart disease.

One of the most revealing reports of this conference resulted from a study of the incidence of occlusive heart disease during a 15 year survey of 5279 men and 5235 women in Israel. All persons studied lived in collective settlements that provided uniform living conditions and standards. Their ages ranged from 41 to 65 years.

Among these individuals, the incidence of occlusive heart disease was found to be 2.5 to 4 times higher in men and women engaged in sedentary work than in nonsedentary workers in the various age

[11]Eckstein, R.: Effect of exercise and coronary artery narrowing on coronary collateral circulation. *Circulation Research, 5*:230, 1957.

[12]Enos, W. F., *et al.*: Coronary disease among United States soldiers killed in action in Korea. *Journal of the American Medical Association, 152*: 1090, 1953.

[13]Glantz, W. M., and Stembridge, V. A.: Coronary artery atherosclerosis as a factor in aircraft accident fatalities. *Journal of Aviation Medicine, 30*:75, 1959.

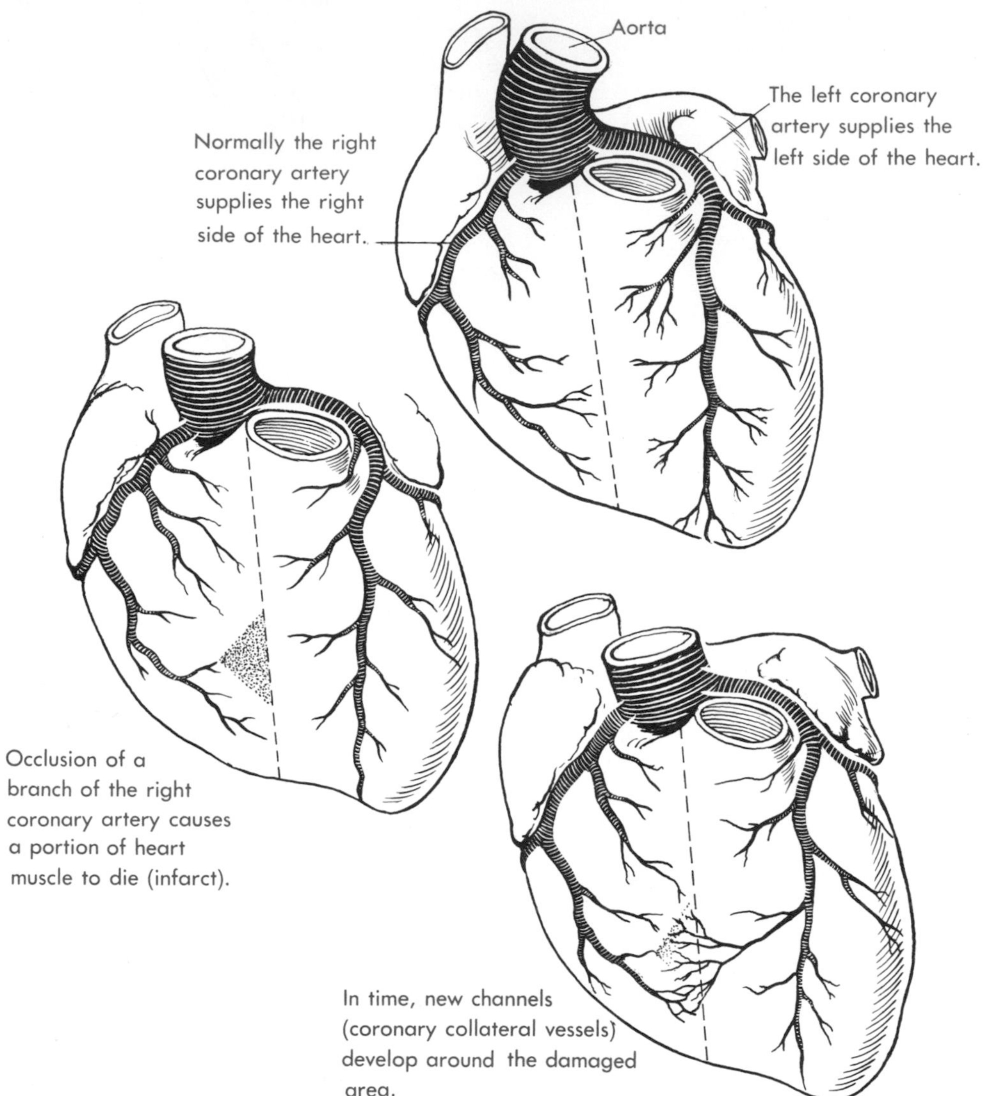

Figure 3–5. Coronary collateral circulation.

groups. Moreover, among those who had suffered a heart attack, the immediate mortality rate was 4.2 per cent for active workers as compared to 17.7 per cent for store clerks and 22.6 per cent for merchants and sedentary professional men. Further, the six-year mortality rate following the initial onset of heart disease was 23.1 per cent for the workers but 54 to 59 per cent for the sedentary individuals. Dr. Brunner, who conducted this research, concluded: "These studies show the effect of physical activity in preventing clinical ischemic heart disease and in improving the course of the once established disease."

In conclusion, a number of points should be emphasized: (1) It is now recognized that coronary artery disease demands a preventive rather than a therapeutic approach. (2) The current theories offered to explain occlusive heart disease indicate that exercise plays a prophylactic role. (3) Although no cause-and-effect mechanism has been elucidated, extensive surveys in England,[14] Austria,[15] Finland,[16]

[14]Morris, N. J., *et al.*: Coronary heart-disease and physical activity of work. *Lancet, 2*:1053, 1953.

[15]Wiener Gebietskrankenkasse, Sterbefalle und Sterbegeld, Jahresbericht d. Weiner Gebietskrankenkasse (Vienna), 1956, p. 168.

[16]Karvonen, J. J., *et al.*: Longevity of champion skiers, *Duodecim., 72*:893, 1956.

Israel,[17] and the United States[18-20] have all demonstrated a lower incidence of ischemic heart disease in persons who are physically active than in sedentary persons. (4) Exercise is rapidly becoming a vital part of the convalescent treatment of the heart patient.

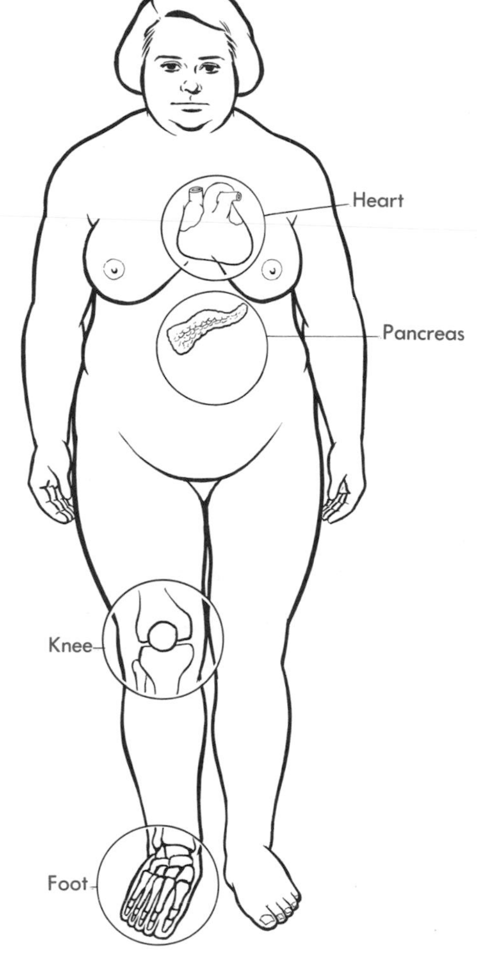

Figure 3–6. Obesity may be harmful to certain organs.

The Effects of Exercise on Weight Control

One of the most frequently discussed problems of our modern society is that of weight control. A concern for personal appearance is probably the primary cause of this widespread preoccupation with the size of the waistline, but an equally important reason for concern may be found in life insurance mortality tables, which reveal that in the age group 45 to 60 years the death rate increases roughly one per cent for each pound of excess fat.

Regardless of motivation, most of the 62 million Americans estimated to be overweight would like to take off a few pounds. Unfortunately, however, it is not an easy matter to lose weight, and all too many persons fall victim to the pseudoscientific faddists who are ready to take advantage of our desire for an easy or trick method.

In discussing weight control, Dr. Jean Mayer of Harvard University wrote:[21] "I am convinced that inactivity is the most important factor explaining the frequency of 'creeping overweight' in modern Western Societies." The American Medical Association states:[6] "There is no longer any doubt but that the level of physical activity does play a major role in weight control."

To be sure, the im ortance of exercise as a factor in weight control has been recognized since antiquity. The practice of penning livestock to fatten them has been employed on an empirical basis for many years, and the lean hunter or soldier has always been contrasted with the fat merchant. In a more scientific study by Green, the cause of obesity in adults was traced to a sudden decrease in activity.[22] Two later investigations of children revealed a direct relationship between obesity and inactivity.[23, 24]

[17]Brunner, D.: The influence of physical activity on the incidence and prognosis of ischemic heart disease. A paper presented to the First International Conference of Preventive Cardiology, Burlington, Vermont, August 24–28, 1964.

[18]Pomeroy, W. C., and White, P. D.: Coronary heart disease in former football players. *Journal of the American Medical Association, 167*:711, 1958.

[19]Luongo, E. P.: Health habits and heart disease – challenge in preventive medicine. *Journal of the American Medical Association, 162*:1021, 1956.

[20]Spain, D. M., and Bradess, V. A.: Relation of sex, age and physical activity to sudden death from coronary arterial occlusion, in Rosenbaum, F. F., and Belknap, E.L.: *Work and the Heart.* Hoeber, New York, 1959, p. 283.

[21]Mayer, J.: Exercise and weight control. *Postgraduate Medicine, 25*:325, 1959.

[22]Greene, J. A.: Clinical study of the etiology of obesity. *Annals of Internal Medicine, 12*:1797, 1939.

[23]Johnson, M. L., *et al.*: Relative importance of inactivity and overeating in energy balance of obese high school girls. *American Journal of Clinical Nutrition, 4*:37, 1956.

[24]Bruch, H.: Obesity in childhood. *American Journal of Diseases of Children, 60*:1082, 1940.

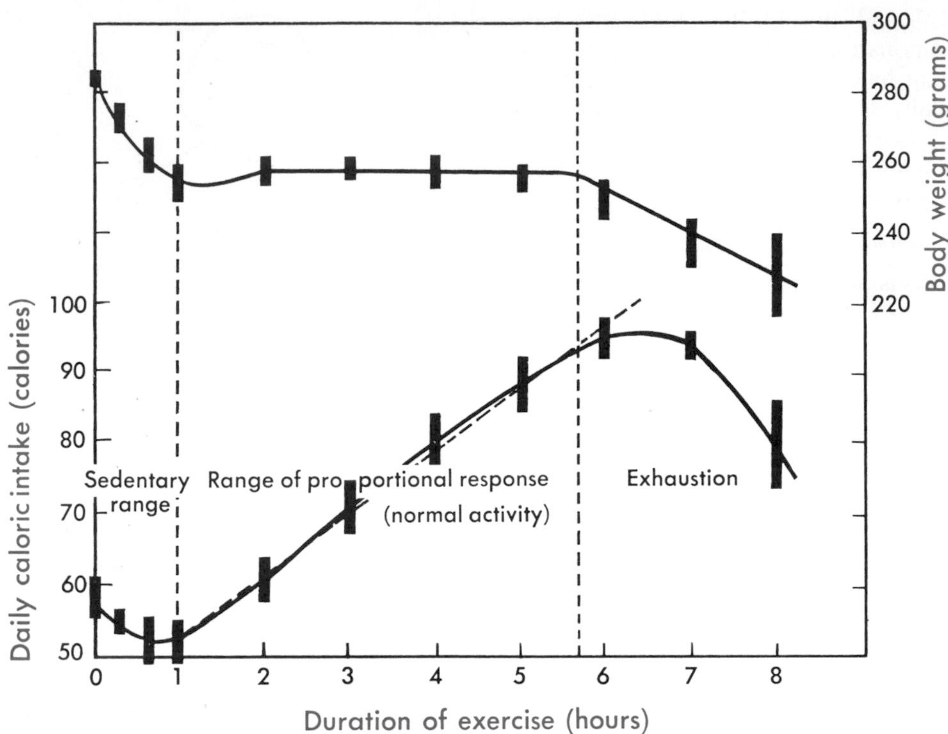

Figure 3–7. A summary of laboratory experiments, this graph shows that food intake does not necessarily increase with exercise in experimental animals. Although rats that have been exercised for three or four hours daily eat more than those exercised for one hour, they maintain their body weight because of their activity. However, rats that have been exercised for less than one hour daily or not at all eat significantly more, and weight accumulates because of the increased food intake and low activity level. (From Mayer, J.: Postgrad. Med., *25*:325, 1959.)

You may have observed that the athlete has little trouble in maintaining a constant weight, and perhaps you have wondered why this is so. Recently, as a result of work by Dr. Mayer, some of the physiological details are beginning to be understood. According to his findings, a physically active animal or person automatically adjusts his food intake to his energy requirements (Fig. 3–7). Consequently, his weight remains constant—that is, unless the activity is extremely prolonged or intense, in which case he may lose weight. But in the case of habitual inactivity, Dr. Mayer found this relationship between food intake and energy requirements does not hold true (Fig. 3–7). He called this lower end of the activity scale the nonresponsive zone. A person who falls in this zone because of occupation and habits may shortly become overweight, for the food intake of such persons is much greater than their needs. (The food intake may actually equal that of physically active workers.) (See Fig. 3–8.) In contrast to this, the active person (even the light worker) maintains a constant weight by adjusting his food intake to meet his energy requirements.

If you remain active, it is relatively easy for you to maintain a constant weight; once overweight, it is rather hard to get rid of extra pounds. It behooves you, therefore, to follow a program of active exercise that will help you to maintain proper weight throughout your life.

Prior to a more detailed discussion of the ways in which exercise may help you control weight, it is helpful to establish a unit of measure by which the amount of food that we take in and the amount that we utilize can be quantified. The unit of measurement most commonly employed is the Calorie. A Calorie is defined as that amount of heat required to raise one kilogram of water one degree centigrade. In physiologic studies, a Calorie represents the energy for heat and physical work that can be obtained from a given weight of food. A pound of fat, for example, supplies about 4000 Calories of potential heat energy. In a practical sense, this means that you would have to burn 4000 Calories in excess of normal food intake (accumulated) to lose one pound of fat. Conversely, it would be necessary to consume at least 4000 Calories more than the body ordinarily requires in order to gain a pound of fat.

How important, then, is the role of exercise in energy expenditure? First, let's examine the caloric expenditure rates contained in Table 3–1. When these rates are compared with the expenditure necessary to burn one pound of fat (4000 Calories), it appears impossible to lose weight through exercise. Would you be willing to walk for 35 hours just to lose one pound, or play tennis for eight hours, or golf for 16.6 hours? It is not surprising, therefore, that the most common conclusion drawn from the examination of caloric expenditure tables is that it is impossible to lose weight by exercise. This is not true. Many athletes regularly train away excess weight before periods of peak performance.

A major misunderstanding of caloric expenditure tables results from the assumption that in order to lose weight all the exercise has to be done at once. Although it is true that you would have to walk 35 miles

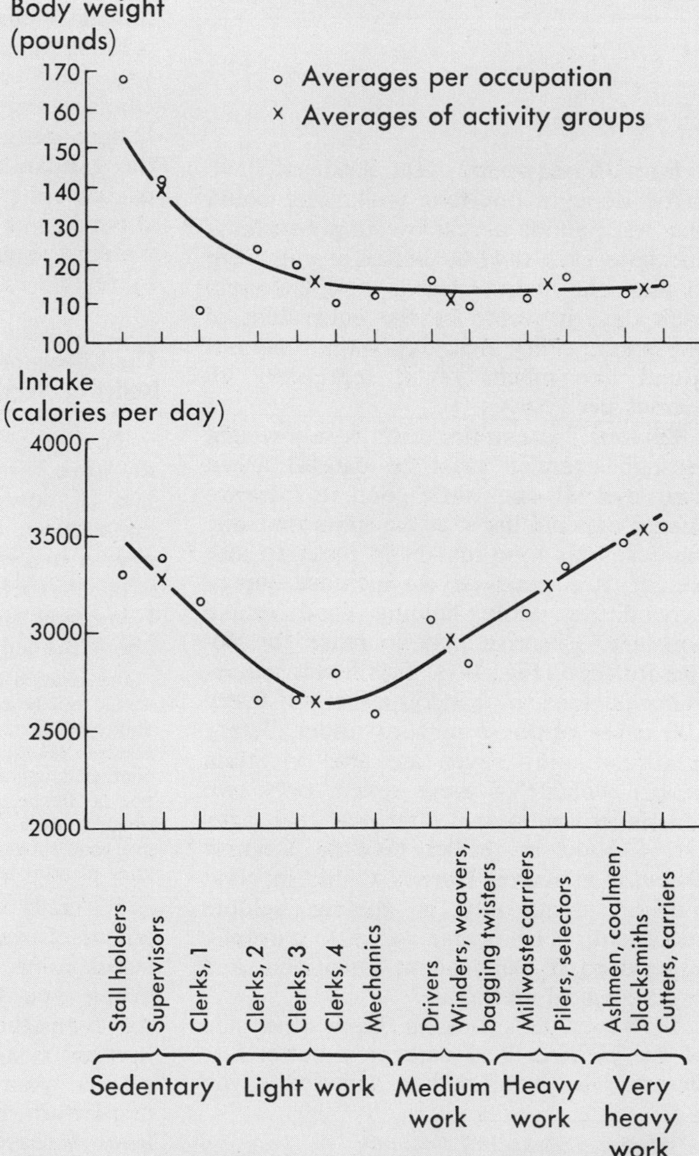

Figure 3–8. Results of a study conducted on a population in India, showing the relation of a wide range of activities to food intake and adiposity. Clerks are grouped according to the daily time spent in walking. As with experimental animals, persons who exercised regularly had the lowest daily food intake. Those who did heavy work ate more to maintain their weight. Inactive persons also ate more and became obese. (From Mayer, J.: Postgrad. Med., *25*:325, 1959.)

Table 3–1. Caloric cost of sports activities

Activity	*Calories per Hour*	*Hours Necessary to Lose One Pound of Fat*
Canoeing (2.5 m.p.h.)	180	22.2
Horseback riding	180	22.2
Volley ball	210	19.0
Bowling	200	20.0
Golfing	240	16.6
Skiing	590	6.8
Squash	620	6.4
Cycling (13 m.p.h.)	660	6.1
Walking	250	16.0
Wrestling	950	4.2
Tennis	500	8.0

to burn off one pound of fat, it doesn't have to be done in one long walk; you could lose ten pounds a year by simply walking one mile each day. Or better, if you were to play one hour of tennis (500 Calories) each day, it would be the equivalent of one pound every eight days—that may not sound like much, yet it represents 46 pounds per year.

Persons attempting to lose weight through exercise must be careful about their diet. It does little good to increase energy expenditure if at the same time one increases his food intake. In order to lose weight, it is necessary to increase energy expenditure while holding food intake constant. Exercise may increase the desire for food (Fig. 3–7). This factor causes many persons to abandon a diet. Of every 100 cases of obese persons under dietary treatment, only seven are able to attain proper weight; of these seven, only two remain at that weight after one year, says Dr. Claude H. Miller (Weight Control Director at Karen Horney Clinic in New York).[25] Not only is dieting seldom successful, but worse, unless carefully supervised it can lead to nutritional and psychological problems.

However, let's look on the positive side of the picture. You deserve a better fate than to join the 62 million Americans who are now overweight. And you can have proper weight, too, if you will think critically about prevention. It should be obvious that weight control is possible by regular physical exercise—once a week or three times per month won't do it. After all, you eat every day. Also, let's consider the situation in which you take in 500 Calories (a milkshake, for example) more per day than you burn. This adds up to a pound every eight days—46 pounds in a year. This might be prevented by one hour of strenuous exercise each day during the year.

In conclusion, exercise is not the only way to control your weight, but it is one of the most effective. To understand why it is the method of choice for so many people, you have simply to compare the discomfort and anguish that accompany the hunger pangs of caloric restriction with the exhilaration and emotional release of participating in an active sport. Worrying about loss of fitness and impending obesity is depressing. They can both be prevented by regular exercise.

The Effects of Exercise in the Relief of Nervous Tension

To live a sane life in our tension-filled world requires a keen insight into the problem of how to handle anxieties. In this connection, the American Medical Association in a joint statement[6] with the American Association for Health, Physical Education and Recreation has this to say about the value of exercise:

> The relation of physical activity to mental health should not be overlooked; from this standpoint, the ability to be engrossed in play is basic. Pleasurable exercise relieves tension and encourages habits of continued activity. In fact, muscular effort is probably one of the best antidotes for emotional stress. Fortunately, such a variety of activities is available that everyone should be able to find some from which he gains pleasure as well as exercise.

To fully appreciate the tranquilizing effects of exercise, it is necessary to understand some of the physiology of stress. When you become angry, for example, the sympathetic division of the autonomic nervous system is strongly stimulated; as a result, your heart beats faster, your respiration increases, your blood sugar level increases and your blood clots faster.

[25] *Medical Tribune,* July 4–5, 1964.

These are a few of the physiological changes intended to prepare the body for fight or flight.

There was a time in our evolutionary development when these responses were essential to the preservation of life. In modern society, however, fight and flight are no longer acceptable responses to the stresses we encounter in our daily lives. Because we are not adapted to this environmental change, our bodies continue to respond in the classic way. Meanwhile, we attempt to compensate with millions of dollars worth of tranquilizers each year.

A more effective way to handle stress is to engage in regular exercise. The additive effects of stressful situations occurring during the day may be dissipated by an hour of physical activity at the end of the day.

In this connection, a recent study revealed that prolonged exercise in rats could deplete the adrenal gland of adrenalin (the same effect produced by some of our more powerful tranquilizers).[26]

[26]Eranko, O., and Harkonen, M.: Distribution and concentration of adrenaline and noradrenaline in the adrenal medulla of the rat following depletion induced by muscular work. *Acta Physiologica Scandinavica, 51*:247, 1961.

The tranquilizing effects of exercise are enhanced if you choose an activity that is pleasurable and requires mental concentration.

The Effects of Exercise on Muscle Tone and Posture

To maintain healthy muscle tone, regular exercise of some kind is necessary.

Digestive processes are aided by exercise. Frequently, vigorous sports and other exercise eliminate constipation by increasing the tone and strength of the abdominal muscles and enhancing completely normal movement of the digestive organs.

Muscle tone is also helpful in promoting good circulation of the blood. Strong abdominal muscles aid the diaphragm in pumping blood to the heart. In the legs, well toned muscles press the blood through the veins, preventing stasis and clotting.

As a rule, a healthy person with good muscle tone automatically assumes a comfortable, attractive posture. Pride and poise are reflective of good postural training, but they are difficult to maintain if physical conditioning is neglected.

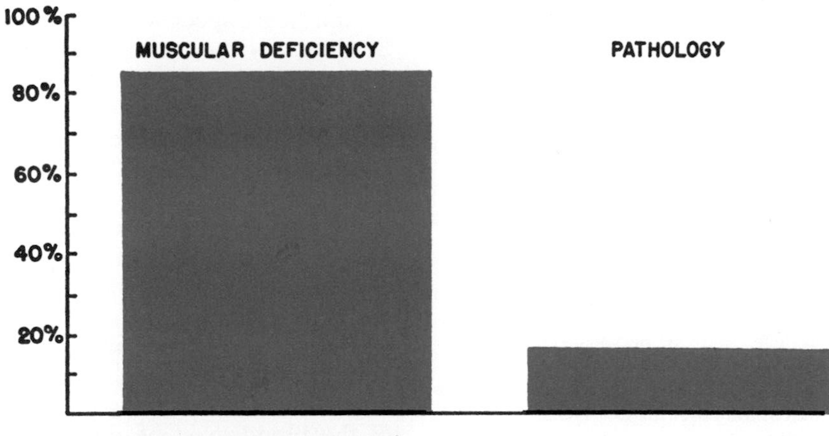

Figure 3–9. Over 80 per cent of low back pain is due to lack of physical activity. (Adapted from Gaston, S.: Preliminary report of a group study of the painful back, presented at a meeting of the Michigan Association of Industrial Physicians and Surgeons, Detroit, Michigan, March 11, 1947; Kraus, H.: Diagnosis and treatment of low back pain, G. P., No. 4, 1952; Stimson, B.: The low back problem, Psychosom. Med., *9*:210, 1947; Thompson, W.: Keeping the patient with low back pain employable. Indust. Med. Surg., *22*:318, 1953.)

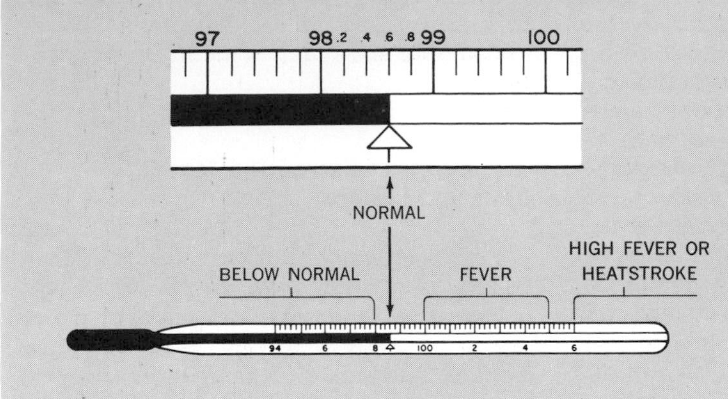

Clinical thermometer measures body temperature to nearest tenth of a degree. The arrows show normal temperature when taken by mouth.

Effects of Physical Fitness on Scholastic Achievement

The results of good physical fitness show up in a variety of areas, some unexpected. For example, there appears to be a definite relationship between physical fitness and academic achievement, according to a study conducted on male freshmen at the State University of Iowa.[27] This study showed that, in general, good grades accompanied good physical fitness. These results were partially confirmed by a second study of the freshmen male students dismissed from Syracuse University because of low grades.[28] H. H. Clarke has concluded that[29] "a person's general learning potential for a given level of intelligence is increased or decreased in accordance with his degree of physical fitness."

The famous psychologist, L. M. Terman, has stated after 25 years of studying the intellectually gifted that:[30]

> "The results of the physical measurements and the medical examinations provide a striking contrast to the popular stereotype of the child prodigy, so commonly predicted as a pathetic creature, overly serious, undersized, sickly, hollow-chested, nervously tense, and bespectacled. There are gifted children who bear some resemblance to this stereotype, but the truth is that almost every element in the picture, except the last, is less characteristic of the gifted child than of the mentally average."

Special Considerations in Exercise

Athlete's Heart. For a long time, it was believed that athletes could endanger their hearts permanently, particularly if they engaged in very strenuous competitive sports. There is absolutely no experimental evidence to support this myth of the pathological *athlete's heart.* Strenuous exercise does not injure a normal heart in any way. That this also holds true for older age groups has been demonstrated by a Miami heart specialist. A study by Dr. E. Sterling Nichol indicated no adverse changes in the electrocardiograms of men aged 65 to 81 years following participation in singles tennis matches.

Exercise in High Temperatures. You have probably noticed that fatigue sets in much earlier when you work in the heat. This is because your blood supply must be divided between the working muscles and the skin. During work, most of the blood is delivered to the muscles to sustain performance; however, when the temperature becomes very high, a large portion of the blood must be diverted to the skin to eliminate heat. Because the muscles are thus robbed of a large portion of their normal blood supply, they may fatigue easily.

If exercise is prolonged before the person

[27] Weber, R. J.: Relationship of physical fitness to success in college and to personality. *Research Quarterly, 24*:471, 1953.

[28] Page, C. G.: Case studies of college men with low physical fitness indices, Master's Thesis, Syracuse University, 1940.

[29] Clarke, H. H.: *Application of Measurement to Health and Physical Education.* Prentice-Hall, Englewood Cliffs, N.J., 1959.

[30] Terman, L. M., ed.: *Genetic Studies of Genius.* IV. *The Gifted Child Grows Up.* Stanford University Press, Stanford, Calif., 1947, p. 24.

becomes heat-acclimatized, the combined needs of the skin and muscles for blood may exceed the capacity of the heart to pump blood. This leads to a type of circulatory shock—not qualitatively different from that suffered in hemorrhage. Fortunately, this usually results in fainting, which terminates the exercise. This condition—known as heat exhaustion—is not serious, and recovery usually follows a period of inactivity. Secondarily, this circulatory inadequacy may lead to a breakdown in the heat regulatory mechanism (heat stroke). This condition—in which sweating stops—is serious, and untreated victims can succumb.

It is important then that you take every precaution to prevent these heat related conditions. The first step in this direction is achievement of heat acclimatization. Given time, your body will adjust to heat, allowing you to work with a lower body temperature and heart rate. This process of acclimatization takes four to seven days. During this period, an hour program of exercise of gradually increased effort should be undertaken. Simply living in a hot environment does not prepare your body for work in heat.

Replacement of fluids and salts lost through normal perspiration is important. Water should be replaced at least each hour, whereas the salt may be replaced at mealtime. Failure to replace salt leads to heat cramps. Both water and salt balance are basic to normal body function.

There are a number of popular misconceptions regarding water replacement. One is that withholding water from an athlete makes him "tough" or better able to do without water. This is not true; furthermore, it may result in heat stroke.

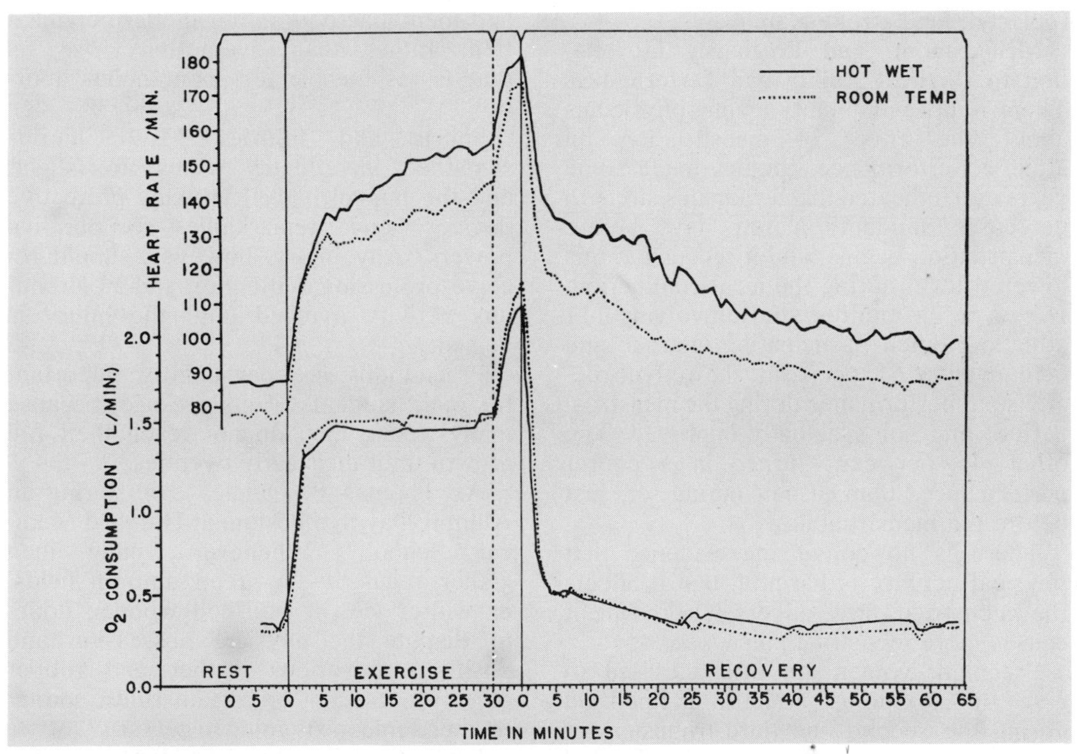

Figure 3–10. Effects of exercise on heart rate and oxygen consumption for six male subjects at normal temperature and humidity (72° F. and 50 per cent relative humidity, dotted lines) and in a hot humid environment (90° F. and 82 per cent relative humidity, solid lines). The exercise consisted of pedaling a bicycle ergometer for 30 minutes at submaximal work (540 kg.m./min.) followed by a 4-minute period of maximum work (900 kg.m./min.). Although a steady state of oxygen consumption was reached at the lower load in both environments, the heart rate continued to increase, particularly with the hot wet environment. Oxygen consumption recovered rapidly after work to the resting level, but even after one hour, the heart rate did not recover, presumably because of an increased skin blood flow. (From Brouha, L., and Radford, E. P., Jr.: In *Science and Medicine of Exercise and Sports* [Johnson, W. R., ed.]. New York, Harper & Brothers, 1960.)

A second misconception is that drinking water before exercise decreases performance. However, a number of studies have disproved this assumption. In one such study, 33 college track men were given one pint of water just prior to running 220-yard time trials.[31] The water had no effect on their times. In a further study, drinking more than a quart of water just prior to exercise had no effect on the ability of college students to run on a treadmill.[32]

A third misconception is that the more you drink, the more you perspire. In the absence of severe dehydration, drinking more water does not affect the rate of perspiration.

In conclusion, it is very important that you drink freely when working or exercising in the heat. Intake of water should be equal to the amount lost through perspiration if you are to maintain maximum physiological efficiency. If water is properly replaced, heat stroke is unlikely.

Menstruation and Pregnancy in Relation to Physical Ability and Performance. There is little unanimity among physicians about the effect of menstruation on athletic performance. Studies made some years ago indicated that a woman's strength decreases suddenly a few days before menstruation begins, and it remains at this lowered level during the menstrual period. However, in another study involving 111 athletic women participating in track and field events, 55 per cent showed no decrease in performance during the menstrual period, and some actually improved. The other 45 per cent turned in a poorer performance than usual during or just before the menstrual flow.

There is no convincing evidence that physical activity is harmful, that it affects the menstrual flow adversely or that it causes more menstrual pain.

Pregnant women are often advised to give up strenuous athletic competition during the second and third trimesters of pregnancy. Particular caution is directed toward horseback riding, high jumping and skating, because a fall might cause malposition of the fetus.

On the other hand, there are very good indications that the better abdominal development of women engaged in regular exercise (and muscular training during pregnancy in general) may shorten the course of labor or reduce the pain. In one of the Olympic Games, a performer who was 3½ months pregnant placed third in the diving competition, and another pregnant athlete was on the skiing team. Both later experienced uneventful deliveries of perfectly normal children. Many top female athletes have reached the peak of their performance just after pregnancy.

There is no scientific evidence to support the belief that overexertion is a cause of miscarriage. Based on a study of the records of 250,000 pregnancies and deliveries in New York City, Dr. Carl Javert concluded: "It is the lack of physical and mental activity in our modern civilization, rather than overactivity *per se*, that is responsible for spontaneous abortion."

Sports and Injuries. Most injuries sustained in athletic games are slight, and the human body has many protective devices and remarkable recuperative powers. Any injury, however, should receive professional attention and all strenuous activity avoided until the injury is healed.

Precautions are particularly important for male students of college age, because many young men do not reach their full growth until their early twenties.

As Thomas B. Quigley said during an Alumni Day Symposium at Harvard Medical School: "Whenever young men gather regularly on green autumn fields, or winter ice, or polished wooden floors to dispute the physical possession and position of various leather and rubber objects according to certain rules, sooner or later someone is going to get hurt."

Proper equipment, knowledge of the basic skills, and proper supervision prevent most situations leading to injury. Safety considerations are discussed in Chapter 19; however, in any activity or sports program the student should be responsible in avoiding action that could lead to injury of himself or others.

---

[31]Blank, L. B.: An experimental study of the effect of water ingestion upon performance. *Research Quarterly, 30*:131, 1959.

[32]Little, C. C., *et al.*: Effect of water ingestion on capacity for exercise. *Research Quarterly, 20*:398, 1949.

PHYSICAL FITNESS AFTER COLLEGE

As early as the 15th century, the artist-scientist Leonardo da Vinci suggested that premature aging was due to lack of exercise. Also, you have undoubtedly observed physically active people who appear to be much younger than their chronological age. Moreover, examination of the internal structures of such persons would reveal the same phenomenon. For example, the surgeon who removed an inflamed gallbladder from Andy Varipapa—a 65 year old competitor in national bowling tournaments—commented: "Observations prior to and after surgery indicated to me that, physiologically, Andy was in the 35-year age classification."

The athletic performance of men in the older age brackets is often astounding. For instance, J. B. Wolffe studied a group of 32 men just before and after they ran a marathon race of approximately 26 miles. Walter Alvarez, Editor of *Modern Medicine,* in commenting on the study, said: "After reading all my life that an athlete is usually 'washed up' by the time he is 35, I was astonished to read that one of the runners was 63 years old, and five were fifty and over. Half the men were 35 and older, and 10 were 40 and over." Perhaps even more astounding is the fact that over 50 men, all more than 70 years of age, competed in a national tennis tournament (for older players) held during 1964.

If you continue to exercise regularly through the years, you too will be able to enjoy many of the active sports in later life. The important thing is *regularity.* Once you become sedentary, it is difficult to get back into the habit of regular exercise. Motivation in middle age is low, whereas the process of rationalization is highly efficient. In this connection, Chauncey Depew, who lived to be 93 years old, is purported to have said that he "got his only exercise by acting as pallbearer for his friends who took exercise."

There are, undoubtedly, a number of persons who scorn exercise and yet live to a ripe old age. Indeed, there are some who have contempt for all the common-sense rules of health and yet live far beyond the average life expectancy. Sir Winston Churchill is a noted example. In addition to brandy and cigars before breakfast, he was famous for his physical laziness.

Although these individual cases may

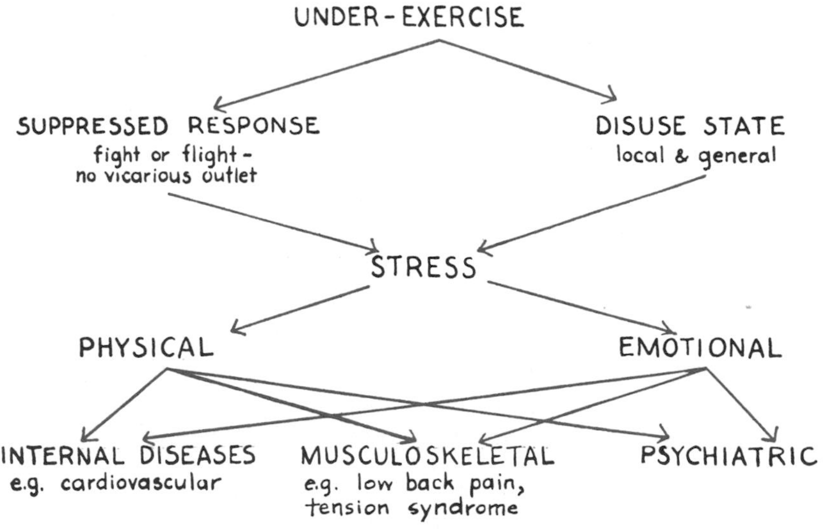

Figure 3–11. After exhibit on hypokinetic disease (A.M.A. Convention, 1956, by Kraus, H., Weber, S., Hirschhorn, K., and Prudden, B., Institute for Physical Medicine and Rehabilitation, New York University, Bellevue Medical Center, New York City: Dr. Howard Rusk, Chairman).

provide solace to those who have uncontrolled appetites and habits, let us be careful of statistics that result from a small sample. The critical person does not ignore the hazards of tobacco on the grounds that his uncle, who was a heavy smoker, lived to reach 95 years of age; or the value of the polio vaccine because his nonimmunized grandmother never had polio; or the hazards of obesity because an overweight in-law is celebrating his 92nd birthday. Neither should the critical person neglect exercise; its obvious benefits and fundamental values in normal body physiology and development are not theoretical but are medical facts.

FUTURE PLANNING

Now is the time to start planning your activity program for the after-college years. One very important consideration in selecting activities for this program is the amount of time they require. Although we hear and read a great deal about the 40 or 30 hour work week, the truth is that in our competitive society it is often necessary to work many extra hours. Indeed, the most frequent excuse for failure to exercise is phrased: "I would like to, but there just isn't time enough." This is also a popular statement with graduate, medical, and dental students and even some physical education teachers. In such cases, it is frequently impossible to engage in activities that make demands on the time schedule. How then does one maintain fitness?

The answer is to select activities that are of short duration but that require intense activity. For example, many business and professional people find it convenient to take a 20 minute swim during the lunch hour, and many YMCA's and YWCA's across the country have organized noon-hour swim clubs for this purpose. Other suitable activities include tennis, badminton, squash, handball and weight lifting. One of the very best activities is running. Running a nine to ten minute mile each day will keep you at a high level of fitness, and it requires very little time and no equipment.

There are also many interesting and challenging calisthenics programs designed to maintain fitness while making only a small demand on your time. One excellent such program has been developed by the Royal Canadian Air Force. It consists of five basic exercises for men (5BX Program) and 10 basic exercises for women (XBX Program). It requires 10 to 12 minutes daily, is a progressive program and can lead to a high level of fitness. An equally good program has been developed by the President's Council on Physical Fitness; it is entitled *Adult Physical Fitness*.[33]

In regard to short intense activity programs, there are several points you should be aware of. First, it is easy to maintain fitness once you have attained a desired level. In view of this, try to avoid becoming discouraged when you first start any program. Second, even though these activities are of short duration, they should not be viewed as drudgery. Try to develop a deeper interest in them by reading some of the references at the end of this chapter. You may also find competition helpful in holding your enthusiasm, even if you are only competing with your own record. With the purchase of an inexpensive stop watch, you can turn almost any activity into an exciting form of competition. Ask yourself the questions: How many laps of the pool can I swim in 20 minutes? How many push-ups or sit-ups can I do in a minute? How fast can I run the mile? Remember, however, that you are not trying for a world record. It may take you 12 minutes to run a mile, but in time you may be able to reduce the time to 10 or 11 minutes.

In planning your activity program for later life, it is also important to remember that activity has a wide range of intensity—from complete relaxation to very intense exertion. Recent emphasis has been directed toward the very intense activities. However, even just being out of bed is beneficial to fitness; early ambulation after surgical operations has resulted in fewer complications, less disability and more rapid convalescence.

[33]For sale by the Superintendent of Documents, U.S. Government Printing Office, Washington, D.C. Publication No. 0-689-764.

According to Dr. R. C. Swan of Ontario, Canada, even the minimal exercise involved in rocking in a chair benefits the body. It increases venous return, stimulates muscle tone, encourages supple joints and helps to avoid lung congestion. A pleasant walk stimulates the appetite, aids digestion, improves circulation and respiration, and eases the tensions of the day.

In view of this, it is very important that you also consider critically the low-intensity end of the activity scale. Activities in the middle of the scale (golf, archery or fishing, to cite a few) may be very important to your health because of their relaxing effect and the opportunity they afford in making new business and social acquaintances whose interests in these activities are common to your own. To be sure, it would be unwise to think that because some activity is beneficial you should exercise as much as possible and to exhaustion each time. The truth is that we have very little scientific information to indicate how much activity a given individual can profit from. It is interesting, nevertheless, to recall that individuals who maintain fitness throughout the years can compete in a 26 mile marathon at 63 years of age, enter a national tennis tournament after 70, and enjoy an active life and good health beyond the span of years of many who will fall victim to diseases or failures of body function because of weakness and inactivity.

Questions

1. How is the need for exercise in modern society related to our evolutionary development?
2. What is the purpose of a college physical education program?
3. What in your opinion should be the content of such a program?
4. How might physical fitness benefit cardiovascular health?
5. Distinguish between sympathetic preponderance and parasympathetic dominance.
6. What advantages does exercise have over other techniques of weight control?
7. What evidence do you think prompted one of our country's leading nutritionists to state: "I am convinced that inactivity is the most important factor explaining the frequency of 'creeping overweight' in modern Western Societies?"
8. How might you use exercise as a tranquilizer?
9. How can exercise serve as a laxative?
10. Why are your sitting habits important?
11. What precautions should be observed when exercising in the heat?
12. What factors should be considered in planning your fitness program for the after-college years?

Topics for Discussion

Exercise and Cardiovascular Health
Role of Exercise in Weight Control
Exercise and Nervous Tension
Exercise and Aging
How to Benefit from College Physical Education
Misconceptions About Exercise

Reading Suggestions

Fitness For the Whole Family, Paul D. White and Curtis Mitchel. J. B. Lippincott Co., Philadelphia, 1964. One of the country's leading cardiologists describes the value and the means of obtaining family fitness.

Adult Physical Fitness, by the President's Council on Youth Fitness. U.S. Government Printing Office, (Publication No. 0-689-764) Washington, D.C. This publication outlines a fitness program for adults.

The 5BX and XBX Program, by the Royal Canadian Air Force. Obtained in this country from *This Week Magazine,* Box 77E, Mount Vernon, N.Y. An interesting and challenging fitness program for both men and women.

Science and Medicine of Exercise and Sports, Warren R. Johnson (ed.). Harper and Brothers Publishers, New York, 1960. An authoritative review of the entire field of exercise physiology.

Hypokinetic Disease. Role of Inactivity in Production of Disease, Hans Kraus and W. Raab. Charles C Thomas, Springfield, Ill., 1961. A well written and clear description of the role of inactivity in the etiology of disease.

Physical Activity in Modern Living, Wayne Van Huss, et al. Prentice-Hall, Englewood Cliffs, N.J., 1960. This book presents the "how" and "why" of physical activity in a lucid but authoritative manner.

Exercise and Fitness, The Athletic Institute, Chicago, 1960. A collection of papers presented on a variety of topics related to exercise and fitness.

Health and Fitness in the Modern World, The Athletic Institute, Chicago, 1961. A collection of interesting papers presented at an International Conference on Sports Medicine.

Sports Medicine for Trainers, Laurence E. Morehouse and Philip J. Rasch. 2nd Ed., Philadelphia, W. B. Saunders, 1963. Excellent discussions of the principles of conditioning for the novice athlete, for the champion and for older adults.

Special section on fitness. *Today's Health,* October 1964, pp. 16–49. This issue contains eleven articles related to exercise and fitness.

"How Your Own Strength Can Hurt You," Kenneth N. Anderson. *Today's Health,* April 1965, p. 19. A well written article on athletic injuries. The illustrations are excellent.

4

FATIGUE, SLEEP AND REST

He that can take rest is greater than he that can take cities.

BENJAMIN FRANKLIN

In Chapter Three, you learned the importance of physical exercise. But inactivity and rest are of equal importance. In fact, every living organism, from the simplest ameba to man himself, shows alternating periods of activity and inactivity in the daily cycle. We may feel very lively at certain times of the day and listless and fatigued at others; everybody seems to have his characteristic cycle.

FATIGUE

Causes of Fatigue. As yet, we do not fully understand the many causes of fatigue, but whatever its origin, it is Nature's cry for rest and diversion. Unlike man-made machines, human machines must occasionally slow down and rest.

If fatigue develops after intense or prolonged physical activity or lack of sleep, it should arouse no anxiety, because this is a normal and natural phenomenon. However, if you constantly feel fatigued even when you should be rested and relaxed, you should suspect some illness or emotional disturbance and consult with your doctor.

In strenuous exercise, the body has a certain limit of endurance, and, past this, we are warned by a sensation of actual pain that fatigue has set in. The pain is probably due to a metabolic disturbance resulting from a lack of oxygen in the overworked muscles.

Sometimes, when the fatigue has not reached too extreme a level, the body succeeds in making the necessary new adjustments in time, and pumps the blood fast enough to take care of the immediate and pressing needs. When this happens, we get our "second wind," and the panting and sensation of extreme fatigue cease temporarily. Because of this physiological adjustment, athletes who feel they are ready to drop often succeed in making the "gears re-mesh" and obtain the energy needed to finish grueling contests.

The capacity of the body to withstand prolonged and extreme fatigue has often been observed in soldiers as well as athletes. Ernie Pyle, the beloved correspondent of World War II, described this very movingly in one of his dispatches to the Scripps-Howard Newspaper Alliance:

> I believe the outstanding trait in any campaign is the terrible weariness that gradually comes over everybody. Soldiers become exhausted in mind and in soul as well as physically. . . . The infantry reaches a stage of exhaustion that is incomprehensible to folks back home. The men in the First Division, for instance, were in the lines twenty-eight days—walking and fighting all that time, day and night.
>
> After a few days of such activity, soldiers pass the point of known human weariness. From then on they go into a sort of second-wind daze.
>
> Have you ever in your life worked so hard and so long that you didn't remember how many days it was since you ate last or didn't recognize your friends when you saw them? I never have, either, but in the First Division, during that long, hard fight around Troina, a company runner one day came slogging up to a certain captain and said excitedly, "I've got to find Captain Blank right away. Important message."
>
> The Captain said, "But I am Captain Blank. Don't you recognize me?"
>
> And the runner said, "I've got to find Captain Blank right away." And he went dashing off.[1]

It is not only physical exertion which brings on fatigue. Excessive noise in the atmosphere of work or play may be very tiring. Also, extreme heat and humidity make the heart pump faster, to evaporate perspiration and cool the skin, and can contribute to fatigue.

Nervousness and psychological disturbance, too, are responsible for some of the fatigue we experience. Tiredness may come on after little or no exertion, and, even after a long night's rest, a person may still complain of listlessness and lack of energy.

Conflicting emotions can disturb the smooth operations of the human body enormously. Doctors say that the majority of patients who consult them because of fatigue are *emotionally* tired and disturbed. Fatigue caused by emotional disturbance is often preceded by feelings of restlessness or nervousness. This is the kind of sensation students often experience when they are studying for examinations, and are anxious about inadequate preparation, lack of time or any other worries.

The converse is also true, however. Fatigue can *cause* nervousness and tenseness, and sometimes they are so intermixed that it's hard to determine which came first.

Most young women feel tired and irritable before or during their menstrual periods, a perfectly normal physiological reaction, brought on by a change in hormonal balance.

Colds, "flu," and upper respiratory infections are usually accompanied by fatigue, which is also one of the commonest warning symptoms of infectious mononucleosis, tuberculosis and a number of other diseases.

Effects of Fatigue. All of us are familiar with occasional episodes of mild fatigue, and what they do to us. We become less attentive, drowsy at lectures or at our work, and a good deal more irritable than usual. Very minor disturbances may be extremely upsetting, and our dispositions and whole outlook on life change when we are tired.

More serious, however, are the effects of fatigue on illnesses and infections, and upon accident proneness. Our resistance to disease may be lowered by fatigue, and the illness prolonged or intensified if we don't obtain adequate rest. This is particularly true of respiratory infections such as colds, flu, pneumonia, and pulmonary tuberculosis. The quickest way to recover from infections of this kind is to keep the body in the best possible condition to fight them, and, above all, to avoid fatigue.

All types of accidents—home, industrial and highway—occur more frequently in people who are tired. This is not unexpected. When we are fatigued, we are less alert than usual to possible hazards: the dangers of laboratory equipment, falling down stairs, tipping over hot teakettles, making a slip with the breadknife.

Anyone who has driven long distances over modern roads, especially the excellent but monotonous turnpikes where the automobile seems almost to drive itself, knows how easy it is to get drowsy and actually

[1]Pyle, E.: *Brave Men,* Henry Holt & Co., New York, 1944.

to fall asleep at the wheel. This may happen because we undertake too long a stretch of driving, so that fatigue is added to monotony.

John A. P. Millet describes such experiences in his book *How Did You Sleep Last Night?*:

> It is possible . . . for certain parts of the brain to be "asleep" while others are "awake." Instances have been recorded of soldiers falling asleep while in the act of marching, and of continuing to march in perfect time while unconscious of all that went on around them. Some of us have had the unpleasant experience of falling asleep at the wheel of a car and of continuing to drive with enough precision to avoid an immediate accident.

What to Do About Fatigue. If you are overly tired, there is only one cure: find the cause and try to correct it. In searching for the cause, you may find a formula suggested by the Canadian medical scientist, Dr. Hans Selye, of value:

$$\text{Stress quotient} = \frac{\text{local stress in any one part}}{\text{total stress in the body}}$$

If there is proportionately too much stress in one part of the body, Dr. Selye says that diversion is needed. For instance, maybe only one part of your body is tired, in which case you should rest this part and use another part. After intensive cramming for an exam, you may feel stale and jaded. A brisk walk can be helpful, because it rests your brain and at the same time stimulates you by exposing you to fresh air, new stimuli and new impressions. If your eyes are tired, stop reading and listen to some music. If your hands feel a little stiff after too much writing, typing or sewing, play a game of cards or engage in some form of athletics in which delicate hand coordination is not required.

If fatigue results from boredom or worry, a change of scene that permits you to forget your troubles is helpful. Athletics, hobbies or almost any form of physical activity is a relief when you work or when studies become too monotonous.

In contrast to local stress, there may be too much stress on the body as a whole; for example, you may suffer from too little or too restless a sleep. In this case, you must rest; exhaustion can be appeased only by adequate rest.

If fatigue persists even after suitable diversion and rest, you should discuss the problem with your doctor. A medical examination may reveal the cause. Remember that your doctor is willing to talk over, in confidence, any problem that may bear on the chronic fatigue. Emotional problems should be mentioned because they often provide the explanation.

A number of stimulants have been used with more or less success to relieve fatigue. Coffee, tea and some cola drinks contain enough caffeine to be a helpful crutch in an emergency, but should certainly not be substituted routinely for adequate rest. The same is true of drugs and medicines such as Benzedrine sulfate, Dexedrine and related stimulants. These substances may stimulate at first, but can also cause nervousness and a jittery feeling. *Never use any medicines* to relieve fatigue or any other symptom, except under a physician's guidance.

Prevention of Chronic Fatigue Through Physical Fitness. One of the most common complaints among modern men and women is chronic fatigue. Indeed, it is this condition that prevents many persons from enjoying what might otherwise be a "good life." It is this same condition that distinguishes the old from the "young at heart."

Too many people come to the end of the workday completely fatigued, although they have performed very little physical work. They are tense and irritable, unable to enjoy the fruits of their work and frequently unable to sleep.

Many cures have been proposed for this "rundown" feeling—especially through television commercials. Unfortunately, most of these cures are of no value; in fact, doctors are frequently unable to find any physical cause of chronic fatigue. Recently, more emphasis has been placed on prevention of this condition. If chronic fatigue is not of pathologic origin or does not result from an emotional disturbance, chances are that it could have been prevented by maintaining a higher level of physical fitness.

The physically fit person comes to the end of the work day with more vigor and zest than his unfit friends. He is able to enjoy recreational pursuits with his family after the workday is finished. He has a sufficient reserve of energy to enjoy a hobby, a book or a dance; when the day ends, he is sleepy rather than tired.

There are a number of physiological explanations for the abundant zest enjoyed by the physically fit individual. Such a person performs his daily physiological tasks with greater efficiency. His heart, circulatory system and muscular system work with less effort. Not only does the fit person work more efficiently, but he also has less work to do – that is, the energy required to complete a given task is proportional to the weight of the individual, and the fit person is less likely to be overweight. The fit person also recovers more rapidly from fatigue and thus is able to continue with his chosen activities after only a brief rest.

SLEEP

Although many theories have been proposed to explain sleep, we are only beginning to understand this extremely important phase of life.

Some of the theories invoke "fatigue toxins"; "wakefulness toxins"; chemical ions, such as calcium, acting on the brain; muscular relaxation; instinct; and lack of sufficient blood flow to the brain.

The part of the brain called the hypothalamus may actually contain the "sleep center." Tumors in this area make people abnormally sleepy, and experimental lesions produced in animals have the same effect. Perhaps there is a "waking center" in the hypothalamus, and when this is inhibited, sleep ensues.

If a "fatigue toxin" were really the cause of fatigue, then we should eliminate this toxin while we slept, and always wake up refreshed and "rarin' to go." Actually, many people awaken very slowly, and don't reach their peak of efficiency until hours after getting up. Some, the real "nighttime people," don't achieve this state until midnight. Body temperature curves help to explain these differences. People who work best early in the day also attain their temperature peak around noon. Others don't reach it until nearly midnight.

We apparently drop off to sleep because of a subtle interaction between our muscles and our brain. Muscular tension stimulates the cortex of our brains, and, in turn, the cortex activates the muscles to activity. When we are tired and lie down, our muscle tone diminishes, and sends fewer messages to the brain. The decreased activity of the cortex lets the muscles relax still further. Finally, we sleep when the cross-stimulation between the brain and the muscles reaches the lowest possible level, like dwindling conversation between two people.

Physiologists have found that we fall asleep in parts. The first to respond are the large muscles which bend the back, legs, arms and neck. Next come smaller muscles, such as those which control the hands, toes, feet and fingers. The smallest muscles, such as the ones around the lips, brows and eyelids, take longest to relax.

Senses relax one at a time, too. First to go is the sense of smell. Vision gets sleepy before hearing, and the sense of touch is the last to give up.

It is now possible, by use of new laboratory devices, to induce a sleeplike state of consciousness by electrical stimulation of the brain. Although these sleep-producing machines are as yet highly experimental, it may some day be possible to completely control sleep. Presently, it is possible to put dogs to sleep in a matter of minutes with this new technique.

How Much Sleep Do We Need? The amount of sleep necessary to maintain good health varies tremendously from person to person. Eight hours appears to be the average, but some individuals require more and others, less. Thomas Edison, for example, apparently managed on only five hours of sleep a night.

In a study conducted by Dr. J. Kamiya of the University of California School of Medicine, a college student slept for only 4 hours a day for a period of one year. He slept from 4 A.M. to 6 A.M. and again from 4 P.M. to 6 P.M. Although this schedule appeared sufficient for the student, Dr. Kamiya says that it cannot be generally recommended until the long range health effects are investigated.

Sleep requirements are greatest at

birth and decline progressively with the years. A newborn infant may sleep 20 to 22 hours a day, although some do well on as little as 15 hours. Between the ages of one and four, about half the day is spent in sleep. For children 4 to 12 years old, about 10 hours sleep are required. Adolescents usually need 8 to 10 hours, adults, 7 to 9 hours, and elderly people, 5 to 7 hours.

College students tend to sleep, on the average, a little less than 8 hours. However, it is important to remember that anyone who is easily fatigued or who engages in strenuous athletics, needs more sleep than the average.

The Soundness of Sleep. The pattern of sleep varies considerably from one individual to another. Some quickly reach a very deep sleep, which becomes more shallow as time passes. Others sleep lightly at first, and then assume a very sound sleep later in the night.

Several methods have been developed to test the intensity of sleep. The simplest one is to determine how loud a sound must be generated to awaken the sleeper. The deeper the sleep, the greater the noise required.

A graph of sleep intensity shows many fluctuations in the course of the night, becoming more and more shallow close to the time of awakening.

Results of Insufficient Sleep. No one has better described the balm of sleep than Shakespeare, and perhaps the most famous are the lines from Macbeth:

> Methought I heard a voice cry, 'Sleep no more!
> Macbeth doth murder sleep!' The innocent sleep.
> Sleep that knits up the ravell'd sleeve of care,
> The death of each day's life, sore labor's bath,
> Balm of hurt minds, great nature's second course,
> Chief nourisher in life's feast.

Shakespeare was not alone in recognizing the tremendous need of the human mechanism for this daily period of rest from the strain and fatigue of everyday life. Insufficient sleep probably means incomplete repair and restoration of body cells. We work at less than maximum efficiency the following day, and may be nervous and irritable.

Long continued lack of sleep, like overfatigue, may be responsible for dizziness, and sufficient mental sluggishness and poor neuromuscular control to cause serious accidents.

Fatigue from inadequate sleep is the most obvious explanation for the large number of automobile accidents which occur at night. Far too many people fall asleep while driving on long trips and may awaken only when the crash occurs. Unfortunately, some never awaken.

An Army experiment showed that it was possible to keep soldiers awake for as long as 98 hours, without drugs or stimulants of any kind. Nathaniel Kleitman extended this figure to a marathon 180 hours (7½ days), and a disk jockey named Peter Tripp stayed awake for 201 hours. This required stimulants, a team of watchers, and constant poking and prodding!

Insomnia. The sound sleeper is a very fortunate person, unfamiliar with all the problems which can interfere with sleep: rolling, tossing, sleepwalking, disturbing dreams which may even awaken the sleeper, and worst of all, insomnia. Fortunately, this is a problem which rarely disturbs college students. A survey made of college students showed that about 80 per cent fell asleep within a few minutes, and about 95 per cent in less than an hour.

The chief causes of sleeplessness or difficulty in falling asleep are anxiety, problems of insecurity and overstimulation.

Anxiety results from our inner emotions and attitudes, and may be very diffuse and generalized. Whatever its nature, it can profoundly affect our ability to relax and fall asleep. It is interesting that feelings of anxiety and insecurity from *specific* causes—such as the dangers of a flood or bombings during a war—may have little or no effect on sleep. For example a study was made during the years of World War II when the people of London were subjected to almost nightly bombings. This very definite physical insecurity, night after night, produced no significant continued ill effects on sleep for most people.

Dreams and Movement During Sleep. Kleitman and his research group have recently shown that dreams and their duration may be timed with electro-oculograms of the eye movements of the sleeper. They can also be studied with the electroencephalograph, because the brain waves change during dreams.

These and other studies indicate that we dream every night, even though we may awaken with absolutely no recollection of dreaming. Most dreaming periods last 10 to 30 minutes, and the end of the night is the busiest time for dreaming.

Also, there apparently is no such thing as motionless sleep. Most people turn as many as 20 to 60 times a night, shifting position so unconsciously that it doesn't disturb the restfulness of their sleep. A surprising amount of time in a perfectly restful sleep will be spent stirring and changing positions.

Sleepwalking. Somnambulists, or sleepwalkers, can engage in numerous activities while they are asleep. They dress themselves, open doors and windows, climb stairs, walk to the refrigerator, and even stroll outdoors.

Dr. Jack Kaplan, writing in the American Medical Association magazine *Today's Health,* gives the following account of some of the activities of sleepwalkers:

> In Enid, Oklahoma, a pretty blond housewife—asleep and completely nude—climbed a tree . . . Another sleepwalker is reported to have written a novel in his sleep. And a civil engineer in Denver, Colorado, stabbed himself while sleeping. In still another case, a mother flung her baby out the window while dreaming that her home was afire. Also, a number of murders have been performed by sleepwalkers.

These daring and sometimes criminal acts are disturbing, until we understand the facts about sleepwalking. The following information, summarized from Kaplan's article, is more comforting:

1. Ordinary sleepwalkers do not act with violence against themselves or others. Nor do they commit crimes. Psychiatrists say that crimes are not committed by simple sleepwalkers but rather by borderline psychotics. It is the opinion of many psychiatrists that sleepwalkers will do nothing to violate their moral code.

2. Most cases of sleepwalking result

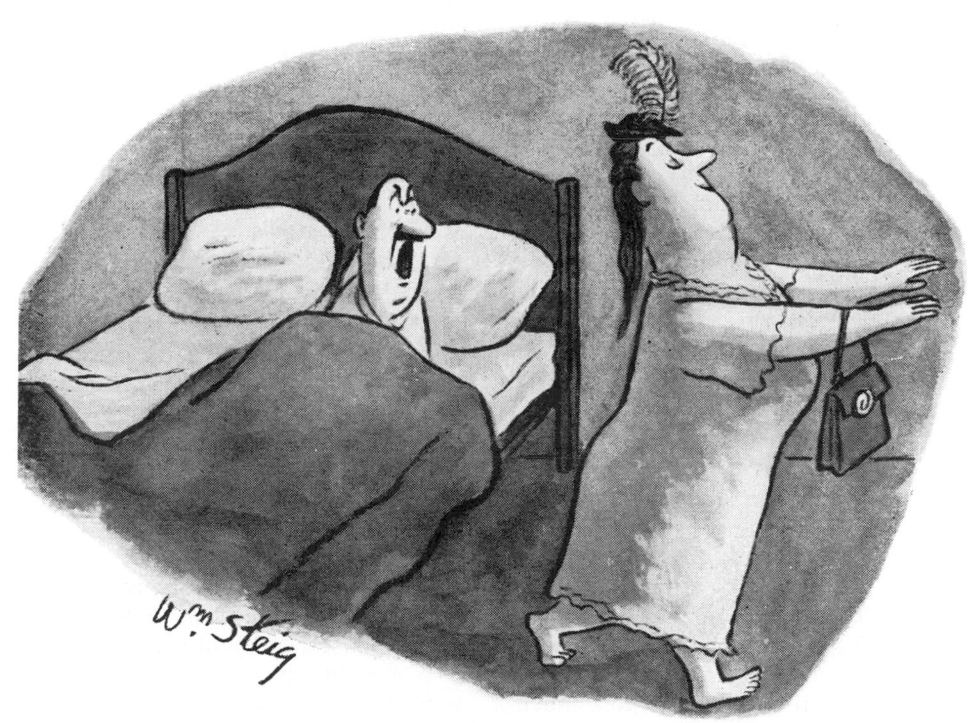

"Macy's is closed!"

(Drawing by Wm. Steig, Copr. © 1949, The New Yorker Magazine, Inc.)

from emotional disturbances that interfere with normal sleeping.

3. Contrary to the popular notion that sleepwalkers never injure themselves, they frequently fall down stairs, trip over objects on the floor and sometimes sustain serious injuries.

4. The normal sleepwalker does not attempt superhuman feats.

5. There is no scientific basis for the notion that a sleepwalker should not be awakened suddenly out of fear that he may go into shock.

6. Sleepwalking occurs more frequently in children than in adults.

7. Since most sleepwalking is an expression of concealed anxieties, the sleepwalker should consult a physician.

Snoring. Everybody jokes about snoring, but the various unpleasant noises which approximately 21 million snorers make can actually be seriously disturbing to their unhappy listeners.

An unidentified wit is responsible for the lines:

> Laugh and the world laughs with you.
> Snore and you sleep alone.

Approximately one out of eight Americans, women as often as men, make some type of unmusical sound nightly. It may take the form of a grunt, hiss, snort, gurgle, or an assortment of noises, and it sometimes assumes a surprising intensity. To indicate the nuisance value of this problem: The United States Patent Office shows patents for more than 300 snore-curbing devices.

Snoring is caused by vibrations in the soft palate and other soft structures of the throat, when they come in contact with inflowing and outflowing air. The position of the tongue, enlarged tonsils or adenoids, a blocked nose, a bent or twisted septum (the septum is the structure which divides the nose into halves), and nasal polyps or growths can all be responsible for snoring. Other common causes are: allergic conditions or colds which cause swelling of the mucous linings of the nose and induce mouth breathing, too much smoking, fatigue, overwork, and general poor health.

Fortunately, many of these conditions can be corrected, either surgically or medically. For example, removal of enlarged tonsils and adenoids or of nasal polyps may give enormous relief. The use of certain drugs—antibiotics to reduce an infection, antihistaminics to shrink the nasal membranes, and steroid hormones—often clear up extreme nasal congestion.

Most people snore only when lying on their backs, and an enforced change in position which prevents the tongue from falling back will prevent the snoring. An old remedy, dating from the eighteenth century, stopped the snorer from sleeping on his back by sewing a hair brush to the back of his nightshirt.

How to Ensure a Good Night's Rest. The best way to guarantee that you will fall asleep—if this is a problem—is to get in the habit of making some kind of ritual out of it. Do the things which you believe make you fall asleep and sleep well: these vary tremendously from person to person and what works wonders for some may be absolutely useless for others. Some of the time-established recipes are: inhaling and exhaling deeply, warm baths, warm drinks, darkness and quiet, and monotonous sounds. Other techniques are: brushing the teeth in a specially vigorous way, laying out the next day's clothes, and undressing in a particular order.

The soundest general advice is to establish regular habits for sleeping, as with everything else. These enhance the quality of one's sleep as well as improve one's performance during waking hours.

Anything which serves to dissipate anxieties or feelings of insecurity—even ritualistic activity—is soothing, and aids sleep. Charles Darwin, a notoriously poor sleeper, carried a compass with him whenever he slept away from home. This enabled him to move the bed around so that his head always faced north.

It is said that Lewis Carroll, the brilliant mathematician who wrote *Alice in Wonderland,* was plagued by anxieties and experienced great difficulty in falling asleep. To divert himself at night and clear his mind of worry, he created mathematical puzzles as he lay in bed. *Pillow Problems* was the book which resulted from these efforts, and other insomniacs also find them a good remedy for sleep.

Nathaniel Kleitman has probably lost

more sleep studying sleep than any other man alive and has exploded many fallacies about the subject. According to Kleitman:

Dreaming doesn't impair sleep. We dream far more than we remember.

No part of the sleep cycle—beginning, middle or end—is any better than any other part. For example, the hours before midnight are worth no more in terms of rest than the hours after midnight.

Deep sleep is not necessarily more restful than shallow sleep.

We shouldn't be surprised if we awaken slowly and listlessly. This is normal and natural for some people.

It is possible to manage for surprisingly long periods of time with much less sleep than we are accustomed to, without endangering ourselves in any way.

Questions

1. Describe some of the causes of fatigue.
2. How do you think the emotions contribute to the sensation of fatigue?
3. What is the influence of fatigue on accident rate, and why? On resistance to infections?
4. Why are stimulant drugs a dangerous crutch in the prevention of fatigue?
5. What determines the amount of sleep we need? How is this modified by such factors as weather, emotional disturbances, and age?
6. What physiological factor differentiates people who wake rapidly and those who awaken and get moving slowly?
7. What are the chief causes of sleeplessness? How can they be eliminated to assure sounder sleep?
8. Describe the causes and prevention of snoring.
9. How are dreams and movements during sleep studied?
10. What do you think the body and the mind achieve through dreaming?

Topics for Discussion

The importance of relaxation in our society.
Body temperature curves.
Current theories and research on sleep.
Methods of avoiding chronic fatigue.
Do dreams have meaning?
Psychologic significance of sleepwalking.

Reading Suggestions

What's in a Yawn? Albert Abarbanel. Today's Health, May 1964, p. 30. An interesting and informative discussion of the physiology of a yawn.

Do You Overwork Around the House? Marvin Weisbord. Today's Health, January 1960, p. 32. Efficiency engineers tell you how to accomplish housework with a minimum of effort.

Sleepwalking: Fact, Fallacy or Fancy? Jack Kaplan. Today's Health, September 1960, p. 33. An authoritative description of the current state of our knowledge regarding sleepwalking.

Do You Need 8 Hours Sleep? Andrew Hamilton. Science Digest, July 1964, p. 23. A very good summary of recent evidence.

The Stress of Life, Hans Selye. McGraw-Hill Co., New York, 1956. The world's most famous stress physiologist describes his theories of stress in a well written and easy to understand manner.

You Must Relax, Edmund Jacobson. McGraw-Hill Co., New York, 1957. The author of this famous book presents techniques designed to help you relax.

Do You Have Trouble Sleeping? Harold L. Williams. *Reader's Digest,* January 1964, p. 117. A psychologist answers some important questions about insomnia.

Sound Facts About Snoring, Noel D. Fabricant. Today's Health, January 1958, p. 18. What causes it and how to prevent it.

Sleep and Wakefulness, Nathaniel Kleitman. University of Chicago Press, Chicago, revised and enlarged, 1963. Probably the most comprehensive volume available on the subject; an accurate and documented account of the physiology of sleep; 4337 references are listed.

Toward an Understanding of Health and Physical Education, Arthur H. Steinhaus. Wm. C. Brown, Dubuque, Ia., 1963. An excellent description of the relationship of exercise and relaxation to good health.

Work and Leisure, Nels Anderson. The Macmillan Co., New York, 1962. The director of research of the UNESCO Institute for Social Research in Cologne, Germany, discusses the creative use of time that advances in technology is giving us.

Of Time, Work and Leisure, Sebastian de Grazia. The Twentieth Century Fund, New York, 1962. A professor of political science at Rutgers University discusses the history of leisure and work. A thought provoking book.

Fatigue Resistance, P. Y. Kravchenko. Pergamon Press, Inc., New York, 1963. Some important tips for living a balanced life are discussed in this well written book.

Anxiety and Tension Control—A Physiologic Approach, Edmund Jacobson. J. B. Lippincott, Philadelphia, 1964. A well known expert in the art of relaxation describes the basis of his time-tested theories.

Women and Fatigue: A Woman Doctor's Answer, Marian Hilliard. Pocket Books, New York, 1962. A sensible discussion of the conduct of life as it relates to fatigue.

Sleep for Sale, Bernard Seeman. Today's Health, September 1964, p. 23. An important evaluation of the remedies for sleeplessness.

SECTION THREE

UNDERSTANDING THE EMOTIONAL LIFE

5

THE HEALTHY MIND

World War II helped strip away the mask of secrecy which has surrounded emotional illness. Selective Service rejected more than a million men because of personality problems or more serious types of emotional disturbance. This represented a large percentage of all rejections; it was higher than the rejection rate for tuberculosis and heart trouble.

The war did not create these cases of mental illness. They had been present long before that time, but the public preferred to take an ostrich-like attitude toward them. Fortunately, we are now becoming more adult with respect to health problems of all kinds. We are learning to talk freely, honestly and sympathetically about emotional illness.

Facing emotional problems honestly is the only way people can understand their own personalities and those of others. This creates better relationships with friends, teachers, and family. It sets a good basis for love and guidance of our children.

Unfortunately, most people have many misconceptions about the emotions. How many of them do *you* subscribe to? Answer *True* or *False* to each of the following statements on the following page.

The correct answer to all these statements is *True*. If you took a long time to decide on most of them, or if you answered eight or more *False*, your attitudes toward mental hygiene need some revision. But don't be discouraged. This quiz was made up by a psychiatrist for doctors, because he found that many physicians still hold completely erroneous ideas in this field.

Our discussion of emotional problems is intended to help you replace threadbare ideas and attitudes with ones that will serve you well in solving problems you may have to face in yourself or members of your family. It will tell you about

1. Only a very few types of mental illness can be inherited. ______________
2. Masturbation does not cause insanity. ______________
3. A certain amount of daydreaming is perfectly normal. ______________
4. Unusual impulses in regard to hatred, murder, or sex—including homosexual ideas—occur *occasionally* in in normal people. ______________
5. Homosexuality is a mental illness, not "degeneracy." ______________
6. A person who is mentally ill should be regarded in the same way as a patient who is suffering from a physical disease. ______________
7. Marriage rarely improves emotional illness. ______________
8. Mental problems are not cured by sexual experience. ______________
9. There are better outlets than anger or temper tantrums for "nervousness," anxiety, or conflicts. ______________
10. Normal young children have considerable curiosity about sex. ______________
11. Even the "ideal child" is occasionally disobedient. ______________
12. Most emotional illness starts early in childhood. ______________
13. Chronic drunkenness is a deepseated psychological illness. ______________
14. Emotional difficulties, rather than inherited criminal tendencies, account for most criminal behavior. ______________
15. Modern psychiatrists deal with many emotional problems that have nothing to do with insanity. ______________

many kinds of mental disorders, how they arise and how some of them can be ameliorated or even cured. It will give you some understanding of *mental hygiene,* fully as important as knowledge of body hygiene (which it can greatly influence, as explained later under *psychosomatic illness*). When the principles of mental hygiene are applied by parents, teachers and doctors, current thinking suggests that many cases of mental disturbance can be *prevented* or *cured.*

WHAT IS NORMAL?

A dictionary defines normal as "in accordance with an established law or principle; conforming to a type or standard," and gives as synonyms: "regular, natural, standard, model, common, ordinary, typical, usual."

According to the law, anyone who is able to distinguish between right and wrong is sane; and normal behavior is regarded as *responsible behavior.*

For centuries it was believed that insanity was due to demons. Even today there is a tendency to define normal as synonomous with "what God intended." According to this vague concept, any behavior departing from Biblical injunctions would be unnatural or abnormal.

Some people define normality as being like the majority. The weakness in this concept is that history has proved that the majority can tolerate astonishingly bestial behavior. Witness the brutally sadistic actions of both men and women in Nazi Germany.

It is also incorrect to equate normality with happiness. Some obviously insane people are "happy."

Maturity is another word frequently used as a synonym for normal. However, adolescents can certainly be normal without being mature.

Actually, all these considerations enter into the psychiatrist's definition of normal. *A normal person is one who adjusts himself to his surroundings—the world he lives in and the people in it—and also to his own potentialities for living. If necessary, he makes realistic efforts to change those aspects of his life with which he is discontented.*

The abnormal person, in contrast, has developed an exaggerated, inappropriate or ineffective method of getting along with people or dealing with life situations. For example, an individual who has fears of being run over by automobiles might refuse to go outdoors, or he might spend his life in bed. This would solve the problem of his fears, but certainly not in a very satisfactory or normal manner.

Personality Structure of the Normal Person

Realistic Attitudes toward Life. The normal, emotionally mature adult faces facts whether they are pleasant or unpleasant. For example, he likes to drive his car, but realizes that there are definite dangers attached to driving. Because he is mature, he takes special care to check the brakes, tires, lights, and all the essential parts of his automobile at reasonable intervals. The immature person may say, "Accidents never happen to me," and refuse to take any precautions. Or he may be the other type of anxious individual who checks his brakes every day and still loses sleep at night worrying about the possibility that "accidents always happen to me."

Independence. The mature person forms reasoned opinions and then acts on them. He is not reckless or headstrong, and seeks a reasonable amount of advice. Once he has the facts, he is capable of making a decision and willing to face the consequences.

On the other hand, the immature person often has difficulty making up his own mind. He wants his relatives or friends or business associates to tell him how to proceed. When he is forced to make decisions alone, he may become upset, nervous, rattled, or even vicious. Many immature people don't want to accept the responsibility of the decisions they have reached, but blame others if something goes wrong, and demand inordinate praise if the decision leads to success.

Ability to Love Others. The mature adult gets pleasure from giving love to children, mate, close relatives, and friends. The mature personality overflows with a storehouse of love in the way water flows from a dam to irrigate and make bountiful the surrounding country. Such a person is selective in his love relationships and doesn't need a huge circle of people to be intimate with. On the opposite side, the immature person finds it difficult to love others and wants always to be loved, to be fussed over, and to be the center of attention. If you observe young children, you will notice that they want to be loved and to be the center of all affection. A little child seldom shows sustained love for others. This is part of normal development in children, but when such traits appear in adults, they interfere with healthy personal relationships. The adult person expects to give more love to a child than the child returns.

Reasonable Dependence on Others. A mature person can give a great deal of affection and love, but he also enjoys being on the receiving end. A good love relation between grownups must be based on the capacity of both partners not only to give love and sexual pleasure, but also to experience pleasure in receiving them. Only in this way can two people build a rich emotional relationship. The ability to share, to give, and to receive love and friendship indicates that a person possesses a reasonable degree of adaptability.

The flexible, normal person will seek advice when important decisions must be made. He will accept just criticism about mistakes or faults.

Moderate Reactions of Anger and Hatred. The normal person gets angry, of course, but he restrains his anger to reasonable limits and doesn't indulge in temper tantrums. At work, or in other situations which he may not be able to control, he may have to curb his temper in the face of petty annoyances because of the long-term values. Yet, even the normal person *can* be stirred to fierce anger when the occasion demands, as enemies of humanity have learned to their own cost. Such anger is a sign of normality and a healthy attitude toward life. It is very different from going into a temper tantrum because a storekeeper can't provide a desired item, or a teacher doesn't give the expected grade.

Ability to Make Long-range Choices. The mature person can forego immediate gratification for the sake of more lasting values. For example, a mature young couple may decide to put off marriage for a few years in order to complete their educations and get started in life. Immature individuals rush into an elopement without thought of the greater happiness which a delay might bring.

A mature student working hard before examinations refuses invitations to the movies and dances, and indulges in these pleasures when the work is finished. He foregoes the immediate pleasures for the deferred gratification of making a good showing in his studies. That would be good judgment and would indicate a flexible, healthy personality.

A Relaxed Conscience. The normal person accepts responsibility, does his job well, but insists on and enjoys his leisure hours and vacations. He and his conscience are at home with each other. The poorly adjusted person always feels driven to "accomplish," and rarely really enjoys his work. This is the unfortunate type who spends Sundays and vacations worrying about how things could have been done better, or about what was left undone. The mature person enjoys his leisure, and returns to work with refreshed strength and interest. He may do many things during his periods of relaxation, but he looks upon them as hobbies, not as more work.

Good Adjustment at Work. A normal person usually likes his work and does good work. He does not change jobs often. When he does, it is on the basis of a realistic appraisal of the job and of the chances of finding something better. He might give up a job if health and accident hazards are not being corrected, or if the rate of pay is substandard. But the normal individual will not change jobs simply because the supervisor has a nasty disposition or a fellow worker is difficult to get along with. He doesn't go from job to job, or from city to city, seeking some other type of employment merely because the "other fellow's grass looks greener."

Love and Tolerance for Children. The mature adult likes children and takes time to understand their special needs. He can almost always take a few minutes off, no matter how busy he is, to build blocks with his 3-year-old or to answer the many questions of an older child.

Good Sexual Adjustment. The normal adult makes a good sex adjustment, without prudishness and with full enjoyment. He or she achieves a pleasantly satisfying orgasm during the sexual act and can relax completely afterward.

Sexual adjustment has broader implications as well. It means accepting oneself as a male or female without conflict about this accident of birth. It includes understanding the special problems of the other sex, and accepting with tolerance and sympathy some of the emotional difficulties these create—in oneself and in others. For example, the still-existing inferior status of women creates problems in certain situations, and the bread-winner role of men engenders tensions in our excessively competitive world.

Capacity for Continued Emotional Growth. The ability to learn and grow emotionally is characteristic of the normal individual. This should express itself not only in sexual love and family relationships, but also as tolerance and understanding of people with different racial, religious, national, and cultural backgrounds. It should also be possible to age gracefully, for understanding can increase even though an aging person has reached or passed his prime in other spheres.

Normality versus Perfection

No one is perfectly normal because perfection is seldom attained by human beings. One does not have to be a complete conformist to be normal. Fears, emotional conflicts, and frustrations are also a part of normal living. Yet the personality structure we have described embodies worthwhile goals to seek throughout life.

It is important to know that even the most normal person has limits which can be strained to the breaking point. The well adjusted individual is still a reactive human being, not a steel automaton. During World War II, for example, it was soon recognized that there was a limit to the number of bombing missions even the most stable pilots could participate in without suffering from combat fatigue. This was the result of continued, unrelieved emotional stress, and fear and sorrow about the loss of comrades. There was a point at which the situation became unbearable. Fortunately, the well-adjusted pilots usually recovered quickly after a rest period, free of responsibility and strain.

Certain forms of stress are difficult for almost anyone to endure for long. When you can't fight back in any way against an unendurable situation, and have to bottle up your fury for very long, it may explode in some other way.

Pressures can be dramatically extreme during military combat, but everyday life can also be frustrating to the point of explosion. The student under pressure to achieve, the businessman forced to make profits constantly, the assembly-line worker facing an inexorable production quota—people in many situations must find acceptable outlets for life's everyday pressures.

All Normal People Are Not Alike. Some forms of pressure can be endured more easily by one normal person than by another. The reason for this is fairly obvious. Human beings are not simply chemical combinations, but are extremely complex, and every human being is different from every other one, except perhaps his identical twin. All well-adjusted people are not equally intelligent, physically well endowed or talented. It definitely takes all kinds to make a world.

You have undoubtedly noticed that there are many different personality types. Psychiatrists have described them in various ways. Carl Jung, for example, classified people as *introverts,* who are absorbed in what goes on inside their own minds, and as extroverts, who are more concerned with life around them than with their own experiences or reactions. Another psychiatrist, Karen Horney, speaks of three basic character types—those who "move toward people," those who "move against people," and those who "move away from people." These might become, respectively, a successful salesman, a competitive athlete, and a philosopher. Under unfortunate circumstances, the same types might produce, respectively, a playboy, a gunman, and a recluse.

Normal People Are Influenced by Unconscious Motivations. People suspected that there was an unconscious part of the mind long before Sigmund Freud, the great Viennese psychiatrist, studied its influence in normal individuals and in emotional illness. Carlyle, for example, wrote in 1838: "The uttered part of a man's life bears to the unuttered, unconscious part a small unknown proportion. He himself never knows it, much less do others."

People noticed, for example, that they sometimes forgot things that they didn't want to remember—even though they *thought* they wanted to remember them.

Even the well adjusted person doesn't, for example, fall in love in a completely conscious manner, although he isn't ruled by his unconscious to such an extent that he falls in love with someone he knows to be completely unworthy of affection.

A well adjusted person may be afraid of a snake even though he knows it is harmless. He may go through periods of emotional distress—as, for example, during puberty when he is faced with the problem of tearing himself away from the dependence of childhood and of solving his sexual needs. He, too, is distressed by tensions, sometimes seeking foolish ways (such as overeating) to relieve them. He even has periods of depression, for example, when he has lost a dear one, or his health is below par. Perfectly normal women may regularly experience a brief premenstrual depression.

Of course, maturity is a relative term—it is not restricted to adults. Teenagers and young adults also are expected to display reasonable maturity for their age, and for the young man or woman in college, a responsible attitude and a readiness to make adjustments are necessary to remain in school and to move ahead.

The Dropout Problem. One of the consequences of immaturity or failure to adjust by a college student is the dropping out of college. This is a particularly distressing problem in the first year, when throughout the country up to 40 per cent of the freshman class leave college. Only one out of five of these dropouts ever returns, even to another school. While the percentage of college dropouts has not significantly increased in proportion to population growth in the last 30 years, the consequences of leaving college are much more serious now than they were a generation ago. Primarily, the reasons for this are that society places an increasing value on higher education and specialized training, and there is correspondingly less room for the under-educated and the underskilled.

There are a number of explanations for the dropout problem, which in many cases can be traced to other difficulties inherent in our times. The affluence of our society had made material things readily accessible to today's parents. A growing number of college students do not know the financial struggle that previous generations have experienced. They do not have to "work their way through college," and they have other economic advantages offered them as a matter of course. On the other hand, the uncertainties of today's times and especially the future make students impatient to start life on their own. Preparation for an economically independent life takes appreciably longer than it did in the past. For example, in many professions an M.A. and even a Ph.D. degree are needed where a B.A. sufficed before. Often the impatience to be on their own causes students to drop out of college and try a job they are not yet qualified for. The sense of failure frequently makes it difficult to return to college and especially to accept the parents' support for an even longer period.

Students who feel the emotional need to leave college should probe this inner drive with a qualified expert. Many colleges have adequate counseling services. If these services are not available, we suggest a talk with a psychologist or psychiatrist before the student makes this potentially dangerous decision.

Because of the inquiries about the dropout problem that the U.S. Office of Education is receiving in large and increasing numbers, this office of the U.S. Department of Health, Education and Welfare has prepared a valuable compilation of the books, reports and studies published since 1960 on the problem, entitled "Dropouts: Selected References."

How to Relieve Emotional Tensions

Almost everybody experiences tensions at some time. In fact, like hunger and thirst, tensions may be a natural, protective reaction when our safety, well-being, or happiness is threatened. However, it is very important to differentiate between occasional periods of anxiety which are quickly dissipated and emotional upsets which come very often, take a long time to wear off and are unduly disturbing.

George Stevenson, a noted psychiatrist, has suggested that you ask yourself the following questions:[1]

> Do minor problems and small disappointments throw you into a dither?
>
> Do you find it difficult to get along with people, and are people having trouble getting along with you?
>
> Do the small pleasures of life fail to satisfy you?
>
> Are you unable to stop thinking of your anxieties?
>
> Do you fear people or situations that never used to bother you?
>
> Are you suspicious of people, mistrustful of your friends?
>
> Do you feel inadequate, suffer the tortures of self-doubt?

If you answered most of these questions with "Yes," it doesn't necessarily mean you need feel great concern. But it does indicate that you have problems you should try to work out. Here are some simple, practical steps you can take:

Talk It Out. Don't bottle up your worries, but discuss them with a sympathetic friend, relative, doctor, teacher, or anyone whose judgment and advice you respect. Talking often helps you see your worries in a clearer light—and gives you clues to eliminate them.

Escape for a While. Do something different, find a real escape from a problem—a movie, a walk, a game of bridge. It may help compose you emotionally, so that you'll be better prepared to return and tackle the problem in a more mature fashion. Sometimes just sleeping on it helps. The philosophers who wrote the *Psalms* were very wise when they said, "Weeping may endure for a night, but joy cometh in the morning."

[1]Stevenson, G. S., and Milt, H.: *How to Deal With Your Tensions.* National Association for Mental Health, New York, 1957.

Work Off Your Anger. If you find yourself using anger as a general pattern of behavior, you may end up by feeling both foolish and sorry. It's much better to try to work the anger out of your system, so that you can deal with a problem rationally and intelligently. A very good way of doing it is to pitch into some physical activity—tennis or handball or a long walk, gardening or carpentry. It is surprising and gratifying to observe how much tension can flow out through the muscles.

Give in Occasionally. Only frustrated children insist that they are always right, and must have their own way. Stand your ground on what your convictions, not your emotions, tell you is right. But be prepared to be found wrong, and to admit your error gracefully. Even if you're sure you *are* right, it sometimes pays to give in to the other person, especially in relieving snarled, tense situations.

Do Something for Others. If you find yourself too preoccupied with yourself and your own problems, try to escape this vicious circle by doing something for others. It has many rewards, not the least of them the warm feeling of improving a human relationship.

Take One Thing at a Time. If you feel you are becoming overwhelmed with the pressures of too much to do, try hard to concentrate on one job, to the exclusion of everything else. All the time that is wasted worrying about having too much to do could be much more efficiently used doing *something*. If you get the harassed feeling that everything is so important that nothing can be put aside, ask yourself if you might not be exaggerating the importance of things you do and have to do—and therefore your own importance.

Watch the Superman Urge. If you're a perfectionist, it's easy to start feeling anxious that you aren't doing as much as you should and as well as you should. Be careful. This way leads to ruin.

You can't do everything, and you can't do everything perfectly. Concentrate on what you can do best, and give everything else as much as you can of yourself—always recognizing that you aren't a superman, and can't do everything, perfectly.

Be Gentle with Criticism. If you expect too much of people you're associated with, you're bound to feel disappointed and let-down when they don't come up to the high standards you are setting. Everybody has a right to develop as an individual, at his own pace, and to his own limits. If you're constantly feeling frustrated and disappointed because of your friends' imperfections, it might actually mean that you're disappointed about yourself in some way. Instead of being too critical about your friends' weaknesses, search out their strong points, and emphasize them. This will give you both deeper satisfactions.

Give the Other Person a Break. Life shouldn't have to be a competitive race, day and night. Cooperation might get you farther—and make you happier—than competition. Nothing can create so many tensions as the competitive struggles of school and of life—the feeling that you have to win all the time, get the highest score, the best grade, the top job. You might reach it, but be so weary and tense when you get there that you won't even enjoy your success.

Make Yourself Available. Often we bring on ourselves the feeling of being neglected or left out. Sometimes we merely imagine that we are. Instead of shrinking away from situations or contact with others, and feeling sorry for yourself, it is a lot healthier and more practical to make the first overtures.

Schedule Your Recreation. Set aside time for activities which will help you forget your responsibilities and worries. If you find it hard to take time out, force yourself to schedule some time for activities into which you can really escape and forget your work.

Questions

1. Discuss some misconceptions about the emotions.
2. What is your definition of a "normal" person?
3. What are some attributes of the personality structure of a normal person?
4. How is it possible for an emotionally healthy person to be both independent and dependent at the same time?
5. Why is a good sexual adjustment such an important component of a normal individual?
6. Can you differentiate between an introvert and an extrovert?

7. Can you find unconscious motivations for at least three things you do regularly, or for attitudes you possess?

8. Under what conditions of stress can normal persons develop temporary emotional breakdowns?

9. Why is it so important to make yourself available, and to do something for others?

10. Why is an understanding of mental health as important as an understanding of physical health?

11. When is it healthy to disagree with the majority?

12. How can you resolve the need to look out for yourself with the need to help others, even at some cost to yourself?

13. Is a normal person a conformist?

14. When does unwillingness to conform become a symptom of a personality problem?

15. Why does physical activity relieve tension?

16. Describe some normal tendencies and activities of the young adult that are inappropriate in a man or woman 10 or 20 years older. What does this tell you about the definition of normality?

17. How does society make it difficult to maintain a condition of mental health?

18. Are guilt feelings about one's emotions and private thoughts a sign of a good conscience or of a personality problem? Is this a question of ethics or of psychology?

Topics for Discussion

The relationship between home atmosphere and mental health.

How group opinions and activities affect one's personality.

Contrasting attitudes toward mental health, today and a generation ago.

The range of normality.

Different concepts of a healthy personality—by age, sex and profession.

When to be concerned about one's own conduct.

Interdependence of the mind and body.

Influence of psychiatry on our penal system.

Difference between mental illnesses and neurological diseases.

Reading Suggestions

How to Deal With Your Tensions, George S. Stevenson and Harry Milt. National Association for Mental Health, Inc., New York, 1957. An excellent informative pamphlet, written at a popular level.

The Conquest of Happiness, Bertrand Russell. New American Library of World Literature, New York (paperback), 1933. A thoughtful book by the great philosopher, with sound practical advice on how to keep a sound mind.

Discovering Ourselves, Edward A. Strecker and Kenneth A. Appel. The Macmillan Company, New York, 1962. An easy-to-read discussion of emotional life, written by two distinguished psychiatrists.

Action for Mental Health, The Joint Commission on Mental Illness and Health. John Wiley & Sons, Inc., New York, 1961. Findings and recommendations, following a five-year study of mental health in America.

Emotional Maturity, Leon J. Saul. J. B. Lippincott Co., Philadelphia, 1960. A calm and thoughtful presentation of a hard-to-define goal.

Mental Health in the United States, Nina Ridenour, Harvard University Press, Cambridge, Mass., 1961. A concise 50 year history of the mental health movement, with the emphasis on "firsts."

The Vital Balance, Karl Menninger. The Viking Press, New York, 1963. A famous physician explains and illustrates the life process as it continues through mental health and illness.

The Tormented Generation, Morton M. Hunt and Rena Corman. The Saturday Evening Post, October 12, 1963. A sympathetic treatment of some problems confronting college students.

You and Psychiatry, William Menninger and Munro Leaf. Charles Scribner's Sons, New York, 1955. A short, absorbing narration of the growing personality from childhood to maturity.

Psychiatry Today, David Stafford-Clark. Penguin Books, Inc., Baltimore, 1959. An account of current theory and practice, taking into account changing social conditions.

Popular Conceptions of Mental Health, J. C. Nunnally. Holt, Rinehart & Winston, 1961.

Dropouts: Selected References, Prepared by Leonard M. Miller. U. S. Government Printing Office, Washington, D.C., 1964.

Emotional Problems of Living, O. Spurgeon English and Gerald H. J. Pearson. Norton, New York, 1963. How, when and why emotional conflicts arise in everyday life, and how they may be avoided. The authors, both prominent psychiatrists, also give an account of the psychological development of the human.

The Dropout: Causes and Cures, Lucius F. Cervantes. University of Michigan Press, Ann Arbor, 1965.

6

EMOTIONAL DISTURBANCES

Diseases of the soul are more dangerous and more numerous than those of the body.

Tuscan Discourses, CICERO

Perhaps you know the remark ascribed to an anonymous old Quaker, who commented to his wife: "All the world is queer but thee and me, dear, and sometimes I think even thee is a little queer." If you look searchingly at people, you might be tempted to conclude that everyone seems to be more or less peculiar. It is actually difficult to find anyone who doesn't have some little behavioral quirk, different from what you consider strictly normal.

Until fairly recently even the medical profession tended to ignore the people who were a "little queer," dividing individuals instead into two arbitrary groups, the *normal* and the *abnormal.* Like the legal profession, medicine was concerned only with the *sane* and the *insane*.

Such a division is scientifically inaccurate. Now we recognize that there are all shades of behavior between the well adjusted and the unbalanced. This range extends from the best-adjusted to those who are only a little upset, such as the maladjusted, "peculiar," troubled, or *neurotic* persons and on to those whose mental condition is such that they cannot function, unprotected, in society. A rough, but valid, analogy would be to compare the best-adjusted to people who possess good *physical* health. Those in the second group, the neurotics, are similar to people whose illnesses, more or less severe, limit them somewhat, but still involve only a part or a few parts of the body. They can usually manage to be up and about, functioning more or less well. Individuals in the third major group, the *psychotics,* are comparable to patients with an incapacitating physical illness.

THE MAGNITUDE OF THE MENTAL HEALTH PROBLEM

It has been estimated that as many as 18 million Americans may be suffering

Table 6–1. Overall annual costs of mental illness in the United States, 1963*

Loss of income from mental illness	$ 1,441,489,524
Total maintenance expenditures of public mental hospitals	1,084,713,981
Costs for care and pensions, U.S. Veterans Administration and other Federal agencies	862,785,970
Cost of public assistance and maintenance of mentally ill and mentally retarded persons	396,106,994
Private hospital and office psychiatric care	186,944,000
Outlays by states for mental hospitals	176,000,000
	$ 4,148,040,469

*From *Facts on the Major Killing and Crippling Diseases in the United States Today,* compiled by the National Health Education Committee, Inc. (1964). "Facts," in turn, drew upon a number of sources, including the American Hospital Association, National Institute of Mental Health, Veterans Administration, Bureau of Census, Budget of the Federal Government, and the Joint Commission on Mental Illness and Health.

from mental illness, mild or severe. There are, perhaps, 1.7 million individuals who are *psychotic,* afflicted with mental disorders which require long, sometimes indefinite care in an institution. About 710,000 of these are hospitalized because they are dangerous either to themselves or to others, or need full-time custodial care for other reasons. At the present time, one out of every two hospital beds in the United States is occupied by a psychiatric patient.

There are probably 10 million persons with emotional disturbances of greater or less degree, which render them unhappy, frustrated, or inefficient. In addition, perhaps as many as 50,000 Americans are narcotic addicts, four million are problem drinkers, and about one million are chronic alcoholics. Suicide, which is almost always motivated by some kind of emotional disorder, ranks eighth in causes of death. More than 20,000 people commit suicide each year, besides the uncounted thousands who make abortive attempts at self-destruction.

Many social problems have their roots in emotional maladjustment—crime, juvenile delinquency, prostitution, industrial absenteeism, and divorce.

Some doctors estimate that 70 per cent of the so-called physical ailments are really psychosomatic (mind-body) diseases, and involve an emotional factor.

It has been stated that emotional disturbances in workers cost industry 3 billion dollars each year in unproductive wages and in injury to workers and damage to their machines. All told, the cost of mental illness is staggering.

The cost of caring for only the seriously ill mental patients is approximately $1.1 billion a year.

The extent of this problem and some recommended approaches for its relief were described in detail by the Joint Commission on Mental Illness and Health in 1961. This group of specialists, representing 36 organizations in the mental health field, proposed a many-sided program in its massive report, *Action for Mental Health.* The recommendations included increased funds for research, especially basic research; greater efforts to encourage young men and women to enter the field; the establishment of mental health research institutes; a scholarship and loan program; community clinics for the mentally troubled; and a program to improve public understanding of mental illness.

The authors of the report stated:

> "This report can succeed in its purpose only if its readers can keep in mind that its primary object is to bring help to the mentally ill that hitherto has been generally denied them. If we are to accelerate the mental health movement, reduce mental illness, and improve mental health, we must rise above our self-preservative functions as members of different professions and different social classes and adherents of different economic philosophies, and illuminate the means of working together out of mutual respect for our fellow man .... We each have one kind of responsibility that is common to all and transcends all others. This is our responsibility as citizens of a democratic nation founded out of faith in the uniqueness, integrity, and dignity of human life."

In light of this eloquent summing up, it is encouraging that in 1964 the Federal Government appropriated $171 million for the National Institute of Mental Health. The sum appears impressive until it is compared with the billions of dollars that mental illness costs every year. The appropriation also is only a tiny fraction of the money spent in research and development activities—in the fiscal year ending June 1963, the Federal Government appropriated $15 billion for these purposes, and industry spent almost another $5 billion.

By way of contrast, the amount spent by the consumer public in the United States is rather discouraging. For alcohol, we spent $10.7 billion in 1962, nearly $8 billion on tobacco, more than $17 billion on new and used cars, and an almost unbelievable $21.6 billion on recreation. Chewing gum alone accounted for about three times the Federal appropriation for mental health research and training. Many authorities have recommended, as a minimum, an effort to double the present national investment in mental health research over the next five years and to triple it within a decade.

BASIC EMOTIONAL NEEDS

By studying the individual as a whole, psychiatrists and psychologists have learned that people have basic needs, involving security, affection, independence, and sexual activity, which vary according to the stage of their development. They have found, for example, that a baby is not "a little vegetable" who will thrive as long as it is kept warm and well fed. On the contrary, a baby may become listless and apathetic, and even die, through lowered resistance to infection merely because he has received *no* affection. They found that a baby can be upset, even though he is given adequate care, if his mother is always tense or "in a state of nerves."

It was clear that a child has to control certain impulses because of their consequences; for example, he must learn to check his desire to touch the pretty flame because it will burn his fingers.

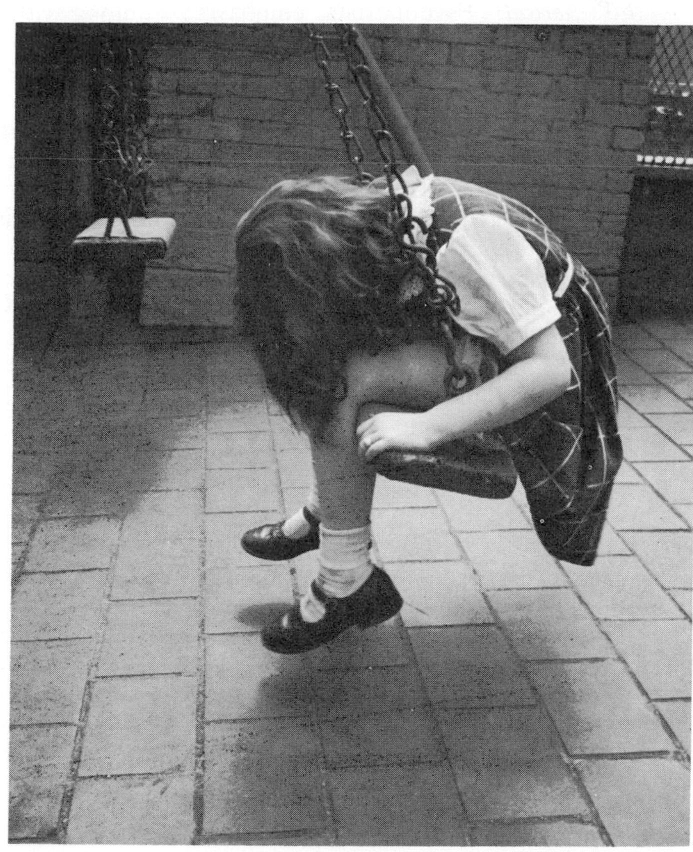

The shy and lonely child. An adjustment problem of the early years. (Ken Heyman from Magnum.)

Certain *inhibitions* are necessary. But if the child's *basic emotional needs* are frustrated, unfortunate repressions and inhibitions result, causing unconscious conflicts. Forbidden impulses are forgotten or excluded from awareness but continue to exert an influence from the unconscious part of the mind. In other words, the child arrives at a solution to his problem that doesn't actually solve it, although it makes things seem bearable. Take a 4-year-old boy whose normal interest in sex is expressed by comparing his own sex organ with that of a little girl. Let us assume he is discovered by horrified parents who tell him he's wicked, punish him, and frighten him with threats that the doctor will cut off his penis. From then on the little boy may indeed "behave properly" by repressing his sexual instincts. Unconsciously, however, they still exist. These unconscious desires conflict with his desire for love and approval, and he feels anxious, afraid and guilty without knowing why.

A great many mental illnesses are initiated or the soil is prepared for them in this period. Psychiatrists emphasize that the child's emotional life—his sense of security, his feeling of being loved—is frequently far more important to his development than the qualities he inherits.

The attainment and maintenance of a healthy emotional life is really a continuous problem. Life is never static. Childhood experiences are extremely important, but everything that happens to us leaves some imprint. Adolescence is also a critical stage in emotional development, just as it is in our physical maturation.

Marriage is another great step forward in helping us attain the fullest emotional life. Although it is a valuable experience for most people, some individuals, unfortunately, are unable to benefit from it or even to accept marriage. Other, earlier and deep-rooted emotional conflicts limit their flexibility in adapting to the new demands of marriage.

THE NEUROSES

Differences between Normal and Maladjusted Individuals

Everyone has fears, worries, tensions and emotional discomfort at certain times. However, those of the neurotic person have special characteristics.

1. They are usually exaggerated, continual, of long duration, or they are not realistic.

Here are some examples. Any normal person may be afraid of catching a disease, being struck by lightning, or run over by a car; the neurotic person may be terrified or panic-stricken. The normal person gets over his fear of being hit by an auto when he reaches the other side of the street; the neurotic person starts immediately to anticipate the next street crossing.

The normal person may worry about failure in business or in love when he has obvious evidence that things are not going well; the neurotic person does so even when things are going beautifully. For example, he may interpret the most casual glance of his loved one at another person as a sign of infidelity.

2. These fears, worries, and tensions prevent the neurotic individual from reacting to his best interests. They interfere with his ability to work and to get along with people.

For example: the fear a normal person experiences on going into battle makes him alert and cautious (i.e., a good soldier); the neurotic person may become panicky and be unable to protect himself. A well adjusted mother knows her older children face certain risks, but she doesn't refuse to let them out of her sight on that account. A neurotic mother may keep her children with her even though she knows it hinders them from developing a healthy degree of independence. A well adjusted person may dislike unfair criticism of his work but he'll put up with a certain amount of it if the job is excellent in other respects; a neurotic individual may quit work because he is spoken to in only a moderately critical tone.

3. Neurotic people experience feelings of fear, anxiety, and depression without knowing why. This sometimes makes them fear they are becoming insane. Quite the contrary, there appears to be some truth to the saying, "The best way to keep from going crazy is to be neurotic." Of course it isn't the *best* way, any more than the best way to avoid breaking your arm is to keep it in a sling.

One explanation of all these neuroses lies in the unconscious mind.

The Tyranny of the Unconscious

Some understanding of the unconscious is necessary for a comprehension of the reasons for the way people think, feel, act and talk. The concept of the unconscious was developed to explain how actions, events, feelings and ideas of very early life seem to disappear into forgetfulness, but in fact influence all of one's remaining years. The unconscious mind may be thought of as a storage place for past thoughts and experiences. This area of the mind releases the past to the present reluctantly and slowly, because the human tendency is to want to forget what has been unpleasant, fearful or otherwise undesirable. For example, a small child whose surroundings seem fearful and who lives in a state of worry may very well become an anxious adult who cannot identify the source of his anxiety. Feelings of guilt or inferiority may determine the behavior of an unhappy neurotic individual who is tyrannized by his unconscious but who can no more peer into that part of his mind than he can look into a mirror to see how he appears when his eyes are closed.

Characteristics of Neurotic Individuals

Personality Disturbances. Some people have no really incapacitating neuroses, but suffer from what might be described as *personality problems*. They do not actually have mental illness, yet they are not in perfect health. The situation is somewhat similar to the man who is 50 pounds overweight and has no serious illness. Still, he's too fat to enjoy really perfect health and comfort.

Such problems result from the exaggeration of some normal personality feature, for example, excessive timidity, shyness, irritability, or melancholy. You have certainly said or heard someone else describe a mutual friend in the following terms:

"Mary would have heaps of boy friends if she could only realize how good-looking she is."

"You get the feeling Jack doesn't quite trust anybody; he always seems so wary."

"Tom's great fun when things are going his way, but he's a very bad loser."

"We really ought to ask Joan because she's so sweet, but she kind of puts a wet blanket on things by always being in the dumps."

"I bet Dick'll be the last one to get a raise even though he's the smartest one in the office."

"It's a shame Dotty flies off the handle the way she does; she feels awful about it afterwards."

"Anne's so jittery she makes me nervous."

People like this have often been described as their own worst enemies. Their problems may be so minor that some friendly discussions with the family physician may relieve them. They may be sufficiently serious to warrant consultation with a psychiatrist.

Varieties of Neuroses. *Anxiety Neurosis.* In this condition a person experiences episodes of anxiety which vary from mild uneasiness to panic. Sometimes they manifest themselves by physical signs such as sweating, dizziness, diarrhea, difficulty in breathing, or a pain in the heart. The individual may feel extremely tense and irritable; he may awaken in the night in a state of terror. The characteristic feeling is one of anxious expectation, as if something dreadful is about to happen, except that there is no idea as to what the dreadful thing might be.

Sometimes the anxiety is "shunted off" by associating it with the situation in which it was experienced. For example, if the anxiety first occurred in an elevator, the individual may blame the elevator, which he then fears and avoids in the hope of preventing anxiety.

This state is often associated with a fear of losing love, as, for example, when there is conflict in the unconscious mind between a desire to hurt the loved one (perhaps to get even for having been hurt) and a desire to win that person's love.

Phobias. These are divided into *common phobias*—the exaggerated fears many people share, such as the fear of death, and *specific phobias*—the fear of things or situations that aren't really frightening to the average person, such as the fear of open fields.

Included in the almost endless list of phobias are *acrophobia,* the fear of high places; *agoraphobia,* of open spaces; *aichmophobia,* of sharp and pointed objects; *anthropophobia,* of people; *astraphobia,* of storms; *batophobia,* of falling objects; *claustrophobia,* of enclosed spaces; *climacophobia,* of falling down stairs; *dromophobia,* of crossing the street; *hypnophobia,* of sleep; *kleptophobia,* of stealing; *mechanophobia,* of machinery; *monophobia,* of being alone; *mysophobia,* of dirt and contamination; *necrophobia,* of the dead; *nychtophobia,* of the dark; *pantaphobia,* of everything; *phagophobia,* of eating; *potamophobia,* of running water; *syphilophobia,* of syphilis; *topo-*

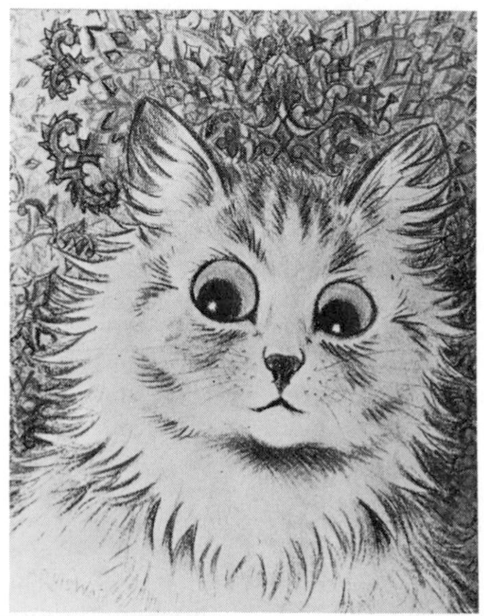

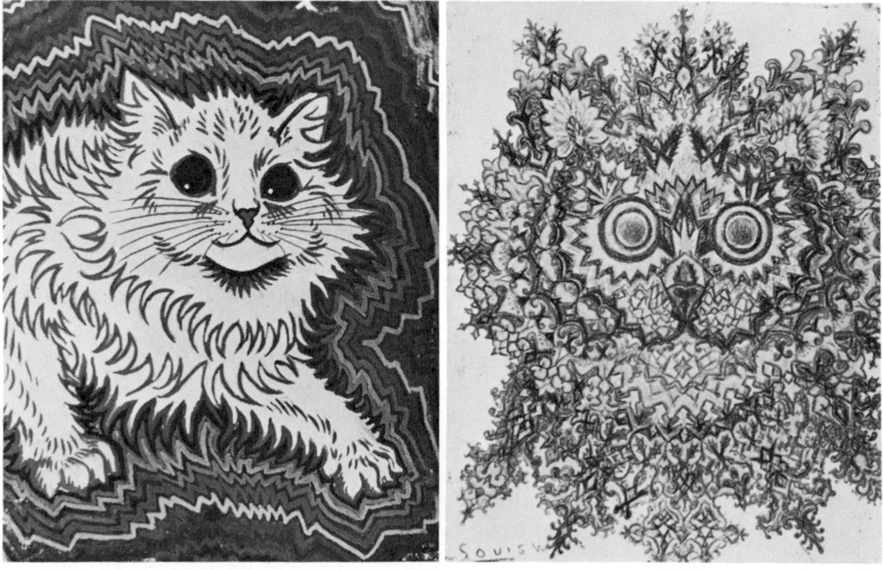

Paintings of a cat by an artist who developed a mental illness. In the early part of the century one of the best known British artists was Louis Wain, an eccentric bachelor who lived surrounded by the cats that he used as models for his popular drawings. In the early 1920's, Wain had a schizophrenic breakdown with intermittent relapses until his death in 1936. This series of cat paintings shows the remarkable style during attacks. (Courtesy of World Health Organization, Guttman-Maclay Collection.)

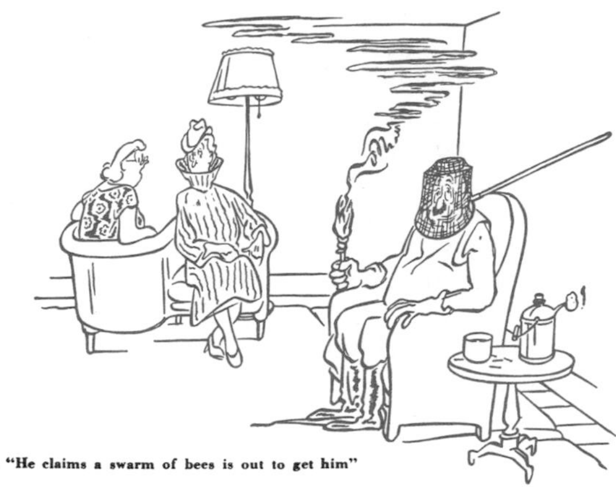

"He claims a swarm of bees is out to get him"

(Copyr. © 1940 by Geo. Price, *Good Humor Man,* published by Farrar and Rinehart, Inc., New York.)

phobia, of situations (stage fright); *xylophobia,* of the forest; *zoophobia,* of animals.

A phobia is a persistent, unreasoning fear of something. It is usually rooted in guilt, in the fear that, because you were "bad," some punishment is inevitable.

Most doctors believe that the essential mechanism in the formation of a phobia is *displaced anxiety.* The anxiety developed in a particular emotional conflict is displaced from its original source to an *external object or situation,* usually related, directly or indirectly, to the anxiety.

For example, Freud described the following typical case:

> A young girl had for many years a morbid fear of running water. Even running water from a hydrant would provoke an almost unbearable anxiety. She was completely at a loss to explain this fear until she was visited by an aunt whom she had not seen since childhood. Shortly after arriving the aunt took her aside and whispered, "I've never told our secret." Upon hearing this, the patient suddenly remembered an incident that had occurred when she was five years old. Against her mother's strict orders she had slipped away to go wading in a stream with a small waterfall. While wading, she lost her footing and was drawn under the waterfall by the current. The aunt happened along and rescued her, then helped her dry out her clothes and agreed to keep the secret so the little girl would not be punished by her mother. With the recovery of this memory, the woman lost her fear of running water. In this case the running water was a sort of abbreviated mental symbol for the original anxiety-provoking scene, the rest of which had been blotted from conscious memory. The emotional response was appropriate enough in the original setting—terror at the near-drowning and fear of the mother's punishment.[1]

[1]Freud, S.: *Collected Papers,* Vol. III, Hogarth Press, London, 1950.

Unfortunately, not all phobias are so readily understood and cured.

Phobias are far more common than you may realize, and can disturb even the most brilliant and creative people. It is said of Tschaikovsky, the famous composer, that he

> lived suspended in a world of phobias. He feared strangers, women, foreign places, conducting, for years lived under a morbid conviction that his head would fall off. Ironically, he dreaded death from cholera, was convinced of this eventual *dénouement* because his beloved mother had died of this disease. Under the pressures of these fears and insecurities, he would swing abruptly from elation to abject depression, was often observed sinking swiftly into weeping melancholy while chattering in animated conversation. He drank heavily, avoided crowds, clung to his devoted family, built a solitary retreat in the small town of Klin where he spent his last years.[2]

Hypochondria. In this neurosis the mind's illness is expressed through a preoccupation with body functions or organs. The patient is afraid of, or believes he suffers from, physical disease. He notices body sensations, such as normal fatigue, that do not concern or bother other people. There is no physical cause for this condition. However, telling him he's all right physically won't cure the hypochondriacal attitude.

Karl Menninger of the famous Menninger Clinic in Topeka, Kansas, described the hypochondriac as a person who unconsciously "cherishes his ailments," his "beloved symptoms," which bring him sympathy and attention.

The cause of hypochondria is not too clear, but it is certainly a widespread illness. Physicians say that their practices include many physically healthy men and women who "enjoy poor health." This "enjoyment" of illness and symptoms perhaps best describes the hypochondriac. For reasons not too clear, such individuals are constantly preoccupied with their bodies and sensations arising from it.

Some psychiatrists feel that, for one reason or another, the hypochondriac as a child, and later as an adult, found the expression of normal feelings of love or hostility too disturbing when they were directed where they should be—toward

[2]*MD Publications,* January, 1959.

teachers, parents, or other authority figures. Or perhaps he lost a loved person. As an alternative, he turned his feelings inward, fastening them onto some innocent organ of the body—the lungs, the heart, a portion of the intestine or some other part of the body. Sometimes a parent shows so inordinate a concern for his own, or the child's, health that the pattern is set for hypochondria.

It almost appears that the hypochondriac has given up hope that he will be accepted as a worthy individual for his own personal qualities and accomplishments. He obtains the social attention and acceptance he feels he has been denied by presenting a recital of his symptoms and complaints. Illness becomes a kind of retreat. He can throw off responsibility, be waited upon by friends and family, and get attention from his doctor.

Walter Alvarez, a noted physician, has pointed out: "Everyone has a touch of hypochondria. But to the vast majority, minor pains are not disturbing. A slight stomach upset, probably a sign of overeating, is simply a signal for investigation, not alarm." To the hypochondriac, however, every symptom is a cause for concern. The slightest sign of nausea represents appendicitis, a gallbladder attack, and even, perhaps, cancer. "He begins to spy on his digestive tract," Alvarez points out, "and he doesn't know that no self-respecting organ does good work when constantly spied upon."

Hypochondria is not confined to ordinary mortals. Some very famous figures in history have been plagued by a variety of imaginary or exaggerated ailments. The eminent scientist, Thomas Huxley, referred to "my constant friend, hypochondriacal dyspepsia." Charles Darwin was convinced that he would die of heart disease, although he was really an organically healthy person who lived to the age of 73. Florence Nightingale returned from the Crimea in 1856, after a remarkable career in nursing, and went to bed with what she called "heart disease." She made her will, and led an invalid's life until she died at the age of 90 in 1910. Elizabeth Barrett Browning went to bed as a young woman, and spent twenty years there with a "spinal ailment." When she was 40, she eloped with Robert Browning, soon forgot her "spinal ailment," and had a son at the age of 43.

Unfortunately, many doctors are not sympathetic to patients who complain of non-organic symptoms and ailments. It's true that hypochondriacs can anticipate little relief from medicines, because they can always imagine a new disease. However, they do need treatment of a special kind. Psychotherapeutic interviews can be very reassuring to such people and help avoid unnecessary surgery and medication. They also deter these individuals from seeking out quacks, who at least listen to their woes.

Conversion Hysteria. This differs from hypochondria in that the mind's illness is expressed in a physical symptom or symptoms, which, although not *real* in one sense of the word, are certainly real to the patient. Hysterical paralysis is an example. A soldier undergoing a severe conflict between his desire to be brave and his desire not to be killed, finds his legs suddenly paralyzed. He is not faking—he actually feels nothing when pins are stuck into his legs. However, there is absolutely nothing wrong with his nerves; usually the loss of sensation is not even anatomically possible, a section of one nerve being "dead" while other sections beyond the "dead" point remain sensitive. When the conflict is resolved, either by circumstances or within the soldier himself, his paralysis vanishes.

Obsessive-compulsive Neurosis. This causes people to perform actions without knowing why, or without wanting to perform them. The impulse stems from an idea or set of ideas that have no relationship in the individual's conscious mind. For example: a person always has to put on a certain undergarment inside out. This is similar to the way some of us feel about having to touch wood. It is a sort of ritual, an appeal to magic powers.

The normal person who touches wood does so as a kind of joke because he has been told it is lucky. However, it is no joke to the victim of such a neurosis. He performs his rituals because he is extremely insecure. As a child, he turned to his own magic in a desperate attempt to cope with problems too great for him to handle.

Neurasthenia. Literally, this word

means nerve weakness. It was once believed that the nerves in the brain could actually get tired, and "brain fatigue" would result. Now we know that, like hypochondria and conversion hysteria, this is a product of the patient's psyche. It is real to him, even though it is medically and scientifically impossible. The patient honestly feels and *is* too weak or tired to get out of bed, or even to think coherently. He can sleep for periods that would be impossible for a well person, or simply lie for hours doing nothing. Yet he is not physically ill. Resting doesn't cure him, but solving his problems does.

Neurotic Depression. It is not neurotic to be unhappy or depressed under certain circumstances, for example, when a beloved person dies. It is certainly quite normal to experience *grief* and to mourn such a loss.

However, well-adjusted people work through their grief so that they can resume their activities and reestablish social contacts. They do not grieve week after week to the point of *melancholia*. This is not because they are insensitive or superficial. On the contrary, their grief is usually more profound than that of badly adjusted people. But when the latter suffer from neurotic depressions, they feel helpless because of their loss or perhaps even because of a change; their low self-esteem convinces them they can never cope with such situations. These neurotic depressions are so closely bound up with feelings of inadequacy and insecurity that they can be brought about by events which well adjusted people accept as all in the day's work. Yet such depressions cause great suffering.

Psychosomatic Illness

In recent years we have heard a great deal about psychosomatic illnesses. Psychosomatic medicine is the branch of medicine which studies the interaction of the mind, the *psyche,* with the body, the *soma,* in the production of disease.

This is not a new science. Ian Stevenson, a well known psychiatrist, has pointed out that Greek, Roman and medieval Arabian physicians understood psychosomatic medicine, and incorporated this knowledge in their teaching.

John Wesley's *Journal*, written in the eighteenth century, had this to say of a patient: "Reflecting today on the case of a poor woman who had continual pain in her stomach, I could not but remark the inexcusable negligence of most physicians in cases of this nature. They prescribe drug upon drug, without knowing a jot of the matter concerning the root of the disorder. Whence came this woman's pain, which she would never have told, had she never been questioned about it? *From fretting for the death of her son. And what availed medicine, while that fretting continued?"*

Many studies in this field have led to the concept that emotional disturbances can produce physical changes in the body. These may be as simple as shivering with fear, blushing with shame or perspiring with nervousness. Or they may be so complex as to cause physiological malfunctioning, and, finally, even to lead to structural changes in the tissues themselves.

Franz Alexander, a leader in this field, believes that it is unrealistic to try to separate emotional and organic factors as causative agents in disease. According to Alexander, "*Every* disease is psychosomatic because both psychological and somatic factors have a part in its cause and cure. This assumption is valid even for such specific infectious diseases as tuberculosis. Apart from exposure to the bacillus of Koch (the tuberculosis germ), the resistance of the organism is an equally important factor in this disease."[3]

A "psychosomatic cold" has been very humorously and accurately described in the song, "Adelaide's Lament," from the musical comedy, *Guys and Dolls:*

Adelaide's Lament

The av'rage unmarried female, basic'lly insecure,
Due to some long frustration may react
With psychosomatic symptoms, difficult to endure,
Affecting the upper respiratory tract.
In other words, just from waiting around for that plain
little band of gold,
A person can develop a cold.

---

[3]Alexander, F., and French, T. M.: *Studies in Psychosomatic Medicine,* Ronald Press, New York, 1948.

You can spray her wherever you figure the streptococci lurk
You can give her a shot for whatever she's got but it just won't work
If she's tired of getting the fish-eye from the hotel clerk,
A person can develop a cold.

It says here the female remaining single, just in the legal sense,
Shows a neurotic tendency: See note*
*Note: Chronic, organic, syndromes, toxic or hypertense,
Involving the eye, the ear, the nose and throat.
In other words, just from worrying whether the wedding is on or off,
A person can develop a cough.
You can feed her all day with the Vitamin A and the Bromo Fizz,
But the medicine never gets anywhere near where the trouble is.
If she's getting a kind of a name for herself and the name ain't "his,"—
A person can develop a cough.
And furthermore, just from stalling and stalling and stalling the wedding trip,
A person can develop La grippe.
When they get on the train for Niag'ra and she can hear church bells chime,
The compartment is air conditioned—and the mood sublime,—
Then they get off at Saratoga—for the fourteenth time,
A person can develop La grippe. (hm!) La grippe, La post nasal drip,
With the wheezes and the sneezes and a sinus that's really a pip!
From a lack of community property—and a feeling she's getting too old,
A person can develop a bad, bad cold.

(From the Broadway Production Guys and Dolls, *by Frank Loesser)*[4]

The influence of the emotions on the formation of stomach and duodenal ulcers is a good illustration of psychosomatic illness. Observations were made by two physicians on the digestive processes of a patient who, because of a previous accident, had to be fed through an opening made directly into his stomach. They could actually see that inflammation occurred when the patient became angry or upset.[5]

When food is present in the stomach, juices are put out to digest it. However, certain emotional reactions can also stimulate the flow of these fluids. If there is no food in the stomach, the acid juices may irritate the stomach itself. In some instances, this may eventually cause an ulcer, or open sore. It is important to remember that the ulcer which is formed is a definite organic disease of the stomach. Unless it is treated by medicine and diet, it may cause a hemorrhage or it may perforate. However, unless the emotional tension is relieved, the patient won't be giving his ulcer its best chance to heal; and he may also have to continue his diet and medicine in order to minimize the risk of getting another ulcer. Thus, *psychosomatic diseases frequently require treatment of both the body and the mind.*

In addition to ulcer of the stomach and of the duodenum, the following are regarded as diseases in which emotional factors may play an important part: migraine headache, mucous colitis, ulcerative colitis, asthma, high blood pressure, hyperthyroidism (overactive thyroid), and arthritis and rheumatism.

Undoubtedly others will be added to this list. As yet the evidence is not so clear-cut in any of these diseases as it is in the case of certain ulcers. We do not know, for example, to how great a degree a patient's asthma is due to his having inherited an allergic constitution and how much to his having emotional problems. However, we do know that asthmatic patients generally improve far more rapidly when their emotional difficulties are relieved at the same time that they are being desensitized to the pollens or other allergens which set off their attacks of asthma.

The effects of stress on the body, with resulting tension, are everyday examples of the relationship between the body and the mind. When a person must make a physical or emotional effort beyond the normal, in response to some difficult situation, he is under stress. This can be a source of worry, fear and anxiety to the point that a mere tendency to illness may develop into an active health problem, or new illnesses may result. Trying to live with too low an income is one of the most stressful situations. A study by Doctors S. H. King and S. Cobb (published in the

[4]Copyright 1950 by Frank Loesser. © Copyright 1951 by Frank Loesser. All rights throughout the world controlled by Frank Music Corp., New York, New York.

[5]Wolf, S., and Wolff, H. G.: *Human Gastric Function,* Oxford University Press, New York, 1943.

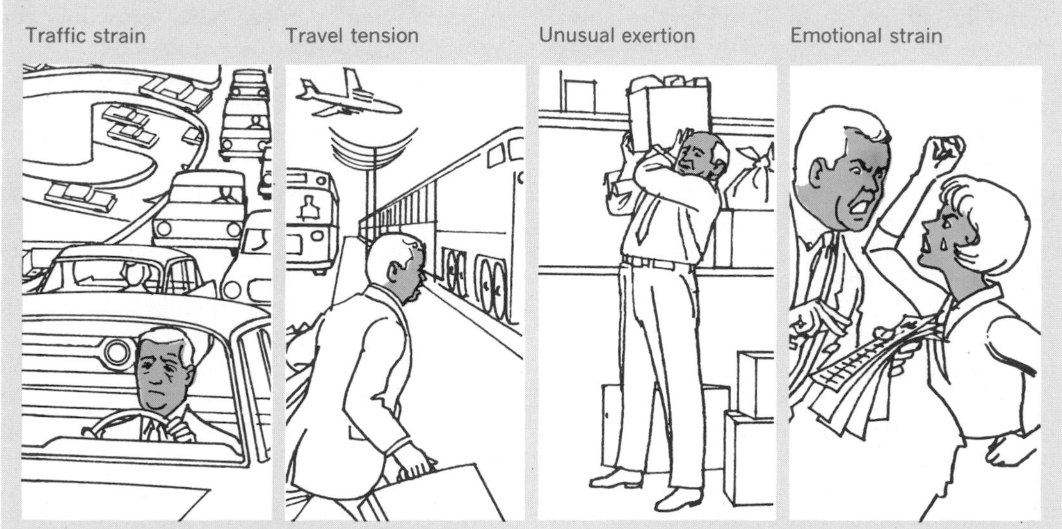

These forms of stress, when prolonged, have been found to have a significant part in the occurrence of coronary thrombosis, or a heart attack caused when a clot blocks an artery to the heart.

Journal of Chronic Diseases, 7:466, 1958) showed 12 times as much rheumatoid arthritis in men whose annual income was less than $3000 than in those earning $4500 or more. In addition to below-par income, other stressful conditions are inadequate education, an overabundance of children, lack of spare time and termination of marriage.

Stress is a highly personal matter. What may be stressful for one person may not be so for another. Also, some men and women are more adaptable to difficult situations than others. Very competitive, ambitious persons may thrive on difficulties. In our complex society, it is not possible to remove all causes of stress, nor is it desirable because the pressure of stress is often necessary for the accomplishment of goals.

The problem of how to handle stress arises. The body has many ways of adapting to pressure situations, such as the discharge of certain chemicals from the adrenal glands, changes in blood sugar levels and alterations in the digestive tract. If bodily tensions and anxieties develop sufficiently in response to stress, the individual may react with any of a vast number of ailments, any of which, as Dr. Franz Alexander pointed out, may be considered psychosomatic.

Therapy

Neuroses can be extremely incapacitating and long-lasting, limiting an individual's happiness and effectiveness in many ways. *Psychotherapy,* which means treatment by psychological measures, is the most successful procedure for the milder emotional problems. The term covers everything from the simplest "spilling out" of troubles to a spiritual advisor or wise friend, to occasional interviews with a sympathetic physician or a trained psychiatrist, to the long, involved process of psychoanalysis.

There are times when simply putting one's problems into words helps clarify them and make them seem less alarming. It may reveal what the real trouble is. Confessing one's weaknesses, failures and errors is valuable, even though it may be painful, provided the person to whom they are confessed understands their importance (however trivial they may actually be). He must also be able to make the person who is confessing feel that he in not being condemned, but that he is still worthwhile, despite his faults and frailties. Doing something constructive to make up for the past is far better than brooding about it.

Receiving information is sometimes most

useful in equipping an individual to solve his own problems, especially if they were due, wholly or in part, to ignorance or misinformation.

Almost every doctor practices some form of psychotherapy, sometimes without knowing it. In dealing with a patient who has an exaggerated fear that he is ill, the doctor's examination, explanation, reassurance, and firmness are forms of psychotherapy. Or when he helps a tense, nervous person find a hobby—that, too, is psychotherapy.

Psychoanalysis. This process consists in uncovering the unconscious forces influencing the patient, which he cannot, simply by will, bring into his consciousness. The patient does this by free associating (saying anything that comes into his head), telling about his dreams, his fantasies, whatever he thinks of. The psychoanalyst makes this as easy as possible by having the patient recline on a couch where he is less aware of the doctor's presence, and by prompting him with an occasional question, such as "What does that make you think of?"

If these sessions are successful, *transference* takes place, and the patient begins to react toward the therapist in the same ways that he reacted, or still reacts, to important figures in his life, usually his parents. Because the psychoanalyst is a neutral sort of figure, the patient can see his own patterns of reaction. For example, unable to find a "reason" for his fear of the analyst, he may discover that it springs from his unconscious mind, and that it actually represents a concealed fear of his father, stemming from childhood days.

Once the unconscious material has been brought out, the patient can develop insight into his problems and overcome some of the power of his unconscious.

Psychoanalysis is usually a prolonged and expensive form of treatment, often requiring three to five sessions a week for several years. The reason it takes so long is that it isn't easy to bring unconscious motivations to light. When a person has been reacting in a particular way for many years, habits are not easily changed even when one understands how they came about, and wants very much to change them. When you've been crawling for years, it's difficult to learn to walk.

Psychoanalytically Oriented Psychotherapy. This is sometimes called *brief therapy* or *analytic interviews.* Some of the techniques of psychoanalysis are used, but this type of therapy is much shorter.

In *group therapy,* four to ten patients may be treated during the same period. Some psychiatrists combine this with individual sessions, others use it alone. It is considered valuable because the patients react to each other as well as to the doctor, and because their self-confidence is increased by being with people whose problems are like their own. For example, obese people who overeat for psychological reasons often respond well to group therapy, and some of its principles are used successfully in *Alcoholics Anonymous* as well.

Narcosynthesis. This treatment is similar to treatment by hypnosis, and was used successfully, for example, on soldiers who "cracked up." Medicines (such as sodium amobarbital) are used to put the patient into a sleeping state, in which he may remember and bring into the open what is troubling him. The trouble in soldiers was often found to be due to guilt feelings connected with the death of a comrade; the incident that caused these feelings had been forgotten (being too deeply disturbing), but it was recalled during the sleepy state. Once brought into the open, these feelings could be coped with.

Other Methods of Treatment. *Rest cures* in pleasant sanitoria used to be widely recommended for neurotic patients, but are suggested less often today because the patient has to adjust to the world as soon as he is discharged. Such treatment may be necessary if the neurotic individual is physically run down, or if the conditions in his home are connected with the patient's specific problems.

Medicines such as the barbiturates and some of the new tranquilizing drugs may be used to relieve tension. Stimulants are also helpful at times. These preparations should be taken only on a doctor's prescription and under his guidance.

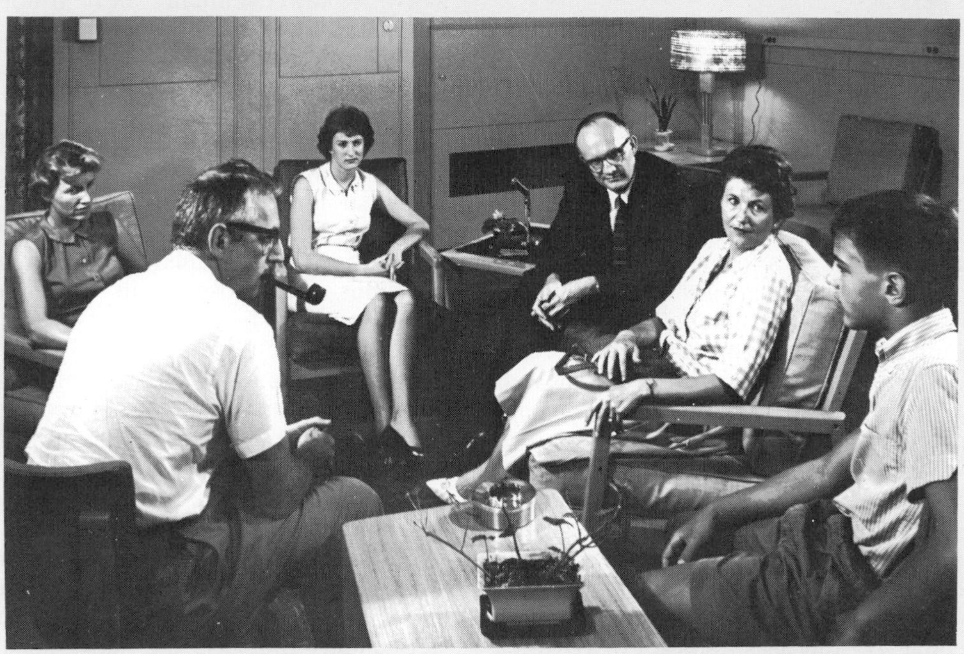

Family therapy under the direction of a psychiatrist is often helpful in easing the tensions that can be created when a member of the family has mental or emotional problems. The family, which often has to live with the disturbed person, can come to understand the patient's problems and help him.

THE DEVELOPMENT OF PSYCHIATRY

For centuries, mental disorders were problems for the devil-doctors, magicians, or priests. This was logical, for all illness was supposed to be of supernatural origin. The supernatural theory of mental diseases persisted long after it was suspected that physical ailments were not caused by forces from the other world. (The word *lunatic,* for example, comes from the Latin word for the moon, which was supposed to cause madness.) Yet even in early days there were indications of some insight into psychology, such as the interpretations of dreams, the treatment of the insane by music, the rituals of mourning for the dead, and the confessing of sins.

As long as people believed that mental disorders were the work of evil demons who inhabited human bodies, the mentally ill were treated with extreme cruelty. Although the supernatural theory has been

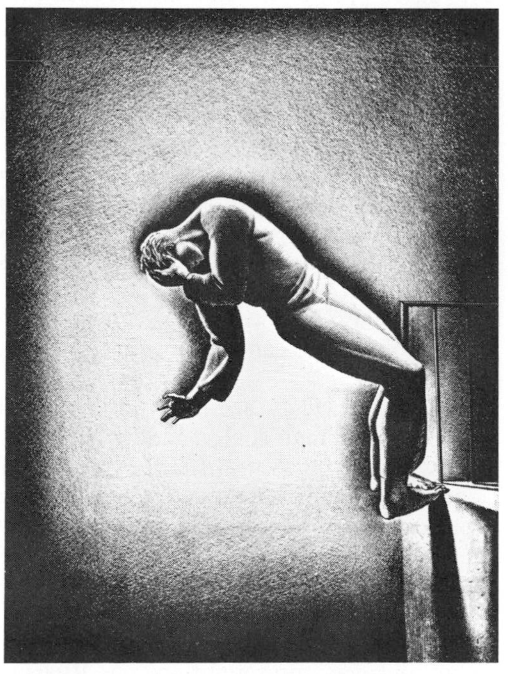

A lithograph by Rockwell Kent, suggesting the fear of falling. (Courtesy of Philadelphia Museum of Art.)

discarded, some traces of the old attitude still persist.

By the sixteenth century, some connection between the human brain and human behavior began to be suspected. But it was not until the French Revolution in 1789, that a French doctor, Philippe Pinel, advanced the revolutionary theory that the *insane should be treated as patients* and not as loathsome or amusing monsters. This idea formed the foundation for modern psychiatry, although it did not of itself explain very much.

Soon after this, two other French doctors made great discoveries. Paul Broca showed that an injury to a portion of the brain (the speech center) caused a man to utter unintelligible sounds, so that he *seemed* to be insane, although he was not. The other doctor, Jean Marie Charcot, showed that he could hypnotize certain patients who would then produce the actual physical symptoms he suggested, such as a swelling of the legs. These discoveries opened the door to an understanding of the relationship between the body and the mind.

Because doctors were learning how to use the microscope, the emphasis during the later years of the nineteenth and the early ones of the twentieth century was placed on studying the *physical* origin of mental disorders, particularly in the nerves. Rapid advances were made in *neurology* (the study of the nervous system). The theory that all mental diseases had an organic-structural origin became popular. A great deal was learned about hereditary defects, head injuries, and bacterial infections. Now it is generally agreed that only a small portion of all mental illnesses can be accounted for in this manner.

In the early years of the twentieth century a German doctor named Kraepelin advanced the *disease-entity theory,* according to which mental diseases differed from one another as much as, for example, measles differs from appendicitis. Kraepelin made an excellent contribution in classifying mental diseases.

The *conditioned-reflex theory* of human behavior was presented by a Russian, Ivan Pavlov. He discovered that dogs could become so accustomed to associating the ringing of a bell with being fed that saliva would eventually flow from their mouths when the bell was rung, even though no food was present. For a time psychologists were inclined to believe that abnormal human behavior could be explained by the theory of conditioned reflexes—the "conditioning" having taken place so long ago that it was forgotten. Modern psychiatrists are not in agreement about how much this can explain the reactions they observe in the mentally ill.

Toward the end of the nineteenth century, Sigmund Freud of Vienna discovered that when he hypnotized an hysterical patient, she talked of things about which she obviously had no conscious knowledge. He worked out techniques for getting at this unconscious material without resorting to hypnosis. One of his methods consisted of getting the patient to say anything that came into her mind—that is, he developed the technique of free association as a form of therapy. By means of his new methods, Freud worked out what was actually the first scientific explanation of the deep roots and motivation of human behavior. He took into account both unconscious and conscious motivation.

His contributions were invaluable. Even though all of his interpretations are not universally accepted today, most modern psychiatry is based on the same general theory to which Freud subscribed, that is, the *functional* theory. This places emphasis upon the patient as a whole—his past life in addition to his present symptoms—the *person* and not just the disease.

More recently, just as Freud emphasized a person's entire life as it related to a present illness, many psychiatrists have looked beyond the patient to the world he lives in. Each of us is a member of a group, often of overlapping groups. Each is subject to group obligations. An individual has a role and a place and is subject to rewards, punishments and other pressures. A well known sociologist, E. W. Burgess, has pointed out: "Mental ill health is a symptom and index of the malfunctioning of society. . . .Perhaps the most important single factor in mental disorders and disturbances is the failure of society to provide adequately for the social roles essential for the mental health of its members." While the Freudians and the non-Freudians disagree among themselves, it is generally true that to understand and treat mental illness the therapist must know and understand as much as possible about the individual—his body, his life and his environment.

Questions

1. Why do you think inhumane treatment of mentally ill people persisted so long?
2. What is the relation of free association, which is used in psychoanalysis, to unconscious motivations for our actions?
3. Would this be a happier world if we had no inhibitions, from infancy on?
4. Can you inhibit a child without causing him severe emotional frustrations that might later express themselves in abnormal behavior?
5. How might a normal and an abnormal person face the following situations: the death of a parent? the theft of a valuable heirloom? signs that a serious disease might be developing?
6. How do psychiatrists believe phobias arise? How could a phobia be cured?
7. Do you think that an over-protective mother might have a better, the same, or a worse influence on her child than a careless, thoughtless mother?
8. Why does the cure of psychosomatic illnesses require treatment of both the body and the mind?
9. How can self-awareness of one's personality problems help bring about improvement?
10. What are some of the dangers of the "stormy" periods of life—for example, adolescence?
11. Should everyone have a psychiatric checkup as routinely as a physical examination? Why, or why not?
12. How do you draw the line between being observant and "playing psychiatrist"?
13. What were some of Freud's contributions toward our understanding of ourselves?
14. Can you define precisely where mental health ends and mental illness begins? If not, what are some of the criteria for deciding that a person is mentally ill?

Topics for Discussion

The contributions of Philippe Pinel to the treatment of the insane.

Some contributions of Adler, Jung, and Meyer.

Attitudes of various religions toward psychiatry.

The concept of maturity as it applies during college years.

Ways to stimulate public interest in problems of the emotionally disturbed.

The possibility that not only the individual but also society is "sick."

The relationship between genius and neurosis.

The possibility of conscious control of emotional disturbance.

Reading Suggestions

Peace of Mind, Joshua L. Liebman. Simon & Schuster, New York, 1946. Thoughtful advice on how to reduce emotional tensions.

Mental Health in the Metropolis: The Midtown Manhattan Study, Leo Strole and others. McGraw-Hill, New York, 1962. This is an authoritative report of a study of the relationship of mental illness to sociological factors.

Social Class and Mental Illness, A. B. Hollingshead and F. C. Redlich. Wiley, New York, 1958. An influential study of the differences in incidence of mental illness and varying treatments, according to the social and economic classes of the patients.

The Psychology of Human Conflict, Edwin R. Guthrie, Beacon Press, Boston, 1962. The conflict of motives and drives within every individual.

Tensions and How to Master Them, George S. Stevenson. Public Affairs Pamphlet, New York, 1960. Advice on a professional level on a subject of immediate interest.

That Wonderful Machine, the Brain, George A. W. Boehn. Fortune, February 1963. A lucid presentation by a well known science writer.

Anxiety, Heiri Steiner and Jean Gebser. Dell Publishing Co., New York, 1962.

The Layman's Guide to Psychiatry, James A. Brussel. Barnes & Noble, New York, 1961.

Mentally Healthy Young Male College Students, Roy R. Grinker, Sr., Roy R. Grinker, Jr., and John Timberlake. AMA Archives of General Psychiatry, June 1962.

Handbook of Community Psychiatry and Mental Health, L. Bellock (ed.). Grune & Stratton, New York, 1964.

The Life and Work of Sigmund Freud, Ernest Jones, edited and abridged in one volume by Lionel Trilling and Steven Marcus. Basic Books, New York, 1961. A remarkable book, as much for its beautiful and readable style as for its accuracy and authenticity.

Abnormal Psychology, Ephraim Rosen and Ian Gregory. W. B. Saunders Co., Philadelphia, 1965. For the undergraduate student, a review of the subject in two parts: one, an introduction to the general principles of abnormal psychology, and two, an application of those principles to the main symptom-systems of abnormal behavior.

Mental Health in Modern Society, In *Mental Health and Mental Disorder* (A. M. Rose, ed.). W. W. Norton & Co., New York, 1955.

7

SERIOUS EMOTIONAL ILLNESS AND MENTAL DEFICIENCY

My pain's past cure, another hell,
I may not in this torment dwell!
Now desperate I hate my life,
Lend me a halter or a knife;
  All my griefs to this are jolly,
  Naught so damned as melancholy.

ROBERT BURTON,
The Anatomy of Melancholy

The problem of mental illness is full of ironies. More than 700,000 patients—half of those in all hospitals in the United States at any one time—are mental patients, and one out of every ten Americans now living will eventually suffer a serious mental illness. Unfortunately, most people look the other way when this problem is mentioned. Mental illness today is often curable, and more often controllable, but ironically, people are more afraid to even think about it than about many other illnesses that are much less able to be controlled.

Many mentally sick people somehow get through life, more or less miserably, without seeking or receiving adequate help. Many others may appear normal in most respects but show bizarre behavior at certain times. They may institute one lawsuit after another out of an unjustified feeling that they have been wronged. They may grate on the nerves of everyone around them without recognizing that they cannot maintain a healthy relationship with anyone. Or they may show little or no emotional response to experiences that would strongly affect normal people.

Serious mental illness involves a range of personality disturbances. One type of disturbed person is called a *psychopath.* He may function without getting into serious trouble, but he may be a problem for other men and women because he has little or no concern for them. An extreme form of mental illness is *psychosis.* Psychotic individuals are out of touch with reality and must be treated, usually in hospitals, for their own protection and the protection of others. Finally, the *mental defective,* who may never develop into normal adulthood at all, requires very special care and education, possibly for his entire life.

THE PSYCHOPATHIC PERSONALITY

No one starts out in life with standards of right or wrong. These must be taught, by parents, by teachers and by friends and associates. Sometimes the lessons are hard to take, and sometimes the lessons make no impression at all, or perhaps they are never given. Those persons who fail to develop a conscience, and who have little or no sense of what is socially acceptable are called psychopaths, or sociopaths.

Psychopaths are generally antisocial, aggressive and impulsive, and they feel little guilt (or none) about their actions. They cannot form strong bonds of affection with others. Thus, the psychopath, free of worry or concern for the present or the future, may lie, cheat, swindle or steal. If he feels hostile, he expresses his feelings freely. He may be quite charming and capable of manipulating other people, and he also may cheat or harm, in one way or another, those he has attracted to him.

Psychopaths may be quite intelligent. Their particular form of personality disorder apparently is not caused by organic damage. However, they have not grown emotionally. In this respect, they are about at the level of a two-year-old, and their lack of concern about their actions may result in their performing criminal acts. In doing so, their only remorse is that they were caught.

Psychiatrists and psychologists have tried to treat psychopaths in many different ways—with drugs, brain surgery, psychoanalysis and family therapy. In some cases, psychopaths abandon their antisocial behavior as they grow older—perhaps because they finally realize their way of life is self-defeating, perhaps because the complex pressures of their world finally force them to become socialized, at least to a degree.

There are many types of sociopaths, but the lack of concern about the results of their behavior characterizes them all. Here are some examples:

William A. met and married a prostitute when he was in the armed forces as a military policeman. After their marriage, both he and his wife continued to be promiscuous, but he began to beat her because of her extramarital activities. When she divorced him, he became depressed and threatened suicide. Finally, when he realized that she would not return, his depression cleared up and he promised to marry another woman with whom he was already living. In fact, he really had no guilt or remorse about his treatment of his first wife, and had no intention of keeping his promise to marry the woman with whom he was living.

Following World War II, Roger E., 37 years old, applied for a medical internship at a Brooklyn hospital. He displayed all the necessary credentials from universities and hospitals, and he was assigned to the staff. He delivered several hundred babies, and participated in other hospital work. After approximately five years, he missed a payment on his car, and in the ensuing credit investigation, police learned that he never had been licensed to practice medicine. He had served in the Army Medical Corps and had read medical books whenever possible. After the war, he forged his credentials. Like many psychopaths, he had a friendly personality, and even after he was arrested, many of the hospital staff had kind words for him.

On Halloween, Mrs. Ethel M. was annoyed by children ringing her bell. She heated pennies in her stove, then threw them on the porch when children arrived for their "trick or treat." Their cries when they were burned, their parents' uproar and the tongue-lashing and sentence she received when she was brought into court never resulted in the slightest expression of regret for what she had done.

Lee Harvey Oswald, accused of the assassination of President Kennedy on November 22, 1963, was a man of above-average intelligence, whose behavior could be described in an oversimplified way as psychopathic. The product of an unhappy childhood and of a disturbed adolescence, during which he was recommended for psychiatric treatment that he never received, Oswald was an alienated person during his brief life. A reporter who interviewed him in Russia reported that he was unconcerned and dispassionate about Kennedy. Apparently, his hatred was directed against the office of President, which happened to be occupied by John F. Kennedy, and was not directed against Kennedy himself. The fact that Oswald himself was killed before he could be brought to trial, of course, destroyed the opportunity for psychiatric and legal analysis of the man and his motives.

SEXUAL CRIMINALITY

There is no clear line, no simple definition, of the differences between mere eccentricity and some forms of mental illness. There is also no easy way to predict when the psychopath may perform a criminal act. Nor is it true that only psychopaths are capable of sexual criminality. Delinquency or outright criminality may be rooted in organic brain damage, family difficulties or an unfortunate neighborhood environment. Some sex crimes may be impulsive, committed as a result of intolerable stress.

However, most persons who commit violent sex crimes, such as rape or murder, are definitely suffering from emotional illnesses or defects, however well concealed these may have been before the crime was committed. Most of us have transient peculiar sex impulses, and many of us have murderous desires, but we generally never carry them out. But in criminals, the *controlling* or *inhibiting* mechanisms are defective, or even absent. In some persons, deep-rooted feelings of guilt, inferiority or insecurity may shunt their sexual instincts in abnormal directions, some of them definitely dangerous to society.

The term *sex maniac* includes people who, like Jack the Ripper, commit violent sex crimes, such as rape and murder. They are definitely suffering from emotional illnesses or defects, however well concealed these may have been before the crime was committed. Many people have transient, peculiar sex impulses or murderous desires, but they never actually consider carrying them out. They are in the same category as any number of notions that may pop into the mind—from jumping off the top of a high building to tripping a pompous fat man. In some sex maniacs, the *controlling* or *inhibiting* mechanisms are defective, or even absent. In others, deep-rooted feelings of guilt, inferiority or insecurity may shunt their sexual instincts into abnormal directions, some of them definitely socially dangerous.

ALCOHOLISM AND DRUG ADDICTION

Some psychiatrists feel that alcoholics and drug addicts are not, strictly speaking, psychopathic personalities, but that the addiction must be attributed to some emotional disturbance. These people differ from other maladjusted individuals in that they have turned to something *outside* themselves to find the characteristic "inadequate but temporarily satisfying solution" to their problems. Alcohol and drugs are used to provide an escape and relief from emotional tensions. Obviously, they have not really found a solution. In fact, they compound the problem because excessive use of alcohol and the intake of drugs have very harmful physical and mental effects.

SEXUAL DEVIATIONS

Sexual deviations of certain types are the symptoms of emotional illnesses, maladjustments or immaturities which reveal themselves in the individual's sexual behavior.

Psychiatrists are not in entire agreement about the exact cause of sexual deviations. People are not sexual perverts because they are too weak to exercise will power. It is now fairly generally accepted that behavior of this type results from emotional difficulties which should, if possible, be corrected. At the same time, the actions of deviates must be controlled in order to prevent them from harming themselves or others.

Peeping Toms are individuals who receive their greatest—or only—sexual pleasure from watching a woman undressed or undressing, or a couple engaged in sexual relations. Such individuals do not experience equivalent pleasure in normal sexual activities.

Homosexuality is the term which was formerly applied only to people who had actual physical relations with members of their own sex. Now, however, it includes those who can form deep emotional or love attachments only with a member of their own sex. This may never be expressed sexually.

In certain rare instances, homosexuality results from definite glandular dysfunction. Usually, however, it is of psychic origin.

A number of theories have been advanced to explain homosexuality, but there is fairly general agreement along the following basic lines:

Children normally tend to identify themselves with the parent of the same sex; a little girl wants to be like (and to rival) her mother, a boy, his father. If, for some reason, the identification is with the parent of the opposite sex, the child may be oriented in the direction of homosexuality at an early age.

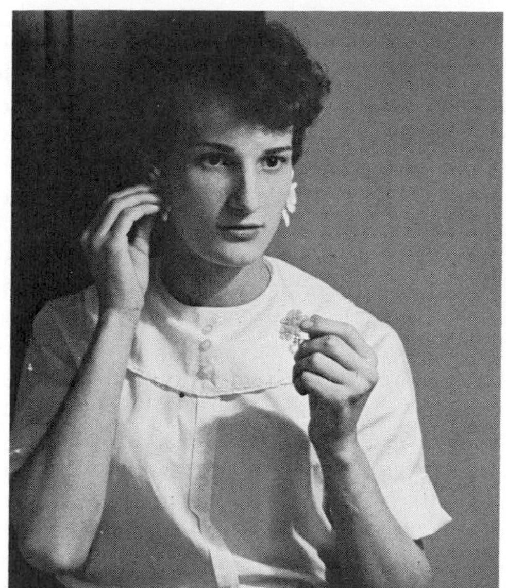

A 17 year old transvestite. While not a professional female impersonator, he occasionally does a "strip-tease" act at private clubs and parties. (From Kisker, G. W.: *The Disorganized Personality*. McGraw-Hill, 1964.)

Homosexuality may also come about in another way. During a certain period (usually shortly before adolescence and in early adolescence) children prefer members of their own sex. Boys look down on girls, have male heroes, and enjoy being together, while girls detest boys, have crushes on girls, and love some best friend intensely. With the coming of sexual maturity, their sexual drives are, not always without conflict, directed toward members of the opposite sex.

During this transitional period, unfortunate sexual experiences may have a devastating effect on young people, especially those who have some conflict in this area. These experiences, whether subtle or obvious, form a barrier on the road to normal sexual development. Homosexuality is a detour on that highway, and some people, tragically, never find their way back to the main road.

As a rule, homosexuals are lonely and unhappy people, often tortured by their inability to find happiness within society's norms. Moral judgments or disapproval of their way of life will not change them. However, every effort must be made to keep them from injuring others who could succeed in finding the road to a normal sex life.

"Amateur psychiatrists" have done a great deal of harm by speaking glibly about "latent homosexuality" or "bisexuality." It should be reassuring to know that: (1) A homosexual experience (or experiences), especially in adolescence, does not mean that an individual is homosexual. Neither do homosexual dreams or fantasies. (2) There are also some holdovers from the period during which the company of one's own sex was preferred. A high-school girl expressed this when she said, "I'd ever so much rather be with girls, except for the fact that men are so attractive!" (3) *There is a variable component of basic homosexuality in every normal individual.*

True homosexuality is a very complicated problem, and usually represents only one aspect of personality maladjustment.

Exhibitionism is the act of revealing one's body, usually the genital organ. In essence, this is similar to peeping. A certain amount of showing off is normal, and should not be confused with the exhibitionism of a truly maladjusted individual. Such a person may be attempting to reassure himself against fears of sexual inferiority. Or he may be expressing his defiance of a supposedly hostile world by shocking people in this manner.

Excessive narcissism or *self-love* is quite different from *self-respect* and from the satisfaction which normal men and women derive from looking their best. The term comes from the name of the Greek youth who, according to the myth, saw his own reflection in a pond and was so enamored of it that he fell in and was drowned while attempting to embrace himself.

Most children go through a period of being attracted to their own images in a mirror, stating frankly, "You're pretty" or "I love you." People who do not outgrow this stage are often basically so insecure that they feel no one else will ever love them. This exclusive preoccupation with self is frequently accompanied by a preference for masturbation to sexual intercourse. Such people are incapable of actually loving anyone else. If they marry, and they often do, it is to conform to society's patterns, outwardly, or to obtain support and money to spend on the beloved person, namely, himself or herself.

Nymphomania and *satyrism* represent the excessive desire for intercourse in a woman and a man. These conditions are rare. Although the terms are often applied to people who are promiscuous or highly sexed, they should be reserved for *compulsive* sexuality, which cannot be satisfied. Like compulsive eating, it often springs from insecurity and may be indulged in to ward off anxiety. Unable to find the hoped-for release in sexual intercourse, such people must desperately try, try again. A nymphomaniac is often unable to experience an orgasm, remaining unsatisfied no matter how often she has intercourse. Usually this is because she is attempting to satisfy a need that cannot be fulfilled by coitus. She may be unconsciously homosexual. If so, she will not find what she is looking for in any man. She may be trying to compensate for feelings of inferiority; or she may feel unconsciously that intercourse is wicked and therefore must not be enjoyed fully.

The male equivalent of the nymphomaniac may be similarly maladjusted, often an unconscious homosexual, or besieged by intense conflicts due to feelings of guilt, fear, or inferiority.

Bestiality is the act of having intercourse with animals. The Kinsey reports indicate that about 17 per cent of all males raised on farms have had some sexual experience with animals. The practice is fairly common among shepherds and others who are isolated from women. However, *preference* for sex relations with animals is due to an emotional maladjustment usually springing from feelings of inferiority.

Sadism and *masochism* mean deriving pleasure from giving or receiving pain. Sadists may inflict pain on animals or upon people, usually their sexual partners. They wish to dominate, to prove their strength or virility by being aggressive or (for example) by being like their dominating fathers who used to punish them. Sadism does not have to be expressed only as a sexual deviation. Teasing and practical jokes can also have sadistic elements.

Children sometimes appear sadistic in their drive to assert themselves. However, the actions of children which are sometimes called sadistic are not necessarily so. They may be due merely to curiosity or lack of understanding. For example, a child who pulls the wings off flies is not necessarily being cruel. He may be impelled by the same impulses that make him examine and study any inanimate object.

Masochists derive pleasure and satisfaction from being treated cruelly, from being hurt physically or emotionally, or from hurting themselves. This usually has its roots in the desire, often unconscious, to be punished for some "sin." Masochism has been called neurotic submissiveness, and sadism, neurotic aggressiveness; but since they spring from similar maladjustments, both may exist in the same person. Masochism appears in a nonphysical form, as a character attitude, far more frequently than it does as a sexual deviation.

There are frequently sadistic and masochistic elements even in normal sexual and love relationships. But these have the mutual consent of both partners, and serve merely to enhance the pleasure and intimacy. They are eventually subordinated to a tender fulfillment.

PSYCHOSES

People suffering from psychoses are called psychotics, or psychotic personalities. To a greater or lesser extent they are out of touch with reality for some, if not all, of the time.

A psychotic individual may live in his own private world, not seeing or hearing anything that goes on around him. He may not even feel it if he is suddenly slapped; or if he does feel it, it may actually bring a happy smile to his face. He may go into a *catatonic* state, standing absolutely motionless for hours in a position no normal person could maintain for more than a few minutes. He may suffer from *hallucinations,* seeing and hearing things that have no existence outside his own mind, or he may experience *delusions,* or unreal beliefs. Such people, for example, may be convinced that they are famous kings or Napoleon. Mental institutions are full of men and women who are certain they represent some of the greatest names in history.

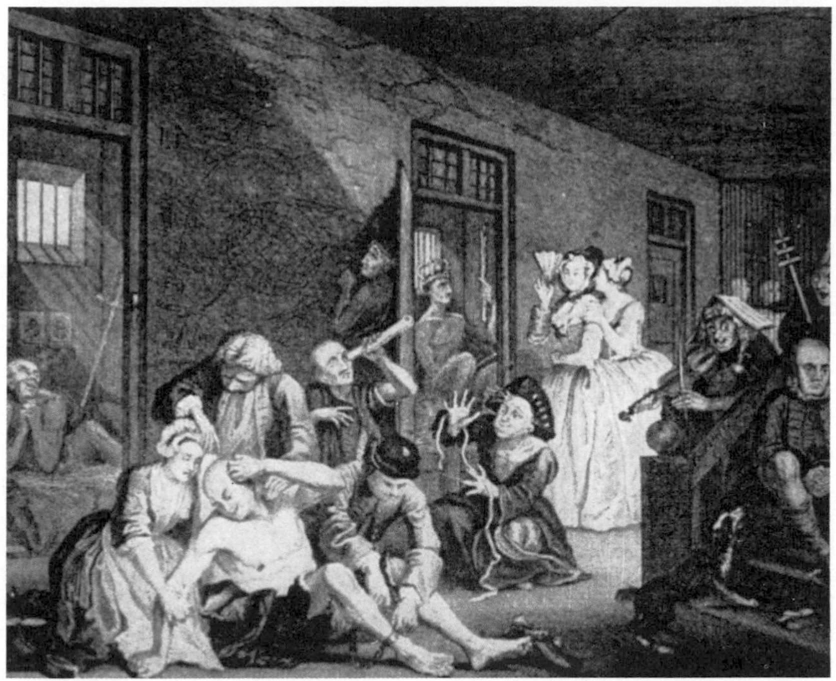

Scene in Bedlam, by Hogarth. Last picture in The Rake's Progress series.

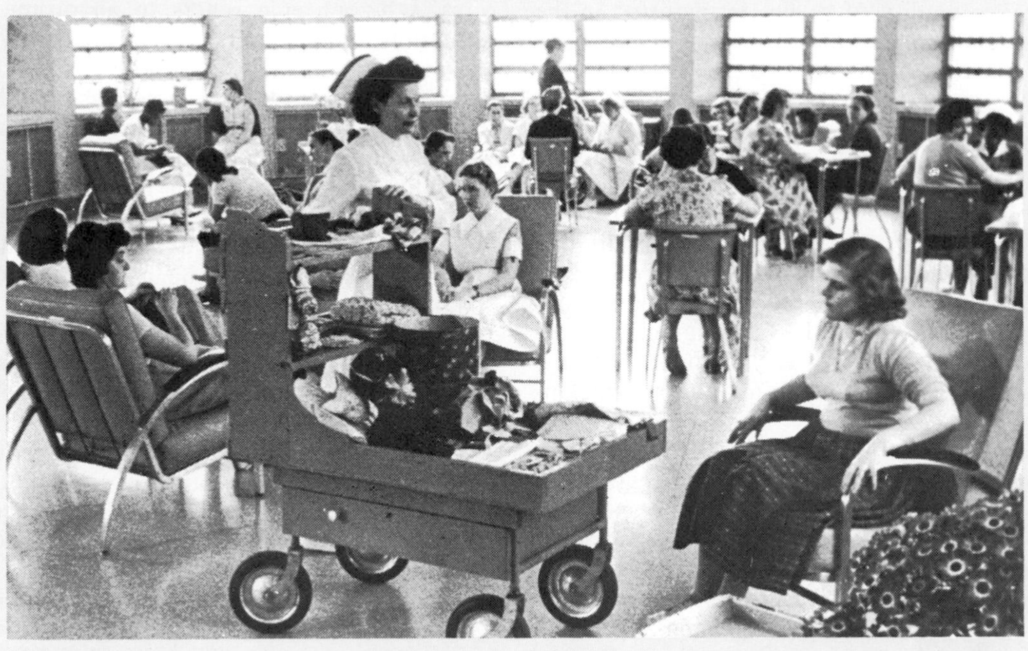

The solarium in the women's wing of a modern mental hospital. Unlike the "snake pits" of fifty years ago, it is clean, spacious, and well staffed, and the patients enjoy occupational therapy and recreation.

This distortion of reality is one of the primary differences between neurotic and psychotic people. A neurotic individual may be plagued by uneasiness or an unreasonable fear of people. He may say he *feels* as if he were living on enemy territory. However, he *knows* exactly where he *is* living. On the other hand, a psychotic person, suffering from the same delusion, would be convinced that he was actually surrounded by enemies who wanted to kill him, force him to do certain things, or "gain control of his thoughts."

The "evidence" which the psychotic presents as proof of his contentions is quite different from that of the neurotic individual. If, for example, a neurotic person believes he is unattractive to women, he may support his theory by pointing out that a girl refused to accept his invitation to go out with him, ignoring the fact that he invited her so late she might well have had a previous engagement. A psychotic person, however, by indicating a television aerial on a neighboring roof, or describing how strangely someone looked at him on a bus "proves" that people are trying to sneak into his thoughts. The entire quality of reality is distorted in the psychotic individual.

Types of Psychoses

The psychoses may be classified in various ways, but they are usually divided into *functional* and *organic* (with brain damage). The functional psychoses are considered under the headings of: schizophrenia, paranoia, and manic-depressive psychoses, including involutional melancholia.

Schizophrenia. This disease was formerly called dementia praecox (early loss of mind), because it usually appears between the ages of fifteen and thirty. It is the type of psychosis most frequently seen.

About one-fourth of the mental patients newly admitted to hospitals each year are schizophrenic. At any one time, about 400,000 schizophrenics are hospitalized. No other illness can match this terrible figure.

Schizophrenia actually means "split mind," and, indeed, the individual suffering from this disease does not appear to be a whole person. The type of child most apt to develop schizophrenia is usually shy, dreamy, bored and lacking in physical and mental energy. A certain amount of daydreaming is perfectly normal, but the incipient schizophrenic, unable to cope with the world, withdraws from it. The added difficulties of adolescence may drive him into a world of his own creating.

Generally, schizophrenia manifests itself slowly, although sometimes it appears abruptly in an acute attack of confusion. The patient becomes more and more withdrawn, listless, eccentric or secretive, or extremely suspicious. He may stay in his room. His emotional responses become dim or somewhat distorted. Often he or she will complain of unusual physical symptoms: one side of his body feels different from the other; something has gotten into his head and is ticking; he is turning into a woman (or, if a woman, into a man); his body is full of electricity or irradiation. The list of symptoms is endless.

A schizophrenic reacts to an ordinary situation in a variety of unusual ways: he may be cunning, or secretive and withdrawn; he may indicate violent, homicidal rage; he may show a trancelike withdrawal. In extreme cases, the patient seems to abandon all contact with the world and assumes a hunched-up position, as if he had reverted to the isolation of the womb. In such circumstances he is helpless and completely unresponsive.

Although certain types of schizophrenia respond more readily to treatment than do others, early diagnosis and treatment are extremely important. Of course, this is highly desirable in all cases of neurotic and psychotic illness, but it is particularly true with schizophrenia, as the chances of recovery appear to be closely related to the duration of the condition.

Paranoia. This psychosis is also called *monomania, delusional insanity,* and *persecutory insanity*. The patient suffering from it may, for example, sound and act fairly normal, although he is very ill. His memory may be adequate, his confusion not apparent, and his reasoning logical,

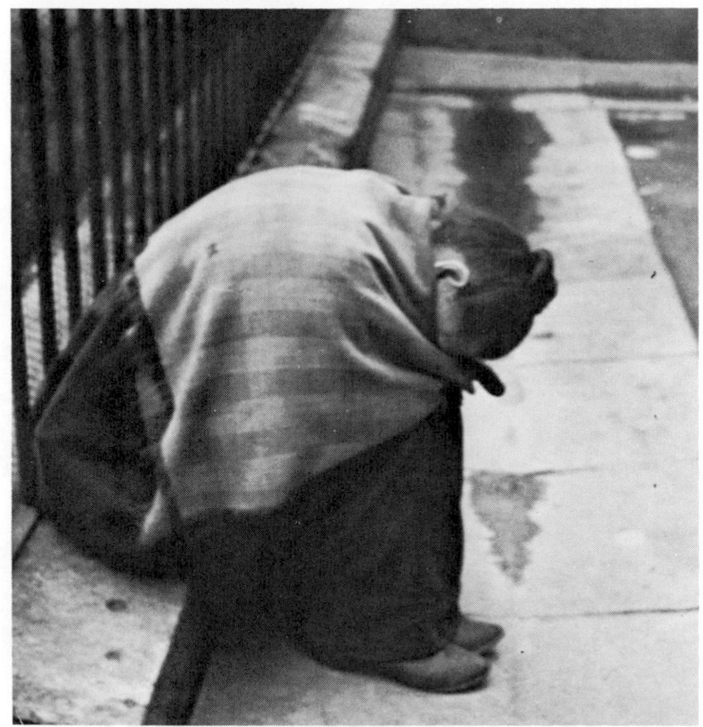

The withdrawn schizophrenic.
(Roger-Viollet, Paris.)

although his premises are false and his judgment impaired.

Paranoia usually develops between the ages of 30 and 50, particularly among people who have always been self-centered, jealous, and suspicious. The individual becomes more and more deluded, seeing hidden meanings to support his conviction that he is being plotted against, perhaps by such means as x-ray or hypnotism. This type of psychotic person feels quite justified in "defending himself" by lawsuits, or antisocial acts, including murder. *Pyromaniacs* sometimes are paranoid individuals who set fire to buildings to "destroy the evil people in it."

A paranoid person is quite different from a neurotic individual who may believe "everyone's against me" or "everything happens to me." The latter merely places undue emphasis on events in his life, whereas the former distorts them completely.

Manic-depressive Psychosis. This is also called *alternating insanity,* because of the alternating period of mania, with exaggerated feeling of elation and well-being, and of melancholia, an equally exaggerated and groundless misery. The term *cyclical insanity* has been used because of the rhythmical nature of these states, which are usually separated by a relatively normal period. During the manic stage, the patient's energy seems boundless; he may dash about talking gaily and wildly for 24 hours at a time without rest or sleep. The term *maniac* is specifically applied to a person whose behavior is very wild at this stage of the psychosis. In his depressed state, he may sit or lie, miserable, scarcely able to move or speak, and wishing for death which he sometimes seeks very cleverly.

The "cyclic personality type" of individual is not to be confused with a person suffering from a true manic-depressive psychosis. Normal people also have their ups and downs, and these may be of a fairly rhythmical nature. Their moods may alternate during the course of a day, and they may feel wonderful (or terrible) in the morning, and quite the opposite at night. Many women are depressed before each menstrual period. Some people feel "blue" in bad, wintry weather while a sunny spring day makes them bubble over with high spirits. These moods are quite different from the periods of wild

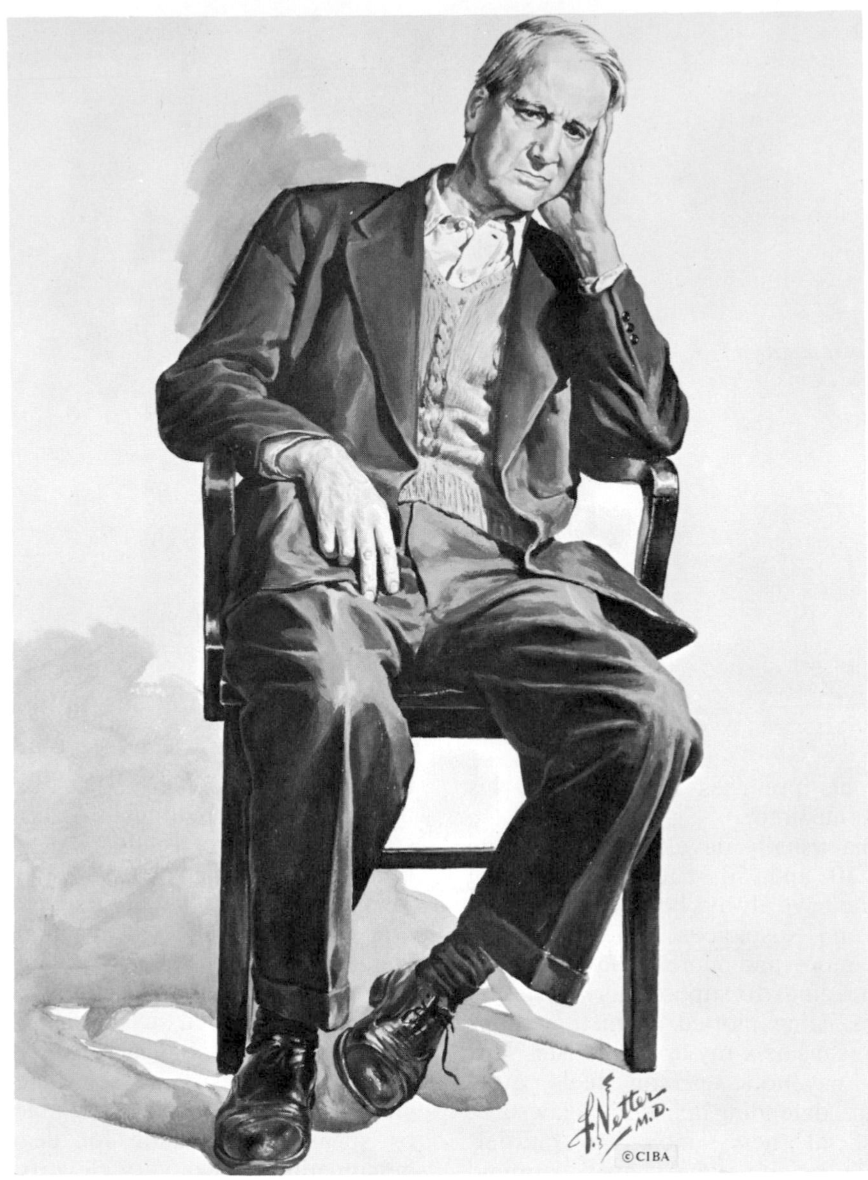

Retarded depression.

elation and profound unhappiness which the manic-depressive psychotic experiences.

Involutional Melancholia. This is a state of depression which may occur in the later periods of life, during the change of life (menopause) in women and its emotional counterpart in men. It is always accompanied by the danger of suicide.

The Causes of Psychoses

The causes of many psychoses are obscure at the present time. However, extensive current research in this field is broadening our understanding tremendously. As far as we have been able to discover, some of them appear to be the result of *functional* disorders. So far, no striking biochemical or physiological changes have been detected. However, improvement in physical and chemical techniques may reveal such changes, once we know what to look for.

Some psychoses do have definite physical causes. These include:

Infectious Diseases. These involve the

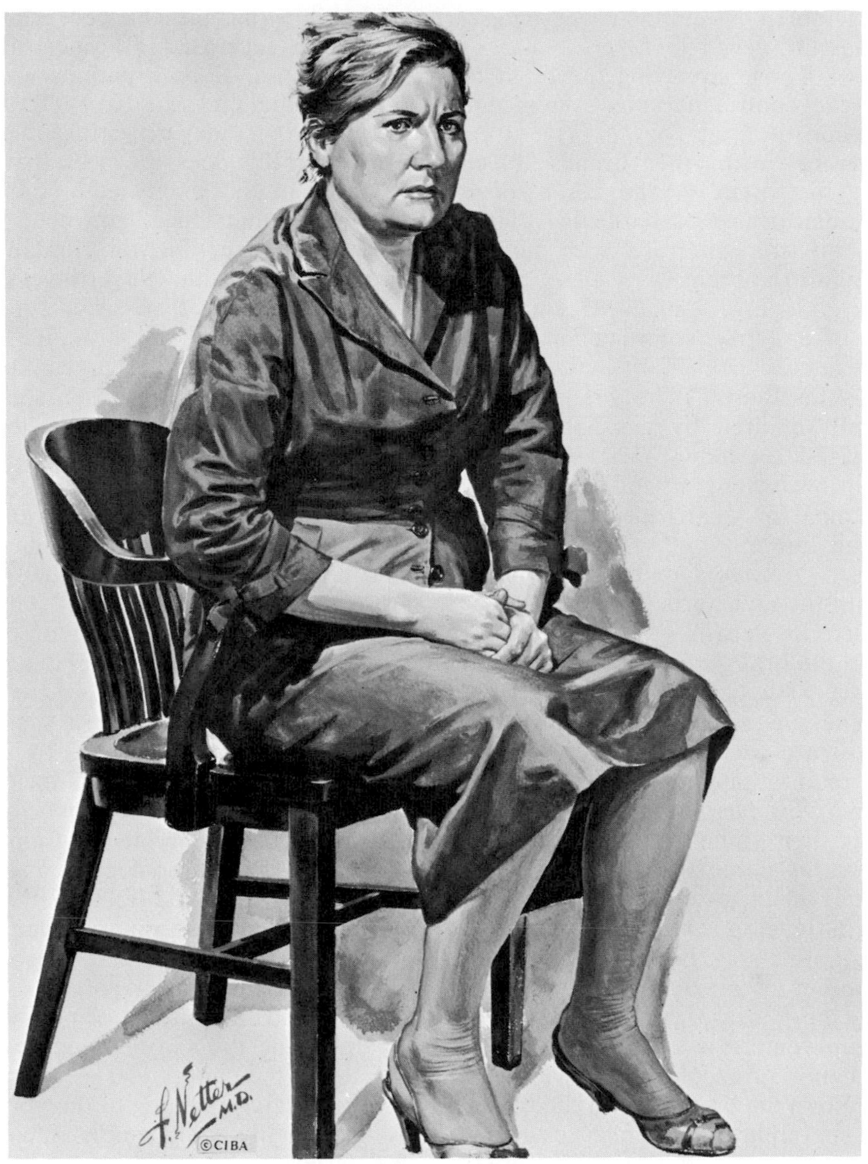

Agitated depression.

brain itself, such as abscesses, encephalitis, tubercular or syphilitic lesions. Today, many infections of the brain can be controlled by sulfa drugs or antibiotics before they can injure it. *Paresis,* an advanced stage of syphilis, causes a form of paranoia which was very prevalent in the past. Today, syphilis can be prevented and cured. In one hospital alone (Central State Hospital of Indiana), the number of men admitted suffering from paresis caused by syphilis decreased from over 30 per cent to less than 3 per cent of admissions. The widespread use of penicillin is credited for this reduction.

Nutritional Deficiencies. Pellagra, a vitamin deficiency, quite common in southern states not too many years ago, can eventually affect the brain. Fortunately, this disease responds very quickly to the administration of one of the B vitamins, nicotinic acid.

Poisons. Certain chemicals, such as lead, can cause brain deterioration. The poisonous toxins formed by some bacteria can bring about delirium, which very much resembles a temporary psychosis, in patients with very high fevers.

Tumors. Those involving the brain or affecting the central nervous system can cause psychoses.

Interference with the Brain's Blood Supply. This often is the result of a cerebral hemorrhage or hardening of the arteries and can interfere with normal functioning of the brain.

Epilepsy. In a very small percentage of all cases of epilepsy, some mental deterioration results.

Wounds or Blows. The brain can be permanently injured by gunshot wounds and damaged by blows. The shambling, incoherent, wornout prize fighter is a good example of what repeated battering to the head can do.

Senility. Psychoses are frequently associated with the aging process. This may be due to arteriosclerosis affecting the vital arteries in the brain.

Heredity. The effect of heredity in mental illness is rather difficult to assess, but there are definite indications that heredity factors may play a role. Franz Kallmann, who has studied 7000 twins, as well as their siblings and half brothers and sisters, has come up with the following statistics: the chance that the average person will develop schizophrenia is about 1 per cent (one in a hundred). However, a half brother of a schizophrenic person, inheriting the genes of only one parent of the schizophrenic, has a 7 per cent chance of also being schizophrenic (seven in a hundred); for a full brother, with genes from the same set of parents, the chances double to 14 per cent (14 out of a hundred). The identical twin of a schizophrenic, who shares the same hereditary factors, has an 86 per cent chance (86 out of a hundred) of developing this disease.[1]

Another indication of hereditary factors involved in mental illness is that the incidence of certain types of mental illnesses is greater in the children if the parents have had mental illness. It is also greater in children whose parents are closely related, for example, first cousins.

If one parent is schizophrenic, the probability that the children will have the disease is increased 19 times, according to Kallmann. If both parents are schizophrenic, the children have 80 times the normal expectancy of getting the disease. However, this does *not* mean that because someone in your family suffered from some type of mental illness you need to spend the rest of your life worrying about your own mental health. Nevertheless, anyone who knows that there is a considerable history of mental illness among his forebears should take the precaution of an honest discussion of these facts with a psychiatrist. The reassurance he obtains, or preventive suggestions, if needed, more than repay the time and expense involved.

Many students of this problem are becoming more and more interested in the concept that mental illness results from a "biochemical defect." This means that some chemical system of the body, responsible for normal behavior, is not functioning properly, and bizarre behavior results. Such an "error in metabolism" might actually be inherited by a certain percentage of children from their parents.

One piece of evidence in favor of this theory has been suggested by Ralph Linton, Professor of Anthropology at Yale. Linton has emphasized the fact that neuroses, psychoses and hysteria are common to all people and all cultures, despite wide differences in cultural patterns, kinds of taboos, and the amount of permissiveness or discipline used in bringing up children. Whatever the pattern and the psychological and cultural upbringing of the young, there is a roughly comparable incidence of mental illness.

Recently, research scientists in this field have studied several chemical compounds, not too unlike compounds synthesized by the body, which produce symptoms closely resembling those found in certain types of mental illness. This, too, has increased the interest in a possible biochemical basis for mental illness.

Therapy

A number of methods are used for treatment of the psychoses. Many of these illnesses are not hopeless although their

[1]Kallmann, F. J.: *Heredity in Health and Mental Disorder,* W. W. Norton & Co., New York, 1953.

FROM TORMENT TO TREATMENT

Highlights in the History of Mental Illness

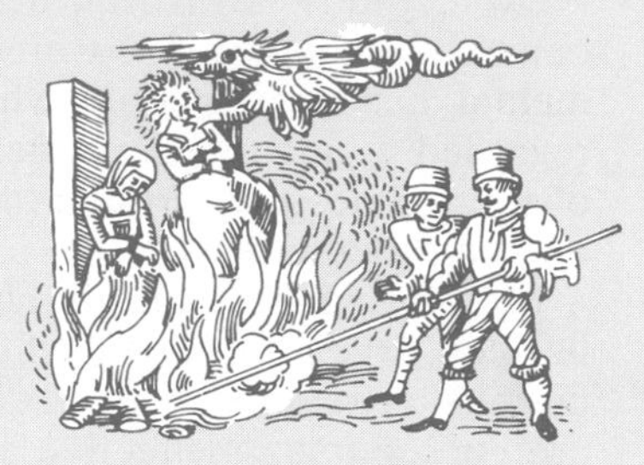

BEFORE THE 19TH CENTURY the insane were locked in dungeons without light. Some, if they were peaceful, roamed from village to village as beggars. During the 16th and 17th centuries they were often burned at the stake as witches.

BEDLAM the popular name for London's first asylum, became a hospital for the insane in 1547. Within a few years it was more like a prison than a hospital. Patients were beaten, caged, and chained. On Sundays families came to watch them as if they were animals in a zoo.

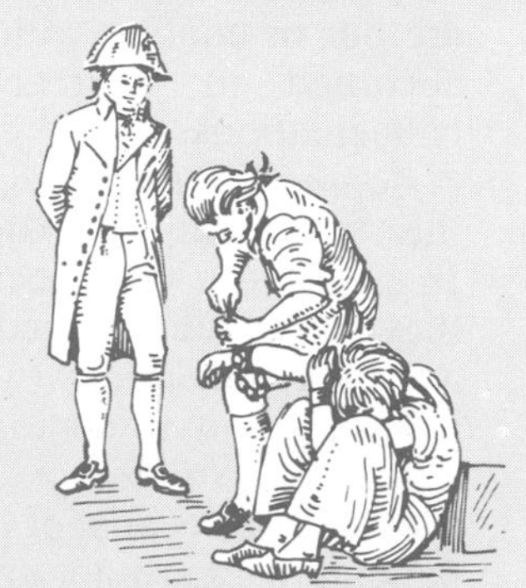

PHILIPPE PINEL a French physician called the Father of Psychiatry, in the 1790's unchained the inmates of the Salpêtrière and Bicêtre hospitals in Paris. He was the first psychiatrist to keep systematic case records based on exact observations of his patients. Pinel felt that treatment must include large measures of sympathy and understanding rather than punishment and cruelty.

DISEASES OF THE BRAIN were better understood as neurology became an important science in the 19th century. Many doctors believed that all mental illness resulted from lesions in the brain and attributed little to psychological disorders. Jean Martin Charcot, in Paris, studied the emotional causes of disease and experimented with hypnotism to treat hysteria.

SIGMUND FREUD the famous Austrian psychiatrist, began treating his patients through psychoanalysis around 1895. This method employs free association of ideas and the interpretation of dreams to uncover troublesome memories and desires locked in the unconscious mind. Freud's concepts of the basic elements of conduct, religion, art, love, and family relations have had an immense influence not only on psychiatry and psychology, but also on literature, art, and social thinking.

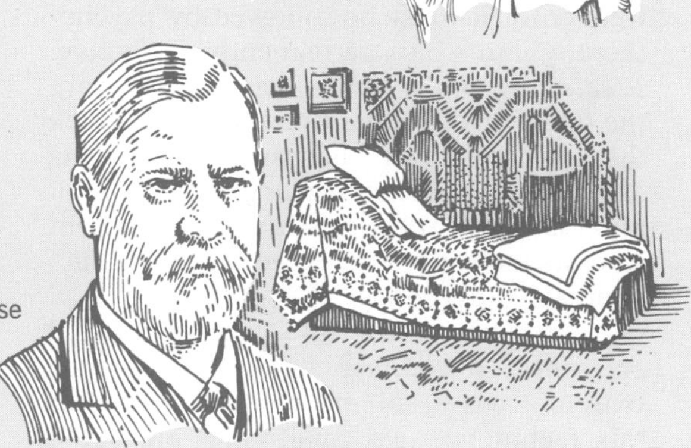

TREATMENT OF MENTAL ILLNESS TODAY has advanced with medicine and psychology. The superstitions surrounding diseases of the mind are gradually being overcome through an understanding of the causes of these diseases. In the United States the state and Federal governments are building spacious, modern hospitals where, with research, medicines, surgery, and psychotherapy, the mentally ill enjoy a greater chance of recovery than ever before.

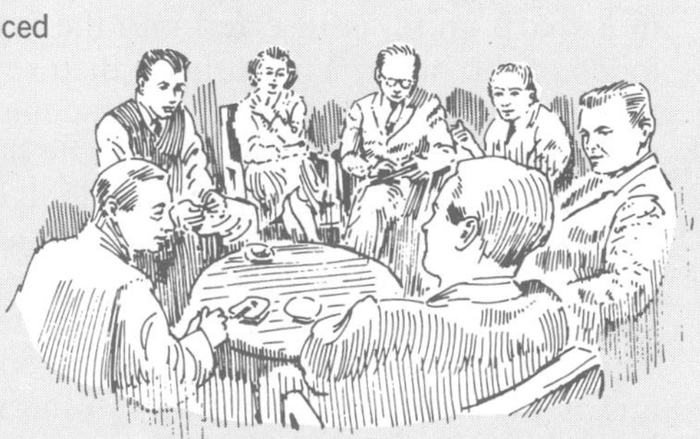

severity may make them appear to be. New methods have been devised and are constantly being discovered to restore mental health to people who used to be regarded as incurably insane. The severity of these illnesses warrants the use of more drastic procedures.

Methods based on *psychotherapy* are used on psychotic patients if their condition permits. Attempts at verbal communication are, of course, ineffective when patients are out of contact with reality, completely absorbed in their own fantasies and hallucinations.

Adjunctive therapies are very useful in the treatment of psychotic individuals. In addition to occupational therapy, they have been helped by *music therapy* and by *hydrotherapy* (wet packs, or immersion in warm water for several hours at a time). *Psychodrama,* like play therapy, provides a means of communication for patients who are not up to the more articulate forms of expression, as well as a way to "get things out of their systems."

Shock therapy is often employed when a psychotic patient remains out of contact with the real world. This method has proven very effective, sometimes bringing about spectacular improvements, although frequently it must be followed by psychotherapy to be permanently effective. *Electrical shock* and *insulin coma* are the ones most frequently employed. Shock therapy has been successful in patients suffering from depressions and schizophrenia. Cure rates as high as 80 per cent have been reported, especially in manic-depressive psychoses.

A special form of surgery, called *prefrontal lobotomy,* has been used in extreme cases of psychotic illness. In this technique, two small holes are bored in the forehead. A slender rod, which ends in a sharp knife, is inserted into the frontal lobes of the brain. The surgeon then severs the connecting nerve fibers and disconnects the frontal lobes from the rest of the brain. Patients who undergo prefrontal lobotomy usually undergo a marked change in personality, characterized by lack of apprehension and indifference to fears. This is a drastic and irreversible procedure, and is probably justified only in otherwise hopeless cases, where there is no response to other forms of therapy, and the patient is in extreme misery.

Deep encephalography is a new therapeutic technique, in which tiny electrodes are implanted in specific regions of the forebrain. These areas are then stimulated electrically, in an effort to alter abnormal circuits in the brain's switchboard.

Drug therapy has opened up an entire new era in psychiatry during the past ten years. (It has also led to the development of a new medical specialty—psychopharmacology.) Physicians in increasing numbers are using tranquilizing agents, for example, not as cures for psychoses, but to make belligerent, overactive patients much more manageable and responsive to other forms of therapy. Depressed patients, on the other hand, may become even more depressed under the influence of tranquilizers. They do, however, react well to another set of medicines—the central nervous system stimulants, or mood-elevating drugs.

This new and effective form of therapy not only has benefited the patients, but it has drastically changed the kind of care given patients in mental hospitals and has steadily reduced the number of such patients.

In 1963, the U. S. Public Health Service reported that the number of patients in state and county mental hospitals decreased for the eighth consecutive year. During those eight years, the total number of patients in public mental hospitals decreased by 54,000, from 560,000 in 1955. This reduction alone saved the taxpayers about $700 million, which is more than the total accumulated appropriations of the National Institute of Mental Health since it was founded in 1948.[2]

The savings were even greater than that, though. In 1955, those 560,000 patients were crowded badly. To replace obsolete beds and add new facilities would have cost about $1.3 billion, at the 1955 hospital occupancy rate. So the total saving in the years from 1955 to 1963 was actually about $2 billion, and the revolution in mental hospital care and occupancy shows

[2]Senate Committee Report No. 383, August 1, 1963, on Department of Health, Education and Welfare Appropriations for 1964.

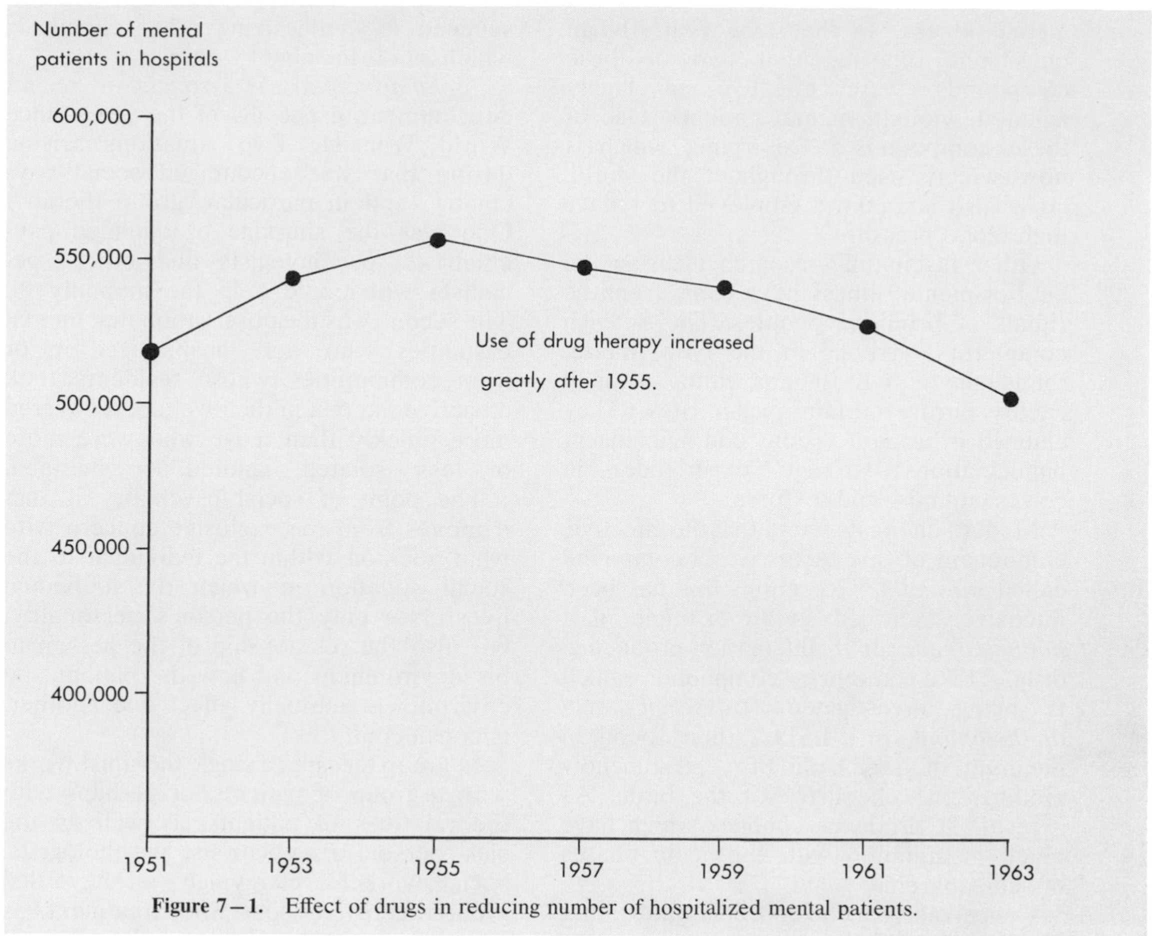

Figure 7–1. Effect of drugs in reducing number of hospitalized mental patients.

no sign of abating. The prospect is that the reduction in the number of patients in mental institutions maintained at public expense (and that is about 98 per cent of all such patients) will be reduced by 50 per cent or more within the next 20 years. Finally, this downward trend in mental hospital population has been accelerating—the total drop of 22,500 patients in 1963 was about double the rate of decrease of the preceding years.[3]

For the individual patient, the possibility of drug therapy can mean the difference between an almost impossible financial outlay and a modest expense. Frank Ayd, a well known Baltimore psychiatrist, has reported that one twin sister who suffered a psychotic episode was hospitalized for six months and received shock therapy, followed by additional treatment for another year. The cost to her was about $3000. Some time later, her sister had a comparable breakdown. She spent a week in a nursing home where she received a tranquilizing drug, chlorpromazine. For 11 weeks, she received the same medication in her own home, and her illness was brought under control at a cost of only $325.

It is interesting that although the intensive study of drugs as an adjunct in the treatment of mental illness is a recent development, it was stimulated by reports of an ancient method. For centuries, *Rauwolfia serpentina,* the snake root plant, was used in India in the treatment of a wide variety of diseases, including mental illness. In 1931, two Indian chemists isolated five crystalline compounds from *Rauwolfia serpentina* and confirmed reports of their effectiveness in

[3]Provisional patient movement and administrative data, Public Mental Hospitals, United States, 1963, Mental Health Statistics, Current Reports, January 1964. National Institute of Mental Health, Bethesda, Md.

mental illness. In the same year, Indian physicians reported that two of these compounds were effective in highly agitated, violent, mental patients. One of these compounds is reserpine, which is now widely used throughout the world. (It is also sometimes employed to reduce high blood pressure.)

Other fascinating research ideas in the field of mental illness have come from the rituals of primitive peoples. The Spanish conquerors, arriving in the New World, found the native Indians eating a small cactus during certain pagan rites. They claimed it brought visions and magnificent hallucinations, strange experiences in colors, sounds, and textures.

Modern chemists found that the effective component of this cactus was a compound called *mescaline*. Recently, this has been intensively studied as an example of a *hallucinogen,* or hallucination-producing, drug. Like another compound which is being investigated, D-*lysergic acid diethylamine,* or "LSD," (first found in the ergot, or green mold, of rye) it somehow modifies the chemistry of the brain. As a result, it produces changes which have much in common with the acute phases of schizophrenia.

Conceivably, schizophrenia and other severe mental illnesses may be due to a derangement in the chemistry of the body, producing a similar compound with tremendous power in deranging the mind. (LSD, for example, is effective in an adult human in amounts as low as 1/10,000 of a gram, or approximately 1/300,000 of an ounce!)

Even our expression, "going berserk," seems to be related to the use of hallucinogens in the past. The word comes from Berserk, who was an ancient Norse hero. In the ninth and tenth century A.D., when the Scandinavian sagas were being written, a group of brawlers emerged, who called themselves "berserkers" after their mythical hero. They were a fierce lot, raiding, looting, robbing and killing—going berserk, in fact—under the influence of hallucinogen-containing mushrooms!

If schizophrenia can be produced chemically, research chemists may also succeed in synthesizing other chemicals which can bring about a cure.

Social psychiatry is a significant recent development, especially of the years since World War II. Two situations arising during that war encouraged social psychiatry, and in particular, group therapy. One was the shortage of qualified psychiatrists, psychologists and other specialists who could help the mentally ill. The second was the observation that mental casualties who were hospitalized in or near communities whose residents took an active interest in their welfare recovered more quickly than those who were more or less isolated, ignored, or shunned.

The point of social psychiatry is that it moves from the exclusive concern with what goes on within the individual to the social situation in which the individual lives. Not only the person's personality, but also the relationship of the person to his environment and how the patient and environment mutually affect one another, is considered.

In group therapy, a single therapist works with a group of patients, or perhaps with the relatives of patients, as well as the sick person. Psychiatrists, psychologists, social workers, clergymen—all have led group therapy sessions. Such treatment has been given in hospitals, clinics, private offices, and even prisons.

Of course, not every patient finds group therapy more helpful than individual treatment. But men and women who have lacked good social relationships find this type of therapy useful because it gives them a chance to test social reactions when they express their feelings and attitudes toward themselves, the therapist, and other members of the group. The individual in a group situation has an opportunity to see immediately how he affects other people and how they regard him. The open give and take of group therapy means that, in a way, every member of the group is in effect a therapist for every other member.

Another type of group therapy is *family therapy*. In this situation, a psychiatrist, perhaps with the assistance of a psychiatric social worker, meets regularly with not only the sick person but with his family. The theoretical basis of this approach is that certain forms of mental illness stem not exclusively from the patient's personality but from a family situation in which a cycle of unhealthful events and relationships has developed. The family environment worsens proportionately with the illness of the patient. Finally, a therapist must intervene to break the cycle, get the family to take a fresh look at one another and the overall family picture, and eventually gain some insights that may help to change an unhealthy situation.

Changes in therapy have led to changes in the hospital setting. Just as drug therapy has brought about a decline in the total mental hospital population, so group therapy and social psychiatry have led to the development of smaller, more flexible, less rigid hospitals. Between the extremes of full-time care in a large hospital and little or no care at home, the mentally ill person in some communities may now be helped in a "halfway house." Just as the name implies, this is a center where the patient may be helped as he travels the road from extreme illness to recovery. He may sleep there and go to a job during the day, or perhaps simply return to this center at regular intervals for the attention and help he needs for continued progress. In such hospitals, there are no barred doors or windows. Rules are much less strict than in the large public mental hospitals, and the atmosphere is friendly and permissive. The nurses do not wear uniforms. The personalities of the attending physicians differ from those of staff members of a general hospital, where much emphasis is placed on the doctor's precise, firm, and directive manner.

Another type of halfway house is not a hospital at all, but a homelike center where former patients can be helped on the road back to full recovery. One of the oldest such centers in the United States is the Rebecca Gratz Club in Philadelphia, where young women discharged from public and private psychiatric hospitals and other women who are having problems of social and emotional adjustment may live temporarily. This interracial and inter-

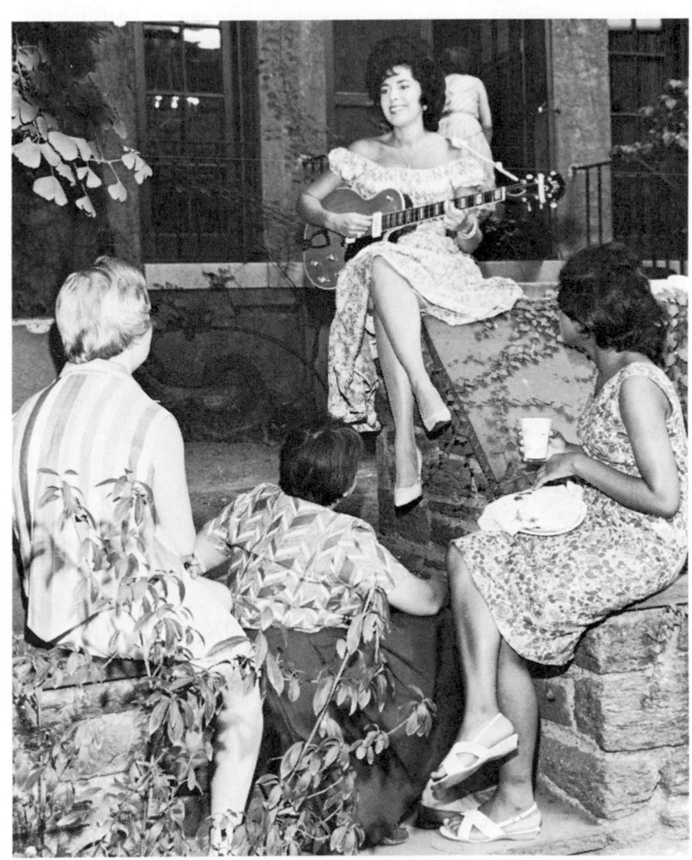

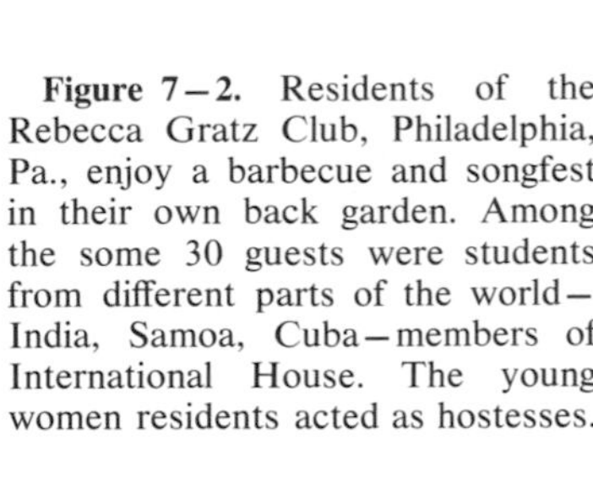

Figure 7–2. Residents of the Rebecca Gratz Club, Philadelphia, Pa., enjoy a barbecue and songfest in their own back garden. Among the some 30 guests were students from different parts of the world–India, Samoa, Cuba–members of International House. The young women residents acted as hostesses.

denominational center provides each girl or woman with a private bedroom plus community living and dining rooms. The staff includes social service workers, housemothers, and medical and psychiatric consultants. The Rebecca Gratz Club stresses the importance of living and working in a group, the group in this case being a special example of the outside world, for which each young woman is preparing to live in a healthy and responsible way.

Whatever form nonindividual therapy takes, the goal is to treat the patient in a social setting. Of course, what goes on in the patient's mind is important, but there is equal concern with the world he lives in and the environment that shapes the man and is in turn shaped by him.

With a variety of methods now showing promising results in therapy, the future in mental illness is far brighter than it has ever been before. According to Karl Menninger:

> Of all the diseases that confront mankind, mental illness is the most hopeful of recovery. Given proper treatment in time, up to 70 per cent of all the patients could be discharged as improved or recovered within a year.

MENTAL DEFECTIVES

Most mental illnesses do not stem from lack of intelligence. However, there are conditions in which the intellect is involved. The term *mental defective* is used to describe individuals whose intelligence is below normal. Lowest in the scale are the *idiots,* who cannot progress beyond the intelligence level of a 3-year-old child. Next come the *imbeciles* with a mentality of, roughly, three to seven years. Finally, there are the *feeble-minded* (also called *retarded* or *morons*) who go all the way up the scale from the mental age of seven to the "low normals."

Idiocy and imbecility are manifested very early in a child's development. However, feeble-mindedness may not become apparent immediately. In fact, it is not always easy to recognize the milder types of feeble-mindedness. Usually we rely upon one of the various *intelligence tests,* but, unfortunately, these don't always tell the whole story, because emotional factors cannot always be easily separated from intellectual ones. There have been many instances in which a child's very low intelligence quotient has "changed." A low level is sometimes due to apathy or to emotional disturbances; it can improve markedly when these conditions are corrected.

Some types of mental deficiency are due to a constitutional defect, and are present when the child is born. Fortunately, such abnormalities are rare, and, when they do occur, may also limit the deformed infant's length of life.

A hereditary defect may be responsible, or some abnormal condition during pregnancy, such as: (1) *excessive exposure of the mother to radiation,* (2) *syphilis,* (3) *German measles* in the first three months of pregnancy, (4) *poor nutrition* during pregnancy.

Mental deficiency can also result from birth injury, *i.e.,* damage to the baby's brain at birth. A small proportion of persons with cerebral palsy, resulting from such brain injury, may be mentally deficient.

Certain defects causing mental deficiency, for example, cretinism due to iodine lack, can be corrected to some degree before any permanent damage is done if the infant is treated early enough. However, even with optimum treatment, the I.Q. of cretins rarely exceeds 70, although their physical development may show remarkable improvement.

Neither mental deficiency nor any other defect in a baby is caused by the mother's smoking cigarettes, taking a drink, eating lobster, having sexual intercourse or being frightened during pregnancy.

A surprisingly high percentage of mental defectives can be trained to be useful people. Of the approximately 11,400 babies born every day, 340 will be handicapped mentally. This figure is based on the fact that there are about 30 retarded individuals among every 1000 persons. With the right training and guidance, 25 of these 30 can become self-supporting adults. Four can be trained to care for their own personal needs, but do little more. Only one of these 30 will be totally dependent throughout life.

Questions

1. Many alcoholics and drug addicts seem perfectly normal in many respects. Why do psychiatrists feel that these addictions must stem from serious emotional disturbance?
2. What are some of the differences between *psychopaths* and *psychotics*?
3. Do you think drug therapy will make other forms of treatment less important?
4. Differentiate *psychoses* from *neuroses* and give examples.
5. Name at least four causes for psychoses and methods for treating them.
6. What is the role of heredity in mental illness?
7. Is there any evidence that chemical defects in body metabolism might cause mental illness?
8. How do you classify mental defectives?
9. Do you think there is justification for so drastic a procedure as prefrontal lobotomy in the treatment of the mentally ill?
10. What are the most effective therapeutic methods in mental illness?
11. How are new techniques, such as group therapy, likely to affect hospital treatment of the mentally ill?
12. What advantages can you cite for the smaller, more flexible mental health centers over the traditional, large hospital?
13. Does the lower patient population in mental hospitals mean the problem of mental health is lessening? Why, or why not?
14. Explain the difference between functional and organic disorders. Give examples.
15. Can an intelligent person also be mentally ill?

Topics for Discussion

Origin of terms sadism and masochism.
Psychodrama.
Current attitudes (social, medical, and religious toward mental illness).
Causes of homosexuality.
Relationship between family environment and mental illness.
Possible dangers of drug therapy.
Advantages of public information about mental illness.
Desirability of greater government contributions toward mental health programs.

Reading Suggestions

Heredity in Health and Mental Disorder, F. J. Kallmann. W. W. Norton Co., New York, 1953. Includes a consideration of inheritance of mental illness.

Live at Peace with Your Nerves, Walter C. Alvarez. Prentice Hall, Englewood Cliffs, N.J., 1958. Describes in simple layman's language how our aches and pains can block happiness and even turn into serious ailments.

Exploring the Cerebral Jungle, John Pfeiffer. New York Times Magazine, May 13, 1956, p. 26. A lucid discussion of recent advances in the chemical approach to the treatment of mental illness.

My Life in Bellevue, S. R. Cutolo. Saturday Evening Post, May 5, 1956, p. 44. Fascinating description by a physician of patients and problems encountered in the psychiatric ward of Bellevue Hospital.

My Husband Came Home (as told to John Toland). Cosmopolitan, March 1956, p. 38. A sensitive discussion by a young wife of her husband's experiences in a mental hospital and of his subsequent recovery at home.

A Mind That Found Itself, Clifford W. Beers. Doubleday & Co., Inc., New York, reprinted 1962. First published in 1908, this was the first significant book on mental illness for the layman. A classic first-person account of illness and recovery.

The Talking Cure, Morton M. Hunt and Rena Corman with Louis R. Ormont. Harper & Row, 1964. An informal introduction to the theory and practice of psychoanalysis today, written in the unusual style of a series of conversations with a psychoanalyst.

An Outline of Psychoanalysis, Sigmund Freud. W. W. Norton & Co., Inc., 1949. Freud says in his foreword: "It is the aim of this brief work to bring together the doctrines of psychoanalysis and to state them, as it were, dogmatically—and in the most concise form and in the most positive terms."

Mental Drugs: Chemistry's Challenge to Psychotherapy, O. A. Battista. Chilton Co., Philadelphia, 1960. A guide to some of the preparations used in treating mental illnesses.

Group Psychoanalysis, Norman Locke. New York University Press, New York, 1961.

Mental Retardation; A Family Study, E. W. Reed and C. S. Reed. W. B. Saunders Co., Philadelphia, 1965.

Family Group Therapy, John E. Bell. Public Health Monograph 64 (PHS Publication 826), 1961.

College Students in a Mental Hospital, C. C. Umbarger et al., Grune & Stratton, New York, 1962.

Family Therapy, George Thorman. Public Affairs Pamphlet No. 356, Public Affairs Committee, Inc., 1964.

Psychiatric Team Comes to Home, P. Rolfe. In *Mental Health and Social Welfare,* Columbia University Press, New York, 1961.

Mental Health Is a Family Affair, Dallas Pratt and Jack Neher. Public Affairs Pamphlet 155, Public Affairs Committee, Inc., 1957.

Studying Personality Cross-Culturally, B. Kaplan, ed. Row, Peterson & Co., New York, 1961.

Family and Class Dynamics in Mental Illness, J. K. Myers and B. H. Roberts. Wiley, New York, 1959.

The Prevention of Hospitalization, Milton Greenblatt, *et al.,* Grune & Stratton, New York, 1963.

The Disorganized Personality, George W. Kisker. McGraw-Hill, New York, 1964. An introductory textbook that includes detailed discussions of many of the recent changes in the field of mental health and mental illness.

After Hospitalization: The Mental Patient and His Family, O. G. Simmons. Hogg Foundation for Mental Health, Austin, Texas, 1960.

Psychosocial Problems of College Men, Bryant M.

Wedge. Yale University Press, New Haven, Conn., 1958. A consideration of many aspects of college life and of students' problems and reactions.

The Layman's Guide to Psychiatry, James A. Brussel. Barnes & Noble, Inc., 1961. A presentation of the highlights of modern psychiatric knowledge.

Psychiatry in American Life, Charles Rolo, ed. Little, Brown, & Co., Boston, 1963. A symposium on the effects and influences of psychiatry on medicine, writing, religion, art, morals, and child care.

Assassination: Psychopathology and Social Pathology, Lawrence Zelic Freedman. *Postgraduate Medicine,* June 1965. An especially lucid portrayal of some of the personality traits and psychopathological characteristics of men who assassinated, or attempted to assassinate, Presidents of the United States.

SECTION FOUR

MARRIAGE

8

HEALTHY ATTITUDES TOWARD SEX

> One touch of Nature makes the whole world kin.
>
> SHAKESPEARE

Of all our human impulses and activities, sex has become surrounded with the most numerous and most complex interpretations, attitudes, rules, and prohibitions. Society in the United States at present appears to be extremely liberal about sex, as compared with earlier periods of history, in participation as well as in discussion. However, even in this time of sex education in public schools and apparent disappearance of any restrictions in books, there is still much ignorance and misinformation about reproduction and sexual activity. Even more serious, beneath our apparent freedom about sexual matters, there is still much hypocrisy, fear, conflict, and guilt. A healthy attitude toward sex does not mean that all rules are out. It means that you learn to understand the significance of sex in everyday life—to see it in perspective. Overemphasis on sex is no healthier than trying to hide it in some dark corner of your mind.

Physically mature young men and women face a painful dilemma. The delights of sex are paraded before them endlessly by every advertising and promotional means of a commercial society, but other forces of that same society act to restrain these youngsters from participation in sex before marriage—and contemporary educational, business, and professional requirements are such that marriage may be years distant from physical readiness.

The current wave of indulgence in sex is discussed in these terms by Dr. Frederick Weiss, member of the Medical Board of the Karen Horney Clinic:

> Overemphasis on sex occurs at times during which anxiety and tension permeate public life, the prospect for full and constructive living appears poor, and the real meaning of life seems to be lost. Where life as a whole seems futile, sex may become an overevaluated substitute, a narcotic agent against anxiety and hopelessness, a stimulant to overcome a feeling of inner emptiness, paralysis and inertia.

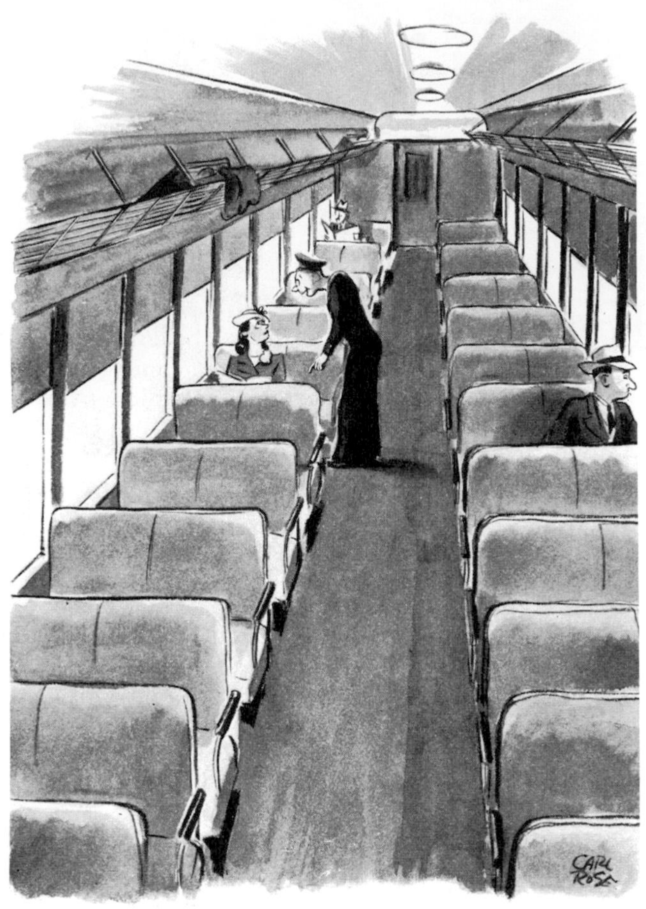

"Is this seat taken?"

(Drawing by Carl Rose, Copr.© 1943, The New Yorker Magazine, Inc.)

The passage from childhood to adulthood has never been easy, but the present great American uncertainty about sex and the resulting painful dilemma for college men and women have made early adulthood particularly difficult. Today's parents tend to encourage independence, to let children grow up, and to abdicate their authority without apparent difficulty. However, the parents' alter egos—the older generation of advisors, administrators, teachers, ministers, and authors—openly or subtly discourage full sexual experience before marriage. Under the circumstances, the questioning and the rebelliousness of the young college generation are not only understandable but inevitable.

These attitudes are illuminated in a poll taken by a psychology professor at a midwestern university. When he asked the men students what sort of relationship they wished to establish with the girls they dated, he learned that within three dates, 79 per cent expected a girl to neck. Further, 52 per cent expected more serious sex play, and 36 per cent of these hoped to progress to intercourse. Continuing, reliable surveys of college students indicate a consistent increase in the number of persons having complete sexual experience before marriage. A 1929 study reported that at the time of marriage, 35 per cent of college women were not virgins; for men, the figure was 50 per cent. By 1938, the figures were 37 per cent for women and 61 per cent for men. Fifteen years later, the figure for women had risen to 50 percent and for men, to 62 per cent. The trend continued into the 1960's, when some school physicians reported that about 60 per cent of the female *high school* student body are no longer virgins.

MATURITY AND THE SEXUAL DRIVE

By 11 or 12 years, most girls have begun to mature. The breasts enlarge, pubic hair develops, and menstruation starts. Boys develop manly characteristics later, generally by the time they are 15 or 16 years old. Their genitals enlarge, pubic hair sprouts, and shaving is in order. Strictly speaking, sexual maturity means that the male is producing sperm and the female, ova. Theoretically, these young people are able to become parents, but obviously, adolescents are far from ready to assume the responsibilities that would accompany the result of this physical maturity.

In the lower biological forms, reproduction occurs without sexuality and without sexual desire. Bacteria and certain other simple forms reproduce by fission or budding. In a sense, they are immortal. But our high degree of development and organ differentation necessitates eventual aging and death. In humans, sexual drive has developed separately from the reproductive function, although many people still do not understand the clear difference. Further, the association of the pleasures of sexual activity with sin and guilt—an association that has evolved over hundreds of years within the framework of Christianity, which frowned upon earthly pleasures that distracted man's attention from heaven and the afterlife—has resulted in a most unfortunate set of conflicting feelings about sex.

Each of us is equipped with a complex

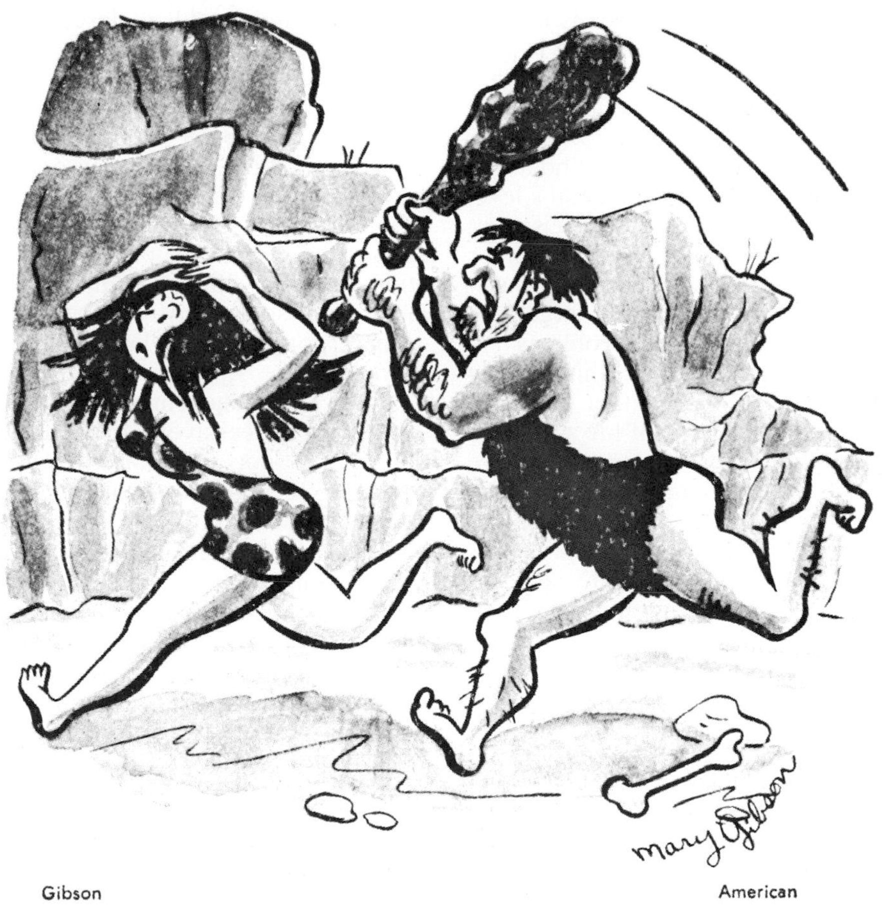

Gibson American

"What's the matter with you—don't you like men?"

mechanism for reproduction (see Chapters 10 and 11). Each of us is also equipped with a very real sexual drive—an intense drive toward pleasure that manifests itself long before we have any awareness or understanding of the function of reproduction. The physical reasons for deriving pleasure from the sexual act are obvious: genital tissue in both the male and the female is richly endowed with a network of nerve receptors, which are extremely sensitive to contact and thus produce very pleasurable sensations.

However, the psychological and social reasons may be even more important in intensifying the sexual drive, perhaps out of proportion to genuine physiological need and response. No other physiological act or drive has such a battery of emotional and moral connotations attached to it. Eating, drinking, elimination, laughing, talking—all are significant, all have some emotional overtones, but all are accepted as part of life, in a way that sex is not. So many prohibitions, regulations, and hypocrisies surround sex from childhood on that it very likely takes on more importance than it deserves.

If the questions children ask about sex were answered frankly, at the child's level of understanding, without embarrassment, and also if sex were treated as another natural function of our bodies, the questions of guilt and shame would largely be wiped out. Of course, the problems associated with sex are not this simply solved, but a society that neither over- nor underemphasizes this part of life would be able to deal with such problems in a more healthful and more rational way.

In the remainder of this chapter, we deal with some of the everyday problems involving the sex drive and with some of the consequences of ignorance and immaturity.

MASTURBATION

Almost every individual has been confronted with the desire to masturbate, and must work out his or her own solution to this question. It is a problem only in the sense that sexual desire is not purely physical. That is, the physical aspects are, normally, closely associated with the desire for intimacy with a member of the opposite sex. This intimacy cannot exist during masturbation, except in the form of fantasy.

These are some real problems of masturbation. Other attitudes have grown up through the years because of groundless superstitions. Although they are not correct, they have caused countless heartaches and even tragedies. The twin specters we have created are the devils—fear and guilt.

Fear is unnecessary because masturbation is not harmful. *It never causes organic or mental sickness, nor does it lead to impotence or sterility.* Guilt is unnecessary because a very large percentage of normal boys and girls have practiced some form of masturbation during their growing years and often into adult life. Fear and guilt cause emotional difficulties that can injure the whole future of a young man or woman.

In childhood and adolescence, masturbation frequently serves as a substitute for normal sexual outlets. This is especially true during adolescence when sexual maturity has been attained, and sexual desire is difficult to master or sublimate. According to the Kinsey report, 88 per cent of single males between 16 and 20 masturbate, and half of the single population continues doing so until the age of 50. Anything so widely engaged in by the general population can hardly be considered abnormal.

The chief danger in masturbation which continues excessively into adulthood is that it is not the normal adult sexual pattern. It may represent an attempt to escape from marriage, for example, because of excessive timidity or because of a more serious emotional maladjustment.

If an individual becomes addicted to masturbation, practicing it—let us say—daily, the problem is an emotional one which should be discussed with a doctor or counselor. Masturbation in this case is a sign, not a cause, of emotional difficulty.

DREAMS AND NOCTURNAL EMISSIONS

This is nature's way of relieving sexual tensions in the male. The fluid containing spermatazoa is stored in the epididymis—a collecting and conducting tube attached to the testes—and is discharged at night, usually accompanied by a sexual dream. The nocturnal emission (it is sometimes called a "wet dream") is a natural part of adolescence, and should certainly not be a cause for shame, pride or concern. Although more frequent during adolescence, they may persist throughout adult life.

Dreams are often wish fulfillments. The sex urge is very powerful, but its gratification and even its acknowledgement are hedged about with prohibitions. It can receive an outlet and relief in sex dreams and nocturnal emissions. Therefore they are apt to be more frequent in individuals who spend a good many daytime hours indulging in sexual fantasy.

Dreams of this type occur in women too, but less frequently. However, they seldom relieve sexual tensions as they do in men.

PREMARITAL SEXUAL RELATIONS

There is no universally complete answer to the difficult question of petting and sex relations for the adolescent. It depends to a great extent on the religious and cultural background of the family and the maturity and personality of the individual.

Contrary to popular opinion, Kinsey believes that petting is actually an attempt to *avoid* premarital intercourse. Many young women enjoy petting but are actually seeking affection rather than satisfaction of sexual desire. They have not yet attained the level of sexual maturity where they would find intercourse pleasurable or desirable. It is interesting that a recent study of sexually delinquent girls showed that most of their sexual adventures stemmed from loneliness, unhappiness and hunger for affection rather than love or intense sexual desire.

Most well adjusted girls can set bounds to petting. They learn to recognize their own melting point and that of their escort, and call a halt before the situation becomes too difficult or unmanageable.

Every woman has to make a decision about whether she will or will not pet, and if so, how far she will go. Withdrawing completely from any sexual contact or the preliminaries to sexual intimacy is certainly an unhealthy situation and an indication of strong puritanical restraint. If a woman has given and received affection freely all her life, she will want to enjoy some form of petting or love-making with a potential mate. In fact, it is almost an essential prelude to the selection of a husband.

Young people marry because marriage promises the special kind of love and happiness family life brings. There is no indication that a man who has had sexual relations before marriage makes a better or a worse husband. It depends entirely on the nature of his sex experiences. If these were only with prostitutes, they may have engendered resentment and contempt for all women because of his own feelings of guilt or distaste. He may spend the rest of his life putting so-called "good women" on a pedestal, and never achieve a happy sexual relationship in marriage.

Our society tolerates premarital sex adventures for the male, but still frowns upon such adventures in young women. Therefore, if she does participate in them, she is breaking certain taboos. There is some rather slight indication that women who have experienced sexual intercourse before marriage have slightly less successful marriages than their virgin sisters. But this is an extremely difficult problem to evaluate. It could be attributed to the fact that such a person breaks these taboos because she *is* a somewhat unconventional person to start with. For the same reasons, she may find difficulty in adjusting to the restrictions and demands of marriage. Or it may be that her husband resents the fact that she was not a virgin when he married her.

The question of premarital relations for young men and women should be examined in terms of the psychological and physical hazards involved. Psychologically, it is perhaps best for both the man and woman—and particularly for the woman—if her first sexual experience is with her future husband. As Brown and Kemptom point out:[1]

---

[1]Brown, F., and Kemptom, R. T.: *Sex Questions and Answers,* McGraw-Hill, New York, 1950.

[In thousands. Beginning 1959, includes Alaska, and 1960, Hawaii. Includes estimates for States in which legitimacy data were not reported. No estimates included for misstatements on birth records or failures to register births. Beginning 1959, based on 50-percent sample of live births in the reporting States]

AGE AND COLOR	1940	1945	1950	1955	1959	1960	1961	1962
Total	**89.5**	**117.4**	**141.6**	**183.3**	**220.6**	**224.3**	**240.2**	**245.1**
Rate [1]	7.1	10.1	14.1	19.3	22.1	21.6	22.6	21.5
By age of mother:								
Under 15 years	2.1	2.5	3.2	3.9	4.6	4.6	5.2	5.1
15 to 19 years	40.5	49.2	56.0	68.9	84.5	87.1	93.3	94.4
20 to 24 years	27.2	39.3	43.1	55.7	67.3	68.0	74.0	77.3
25 to 29 years	10.5	14.1	20.9	28.0	32.0	32.1	33.7	34.0
30 to 34 years	5.2	7.1	10.8	16.1	19.0	18.9	19.8	19.8
35 to 39 years	3.0	4.0	6.0	8.3	10.5	10.6	11.1	11.1
40 and over	1.0	1.2	1.7	2.4	2.8	3.0	3.2	3.2
By color of mother:								
White	40.3	56.4	53.5	64.2	79.6	82.5	91.1	[2] 93.5
Nonwhite	49.2	60.9	88.1	119.2	141.1	141.8	149.1	[2] 147.5

[1] Rate per 1,000 unmarried (never married, widowed, and divorced) women aged 15 to 44 years enumerated as of April 1 for 1940 and 1950 and estimated as of July 1 for all other years.
[2] Excludes data for New Jersey since this State did not require reporting of color.

Source: Dept. of Health, Education, and Welfare, Public Health Service; unpublished data.

Figure 8–1. Illegitimate births in the United States. Rate per 1000 unmarried (never married, widowed, divorced) women, aged 15 to 44 years. (From Statistical Abstract of the United States, U.S. Health, Education, and Welfare Trends, 1964.)

Loyalty to the husband and love for him is greatly dependent upon his skill as a lover. If he has initiated her into the realms of sexual pleasure and has done so with beauty and tenderness, she will remain deeply grateful to him. Much of a woman's self is surrendered in the love she offers a man in her first sex experience. Psychologically, it is best if this emotional outpouring and complete surrender of the ego serves as the foundation upon which marriage is built. When this experience is only one of many, there is the risk of emotional fatigue when marriage takes place, an absence of that freshness and vigor which would otherwise give impetus and momentum to the marriage. As in the fairy tale, it is the prince who first kisses the princess out of her long sleep who is always regarded as her deliverer.

Physically, the unmarried woman is at the mercy of the man with whom she goes to bed. Although the man can protect himself quite easily . . . the woman's resources are more limited. If the man prefers not to use a contraceptive, she risks disease or conception.

The concept of trial marriage to test sexual compatibility with one's future mate has received considerable attention. It may have certain beneficial aspects. But many young women who experience premarital relations suffer considerable guilt later. The male partner may also feel guilty because he, too, has been brought up in the same society—which countenances one standard of behavior for the male, and another for the female. He often projects his own guilt feelings upon his sexual partner, which can and has introduced serious difficulties into many marriages.

Another factor which must be considered is that the conditions under which premarital sexual relations are consummated are far from the best. Parked automobiles, cheap hotels, and second-rate tourist courts lend an atmosphere of sordidness to a potentially beautiful relationship. These arrangements are certainly not conducive to perpetuating feelings of love and romance. Often the strain is so great that it prevents the attainment of sexual harmony, and leaves both partners with a sense of unhappiness and distaste.

In a fine book, *The Happy Family,* the psychiatrist John Levy[2] writes:

Advising adolescents about their sex life is a highly personal and individualized problem. You cannot recommend the same behaviour for all of them indiscriminately. I rather hope that my own daughter will pet or neck, or whatever the proper term may be, preferably with boys she knows well and likes, and only with her contemporaries. Love-making of this type is a healthy preparation for marriage. I hope that she will not have intercourse or end up merely a technical virgin. Quite aside from any moral implications, such a step is risky. . . . If she does have a complete relationship, though, I most earnestly hope that she will know what she is about, that she will not go into an affair because she happens to be tight, or thinks it's "the thing," or wants to prove that she can carry it off. These are my hopes. They are based on my observation of the kind of behaviour least likely to cause trouble in our particular social group. But she may order her life quite differently and be none the worse for it. If she is neither afraid of sex or bamboozled by its glamour I shall be very content.

[2]Levy, J.; and Munroe, R.: *The Happy Family,* Knopf, New York, 1938.

ILLEGITIMACY AND VENEREAL DISEASE

Exactly as one would expect, the increase in sexual freedom has been accompanied by a rise in both the number of illegitimate births and in the incidence of venereal disease.

Between 1940 and 1960, the rate of illegitimate births in the United States more than tripled (Fig. 8–1). By 1963, it had risen again, although not so sharply as during the post-World War II years. Currently, the estimated annual total number of illegitimate births to girls less than 15 years old is 5000.

During the mid-1950's, not only in the United States but throughout the world, venereal disease rates fell sharply. Then, they began to rise again, and the increase in some countries, among them the United States, has been rapid (Table 8–1 and Fig. 8–2). In this country, 56 per cent of the

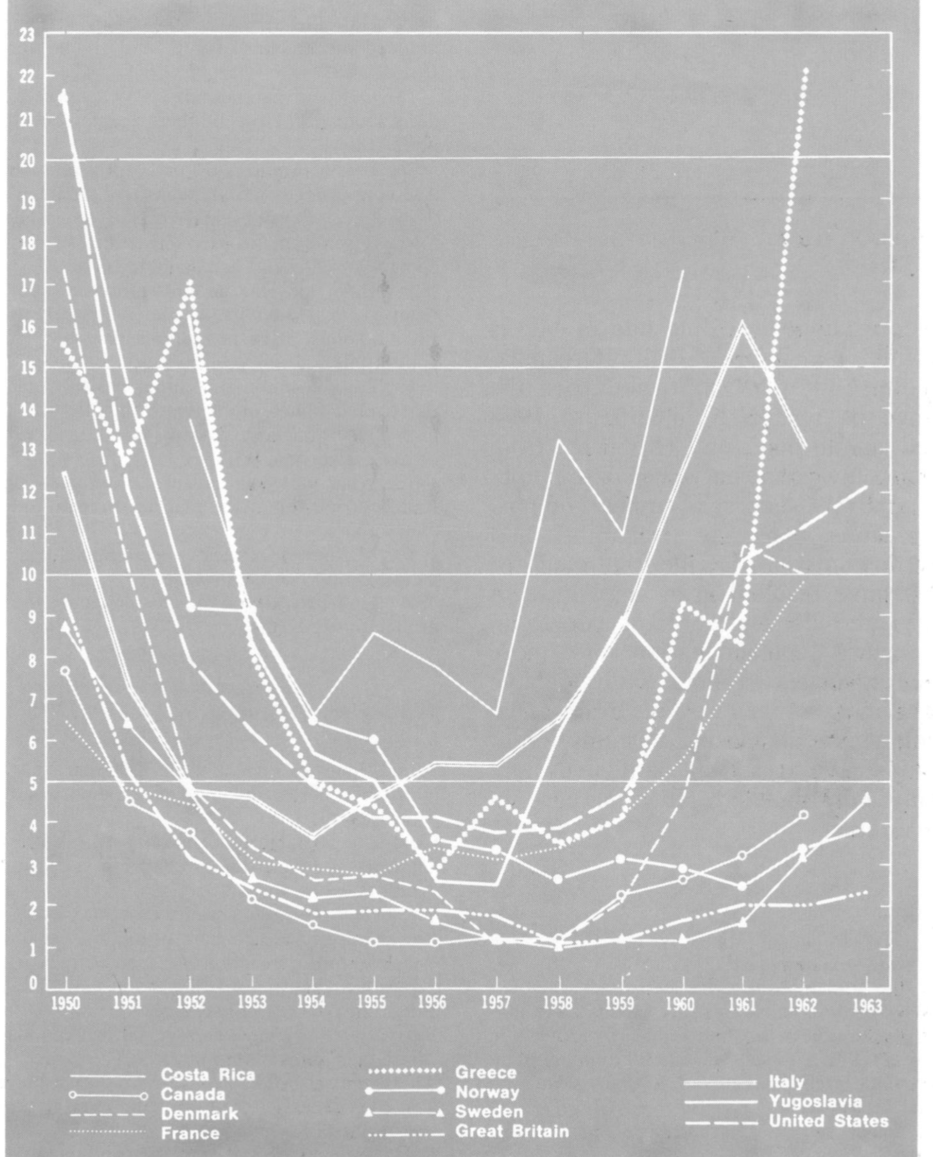

Figure 8–2. Ten years after the end of World War II, the incidence of syphilis had fallen to record lows throughout the world. During the next decade, however, this disease once again became a serious problem, as these curves show. (World Health Organization statistical compilation.)

new cases of venereal disease reported during the first half of 1965 were from persons less than 20 years old—1300 cases daily.

Table 8—1. Incidence rate of syphilis per 100,000 persons, 15—19 years old*

Year	*Percentage*
1956	10.1
1957	10.5
1958	10.2
1959	12.9
1960	19.9
1961	24.2
1962	24.8
1963	22.8

*From U.S. Health, Education and Welfare Trends, 1964.

Concern about the rising tide of VD is worldwide. The World Health Organization points out that in 76 countries the incidence of syphilis from 1955 to 1958 reached an all-time low. However, from that time onward the curve began to climb. WHO analysts suggest a number of possible reasons: the easy availability and relative low cost of penicillin treatment for syphilis have resulted in a false sense of security; the concentration of people in cities makes contact easier and more frequent; changes in moral outlook have removed many of the restraints from sexual intercourse; the increasing consumption of alcoholic beverages has paralleled, and probably contributed to, the increase in sexual contact.

Questions

1. Define sexual maturity.
2. Is the human sexual drive an instinct?
3. Why do you think so many taboos have surrounded discussion of sex and sexual exploration in our society? Can you see how such attitudes might cause extreme prudishness about, or unusual interest in, sexual activities?
4. At what age do girls and boys reach sexual maturity?
5. What is a nocturnal emission? Is it a natural event?
6. Would masturbation have so much guilt and fear associated with it if parents of very small children realized that discovery of the genitals and the pleasure associated with this was no less innocent than discovery of any other part of the body?
7. Do you plan as a parent to answer or ignore questions about sex asked by your children?
8. Do you agree with Kinsey that petting may actually be an attempt to avoid premarital intercourse?
9. What do you think are the major hazards in pre-marital sexual relations?
10. Do you think it is conceivable that there could be a stable society which tolerated such relations?
11. Differentiate between sexual drive and sexual mechanisms.
12. Has the freedom of sexual self-expression reduced the amount of guilt and shame about sex? If not, why?
13. Did your parents answer or ignore your questions about sex? How did their reaction help or hinder you?
14. If you refrain from premarital relations, why? Are your grounds moral, protective, or religious?
15. Legal abortion has frequently been advocated. Discuss some of the probable effects if abortion by competent persons were made legal.
16. How does the administration of your college react to sexual activity on the campus? Do you consider administrative regulations necessary, fair, and appropriate?
17. Do you think some other basis for marriage in the United States other than romantic love (such as marriages arranged by parents) would make for fewer or more divorces? Why?
18. What do you consider the most significant traits to look for in the man or woman you wish to marry?
19. Make some suggestions for combating the rising incidence of venereal disease.
20. How would you suggest reducing the number of illegitimate births?

Topics for Discussion

Appropriate sex education in the home.
A program of sex education in elementary and secondary schools.
Contrasts in public and private attitudes about sex.
The role of advertising in changing sex attitudes and practices.
The extent of sexual activity on your campus.
Sex as a legitimate concern of the college authorities.
Possible future reaction to sexual freedom, and a return to restraints.
Importance of sex in marriage.
Sexual relations between men and women of different religious faiths, different races.
The extent of prudery still existing in American life.
The coexistence of sexual freedom and hypocrisy.
Justifications for abortion.
Relate premarital sexual freedom and the divorce rate.
Colleges' responsibility to help control venereal disease among students.

Reading Suggestions

Sex Questions and Answers, Fred Brown and R. T. Kemptom. McGraw-Hill, New York, 1950. A forthright and lucid book with correct information presented in an easy-to-read style.

Sexual Behavior in the Human Male, A. C. Kinsey, W. B. Pomeroy and C. E. Martin. W. B. Saunders Co., Philadelphia, 1948. A scientifically detailed account of sexual behavior and probably the most frequently quoted book of its kind.

Sexual Behavior in the Human Female, A. C. Kinsey, W. B. Pomeroy, C. E. Martin, and P. H. Gebhard. W. B. Saunders Co., Philadelphia, 1953. A companion book to the studies of male sexual behavior, using the same statistical techniques.

The Sex Age, Howard Whitman. Bobbs-Merrill Co., New York, 1963 (paperback). A facile and witty discussion of the sex revolution in the United States. Discussions of numerous topics, including pornography, sex in advertising, free love, homosexuality, and the sex needs of college men and women.

Sex in America, Henry A. Grunwald, (ed.) Bantam Books, New York, 1964 (paperback). A good collection of articles by authorities in the field of sex education. Recommended reading for college students.

Human Reproduction and Sex Behavior, Charles Lloyd (ed.) Lea and Febiger, Philadelphia, 1964. For parents and educators as well as students. Includes discussions of contemporary attitudes toward sex.

Reproduction, Sex, and Preparation for Marriage, Lawrence Q. Crawley and others. Prentice-Hall, Englewood Cliffs, N.J., 1964. Comprehensive and factual; particularly appropriate for young people.

Release from Sexual Tensions, Toward an Understanding of Their Causes and Effects on Marriage, Mary S. Calderone. Random House, New York, 1962. A discussion of the problems, complexities, and rewards of the sex relationship.

Premarital Intercourse and Interpersonal Relationships, Lester A. Kirkendall. The Julian Press, New York, 1961. Significant questions and some attempts to answer them. The author is Professor of Family Life, Oregon State University.

Sex and Morality, Abram Kardiner. Bobbs-Merrill Co., New York, 1962 (paperback). Stimulated by the Kinsey report, this discussion of sexual behavior was written by a clinical professor of psychiatry at Columbia University.

Sex Histories of American College Men, Phyllis and Eberhard Kronhausen. Ballantine Books, New York, 1960.

Common Sense about Sexual Ethics, Sherwin Bailey. Macmillan, New York, 1962. Ethical aspects of the sexual relationship, treated from the standpoints of history, principles, and practical considerations.

The Hypocritical American, James Collier. Bobbs-Merrill Co., New York, 1964. The sharp and erratic contrast between sex practices and our laws and attitudes is examined critically.

Men, Women and Marriage, Ernest Havemann. Doubleday, Garden City, N.Y., 1962. Not a rulebook for a happy marriage, but a book of information about some of the problems and intricacies of the wedded state.

Too Much Sex on Campus, Jennie L. Baron. Reader's Digest, May 1964, p. 59.

Must Colleges Police Sex?, John T. Rule. Atlantic Monthly, April 1964, p. 55.

Love and Sex, Mary S. Calderone. Redbook, February 1964.

Sex on the Campus: The Real Issue, Margaret Mead. Redbook, October 1962.

9

MARRIAGE: EMOTIONAL ATTITUDES AND HEALTH PREPARATION

It is normal and natural for young people to be thinking seriously of marriage, because marriage is a way of rounding out and completing our lives. Most of us desire the pleasures and fulfillment that marriage can bring. Unfortunately, marital happiness cannot be achieved automatically by the process of two people living together. It is important to understand *why* people want to marry, and *what factors* contribute to a good and stable marriage.

WHY MARRY?

Today about 92 per cent of all men and women are or have been married by the end of the childbearing age, the highest record in American history. Nearly 70 per cent of the population over 15 years of age are married. There are many reasons for this, for marriage is the culmination of many separate drives.

Nearly all of us need emotional warmth and a sense of belonging to someone. We seek a special kind of happiness in marriage, often centering about a longing for the home and family of our childhood. By establishing our own homes, the cycle can be completed; we recover, in new form, what we lost when we grew up and became independent.

The need for companionship, for someone to share our interests and ambitions, hopes and disappointments is equally important. In today's complex world it may be more desirable than ever before to find a sympathetic mate with whom one can discuss all problems and find understanding and sympathy and even acceptance of one's faults and weaknesses.

Sexual gratification, too, is a fundamental and natural goal of marriage. Marriage sanctions and endorses the fullest expression and gratification of sexual needs and the desire for physical closeness with another person.

There was a time when love and happiness were not the major goals of marriage. Young people married primarily for economic reasons, and the family represented a survival unit. Mates were chosen for steadiness, and both had many duties in the rigorous, early days on the farm and the frontier. Every step, from finding a mate to the wedding ceremony, was frequently controlled by the families of the young couple. In many parts of the world this is still the accepted procedure.

However, in America today, people usually marry because they have fallen in love, and the choice of a spouse is up to the individual. We dare to make personal happiness and companionship major goals in marriage today, because life is more secure and less rigorous than it was for some of our ancestors. These are worthy goals, and perhaps represent much higher human aspirations. Unfortunately, important as it is, love by itself cannot guarantee a happy marriage.

WHAT FACTORS CONTRIBUTE TO A SUCCESSFUL MARRIAGE?

Experts in the field of marriage list the following as the most essential factors in choosing a mate. Because falling in love is an emotional process, no one is likely to go around with this list in hand, and check off every item. However, it is a good and sobering idea to consider these factors *before actually marrying,* because a really successful marriage results only if the husband and wife can satisfy each other's psychological, emotional and companionship needs.

Emotional Adjustment

Normal, well adjusted individuals have the best chance for successful lives, which naturally includes happiness in marriage. Certain characteristics should be sought for, or avoided, when considering marriage, and at least two of the *good* characteristics listed below should be present.

Good

Optimistic personality
Cooperativeness
Consideration and sympathy
Some degree of emotional dependence

Bad

Pessimistic personality
Dominating personality
Inconsiderate and unsympathetic
Too self-sufficient emotionally; too much self-love
Excessively dependent personality; too strong an attachment to parents

Cultural, Religious and Racial Background

You will have a greater chance for a successful marriage if you find a mate of the same race, philosophical outlook or religion, and economic or social class. Husbands and wives who have had a similar childhood and have developed comparable customs, manners and tastes are more likely to "mesh" during the long years of marriage.

While marriages between individuals from different backgrounds can be successful, these unions often face additional problems because of social disapproval or the number of adjustments that must be made. Serious tensions and irritations sometimes result.

Diverse *religious* backgrounds, for example, can affect almost all aspects of family life—meals, holidays, recreational life, the education of the children, even conduct in the marriage bed. Divorce rate is apt to be higher in mixed marriages, a sure sign of incompatibility. A study of 4018 marriages[1] by Judson R. Landis, an expert in this field, showed that the divorce rate declined in the following order:

Highest: the parents of both couples professed no religion

Second: Catholic—Protestant marriages. When the wife is Protestant, the rate became twice as high as when she is Catholic, and the husband Protestant.

[1] *Marriage and Family Living,* IX, May 1947, p. 32.

Third: Both Protestant
Fourth: Both Jewish
Fifth: Both Catholic

Because the Catholic Church makes divorce—and subsequent remarriage—extremely difficult, this list is not necessarily an accurate reflection of happiness in marriages.

Also there is a lower birth rate and higher rate of childlessness in mixed marriages. This is undoubtedly a deliberate action on the part of the parents, who recognize that children of such unions may *cause* problems or *develop* problems.

Although it is difficult to obtain accurate figures for all religious groups, numerous studies show that the number of mixed marriages is steadily increasing. During the last two decades, mixed marriages accounted for one-fourth to one-third of all Catholic marriages. A study by the Lutheran church showed that in a recent five year period, 58 per cent of their members married outside this denomination. One of five married a Roman Catholic, one of five, a nonchurch member, and three of five in other Protestant faiths.[2]

It cannot be said arbitrarily that mixed marriages will not be happy ones. All of us have seen extremely successful examples. But the chances for individual happiness are far greater if all possible problems are faced squarely, well in advance, and are greatest if one mate can accept the faith of the other.

Even in marriages within the same faith, it is important to recognize the dominating influence of *national* cultural traditions. For example, Irish, Italian and German Catholics will have very different backgrounds. The same may be true for Jews of Russian and German origin, and for Northern and Southern Baptists.

Educational Level

School provides experience in learning and in living with others. This can be extremely helpful in smoothing over marital adjustments. It is desirable for both partners to have approximately the same degree of formal education or its informal equivalent. Otherwise, there may be inadequate or unsatisfactory communication on issues which are vital to the other partner.

Economic and Job Status

More important than the size of a man's income is the fact that he is steady and reliable, and that his work does not require him to move about too much, leaving his wife and family for too prolonged periods of time. Also, the more educational preparation and professional training he has had, as a general rule, the better candidate he is for marriage.

Number of Friends

Generally speaking, men and women who are capable of solid friendships with both sexes will make satisfactory mates. It indicates a greater ability to make some of the adjustments necessary to marriage. For the same reason, membership in social or religious organizations and clubs may be a good omen, indicating that the individual is accepted by and accepts—or is tolerant of—many kinds of people. This does not mean that excessive socializing is necessary to a happy marriage.

THE COURTSHIP AND ENGAGEMENT PERIOD

No matter how fast your pulse beats at the sight of your beloved, don't rush into marriage. Get to know each other first. It saves trouble later on.

Don't marry anyone with the idea of reforming him (or her). Remember that you are marrying an adult, whose tastes and habits are fairly well established.

Try to use this valuable period before marriage to understand each other, and to settle the really important issues. Questions of the type: *Shall the wife work? For how long? Can you live on the husband's earnings? How many children? How should they be brought up? Who will manage the family finances?* should all be worked out, if possible, before marriage.

[2]Bossard, J.H.S., and Boll, E.S.: *One Marriage, Two Faiths*, Ronald Press, New York, 1957.

Engagements today don't have the finality nor even the same meaning they had in earlier times. One hundred years ago, a broken engagement was almost as rare as a divorce. Marriages were carefully arranged by parents or marriage brokers. The dowry and other financial arrangements had to be settled, and churches required publication of banns. There was even legal recourse for a broken engagement: the law granted damages to the jilted person in a breach of promise suit.

Today, the engagement period is not merely the formal waiting period it once was for completing the arrangements necessary to the marriage ceremony. Instead, it has come to represent a trying-out period for the realities and responsibilities of life, and the opportunity to become better acquainted with each other and with prospective parents-in-law.

One result of the new attitude toward engagements is the large number which are broken today. According to one college student "an engagement ring only lets you qualify for the finals." Professor Ernest Burgess and Paul Wallin surveyed this problem among a group of engaged couples and found that 24 per cent of the men and 36 per cent of the women questioned reported that earlier engagements had been broken. Subsequently 15 per cent of these engaged couples broke off *their* engagements. This meant that by the close of the study, nearly two fifths of the men and half of the women could report broken engagements.

Perhaps in these days of early marriages, more flexible engagements constitute a healthy release valve. Marrying in haste, it has been said very often, means repenting in leisure! An old African proverb put it even better: "Quick loving a woman means quick not loving a woman."

The well known writer, Will Durant, spoke against hasty marriages and urged a "de-emphasis of sex" in our lives:

> Sex, after hunger, he pointed out, is our strongest instinct and greatest problem.... Our civilization has unwisely stimulated this sexual impulse. Our ancestors played it down. We have blown it up ... and ... armed it with the doctrine that inhibition is a mistake—whereas inhibition—the control of the impulse—is the first principle of civilization.
>
> Marry as soon as you can; keep the wolf from the door, but don't let your choice of a mate be determined by the accident of association at a time of physiological needs; don't buy a grab bag in a coma. Let at least three months intervene between acquaintance and betrothal, and between betrothal and marriage.[3]

LOVE VERSUS INFATUATION

Many people ask "Shall I marry for love?" or "I am very fond of someone who, I feel, would make a good husband (or wife). But I am not in love. Should I marry anyway?"

A strong sexual attraction is often mistaken for love. When this feeling is not accompanied by other sentiments such as sympathy and tenderness, psychologists and marriage counselers call it "infatuation." In adolescents, it is "puppy love," and is usually outgrown in time.

An adequate definition of love has troubled poets and philosophers from time immemorial. Erich Fromm, the distinguished psychiatrist and philosopher, has given a beautiful one:

> The deepest need of man is the need to overcome his separateness, to leave the prison of his aloneness. The full answer to the problem of existence lies in true and mature love.
>
> What is mature love? It is union under the condition of preserving one's integrity, one's individuality. Love is an active power, a power which breaks through the walls which separate man from his fellow man. Love overcomes the sense of isolation and separateness, yet it permits you to be yourself. In love the paradox occurs that two beings become one yet remain two.[4]

If you wish to achieve a successful marriage, you might ask yourself these questions:

1. Do you feel a sense of oneness, each with the other? That is, do you consider the other person a part of yourself?
2. Do you feel you can trust the other person? Does he or she give you an added sense of security and completeness?
3. Are you concerned about his or her welfare and well-being? Do you try in all ways to make the other person happy?

---

[3]From commencement address delivered in June, 1958, at the Webb Preparatory School, Claremont, California.

[4]Fromm, F.: *The Art of Loving*, Harper & Bros., New York, 1956.

4. Have you found that when you are separated for a period of time, you still feel the same strong emotional attachment?
5. Do you find that the desire to stay together grows greater the longer you know each other, and that you do not grow bored as time goes by?

If you have answered "yes" to all these questions, you may safely say you are in love. These attitudes embrace far more than mere infatuation and describe the desire for true companionship. Sexual attraction is an important part of the sturdy foundation on which the house of marriage must be built, but alone it is not enough to guarantee a happy marriage.

The following questionnaire is a guide to help you judge marital compatibility:

1. Do you like to spend most of your leisure time together?
2. Do you agree on whether to have children? Agree on their upbringing?
3. Do you enjoy the same friends?
4. Do you have similar tastes in books, movies, art, and the kind of home you want?
5. For the prospective husband: Do you like to putter around the house, build and fix things, do gardening? For the prospective wife: do you like to cook, sew?
6. Do you both have the same basic philosophy of life? Same religion—or agree on attitudes toward religion?
7. Do you like—or share his attitude toward—his parents? Her parents? Is there agreement on ways to deal with them, and a plan for their old age?
8. Will you love each other when you are old?

Don't be surprised if you find yourself answering "no" to some of these questions. You should neither expect nor desire to marry a carbon copy of yourself; disagreement on minor matters makes for stimulating conversation. But *basic antagonisms represent danger signals.*

WHAT IS THE BEST AGE TO MARRY?

Although it is commonly believed that our grandparents and great-grandparents married at a very early age, the truth is that today we have more early marriages than ever before. In 1890, the average young woman married when she was 22.0 years old, and the average young man, at 26.1 years. By 1951, this figure had dropped to 20.4 years for women, and 22.6 years for men. In 1963, 40 per cent of all marriages involved teen-age individuals.

In no other country of the Western world do people marry so young. We not only marry early, but, unfortunately, with greater haste and less preparation than do people of most nations. Many experts in this field believe that there are fewer chances of happiness in early marriages than in late ones. For example, the divorce rate is six times as high when both mates are under 21, as when they are 31 or over at the time of marriage.

Of course, age alone is not responsible for the failure of so many early marriages. Many other factors must be considered. If young people marry because they are in revolt against their parents, because they are bored, or because they are too impetuous, their marriages are shaky from the very start. Marriage requires stability, economic as well as emotional, or it may encounter serious difficulties. *The best age to marry is when you have reached physical and emotional maturity.* But it is reassuring to recognize that even relatively young people *may* be mature enough for happy, stable marriages.

The life history of a prospective partner should also be considered carefully. Most people postpone marriage for economic reasons, until they are able to manage and support their own households. This pattern is changing somewhat today with many student marriages, subsidized wholly or in part by the parents. But be careful about marrying a *confirmed* bachelor of either sex. Many people who marry for the first time when they are over 35, long past the period when they have developed economic independence, are so fixed in their way of life that they may be unable to adjust to the demands of marriage and the amount of give and take it requires.

Also, previous divorces should be carefully evaluated. Don't dismiss the fact that a prospective mate has been divorced with "It wasn't his—or her—fault." Be certain you have a good reason for believing that history won't repeat itself. Men and women who have been married and divorced several times are not usually good marriage risks.

MARRIED LOVE

Love between a man and woman can be one of the most beautiful and ecstatic experiences. If we were to define married love in its simplest terms, we would stress *sexual attraction, a deep feeling of companionship,* and *the desire for parenthood* as the three most important aspects. The first two are essential, and the third, very valuable for emotional fulfillment and complete, enduring happiness.

Most of us have experienced the joys (and of course, the problems) of companionship. We have been close to our parents, brothers, sisters and friends, and may even have felt a parental emotion toward the baby in our own or another family. These relationships are vitally important in preparing us to make good homes of our own.

But the sustained physical intimacy between a man and a woman, which is so important in marriage, is essentially a closed book for young people. This new and crucial factor is, unfortunately, the one for which they have been least prepared by other relationships and observations.

Even in this enlightened day and age, many people—young and old—are troubled by questions about sexual relations. A surprising amount of ignorance and misunderstanding still persists under the taboos of our society. How tragic it is that the act of sexual intercourse should be clouded by fear and darkened by shame.

The sexual relationship should be the perfect physical expression of love and lead to great happiness. Unfortunately, it often produces only misery. It is highly important that both husband and wife understand what this relationship really means.

Biologically speaking, the purpose of sexual intercourse is reproduction, the means by which new life is created. Most people who feel that life is worth living want to pass on the precious gift of life. But sexual intercourse is far more than that. It is also the intimate expression of love. Giving and receiving the greatest pleasure and experiencing the release which accompanies it are natural and healthy desires. A man and woman are bound to each other most securely when they share this intensely close attachment.

In Chapter Eight we discussed many of the questions which trouble men and women who are thinking seriously of marriage, such as: *Should a couple have sexual intercourse before marriage in order to find out whether they are compatible? Does youthful "petting" interfere with satisfactory sex relations later on? Is sexual experience with others in the past helpful (or harmful) to the establishment of successful sex relations with one's spouse?*

Another major question always arises as the marriage day grows closer: *Is the wedding night a crucial one in the establishment of satisfactory sexual relations?* The answer is that it can be. The bride is usually tense and overwrought, especially if the wedding was a large one, and often she requires the utmost consideration from the groom, who is usually fairly nervous himself.

However, far too much attention is paid to the significance of the "crucial first night of marriage." According to the article "How to act on your honeymoon," young modern couples need to know that:

> The honeymoon should be a lark, a picnic, a holiday from reality for two, an escape from accountability to anyone but each other. It should be a retreat to a limbo of directionless joy where the deepest intimacy between bride and groom may be experienced.... Sexual experience on the nuptial night and the honeymoon has no bearing on the emotional health, the physical well-being or the social relationship of the partners, even if physical culmination is less than perfect, or if it is delayed, halting or inexpert. The intimacies of the honeymoon are events in themselves, insulated by the special climate that is natural to the honeymoon holiday. To many, the joys of simple physical embrace and nearness to each other, without fear of intrusion, are in themselves a culmination.
>
> There are months, years, a lifetime ahead for the cultivation of sexual technique. This is one thing that can be counted on to improve with time and deepening love.[5]

[5]Rainer, J., and Rainer, J.: How to act on your honeymoon, in *Modern Bride,* Early Spring (1959).

HEALTH PREPARATION FOR MARRIAGE

When two people marry, they promise to live together in sickness and in health. But they have every right to believe that neither will endow the other with a serious, preventable illness. This is bound to happen if one of them suffers a venereal disease, and it is almost as inevitable if the disease is active pulmonary tuberculosis.

Many states require a blood test, such as the *Wassermann test,* before issuing a marriage license. This should be mandatory in order to detect syphilis which can and should be cured before anyone has a right to marry. Unsuspected syphilis in a woman can cause her to give birth to children who are blind or deformed.

It would be extremely desirable if the law also required an examination for gonorrhea and tuberculosis.

HEREDITY

Many young people thinking seriously of marriage are concerned about the possibility of their children inheriting some physical or mental defect they know to be present in one of the families, or how much danger results when close relatives—cousins, for example—marry. A number of cities now have heredity clinics, usually connected with medical schools, which can advise young couples about their prospects for the future, and in all probability, we will some day have such clinics in all major population centers.

Transmission of Hereditary Characteristics

To understand how hereditary characteristics are transmitted, it is necessary to know certain facts about the living cell. Each cell contains a nucleus, and each normal nucleus contains a specific number of chromosomes. The number varies with the type of animal—cats normally have 38, dogs 78 and humans 46. The chromosomes are made up of three kinds of chemicals—protein, deoxyribonucleic acid (DNA), and ribonucleic acid (RNA). Of these components, DNA appears to be the one most concerned with heredity.

The importance of DNA is related to the fact that, when it is given proper "food," it can reproduce itself down to the last atom. Not only can it reproduce an identical DNA molecule, but it now seems certain that it controls all cellular activity. For example, when the DNA of a polio virus gains entrance to a human cell, that cell suddenly begins to manufacture polio viruses at a rate of 100,000 every few hours. It is thus obvious that the polio virus DNA takes over the cell and puts it to work for a "subversive" purpose.

Normally, however, our inherent DNA controls the body cells to accomplish the functions necessary to life. For example, it is the DNA contained in the nucleus of the cell that determines the individuality of the cells so that one will transmit a nerve impulse, others will aid in a muscular contraction or produce a digestive enzyme. This amazing blueprint for cellular growth, reproduction, and function is completely transmitted at the time of conception.

Human cells normally contain 46 chromosomes, except for the germ cells, the egg and the sperm. Each of these has only half that number, but when the sperm fertilizes the egg, it adds its complement of chromosomes, and the fertilized egg then has the complete number. Half your genetic characteristics were thus passed on from your father, and half from your mother. Every time the fertilized cell divides, the chromosomes duplicate themselves and divide too, so that each daughter cell will possess a full set of chromosomes.

A cat and a rabbit are unable to mate because they are two different species, and their chromosomes are incompatible, differing in kind and number. A horse and a donkey can mate, but their offspring is a mule. Because the chromosomes of the horse and donkey conflict and do not match, the mule is sterile.

On the other hand, two of the most widely differing human beings—the smallest, darkest African pygmy and the tallest blond Nordic, for example—could produce a normal offspring because both are of the human species and have the same number and kinds of chromosomes.

Every chromosome contains several

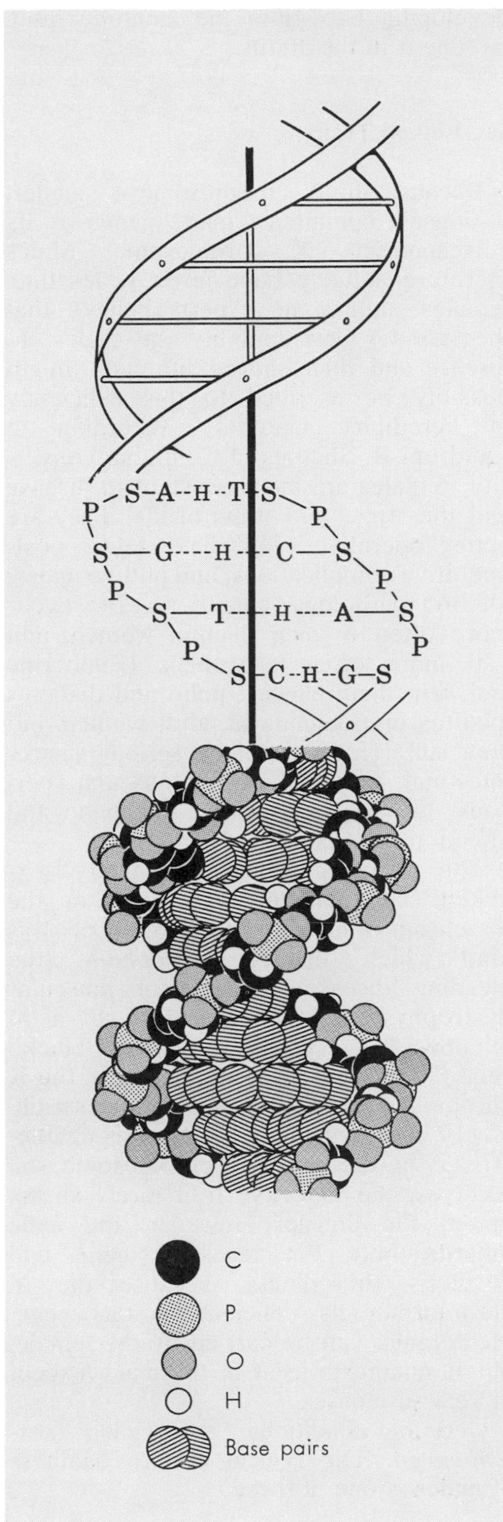

Figure 9–1. The DNA helix. (From Swanson: *The Cell,* Englewood Cliffs, N. J., Prentice-Hall, 1960.)

DNA molecules. These large molecules have the appearance of a twisting spiral ladder. The cross bars on this ladder consist of four chemical substances – adenine, cytosine, guanine, and thymine. These four substances constitute a four-letter alphabet (the first letter of each substance) from which our genetic recipe is prepared. For example, ATGA–CTGA–AGCT might represent the genetic code for a given physical characteristic. In like manner, instructions for any physiological function could be written. A gene consists of a series of genetic directions, such as the one just described (ATGA–CTGA-AGCT).

The chromosomes of each cell contain a large number of genes (500 to 600), and these are the final biological architects, determining the color of your eyes, "slanty" or straight eyes, the color and texture of your skin and hair, body build and structure, head and nose shape, and innumerable other obvious and hidden characteristics. We have an estimated 30,000 genes. The development of certain parts of the body is complex and may require many genes; the construction of the eye, for example, needs at least 150 different genes.

Some genes are called *dominant* and others *recessive:* this simply means that one is stronger than the other and overpowers it. Curly hair is dominant over straight hair, blond hair over red, brown eyes over blue or gray, and freckles over unspotted skin. If you inherit a gene for curly hair from one parent and one for straight hair from the other, the dominant gene will win out, and your hair will be curly. In order to have straight hair, you must inherit the recessive genes for straight hair from both parents.

A tremendous number of traits are known to be inherited or to have some hereditary factor influencing their development. Table 9–1 lists some of these traits and shows which is the dominant or recessive member of a pair.

Sex Determination

A baby's sex is determined by his father, and only by his father. Human eggs usually

Table 9–1. Inherited traits

Dominant	*Recessive*
Dark hair	Blond hair
Nonred hair	Red hair
Curly hair	Straight hair
Abundant body hair	Little body hair
White forelock	Normal hair pigmentation
Normally pigmented hair, skin, and eyes	Albinism
Brown eyes	Blue or gray eyes
Hazel or green eyes	Blue or gray eyes
Near-sightedness	Normal vision
Far-sightedness	Normal vision
Astigmatism	Normal vision
Normal hearing	Congenital deafness
Broad lips	Thin lips
Large eyes	Small eyes
Roman nose	Straight nose
Short stature	Tall stature
Hypertension (high blood pressure)	Normal blood pressure
Migraine headaches	Normal
Normal insulin production	Diabetes mellitus
Stable emotional development	Dementia praecox
Normal clotting of blood	Hemophilia ("bleeder's disease")

contain 46 chromosomes, fairly well matched in size and shape, including a rather large one shaped like an arrowhead, and called the X chromosome. However, only 50 per cent of the sperm possess the X chromosome. The corresponding structure in the remaining sperm is much smaller, and is called the Y chromosome. When a sperm containing an X chromosome fertilizes an egg, the fertilized egg will have the X–X chromosome pair and will develop into a girl child. However, if the other type of sperm with the Y chromosome does the fertilizing, the pattern will be X–Y and the baby will be a boy.

About 105 boys are born for every 100 girls. One explanation for this preponderance of males over females at birth is that sperm with Y chromosomes may be a little lighter in weight and able to swim faster, which would give them a slight edge over their X chromosome mates.

Experts can even predict the sex of the unborn child from these chromosomal differences. This is done by examining cells which have been shed by the developing baby into the amniotic fluid, bathing it in the uterus.

Sex-Linked Traits

Because the Y chromosome is smaller, it doesn't contain as many genes as its corresponding X chromosome. Males therefore actually have fewer genes than females, and some experts believe that the greater susceptibility of males to disease and their shorter life span, might possibly be ascribed to this deficiency in hereditary material. According to Landrum B. Shettles of Columbia University, females are more resistant to disease and the stress and strain of life. They are better operative risks, have fewer postoperative complications, and outlive males. Of 365 pathologic conditions, 245 occur more often in men than in women, and 120 more often in women. (Endocrine and skin disturbances, polio and diabetes mellitus predominate in adult women, but men suffer from the more serious gastrointestinal, vascular, skeletomuscular, nervous, urinary, respiratory, metabolic and infectious diseases.)[6]

The diseases which are called "sex-linked" can definitely be blamed on the Y chromosome. In conditions of this kind—which include *hemophilia* (the bleeding disease), a type of muscular dystrophy, and a peculiar form of night blindness—a recessive, defective, "black" gene is inherited from the mother in the X chromosome. Because she will generally inherit the dominant gene for this characteristic in the other X chromosome she receives, the defective trait rarely shows up in the female. However, the male inherits only the recessive gene and develops the illness, because the Y chromosome is deficient in this gene. Hemophilia can be carried by the female, but it manifests itself in the male, except in very rare cases.

Certain conditions are called *sex-influenced*. The typical pattern baldness of males is one of these.

[6] *Journal of Obstetrics and Gynecology of the British Empire,* February 1958.

First-Cousin Marriages

The danger in first cousins or other close relatives marrying is that both may carry a recessive gene for the same defect, and their children may inherit the recessive gene from both parents and develop the defective trait. However, a knowledge of family background and health may assure the young couple that they have as good a chance as any other pair of people of having normal, healthy children.

It is also important—and sometimes reassuring—to differentiate congenital malformations and defects arising from *hereditary* causes from those which develop because the baby is *exposed to some abnormal situation* during its development in the uterus. We are gradually becoming aware of more and more conditions during pregnancy, like German measles, syphilis, diabetes, polio, treatment with steroid hormones, and certain kidney and other diseases, which adversely affect the development of a baby. Defects produced in this way are not usually hereditary.

Inheritance of Intelligence and Special Abilities

Whether intelligence can be inherited is a very difficult question to answer. Feeble-mindedness *may* be caused by diseases like syphilis and meningitis, or by birth injuries, so that environmental factors during pregnancy and delivery can be very important. Parents of high intelligence usually have bright children, and very stupid people rarely have brilliant ones. However, environmental influences after birth may be extremely important in molding a child and his interests and in developing latent intelligence, and the average intelligence quotient tests are sometimes very misleading. Geniuses can and do arise in families where the parents show only very average intelligence.

The inheritance of musical, artistic, mechanical and mathematical talents seems to be fairly clear-cut. It is interesting that some of these characteristics are relatively independent of general intelligence. Some feeble-minded individuals have very unusual musical and mechanical abilities.

Mutations

Genes normally duplicate themselves with great fidelity. This is the reason you might find that you have a striking resemblance to a relative five generations back. However, every now and then a gene changes and a defective one develops in the process called a *mutation*.

Geneticists estimate that a relatively large number of altered genes are constantly being produced. Yet we inherit surprisingly few unusual characteristics. In all probability, the altered genes which are responsible for really serious defects or malformations are lethal and cause the developing embryo to be aborted.

Cosmic rays and other natural radiations are responsible for about 1 per cent of the mutations. However, x-rays, ultraviolet light, and the newer radioactive elements can increase mutation rates hundreds of times. Three hundred and twenty-five children were born of mothers who were pregnant at the time of the Hiroshima bomb explosion and were within a radius of 2500 miles of the explosion center. Nineteen of these children showed physical or mental retardation or defects. Unfortunately, many more defects may show up in the next generation, because mutated genes are passed on by both the father and the mother, and the progeny may receive a double portion of defective genes. This is one of the reasons for our great concern about radioactive fall-out.

Questions

1. What are the major factors contributing to a successful marriage?
2. It is considered desirable for both partners in a successful marriage to have roughly the same degree of education. Yet you have probably known happy couples in which one was far better educated than the other. How do you think they have managed despite this difference?
3. Differentiating between love and infatuation is very difficult for young people. How would you go about doing this, to prevent jumping into a hasty—and insecure—marriage?
4. What factors should determine the age at which people marry?

5. Do you think the current trend of parents' supporting their children completely during the early years of marriage contributes to the development of stability and responsibility in the marriage?

6. What is the role of DNA in heredity?

7. What is a chromosome? a gene? Define and give an example of a dominant and a recessive trait.

8. What determines a child's sex?

9. Why are certain hereditary conditions called "sex-linked"?

10. What is a mutation? How might it occur?

Topics for Discussion

Religious attitudes toward contraception.
Some practical difficulties in mixed marriages.
Late versus early marriages.

Reading Suggestions

Too Young to Marry? Public Affairs Pamphlet No. 236, Public Affairs Committee, 22 East 38th Street, New York 16, N.Y., 1956. A well-written informative pamphlet.

Apprenticeship for Marriage, Margaret Mead. Redbook Magazine, October 1963, p. 14. An interesting discussion of preparation of today's young people for marriage.

A Man to Marry, W. W. Bauer and Florence Marugne Bauer. Today's Health, April 1965, p. 38. An informative article for college students.

Marriage Counseling in Medical Practice, E. M. Nash, Lucie Jessner, and D. Wilfred Abse, eds. University of North Carolina Press, Chapel Hill, 1964. A medical symposium on marriage counseling. Although written for the physician, it is an excellent reference for college students.

Marriage: An Examination of the Man-Woman Relationship, Herman R. Lantz and Eloise C. Synder. Wiley & Sons, New York, 1962.

All About Love, Julian Huxley. Readers Digest, July 1964, p. 127. A thought-provoking article for the college student.

Husbands and Wives: the Dynamics of Family Living, Robert O. Bloak. The Free Press of Glencoe, New York, 1960. A frank discussion appropriate for those making preparation for marriage.

Handbook of Marriage and the Family, Harold T. Christensen, ed. Rand McNally Co., Chicago, 1964. This authoritative book written by experts in every phase of marriage and the family should be studied by every college student. It is an up-to-date and comprehensive volume.

Love and the Facts of Life, E. M. Duvall. Association Press, New York, 1963.

Emotional Maturity in Love and Marriage, Lucy Freeman and Harold Greenwald. Harper, New York, 1961.

Love on the Campus, J. Poppy. Look, August 1963. The college student will find this to be an interesting article.

The Sex Age, Howard Whitman. Bobbs-Merrill, Indianapolis, 1963. Discusses twentieth century problems.

Counseling in Medical Genetics, S. Reed. 2nd Ed., W. B. Saunders Co., Philadelphia, 1965. A text for the general practitioner of medicine concerning the counseling of his patients.

Today's Health, April 1964, contains a series of articles dealing with love and marriage. These are very well written and especially useful to the college age person.

1. The Real Intimacy in Marriage, p. 18.
2. Why Women Can't Talk to Their Husbands, p. 28.
3. Why Men Don't Talk to Their Wives, p. 28.
4. All Things Special for Your Honeymoon, p. 34.
5. What Every Husband Should Know, p. 48.
6. The Importance of the Premarital Examination, p. 50.
7. Should Newlyweds Live with Their Parents, p. 54.
8. What Newlyweds Should Know About In-laws, p. 56.
9. Do You Dare to Be Honest in Marriage, p. 58.
10. Marriage is Neither Heaven or Hell, p. 60.

SECTION FIVE

HUMAN REPRODUCTION

10

THE FEMALE REPRODUCTIVE SYSTEM

The female reproductive system, located primarily within the pelvic cavity, is an intricate and efficient mechanism that serves a dual purpose—to produce mature ova, with which the male sperm can join and thus conceive a new life, and to shelter and nourish this creation until it is ready to come into the world. Much of the philosophy, poetry, folklore, legends, superstitions, fears, and body of knowledge surrounding woman centers on this essential purpose, which so completely affects and involves her life.

The role of the male in creating a new life is described in Chapter 11. Some of the changes in a woman's body during pregnancy and the development of the child within the womb are discussed in Chapter 13. The major components and functions of the woman's reproductive system—those interrelated structures that produce ova, receive sperm, and manufacture hormones—and the cycle of menstruation are discussed in this chapter.

THE ORGANS OF REPRODUCTION

The woman's reproductive system includes a pair of ovaries, a set of fallopian tubes that lead from the ovaries to the uterus or womb, associated glands, and the external genitals. The breasts are not usually considered part of the reproductive system, although they are intimately affected by changes during sexual development, menstruation, and pregnancy.

The *ovaries* are glands located in the pelvic cavity just below the navel and about 3 inches to the right and left. Each measures approximately 1 inch wide, 1½ inches long, and ⅓ inch thick. These glands have two prime responsibilities—to produce the *ova,* or eggs, making them

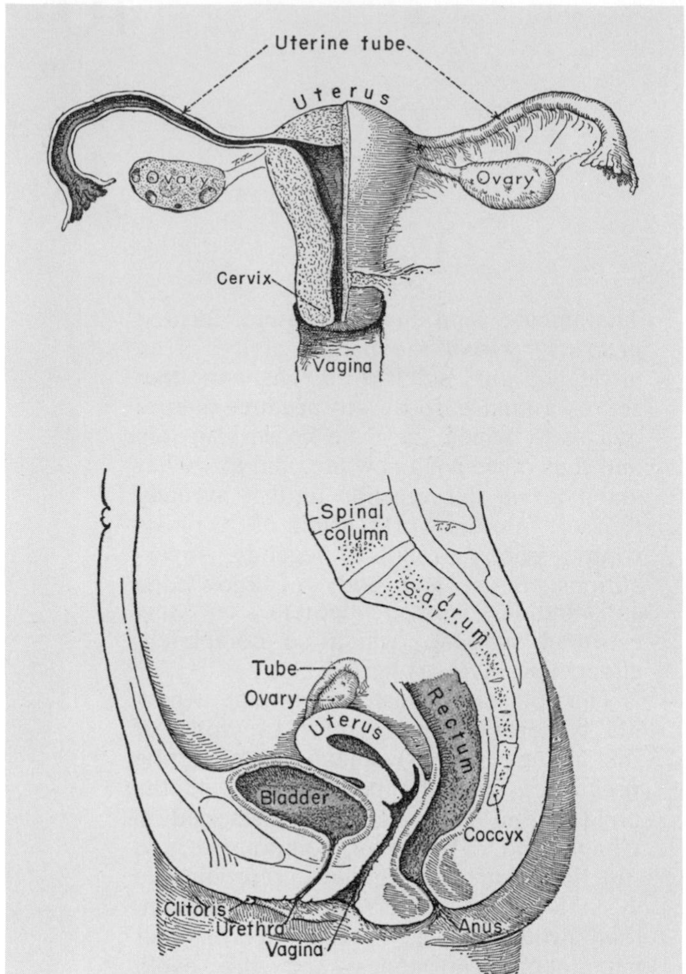

Figure 10–1. The female reproductive system. (From Dowling and Jones: *That The Patient May Know*. Philadelphia, W. B. Saunders Co.)

ready for impregnation by the male sperm, and to secrete hormones that further regulate the reproductive process. When a girl is born, her ovaries already contain an estimated 400,000 primary, immature cells called *follicles,* each of which can ripen and produce a mature ovum after puberty. This is about 1000 times more than she will ever need, for the body produces only one ovum each month between puberty and menopause (two or more only in infrequent cases in which double or multiple pregnancy can occur). Three hundred to five hundred mature ova are the average lifetime quota. Normally, only one ovary releases an egg each month. There is no apparent preference or pattern of alternation between the two identical glands.

The second function of the ovaries is to produce hormones, which is discussed in greater detail on page 183 in the section on menstruation. Both ovaries receive and release hormones, thus governing the monthly menstrual cycle. These hormones, including estrogen, also trigger and control the development of the female secondary sex characteristics, including enlargement of the breasts, development of the female contour of waist and hips, and appearance of pubic and axillary hair. (Table 10-1).

The *fallopian tubes* serve as corridors from the ovaries to the uterus, a passageway for the mature ovum. If fertilization is to take place, it usually does so within the fallopian tube. The egg then continues on its way until it becomes embedded in the wall of the uterus. Each of the fallopian tubes is 3 to 5 inches long. Although its lower end opens into the uterus, its upper end is not connected directly to the ovary at all. The far end, lying close to the ovary,

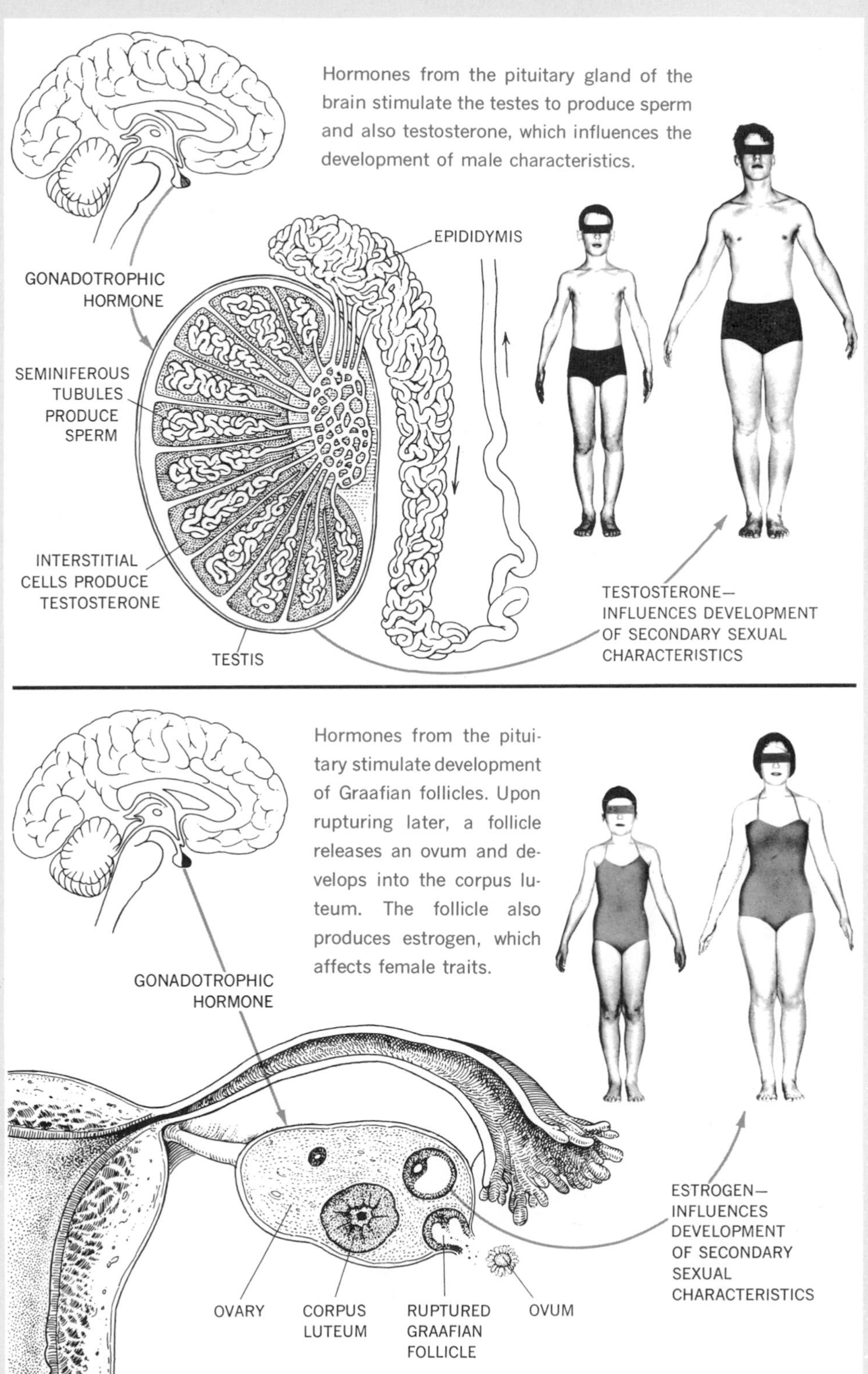
Hormones from the pituitary gland of the brain stimulate the testes to produce sperm and also testosterone, which influences the development of male characteristics.
GONADOTROPHIC HORMONE
EPIDIDYMIS
SEMINIFEROUS TUBULES PRODUCE SPERM
INTERSTITIAL CELLS PRODUCE TESTOSTERONE
TESTIS
TESTOSTERONE—INFLUENCES DEVELOPMENT OF SECONDARY SEXUAL CHARACTERISTICS
Hormones from the pituitary stimulate development of Graafian follicles. Upon rupturing later, a follicle releases an ovum and develops into the corpus luteum. The follicle also produces estrogen, which affects female traits.
GONADOTROPHIC HORMONE
ESTROGEN—INFLUENCES DEVELOPMENT OF SECONDARY SEXUAL CHARACTERISTICS
OVARY
CORPUS LUTEUM
RUPTURED GRAAFIAN FOLLICLE
OVUM

Table 10–1. Time of appearance of sexual characteristics in American girls*

Pelvis	Female contour assumed and fat deposition begins at 8–10 years.
Breasts	First hypertrophy or budding at 9–11 years. Further enlargement and pigmentation of nipples, 12–13 years of age. Histologic maturity, 16–18 years.
Vagina	Secretion begins and glycogen content of epithelium increases with change in cell type, 11–14 years.
Pubic hair	Initial appearance, 10–12 years; abundant and curly, 11–15 years.
Axillary hair	Initial appearance, 12–14 years.

*From E. H. Watson and G. H. Lowrey: *Growth and Development of Children.* Year Book Publishers, Chicago, 1952.

consists of a fringed area *(fimbria).* These tiny projections extend themselves when the mature egg is ready, embrace it, and pull it into the fallopian tube. The egg, having no means of self-locomotion, is moved down the tube by hairlike *cilia* that line its inner wall.

The *uterus,* or womb, is a hollow, pear-shaped, muscular pouch, about 3 inches long and 2 inches wide at the top, narrowing down to the *cervix,* or neck, where it is normally about ½ to 1 inch in diameter. The uterus is one of the strongest and most flexible muscles in the female body, by necessity, since it must be able to hold and nourish a new human for 9 months, until it reaches a weight of approximately 7 pounds, then expel it through the vagina. The uterus is loosely held in place by ligaments, enabling it to expand and move when the woman becomes pregnant.

The inner lining of the uterus *(endometrium)* is a soft tissue, richly supplied with blood vessels. This lining grows each month in depth and is prepared to serve as a home for the fertilized egg. If conception does not take place that month, the

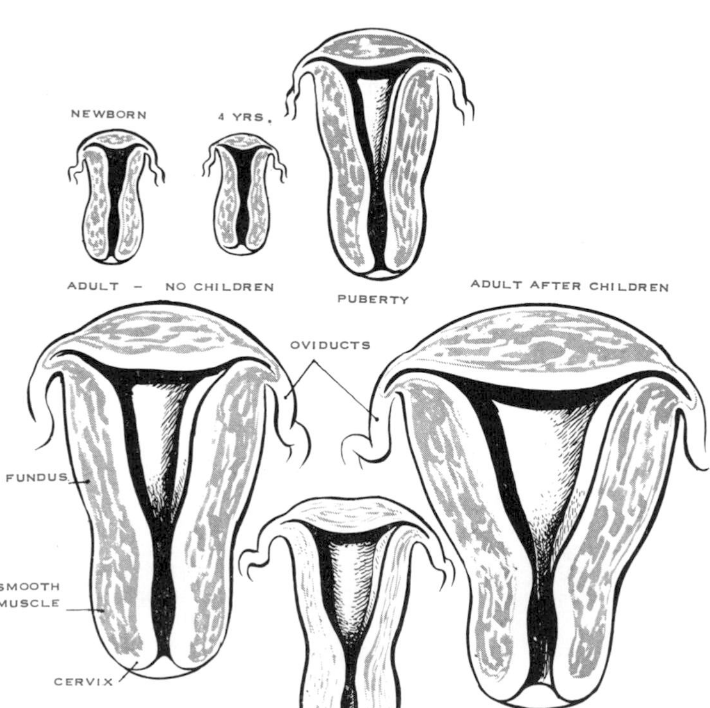

Figure 10–2. Variations in size and shape of uterus accompanying various ages. (From Martin, P. C., and Vincent, E. L.: *Human Development.* New York, Ronald Press, 1960.)

excess material is shed and passes from the body in a discharge of blood and other substances. The appearance of this material constitutes the beginning of a woman's period, or menstrual cycle.

The cervix extends downward into the *vagina,* a tube 3 to 4 inches long, which serves as the female organ of intercourse, a passageway for the arriving male sperm, and the canal through which a baby is born. The lining is a soft membrane, and the tough muscles that constitute the vaginal passage are extremely flexible, sufficiently so that it can extend to four or five times its normal size when a baby must make its way down from the uterus. The *hymen,* or maidenhead, is a thin membrane that stretches across the opening of the vagina. It is not always present, and in many women it varies in thickness and extent. Contrary to ancient (and modern) beliefs, its absence is not a sign that a girl is no longer a virgin, nor is its presence an absolute sign of virginity. It is usually broken by the first intercourse, but it may be torn in other ways while a girl is still virginal—for example, through strenuous athletics, the use of tampons, or by masturbation.

The external genitals comprise the *vulva* and the *clitoris.* The vulva include two pairs of lip shaped skin that surround the external opening of the vagina: the *labia minora*—thin folds of tissue covered with mucoid membrane—and the *labia majora*—larger and heavier folds of skin that in the mature woman are covered with hair that extends in an inverted V up toward the abdomen. Located where the labia unite is the highly sensitive clitoris, composed of tissue that fills with blood and becomes erect when the woman is sexually excited. Other physiological activity during sexual stimulation includes the secreting of lubricating fluids by *Bartholin's glands* and *Skene's glands,* which are near the opening of the vagina. Aside from the emotional connotations, it is important for a man to stimulate a woman sexually before intercourse begins because these lubricating agents help prepare the narrow vagina to receive the penis. In this way, as in so many others, what a man can do during sex play to please and stimulate his partner turns out to make the situation more pleasurable for him too.

THE MENSTRUAL CYCLE

As early as age 10, although usually between the ages of 12 and 14, most girls begin to develop typical secondary sexual characteristics. Their breasts gradually enlarge, their feminine hip contour begins to form, and pubic hair appears. These results are dependent on the release of female sex hormones by the maturing ovaries. The monthly menstrual discharge begins and will continue for 30 or 40 years. The girl's reproductive system is maturing. She is becoming a woman, capable of having children.

Menstruation is the mechanism for eliminating from the body the extra blood and tissue which have been built up in preparation for a baby and have not been used. Menstrual cycles vary, but the average interval from one menstrual period to the next is about 28 days. Differences in the length of the cycle are not unusual. The period lasts three to five days on the average.

During the first 14 days of this cycle, counting the first day of menstruation as Day 1, the ovary contains a *follicle*—a small hollow ball the size of a pinhead. Within it lies an egg. This follicle grows during these 14 days until it is several times its original size, becoming as large as a pea. While it is growing, the follicle makes the hormone *estrogen.* The menstrual cycle and the growth of the follicle are under the control of the pituitary gland. On about the fourteenth day, stimulated by secretions from the pituitary gland, the follicle bursts and the egg is discharged from the ovary. The discharged egg enters the tube on its way down to the uterus. If any sperm are present in the fallopian tubes at that time, fertilization may take place in the tube. The fertilized egg continues its journey to the uterus. Once there, it plants itself in the wall of the uterus. If the egg is not fertilized, it passes out of the body along with the unneeded lining of the uterus. Meanwhile, the ruptured follicle from which the egg was discharged is transformed into a yellowish, solid ball now called the *corpus luteum* (Latin: yellow body). The corpus luteum produces a second hormone, *progesterone.* Let us now examine all this in more detail.

The intricate job of hormone production

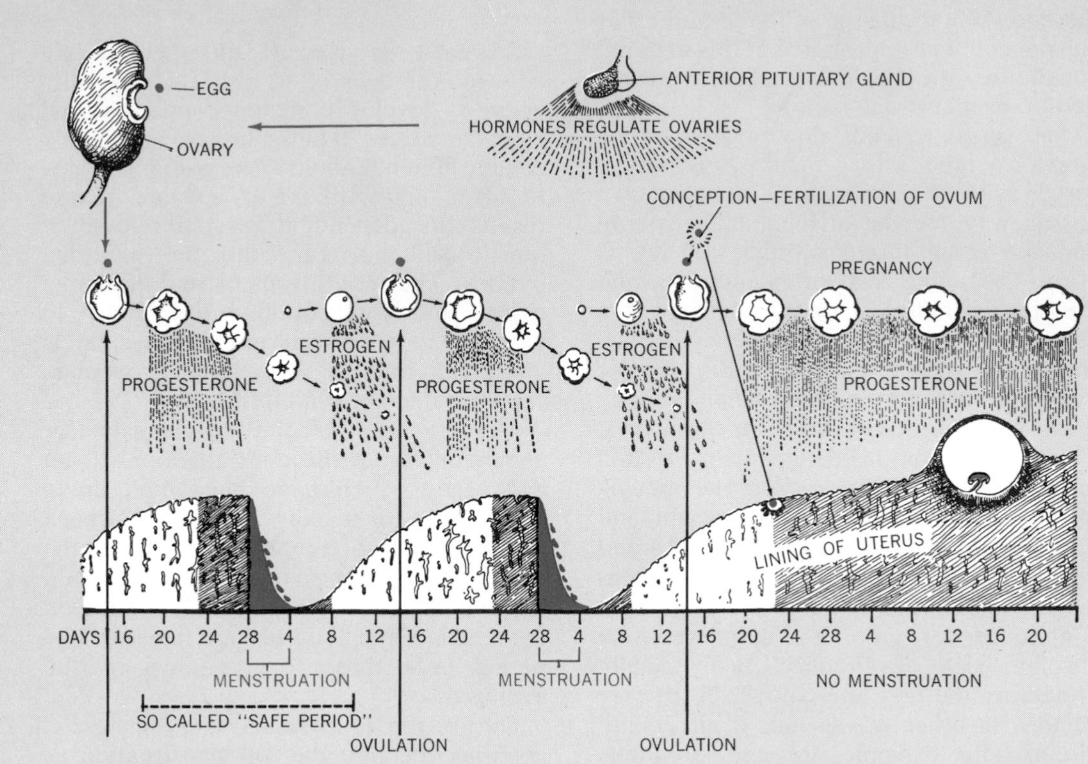

Diagram shows the chain of events that occur during the average 28-day menstrual cycle. The cycle begins when hormones from the pituitary gland stimulate the development of an egg in a follicle inside one of the ovaries. About the 14th day, ovulation occurs: The follicle bursts, and the egg is discharged from the ovary. Three successive ovulations are shown here. After the first two, the egg is not fertilized, and the cycles end in menstruation on the 28th day. After the third ovulation, the egg is fertilized, and pregnancy begins.

and the relationship between the pituitary and the ovary are extremely important. The entire female reproductive cycle is under the control of the pituitary gland, which is located at the base of the brain. This gland secretes hormones that influence other glands in the body, including the ovaries. One of the *gonadotropic* hormones is secreted by the anterior lobe of the pituitary and is transported by the blood stream to the ovaries. This hormone stimulates activity in the egg follicles in the ovary and is known as the follicle-stimulating hormone (FSH).

FSH influences the microscopic follicle to grow into the much larger *graafian follicle*. Eventually, it becomes nearly one-third inch in diameter, millions of times larger than the original single-celled follicle. This structure not only becomes the mature egg, but also begins to secrete estrogen, which causes the lining of the uterus to thicken and its blood supply to increase. Estrogen also causes suppression of further FSH secretion by the pituitary gland.

About 14 days after the period begins (assuming a 28 day cycle), the graafian follicle is fully mature. It ruptures and releases the ovum. The fimbria of the fallopian tube trap the ovum and move it into the tube, then down to the uterus, as previously described. After ovulation, the empty follicle is transformed into a yellowish structure called the *corpus luteum.* This process is regulated by another hormone from the pituitary gland, the luteinizing hormone (LH). The corpus luteum now becomes a gland itself and secretes the second hormonal substance produced by the ovary—*progesterone*—as well as a continued supply of estrogen. Meanwhile, the lining of the uterus continues to be enriched. The two hormones suppress further follicle development and ovulation until the previously released ovum has had time to become fertilized and implanted in the rich endometrium.

If pregnancy occurs, the corpus luteum continues to secrete its hormones for about 9 months, thus suspending any further ovulation and menstruation. Within 10 days after ovulation, the impregnated egg is firmly embedded in the wall of the uterus, and the process of pregnancy (described in Chapter Thirteen) is underway. If the egg is not fertilized, the work of the corpus luteum comes to an end. The endometrium begins to slough off and passes through the vagina along with some blood. This discharge is known as menstruation. It marks the end of the menstrual cycle and the beginning of a new one.

Less than 75 years ago, doctors almost universally agreed that menstruation was an illness. Because of it, women were considered incapable of sustained physical or mental efforts—especially mental efforts, since menstruation was regarded as a temporary insanity.

Some of these attitudes persist even today. There are still many women who avoid touching a flower when they are menstruating because they are sure it will promptly fade. Even well educated women seem to be reluctant to accept menstruation as a natural part of life. They call it "the curse," "the cramps," or "falling off the roof."

The true facts are these:

Menstruation is a completely normal phenomenon.

Menstruation does not preclude engaging in any sport or activity you enjoy when you are not menstruating. This includes swimming, horseback riding, tennis, skiing, and skating.

It is perfectly safe to bathe or shower while you are menstruating.

A woman does not emanate any evil "vapors" during menstruation.

MENSTRUAL ABNORMALITIES

Amenorrhea means absence of menstruation.

It is called *primary* amenorrhea if menstruation has never occurred, and *secondary* if it has begun and then ceases. Secondary amenorrhea is, of course, normal during pregnancy and often while the mother is nursing. It is quite apt to occur sporadically in the first and last months of a woman's childbearing years.

Primary amenorrhea may result from various causes—malformed or underdeveloped female organs, glandular disorders, general poor health, and even emotional factors. Both the fear and the hope of becoming pregnant have been known to stop the periods.

Scanty menstruation, menstrual flow which is so slight as to amount to little more than "staining," may result from the same causes. It is frequently due to anemia.

Menorrhagia means that there is an exceptional amount of menstrual flow at the regular periods. If ordinary pads do not afford protection, or *if the menstrual blood forms into large clots,* medical care is indicated. Tumors, polyps, cancers, inflammations, certain diseases such as rheumatic fever, endocrine disorders, abnormalities of the organs themselves, and emotional factors can all cause excessive bleeding.

During the childbearing years, menstruation usually occurs at definite intervals, starting almost exactly the same number of days apart. *Irregularity* may be due to a harmless change in nature's timing, which will correct itself spontaneously. On the other hand, it may also result from a disease in some other part of the body, such as the thyroid gland, or from a tumor of the womb or ovaries. Most important of all, bleeding between periods can be a warning of cancer.

Dysmenorrhea is the term for painful menstruation. Many, if not most, women experience some discomfort at the onset of their menstrual periods. It is very difficult to draw a boundary between this and pain, since individual reactions vary tremendously. For practical purposes, dysmenorrhea probably is present if a woman's menstrual cramps do not yield to mild pain-killers, and if they prevent her from engaging in her work or social life.

Painful menstruation can be due to physical causes such as an inflammation or *endometritis,*[1] which require treatment. In many instances it is associated with constipation, and vanishes when this condition is corrected. In the past, there was a tendency to believe that cramps were always due to some organic cause, usually the fact that the cervix, the mouth of the womb, was too narrow and needed to be stretched, or that the uterus itself was not in the proper position. Operations were frequently performed to correct this, but in most cases the pain was not relieved.

In general, dysmenorrhea cannot be accounted for by any organic condition, and is therefore called *functional.* It occurs most often in young girls and in women who are unmarried, and is found only occasionally in married women, and rarely in women who have had children. In many cases, there is conclusive evidence that it is caused by emotional factors.

Intermenstrual Pain

Some women experience pain approximately midway between periods, at the time of *ovulation.* This may be accompanied by *leukorrhea,* a white discharge, or a slight show of blood. As a rule, the pain is brief and moderate, but sometimes when the ovum breaks through the wall of the ovary to start its journey toward the uterus, it may cause quite severe pain. When it is located in the right ovary, which lies near the appendix, the pain is so severe that appendicitis is sometimes suspected. This pain may be turned to advantage by women using the rhythm method of birth control. It serves as a signal that ovulation has begun and the "unsafe" time for intercourse has arrived (See Chapter Twelve).

Premenstrual Difficulties

Headache, depression, irritability, slight nausea, and puffiness of the abdomen, skin and other parts of the body may precede menstruation. The reasons for premenstrual tension are not fully understood, but we know that they are associated with a disturbance of the salt balance, resulting in the accumulation of water in the tissues. Often these symptoms vanish with medication or a salt-free diet.

DISEASES OF THE FEMALE REPRODUCTIVE SYSTEM

Infections, including venereal ones (syphilis and gonorrhea), can seriously damage the female genitals. A sudden, profuse, odorous, colored, or painful discharge may indicate a potentially serious infection that may affect not only the vaginal passage but also the uterus, the tubes, and ovaries as well. If such a discharge is accompanied by chills and fever, real trouble may be developing. Fortunately, such infections can be healed by penicillin and similar medicines.

Leukorrhea is a vaginal discharge, but it is not necessarily serious. A certain amount of fluid is normally produced to keep the tissues moist. It is practically odorless and colorless, and is not irritating. Congestion, tension, and minor inflammations can increase this discharge. Germs far less dangerous than those causing syphilis and gonorrhea can cause infections which may become troublesome unless they are cleared up. Your doctor must find the cause of the infection before he can prescribe the right treatment.

The female organs are also subject to tumors and cancers, and should be examined regularly at every complete medical checkup. Any change in menstruation and any unexpected bleeding or discharge, especially after the menopause, should be immediately reported to a physician.

[1]This is an inflammation of the endometrium, the membrane lining the uterus.

FEMININE HYGIENE

Nature has provided very well for the cleansing of the internal passages, and feminine hygiene does not require douches. Altogether too many women have been persuaded by frightening advertisements that frequent douches are indispensable, and that no woman can be clean or dainty without them.

Douches *can* be extremely irritating, unless they are of the mildest type, imitating nature's own secretions, and given under very gentle pressure. The safest douche is a physiologic salt solution, made by dissolving two level teaspoons of salt in a quart of moderately warm water.

FEMALE CLIMACTERIC

Menarche is the term applied to the first menstrual cycle in the female. *Menopause* is the term for the end of this periodic bleeding. The average American woman is 47 to 49 years old at menopause. Almost 75 per cent of all women reach the menopause when they are in their 40's, and about 99 per cent reach it when they are between 35 and 55. In general, the younger a woman is at the onset of menarche, the older she will be at menopause.

Several physiological changes follow menopause; collectively, these changes are called the female climacteric. The climacteric may include changes in primary and secondary sex characteristics, diminished vaginal secretions, atrophy of the breasts, and a change in the distribution of hair. Some women experience "hot flashes" and mild psychological disturbances. Relief is often afforded by the administration of estrogen.

The mental attitude of the woman approaching menopause is most important. It is a perfectly normal event in human life, and although it closes the period of childbearing, it does not mean the end of sexual activity. For some women, the menopause turns out to be the beginning of heightened interest in sex, for birth control is no longer a consideration in intercourse.

Questions

1. What are the major structures in a woman's reproductive system? Describe what they do.
2. Describe in detail all the functions of the ovaries.
3. What analogies can you see between the female and the male organs of reproduction?
4. Why do you suppose that women are given so many more potential ova than they will ever need?
5. Where does conception actually take place?
6. Considering what you know about the functions of the ovaries and the uterus, how do you suppose that surgical removal of the uterus would affect a woman's sex characteristics (aside from her ability to bear children)? Also, the effects of surgical removal of the ovaries?
7. What superstitions, ancient and contemporary, about menstruation can you cite? Are any of these based on fact?
8. What is your own attitude toward and feeling about menstruation? Are they entirely rational?
9. Why do some women fear menopause? How can you explain these fears?
10. Why might the postmenopausal time be enjoyable?
11. How can a husband help his wife during the difficulties of menstruation? of menopause?
12. Define the menstrual cycle, considering the first day of the menstrual period as day one.
13. What is the source of *estrogen?* of *progesterone?*
14. What are the functions of these two hormones?
15. Define *amenorrhea, menorrhagia,* and *dysmenorrhea.*
16. What are some symptoms of "premenstrual tension"?
17. Describe some causes of painful menstrual periods.
18. What is meant by "intermenstrual pain"?
19. Is "feminine hygiene" by regular douching a necessity?
20. When does menopause occur, and what happens at menopause?

Topics for Discussion

Primitive and modern taboos in regard to menstruation.

Factors involved in implantation of fertilized egg.

Premenstrual tension.

Possible sources of superstition and fear about menstruation.

Importance of a prepubescent girl's understanding the forthcoming process of menstruation.

How seriously menstruation should affect physical activity.

Menstruation as an illness or as only an accepted physiological process.

Men's attitudes toward menstruation.

How knowledge of the reproductive system can affect attitudes toward birth control after marriage.

Importance of men and women understanding the details of each other's sexual development.

Irregularities and problems of the menstrual cycle.
Reasons for regular physical examination, especially of the pelvic area.

Reading Suggestions

Facts of Love and Marriage for Young People, Aron Krich, ed., Dell, New York, 1962 (paperback). The emphasis is on successful family living in this informative and factual book.

Women, Aron Krich, ed., Dell, New York, 1960 (paperback). Some enlightening discussions of women's varied sexual experiences.

The Human Body: Its Structure and Operation, Isaac Asimov. Houghton Mifflin, Boston, 1963. A contemporary scientist who is also an outstanding writer offers a clear and well organized presentation for the undergraduate.

The Machinery of the Body, Anton J. Carlson, Victor Johnson, and H. Mead Cavert, 5th Ed., University of Chicago Press, 1961. How the human body works, in health and in illness, with information on recent advances in medical knowledge and techniques.

Function of the Human Body, Arthur C. Guyton. W. B. Saunders, Philadelphia, 1964. This book includes an authoritative chapter on, "Sexual Functions of the Male and Female and the Sex Hormones."

Human Sex Anatomy, Robert L. Dickinson. 2nd Ed., Williams & Wilkins, Baltimore, 1949. The authoritative book on the human reproductive systems, superbly illustrated.

Atlas of Human Anatomy, Franz Frohse, Max Brodel, and Leon Schlossberg. 6th Ed., Barnes & Noble, New York, 1961.

Sense and Nonsense about Sex, Evelyn Millis Duvall and Sylvanus Milne Duvall. Association Press, New York, 1962.

The Genetic Code, Isaac Asimov. Orion Press, New York, 1963. (Also, New American Library paperback.)

Sex and the Adolescent, Maxine Davis. Dial Press, New York, 1959. Accuracy and frankness are combined in this discussion of many aspects of sexual development and activity.

Attaining Womanhood, George W. Corner. Harper, New York, 1952. A distinguished physician and anatomist has prepared this fine presentation of sexual development and reproduction for young girls. A companion book to Dr. Corner's volume for boys.

11

THE MALE REPRODUCTIVE SYSTEM

The male reproductive system is designed primarily for one purpose—to manufacture sperm and to deliver it to the female, so that an egg may be impregnated and a new life conceived.

The major structures of this system are the testes, scrotum, epididymes, vas deferens, seminal vesicles, prostate glands, urethra, and the penis. They interact toward their common goal, but for clarity, they are discussed separately. Although the function of eliminating waste shares part of this genitourinary system, that phase of human activity is discussed in Chapter 2.

THE MALE SEX ORGANS

The two *testes,* each about the size of a walnut, are responsible for the production of *spermatozoa,* or sperm, and of sex hormones. Manufacture takes place in a series of twisted tubules where the sperm develop from immature cells created there early in the life of the embryo. The sperm do not appear until puberty, just as the woman's undeveloped ova wait quietly in the ovary until she reaches sexual maturity. At puberty, the sperm become capable of fertilizing the ova. In some men, this ability continues into old age.

The testes develop before birth inside the abdominal cavity, just below the kidney. During embryonic and fetal life, they gradually descend from this position through the abdominal cavity and reach their eventual destination, outside and below the pelvic area, usually during the seventh month of prenatal life. Sometimes one or both testes fail to descend, a condition called *cryptorchidism.* If both testes remain inside the body, they will fail to produce sperm because of the body's higher internal temperature. As a result, the male becomes sterile, although he may be completely masculine in all other respects, including the ability to have sexual intercourse. However, just one healthy descended testis will produce adequate sperm to ensure male fertility. Undescended testes can usually be placed in their normal positions by surgery and sometimes by the use of hormones.

The production of sperm is called *spermatogenesis*. This process begins around 14 to 15 years of age (Table 11–1 and illustration, p. 123) as a result of stimulation of the testes by a hormone released from the pituitary gland. Following production, mature sperm are stored in fluids within the vas deferens and the ejaculatory duct. They are able to live for several weeks in the body. They may live even longer outside the body, if they are stored in a suitable and cool environment. It is believed that sperm live for about 48 hours inside the female vagina, although human sperm have been observed to remain active after being deposited in the woman for as long as seven days. That they can actually impregnate an ovum after 48 hours appears doubtful.

Transfer of sperm from the ejaculatory duct through the urethra is accomplished by a series of muscular contractions occurring almost simultaneously throughout the male reproductive system. Sperm and supporting fluids are forcibly ejected through the opening in the glans penis by these contractions, summarily called ejaculation. There is a wide variation in the number of sperm contained in each ejaculation; the normal range is 300 to 400 million. If the individual ejaculation contains less than 150 million sperm, the male is often sterile. The reason for this is not clear, for only one sperm is required to fertilize one ovum. One theory offered to explain this suggests that a certain number of sperm cells are required to produce the enzyme hyaluronidase which may be needed to break the outer cover of the ovum so that one sperm can finally fertilize it. A second theory is that hyaluronidase is required to allow successful passage of spermatozoa through the cervical canal.

Table 11–1. Time of appearance of sexual characteristics in American boys.*

Testes and penis	Increase in size begins, 10–12 years. Rapid growth, 12–15 years.
Pubic hair	Initial appearance, 12–14 years. Abundant and curly, 13–16 years.
Axillary hair	Initial appearance, 13–16 years.
Facial and body hair	Initial appearance, 13–16 years.
Mature sperm	Average, about 14–16 years.
Breasts	Some hypertrophy, often assuming a firm nodularity, 12–14 years. Disappearance of hypertrophy, 14–17 years.

*From Watson and Lowrey: *Growth and Development of Children,* Year Book Publishers, 1952.

The testes also produce *testosterone,* a hormone that initiates the development of male secondary sex characteristics. When this hormone is released into the blood stream, it promotes the growth of pubic and body hair, the beard, and wide shoulders. It also increases the size and strength of the large muscles and leads to the development of the male's deep voice. In later life, it may be responsible for a receding hairline, or even baldness.

It is interesting to note that in some animals, such as the rabbit, the testes remain inside the body except at breeding time, when they emerge. This is a more efficient system than that of the human, because the testes are better protected against injury.

The *scrotum* is a saclike structure that contains the testes. In addition to serving a protective and supporting function, the scrotum regulates the temperature of the testes. This is most important, because sperm cannot live at high temperatures. To regulate temperature, the scrotum perspires freely, raises the testes toward the warm body under cold environmental conditions, and lowers them when the ambient temperature increases.

The *epididymides* are collecting and conducting tubes that are attached directly to the testes. Inside these tiny tubes, which are actually several feet long, the sperm become mature and motile (capable of

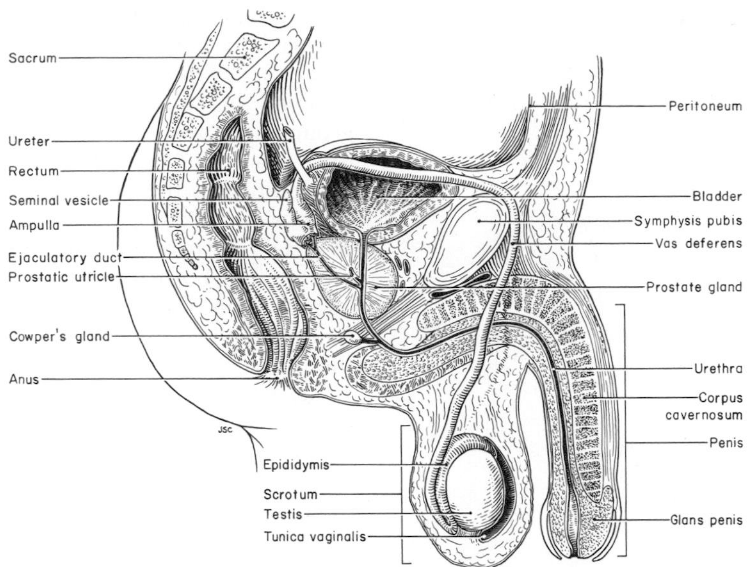

Figure 11–1. Schematic sagittal section of the pelvic region of the male human, showing the organs of the reproductive tract. (From Villee: *Biology*. 4th ed., Philadelphia, W. B. Saunders Co., 1962.)

moving under their own power), although they do not move until they are discharged from the body.

During coitus, the sperm are moved from the epididymides along the spermatic cord, or *vas deferens*. (Each of these structures is duplicated, one from each testis, along each side of the reproductive area.) The vas deferens passes in front of the pubic bone, then loops back into the body around the ureter (the tube connecting the kidney to the bladder) and acquires along the way the secretions of several other structures. Surgical cutting of this tube *(vasectomy)* makes the male sterile, although it does not affect his potency. It is a form, certainly a drastic form, of birth control. An analogous, but more complex, operation can be performed on a woman for the same purpose.

Three structures inside the abdominal cavity discharge components of semen into the vas deferens. They are the *seminal vesicles,* the *prostate gland,* and *Cowper's glands*.

The seminal vesicles secrete a mucoid material containing an abundance of fructose. This secretion is thought to serve as nutrition for the sperm en route to the ovum. The seminal vesicles eject their secretions into the ejaculatory duct at the same time that the vas deferens discharge the sperm. It is a common misconception that sperm are stored in the seminal vesicles.

A nerve reflex, associated with the sensation of orgasm, results in the ejaculation of semen, the nerves responding to both physiological and psychological stimuli. A prime example of psychological prompting of this reaction is the discharge of semen during nocturnal emission.

The prostate gland—a structure the size of a chestnut—is just below the bladder and seminal vesicles and surrounds the *urethra,* which is the tube leading from the bladder down through the penis. The urethra carries urine from the bladder or semen from the reproductive organs but never both at the same time, for the passage from the bladder automatically closes when the penis becomes erect. Not all the functions of the prostate are well understood, but this gland is known to secrete a thin, milky, alkaline fluid that neutralizes the medium in which the sperm float. In an acid environment, such as that of the vaginal tract, the sperm could live for only a few minutes.

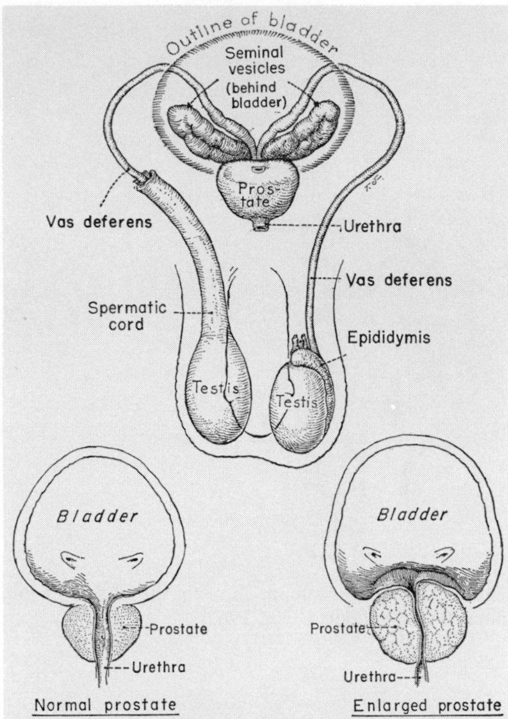

Figure 11–2. Internal genitalia and bladder of the male; prostatic hypertrophy. (From Dowling and Jones: *That the Patient May Know*. Philadelphia, W. B. Saunders Co.)

When the penis is not erect, it is partially covered by a fold of skin called the *foreskin* or *prepuce*. Circumcision is the removal of this foreskin. Among certain groups, circumcision has been customary for many centuries; the Egyptians practiced it even before the Hebrews made it part of their religious customs. Today circumcision is widely performed, regardless of religious preference, both for hygienic reasons and because this minor operation is an important prophylactic measure against cancer of the penis.

An increase in the size of the penis is one of the landmarks of puberty. At maturity, the penis is approximately 2½ to 4 inches long at rest, and about 6 inches long when erect. The size varies widely, but there is no correlation between penis size and body size, nor between penis size and virility, contrary to popular opinion and fraternity house jokes. Inevitably, because of the extremely significant nature of sex and the sex act, a great body of superstition, fear, pride, and humor has grown up around the subject of penis size, virility, and sexual performance, but acceptance of such superstitions by educated men is more a reflection of their

The prostate gland is that part of the male reproductive system most susceptible to disease and loss of function, but such problems almost always are confined to late middle age and old age.

Cowper's glands—each about the size of a pea—are located near the base of the penis. They open into the urethra to discharge a clear, oily lubricant into the seminal fluid. Sometimes, a few drops of this fluid may be discharged from the penis at a time of sexual excitement, not carried to the point of orgasm.

The *penis* is extremely rich in blood vessels, which become engorged to produce erection. The erect penis then can be injected into the vagina to carry the sperm to the ovum. The shaft and head (*glans penis*) of this organ—composed of a cavernous, spongy tissue—not only fill with blood during erection but hold the blood from the body's circulatory system until the semen is discharged or until the erection simply subsides.

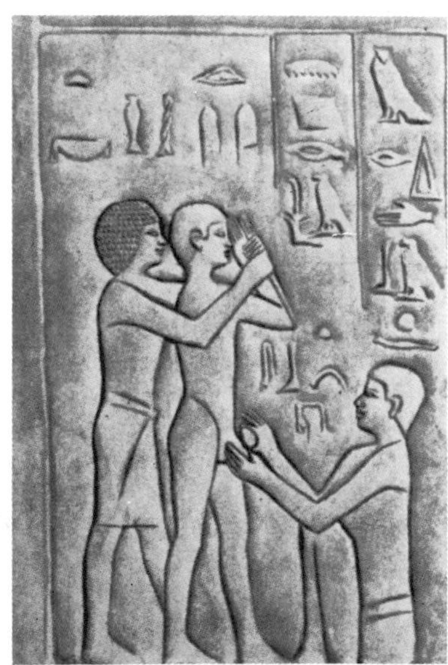

Figure 11–3. *Circumcision.* Mural bas-relief in the tomb of Ankha-Hor, at Sakkara, the most ancient of the pyramids (3000 B.C.) and the oldest structure now in existence. It shows preputiotomy, the early Egyptian variation of circumcision.

bondage to ancient tales and emotional quirks than of their knowledge.

The erection of the penis is the first step in transferring sperm to the ovum. The erection itself results from a parasympathetic nervous action that dilates the arteries of the penis while constricting the veins. Blood under pressure then fills the tissues, causing erection. The second stage involves lubrication of the urethra by the Cowper's glands. The final stage begins during the orgasm as a peristaltic contraction in the testes that spreads quickly to the epididymides and vas deferens. Simultaneously, the seminal vesicles and the prostate gland contract and discharge their secretions. Also, occurring at this time, there is a contraction of some of the muscles of the pelvic area. Finally, about 3.5 ml. (about one teaspoonful) of the liquid semen is discharged. Semen contains, in addition to 300 million to 400 million spermatozoa, the secretions from the seminal vesicles, the prostate glands, and Cowper's glands.

PROBLEMS OF THE REPRODUCTIVE SYSTEM

Male Climacteric. Many men continue to secrete normal quantities of testosterone up to an extremely old age, while others show a decrease in their 40's and 50's. This period, somewhat similar to the menopause in women, may involve "hot flashes," a feeling of suffocation, and psychological disturbances. These symptoms, however, can sometimes be relieved by the administration of testosterone.

Eunuchism and Castration. A male who loses his testes before puberty is called a *eunuch*. Although normal in most respects, such a man may have weaker bones, less muscle mass, underdeveloped sexual organs, and fewer of the other male secondary sex characteristics. If castration (removal or loss of testes) occurs after puberty, some of the secondary sex characteristics may revert to those of a prepubescent child. The sexual organs and voice revert only slightly, however. Sexual desires decrease but may not be totally lost if there has been previous sexual experience. Erection and ejaculation are still possible, although the ability to become a father is lost.

Sterility and Impotence. Sterility and impotence are two separate conditions, unrelated, although many persons confuse them. Men concerned about the possibility of either condition should consult a physician for advice and treatment. Sterility in the male involves a deficiency of normal, motile sperm, for any of several reasons, and therefore is the inability to become a father. Impotence refers to the inability of the male to have an erection, although he may physiologically otherwise have the full potential to become a parent. Impotence may be caused by pathological or endocrine disorders, but usually it is the result of psychological problems. Such problems are amenable to treatment. The male who suffers from impotence, always or occasionally, should not be fearful or despair, but he should realize that this problem has been overcome by many other men through medical or psychotherapeutic help.

Diseases of the Reproductive System. The prostate gland frequently becomes enlarged after 50 years of age, and it may obstruct the urethra and interfere with urination. The cause of this enlargement, or *hypertrophy*, is not well understood.

Cancer of the prostate gland is also frequent in older men. In fact, 2 to 3 per cent of all male deaths are attributed to cancer of the prostate gland. Moreover, among all men autopsied, for any cause of death, 9 per cent have had a malignancy of the prostate.

The testicles are not often affected by illness. They may be involved, however, in the course of mumps, undulant fever, and gonorrhea. The cord that supports them may be invaded by an extension of a hernia, or there may be enlarged veins. The epididymides may also become diseased.

Any swelling, lump, or congestion of the scrotum or testes should be examined by a physician. Also, the skin in and around the scrotum may be infected by ringworm fungus. Keeping these areas clean and dry helps to prevent fungus infections. In addition, the penis can be affected by a number of venereal diseases, the most serious of which is syphilis (see Chapter 8 on venereal diseases).

Questions

1. What are the functions of the testes?
2. Where are the male spermatozoa manufactured?
3. How many sperm are contained in a typical ejaculation? How many are required for conception?
4. What are the secondary male characteristics? What body mechanism triggers development of these characteristics?
5. Describe the purpose and functions of the scrotum.
6. Describe the position, size and function of the epididymides.
7. What is the route of the sperm from the testes to the penis?
8. What other structures contribute to the contents of the semen? Where is each structure located, and what does it do?
9. Physically, what causes an erection?
10. How does the body prevent urine and semen from simultaneously going through the urethra?
11. What is circumcision? Describe some of the reasons for circumcision, aside from the religious aspects.
12. What are the physiological effects of castration before puberty? After puberty?
13. Distinguish between impotence and sterility.
14. Is impotence primarily physiological or psychological? Describe some of the childhood situations and emotional problems that might result in impotence.
15. List some of the disturbances and diseases of the male reproductive system. What measures may be taken to prevent some of them?

Topics for Discussion

Interest in sex at various times of life, including childhood.

Sources of fears and guilt about sexual development.

Need for sex education in primary and secondary schools and in college.

Relationship between genital size and virility.

Reasons for the prominence of fables and jokes about sexual development and practices.

Universal circumcision.

Significance of nocturnal emissions.

Relationship of masturbation to physical and emotional health.

Effects of sex development on personality.

The choice between continence and sexual activity, and the reasons.

Relationship of male personality characteristics to development of sexual characteristics, primary and secondary.

How sexual development may affect scholastic progress.

Reading Suggestions

The Human Body: Its Structure and Operation, Isaac Asimov. Houghton Mifflin, Boston, 1963. A contemporary scientist who is also an outstanding writer offers a clear and well organized presentation at the undergraduate level.

The Machinery of the Body, Anton J. Carlson, Victor Johnson, and H. Mead Cavert. 5th Ed., University of Chicago Press, 1961. How the body works in health and in illness, with considerable information on recent advances in medical knowledge.

Function of the Human Body, Arthur C. Guyton. W. B. Saunders, Philadelphia, 1964. This book includes an authoritative chapter entitled, "Sexual Functions of the Male and Female and the Sex Hormones."

Human Sex Anatomy, Robert L. Dickinson. 2nd Ed., Williams & Wilkins, Baltimore, 1949. This authoritative book is superbly illustrated and discusses the anatomy of the human reproductive systems.

Atlas of Human Anatomy, Franz Frohse, Max Brodel, and Leon Schlossberg. 6th Ed., Barnes & Noble, New York, 1961.

Sense and Nonsense about Sex, Evelyn Millis Duvall and Sylvanus Milne Duvall. Association Press, New York, 1962.

Men: Variety and Meaning of Their Sexual Experience, Aron Krich, ed. Dell Publishing Co., New York, 1960 (paperback).

The Genetic Code, Isaac Asimov. Orion Press, New York, 1963 (also New American Library paperback).

Sex and the Adolescent, Maxine Davis. Dial Press, New York, 1959. Accuracy and frankness are combined in this discussion of many aspects of sexual development and activity.

Attaining Manhood, George W. Corner. Harper, New York, 1952. A physician and anatomist has written this book for boys with questions about sexual development and the process of reproduction.

Sexual Hygiene and Pathology, John F. Oliven. J. B. Lippincott, Philadelphia, 1965.

12

FAMILY PLANNING

Now I would request your kind help in the matter of a birth-control method, which may be 100% effective and noninjurious to health, which may not interfere with the act of coition and the pleasures and benefits to be derived therefrom, and at the same time it must be least expensive so that I may be able to afford it, especially for habitual adoption.

From a letter by a man in Lucknow, India, to the Margaret Sanger Research Bureau, asking for information on birth control.

Nature's methods of ensuring a balance of all forms of life are intricate and marvelous, and many of them still are beyond our understanding. Equally impressive are the ways all varieties of life can reproduce in sufficient numbers to guarantee survival of the species.

Nature is no less generous with humans. Men and women are so constructed that many children may be born to ensure that enough will survive to continue the race. But with his own numbers, as with other aspects of life in which he has interfered, man has created a new problem while solving old ones. For most of history, disease, natural hazards and man's tendency to destroy himself by warfare and accidents has meant that the world's population has risen rather slowly. By the twentieth century, as diseases and other natural hazards began to be controlled, the rise in population became more rapid. In the 1960's, the rate of global annual population growth reached 2 per cent, according to the demographic division of the United Nations. (It was 1 per cent as recently as 1940.) The current population of more than 3 billion will double by the year 2000 at this rate and will double again soon afterward.[1]

The control of the family size is not a new idea; what is new is the magnitude of the problem. Localized areas of the ancient world, such as imperial Rome, had problems of overpopulation, but most of the earth most of the time has been thinly settled. Even so, contraception was practiced in ancient Egypt. One of the oldest written contraceptive recipes dates back to 1550 B.C. The ancient Hebrews and Greeks

[1]For a more detailed discussion of the population problem, see Chapter 31, Community Health, page 442.

knew of and described several birth control techniques, and their knowledge was amplified by the physicians of Arabia and Persia. Pressure for birth control in the United States dates from approximately 1830, and as knowledge increased during the nineteenth century, the movement grew. Today, of course, it is a subject of serious and intense scientific study. Many national governments support birth control studies and dissemination of information. In 1965, when a papal commission of scientists, clergy and laymen was studying birth control, two groups of Nobel Prize winners, 78 distinguished persons altogether, petitioned Pope Paul VI, urging that the Roman Catholic Church change its traditional opposition to birth control.

For the individual family, the question is vital. It is a matter of deciding how many children the parents can provide for adequately and prepare for full participation in a complex and difficult world. Devices, chemical substances, and techniques are now at hand to enable a couple to have the number of children they want, spaced as they wish, according to their beliefs, their desires, and their economic situation.

In 1965, the United States Supreme Court struck down a Connecticut law dating back to 1879 that forbade the use of contraceptive devices or materials, with fines or imprisonment as the penalty. In the majority opinion, Justice Douglas commented, "We deal with a right of privacy older than the Bill of Rights—older than our political parties, older than our school system. Marriage is a coming together for better or for worse, hopefully enduring and intimate to the degree of being sacred." In its decision, the Supreme Court rejected compulsion for or against any method on the grounds of what one denomination holds to be morally right. Its opinion meant that each married couple should have the freedom, within the right of privacy, to choose whether to practice birth control or not.

This chapter is concerned with several methods of birth control, including contraception. Unlike abortion, birth control does not end a life—it prevents a life from being created. One method of birth control—the method approved by the Roman Catholic Church—does not interfere with conception at all. The rhythm method calls for coitus only at times when conception cannot take place. Most other methods are truly contraceptive—that is, at the crucial moment in the long and intricate physiological processes that can culminate in conception, they prevent the male spermatozoon from penetrating the female ovum. One newer method—the oral contraceptive—prevents conception by suppressing the release of eggs by the ovary.

THE RHYTHM METHOD (SAFE PERIOD AND TEMPERATURE METHOD)

The existence of a safe, or sterile, period during a woman's monthly cycle has been the subject of physicians' conjectures and investigations for thousands of years. Based on the current theory that such a safe period does in fact exist, the rhythm method involves these facts in normal physiology:

1. A woman ovulates only once during her menstrual cycle—that is, one egg is released from one ovary and is available for impregnation.[2]
2. Ovulation occurs at a fairly definite time during the cycle—from 14 to 16 days before the *next* menstrual cycle begins.
3. Once released from the ovary, the egg lives for only 24 to 48 hours. Conception can occur only if the egg if fertilized by the male spermatazoon during that time. After this period has passed, conception is impossible until another ovum is released during the next menstrual cycle.
4. The male sperm is capable of fertilizing the female ovum for only about 48 hours, although the sperm may actually remain in motion in the uterus for several days after intercourse.

From these facts, one may conclude that a woman may conceive from intercourse occurring only around the time of ovulation—two or three days before and two or three days after the ovum is discharged from her ovary. Presumably, on all the

[2]For details of the female reproductive system and the menstrual cycle, see Chapter 10, page 121.

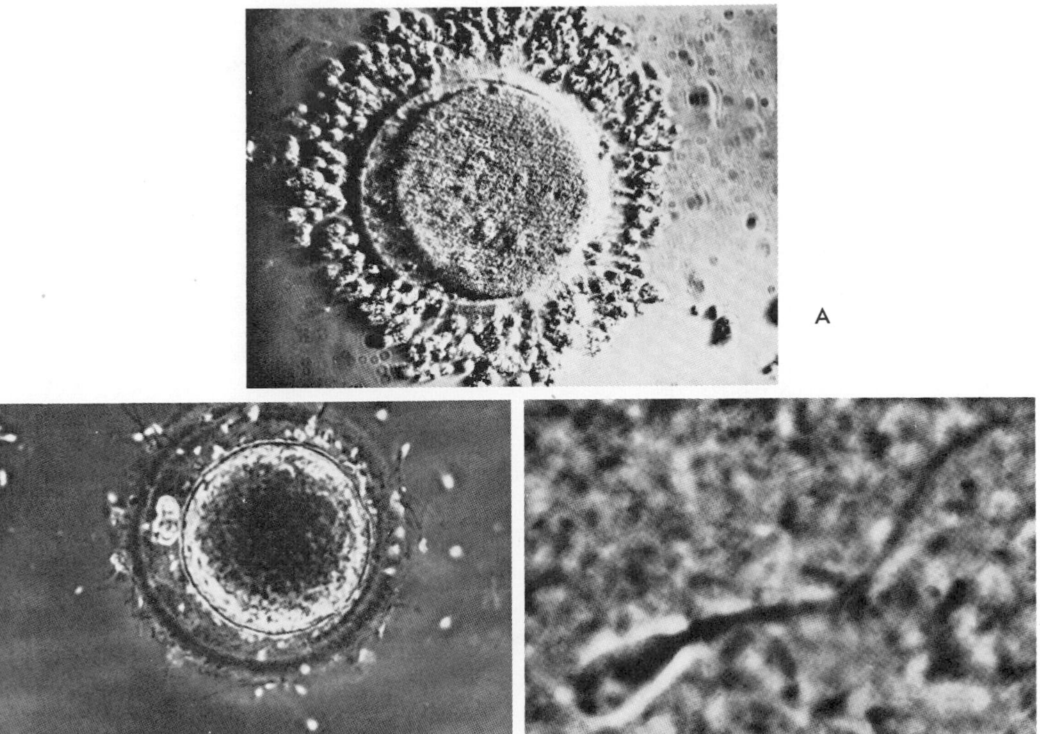

Figure 12–1. Photomicrographs of living human ova and sperm. **A,** The ovum at the time of ovulation. It is surrounded by 3000 to 4000 corona radiata cells, which feed it as it moves along the fallopian tube. **B,** The sperm reach the egg. Several spermatozoa have penetrated the zona pellucida–the outer transparent covering–but only one will reach the nucleus to accomplish fertilization. **C,** The entire sperm is shown penetrating the egg. This photograph is magnified many more times than the others. (Courtesy of Landrum B. Shettles, of Columbia-Presbyterian Medical Center, New York City.)

other days of her cycle, she is infertile and safe from conception. The timing of intercourse *only* during the safe days is the technique of conception avoidance known as the rhythm method.

The advantages of this system of birth control are that it requires no devices or medical preparation, it involves no cost, and it needs little medical supervision (except that in determining the safe period, a physician should be consulted. The major disadvantages are that it depends on a woman's having a dependable, clocklike menstrual cycle (most women do not), and on her (and her husband) maintaining a precise set of calculations.

For practical purposes and as a very rough estimate, a couple may consider that the first third of a woman's menstrual month is relatively safe, the middle third is the fertile (or unsafe) time, and the last third is quite safe from conception. But for more precise control, the following methods of calculation have been suggested.

The Calendar Method. A written record should be made of the menstrual cycle for 12 consecutive months. Day 1 of the cycle is the first day of menstruation, and the day before the next menstruation starts is the last day. Determine the number of days in the shortest and in the longest of the 12 cycles. Subtract 18 from the number of days in the shortest cycle; this establishes the first fertile day. Given a 26-day

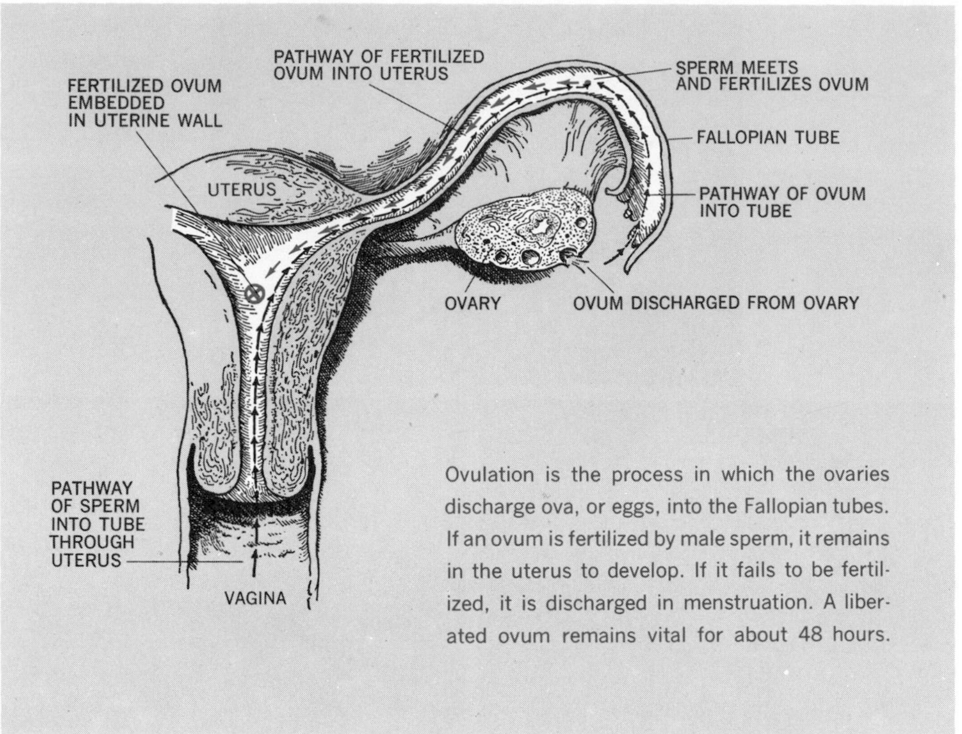

Ovulation is the process in which the ovaries discharge ova, or eggs, into the Fallopian tubes. If an ovum is fertilized by male sperm, it remains in the uterus to develop. If it fails to be fertilized, it is discharged in menstruation. A liberated ovum remains vital for about 48 hours.

short cycle, day 8 would be the first fertile day. Subtract 11 from the number of days in the longest cycle; this establishes the last fertile day, or the end of the period during which it is unsafe to have intercourse. Given a 30-day cycle, day 19 would be the last fertile day. Therefore, in this instance, days 8 through 19 would be fertile, or unsafe for coitus.

This calendar should be maintained indefinitely, so that a record of the 12 most recent cycles is always available. Women whose periods are highly irregular should not use this system (even though it takes irregularities into account) without consulting a physician skilled in advising on the rhythm method. This is so because menstruation is not a simple mechanical function but is easily affected by many other conditions, including the general state of health, tensions, and the woman's emotional tone.

Special slide rules, clocks, and other devices for timing the cycle have recently come on the market, but the crucial element in a rigorous observation of the menstrual calendar is the woman's own caution and accuracy in recording the events of her period.

The Temperature Method. Whatever a woman's normal temperature, a small but measurable increase occurs monthly during the time of ovulation, following a brief, small decrease. Her body temperature then stays at the higher level until the next menstruation begins. By recording these changes carefully every day, a woman may determine when the egg is released from the ovary and thus know approximately when she should and should not have intercourse. A special thermometer, measuring only temperatures from 96° to 100° F., with widely spaced graduations of one-tenth of a Fahrenheit degree, may be used. The woman's temperature should be taken rectally in bed, before she is involved in any activity, even talking. At this time, the body temperature is at its lowest; it is known at this point as the basal body temperature (BBT).

A woman using this system should make an accurate daily record of her BBT for at least three months, so that a recognizable pattern becomes apparent. Figure 12–1 shows a typical temperature chart, with the characteristic increase during ovulation, lasting until the cycle begins again. Again, because menstrual cycles tend to vary and

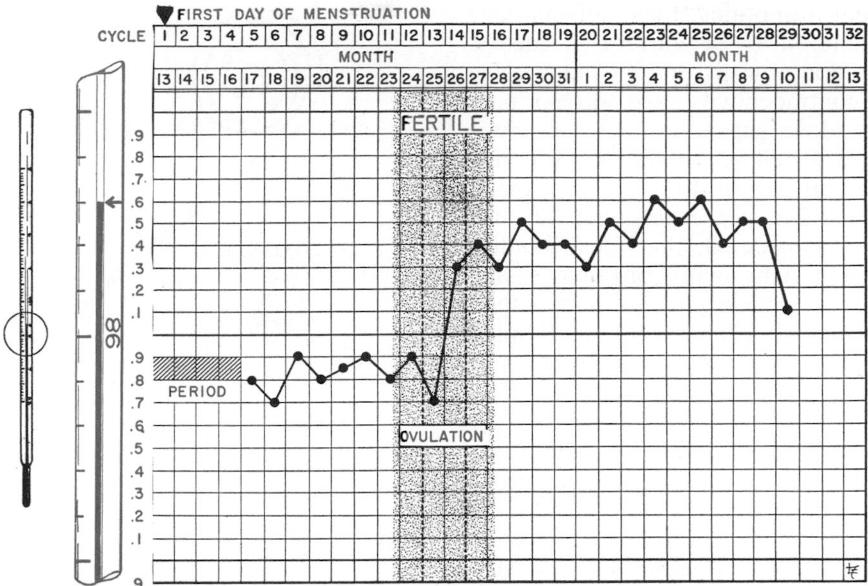

Figure 12–2. Temperature method for determining ovulation.

because many factors can cause slight changes in body temperature, this method should be used only with a physician's guidance.

The Intermenstrual (Mittelschmerz) Method. For some women, probably a minority, ovulation is accompanied by cramplike feelings in the lower abdomen and possibly spotty bleeding. If such reactions occur regularly midway during the menstrual cycle, they may constitute a rough gauge of the ovulation time. Even women who have these sensations regularly should nevertheless use the calendar, thermometer, or both, if they are going to depend on the rhythm method for avoiding conception.

CONTRACEPTIVE METHODS

For Women. The *oral contraceptive tablet,* or "the pill," represents a new approach to contraception. While the older methods depend on preventing the sperm and egg from meeting at coitus, the contraceptive pill is a means of preventing ovulation, thus making conception impossible. The oral contraceptive became possible when scientists learned the relationship of certain chemicals called *progestins* to the secretion of the female hormone *progesterone* by the pituitary gland. Progestin suppresses the activity of the pituitary gland in the release of a hormone which regulates growth and discharge of ova from the ovaries. At the same time, progesterone release, which inhibits the normal pattern of follicle growth and development, is stimulated in the pituitary gland. This contraceptive is a powerful synthetic substance that is very close to 100 per cent effective, if used exactly according to instructions.

The tablets must be taken daily for 20 consecutive days, starting on the fifth day of the menstrual cycle. One to three days after the last tablet is taken, menstruation begins and the count is started again. The first tablet must always be taken on schedule, and no day may be missed. Once the tablets are discontinued, pregnancy again becomes possible.

Some women have experienced side effects from these tablets, but none of these effects have been reported as dangerous. The side effects include nausea, fluid retention, changes in the menstrual cycle (actually "regulatory" changes), or intermenstrual bleeding. During the decade it has taken for this pill to be approved for use by medical and government authorities, these effects have been countered by a variety of means. However, it is obvious that a woman using an oral contraceptive must do so only under the close supervision of her physician, who will tell her of the possible side effects and be prepared to deal with them.

The use of a *diaphragm and jelly* (or cream) is considered the ideal contraceptive method by many physicians, and it is the most frequently prescribed method in birth-control clinics in the United States. The diaphragm, made of soft rubber and resembling a ball cut in half, is designed to lie diagonally across the vaginal canal. It then closes off the upper part of the vagina, including the opening to the uterus. The woman applies a spermicidal jelly or cream to both surfaces of the diaphragm before inserting it. The diaphragm then constitutes an effective mechanical and chemical barrier to the male sperm. Vaginal diaphragms are made in many sizes, and they differ in the type and thickness of the rubber and in the thickness and tension of the rim. A woman who prefers this method of birth control should be fitted by her physician, and she should be rechecked for size every few years.

Next in value to the diaphragm-and-jelly method is the use of the *cervical cap.* This device may be made of soft or hard rubber, plastic or metal. It is designed to fit snugly and directly over the cervix. Like the diaphragm, the cap also should be used in combination with a jelly or cream that will chemically attack the sperm. A physician should advise the woman on the size and type of cervical cap she should use and carefully help her learn to insert it. While this method is similar to that of the diaphragm, the use of the cervical cap is less common because it is more difficult to insert correctly.

About 40 years ago, a German physician developed an *intrauterine contraceptive device,* which, after considerable modification, has recently received limited but growing acceptance in the United States. Generally, this device consists of a stem, button, ring, or star-shaped piece of hard rubber, plastic, or metal. It is designed for placement in the uterus, where it prevents pregnancy by keeping the fertilized egg from embedding itself in the uterine wall.

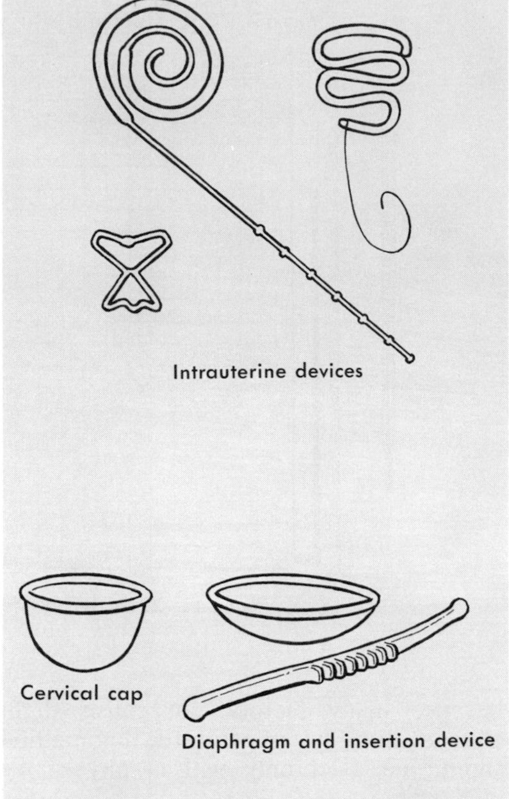

Figure 12–3. Contraceptive devices.

The early intrauterine devices were uncomfortable or dangerous, or both. Constituting a foreign object in the body, they sometimes caused bleeding and abdominal pain. Furthermore, they could slip out without the woman knowing it. Their final danger was that if pregnancy took place even with the device in place, the effect of the object was unpredictable.

Recently, new synthetic materials that are better tolerated by the body have been developed. Intrauterine devices constructed of these materials can be left in place for months or years and are causing new interest. The use of intrauterine devices is now becoming much more widely accepted in this country and elsewhere. In addition to the previously noted problems they may present, however, they are also under close scrutiny as possible causes of cancer. Most physicians feel that not enough experience has been gathered or reported and that great caution should be exercised in the use of the intrauterine devices. Although they hold great promise and are cheap and easy to use, they must still be considered experimental. A physician may suggest their use, but only with a full explanation of their limitations.

Douching, one of the oldest popular methods of contraception, consists of flushing the vaginal area as soon as possible after intercourse. Either plain water (at body temperature) or water plus a spermicide may be used. Douching is the least effective of all contraceptive methods, and it has the added disadvantage that the woman must use it *immediately* after intercourse if it is to accomplish anything at all. It has a special appeal to overly fastidious women for whom the cleansing action is important, but its efficacy in removing sperm (which may arrive at the cervix within 90 seconds after climax) is dubious.

For Men. The most common, and by far the most effective male device, is the *condom*—a soft, thin tube of rubber designed to fit over the erect penis and to contain the sperm. It is harmless, simple to use, and, assuming that it is manufactured without defects, reliable and effective. Action in recent years by the Federal Food and Drug Administration has had a good effect on manufacturers, most of whom now select condom material carefully and test the sheaths before distributing them. Breakage or leakage during intercourse is less likely than it was before manufacturing procedures were improved, but some men still take the additional precaution of placing a bit of contraceptive jelly or cream in the tip.

Many married couples prefer the use of the condom to any other device, especially if the woman finds the diaphragm-and-jelly method cumbersome or unpleasant. Some men object to it, however, on the ground that it diminishes the sensations of intercourse. Of course, it also takes control of the situation away from the woman, who must carry the burdens of childbearing in case of an accident.

A variation on the standard condom is the short type that covers the tip of the penis only. It is much less commonly used, primarily because it is too easily dislodged.

Another birth control practice is *withdrawal* or *coitus interruptus.* In this method, the man withdraws his penis from his partner just prior to ejaculation. It is a method reported in the Bible, used in ancient times in many parts of the world, and still practiced extensively. It requires no apparatus, no chemicals, is always available, and is free. Its one disadvantage is so great, though, that most young men in America are not likely to consider it. The sudden interruption of the sex act, precisely at the moment of climax, is unnatural. It can lead to emotional disturbances and to such physiological complications as congestion of the genital organs. For the woman, this sudden interruption also is disturbing and unsatisfactory, and her own sexual responses are upset.

Finally, it is not quite so safe as it sounds. A delay of even a fraction of a second may leave enough sperm deposited in the vaginal tract to result in conception, even though the man thinks he has withdrawn in time. All in all, in spite of its historical record, *coitus interruptus* is not likely to be recommended by a physician or birth control specialist today.

For maximal safety—when, for example, pregnancy would constitute a serious threat to health or life—couples whose religious convictions do not prohibit contraception should use a combined technique, the male partner employing the condom, the female using the diaphragm, intrauterine device, or contraceptive pills. Also, intercourse should be performed only during the non-fertile period. This combined method reduces the chances of conception to less than one in a million.

Other birth control techniques, devices, and preparations exist, but those described in this chapter are the most common. Clearly, every family must make its own decision about which, if any, method to use. Young couples who have decided to limit and space their family should not make a hasty decision but should discuss the subject with their physician or with a qualified person at a birth control or family planning agency. (Most large cities and several smaller ones offer such services.) Some experimentation probably will be in order, that both husband and wife may learn what is most comfortable, convenient, and acceptable to them. Like all other important aspects of a happy marriage, the details of a subject as intimate as this require time to be worked out to the satisfaction of both partners. They are certain to find that the effort has been worth while.

Questions

1. What is the current worldwide rate of population increase?
2. At that rate, barring catastrophes, what will the population be in the year 2000? In the year 2050?
3. What are some of the problems raised by great increases in population?
4. Why should the size of the family be limited?
5. What is the physiological basis of the rhythm method?
6. What are a woman's "safe days?" In what ways may they be determined?
7. How does the rhythm method of birth control differ basically from contraceptive methods?
8. Describe the changes in body temperature during a woman's menstrual cycle. What do these changes tell her about her fertility?
9. How long does the female egg remain alive to accept sperm for conception?
10. How long does the male sperm remain able to impregnate the egg and bring about conception?
11. What are the limitations of the rhythm method so far as reliability is concerned? Comment on the effectiveness of this system versus methods of contraception.
12. What does the oral contraceptive do in the body to prevent a woman from becoming pregnant?
13. What are some of the side effects of "the pill?" Are these side effects considered dangerous?
14. Why is the diaphragm-and-jelly method most frequently prescribed by birth control clinics?
15. Describe some of the drawbacks of using the intrauterine device.
16. What would you recommend as the one "best" contraceptive, assuming equal protection?
17. Would you prefer that you or that your partner take precautions to space your family? Why?
18. What do you consider to be desirable properties (in addition to effectiveness) of a contraceptive that may be recommended worldwide? Remember that, in many places, educational, social, and economic circumstances are limited.
19. Are there any elements in the question of birth control you consider too private to discuss with a physician? What are they, and why are they too personal?
20. How would you discuss birth control with children of your own, if they ask questions about sexual activity?

Topics For Discussion

Magnitude of the problem of overpopulation.

Everyday problems of living in an overcrowded world.

The right of government to study birth control, disseminate information, and encourage contraception.

Birth control as a religious issue and as a question of social policy.

Whether one religious denomination should seek to impose its moral views on other people.

The moral question of contraception—preventing a life from being created.

Surgery (sterilization) as a method of birth control.

The possibility of enforced birth control by government edict in an overcrowded world.

Countries in which a stable population has been achieved through official encouragement of contraception.

Reading Suggestions

Overpopulation.

Reading suggestions on the problem of overpopulation appear at the end of Chapter 31, Community Health, p. 473.

Birth Control.

Medical History of Contraception, Norman E. Himes. Gamut Press, New York, 1963.

The Control of Fertility, Gregory Pincus. Academic Press, New York, 1965. A technical study, including detailed accounts of animal studies and clinical examinations of men and women.

Science and the Safe Period, C. G. Hartman. Williams & Wilkins, Baltimore, 1962.

Human Reproduction and Sex Behavior, C. W. Lloyd. Lea and Febiger, Philadelphia, 1964.

Planned Parenthood, Abraham Stone and Norman E. Himes. Collier Books, New York, 1965 (paperback). Not only a practical guide to birth control methods, but a historical review of birth control and a careful consideration of its social and legal aspects. Also includes a listing of planned parenthood and family planning services in the United States and abroad.

Birth Control and Catholic Doctrine, Alvah W. Fulloway. The Beacon Press, Boston, 1959.

Jewish Medical Ethics, Immanuel Jacobovits. Bloch Publishing Co., New York, 1959.

Morals and Medicine, Joseph Fletcher, Princeton University Press, Princeton, N.J., 1954.

The Consumers Union Report on Family Planning, Alan F. Guttmacher and the editors of Consumers Union. Mount Vernon, N. Y., 1962. Presented in clear and understandable style, an account and illustrations of contraceptive methods and devices, as well as a section on improving fertility.

Babies by Choice or by Chance. Alan F. Guttmacher.

Doubleday, New York, 1959. Formerly obstetrician and gynecologist-in-chief at Mount Sinai Hospital, New York, and now president of the Planned Parenthood Federation of America, Dr. Guttmacher has written and spoken extensively on family planning and birth control. This book is an excellent presentation of his special subject.

The Complete Book of Birth Control, Alan F. Guttmacher. Ballantine Books, New York, 1961. A full description of the acceptable techniques of birth control.

Modern Science and the Human Fertility Problem, Richard L. Meier. Wiley, New York, 1959. The major premise of this book is that, except for war, population growth is the greatest single deterrent to improvement in living standards, especially in the poorer nations. The author examines new possibilities for controlling fertility and their potential social and economic impact.

Research in Family Planning, Clyde V. Kiser, ed. Princeton University Press, Princeton, N.J., 1962. A compilation of papers on the subject from many countries: a good review of international activity in research, data collection, and problems of popular acceptance of birth control information and services.

Contraception: A History of its Treatment by the Catholic Church Theologians and Canonists, John T. Noonan, Jr. Harvard University Press, Cambridge, Mass., 1965.

Why Americans Must Limit Their Families, Margaret Mead. Redbook, August 1963.

Is "The Pill" the Answer? Kenneth N. Anderson. Today's Health, June 1965.

Ultimate Failure of Rhythm, G. Hardin. Science, Vol. 143, 1964.

Catholics, Birth Control, and Public Policy, Robert F. Drinan, S. J., U. S. Catholic, May 1965.

The Court and Birth Control: a Decision for Privacy, William B. Ball. Commonweal, July 9, 1965.

Bustle About Birth Control, editorial, New Scientist, July 1, 1965.

13

PREGNANCY AND CHILDBIRTH

Most married couples want and expect to have children, and bigger families are again in style. A tremendous upsurge in the number of births started after the end of World War II, with a sharp rise in the number of families having their first child. This has levelled off, but more and more families are having their second, third, fourth, and even fifth child.

Pregnancy is safer than ever before in history. If the downward trend in maternal deaths and the upward trend in automobile accidents continue, pregnancy will soon be less dangerous than crossing the street! In 1915, 61 women died for every 10,000 live births in this country, but by 1962 there were only 3.4 deaths per 10,000 births. This greatly improved situation can be ascribed chiefly to good prenatal care, more births attended by qualified physicians, and control of infections by better antisepsis, sulfa drugs, and antibiotics. Advances in maternal nutrition, obstetrical surgery and anesthesia have also added their part.

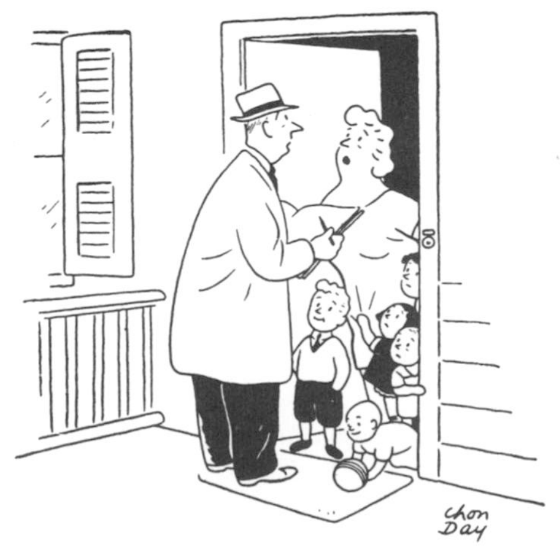

"Occupation?"
"Woman."

(Drawing by Chon Day, Copr. © 1948. The New Yorker Magazine, Inc.)

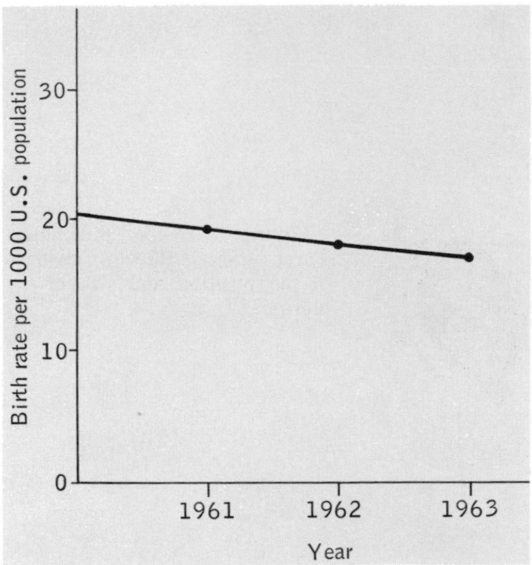

Figure 13–1. The birth rate in the United States rose steadily until 1960 and has since decreased slightly year by year. However, as Figure 13–2 shows, the maternal death rate has dropped sharply.

CONCEPTION AND THE COURSE OF PREGNANCY

Conception, the act of becoming pregnant, has all the ingredients of an exciting drama, carried out on a microscopic scale. During sexual intercourse, the male instills about a teaspoonful of semen into the vagina of his mate, containing 300 million to 400 million spermatozoa. Any one of these millions has the power to fertilize the egg cell of the woman, but only one actually does so.

The spermatozoa face their first hazard in the vagina, whose acid secretion kills millions. However, many escape and swim up through the vagina, propelled by their whiplike tails. Those with sufficient energy proceed through the cervical canal into the womb, and on into the fallopian tubes.

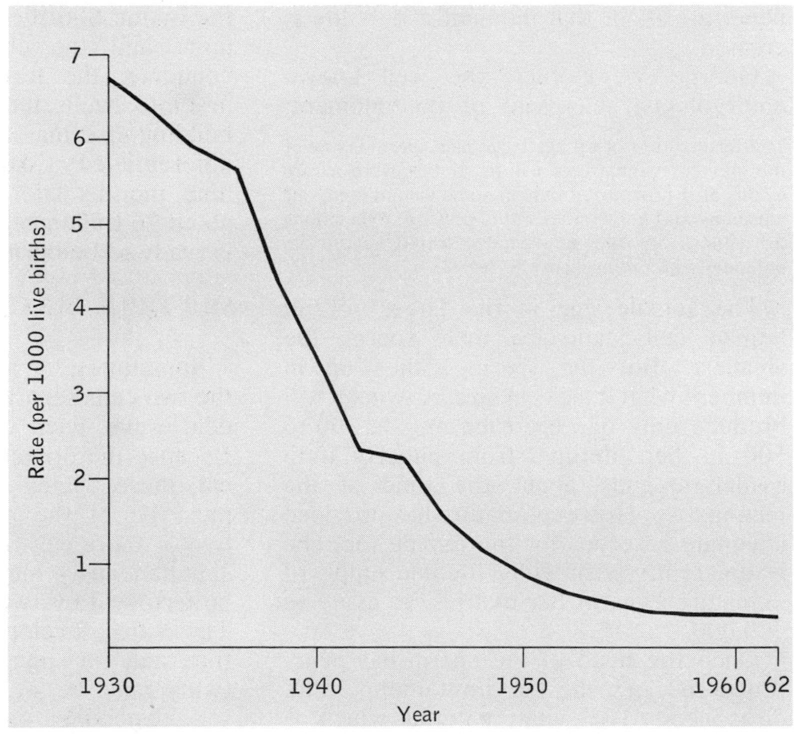

Figure 13–2. The effectiveness of new medical techniques and new drugs is reflected by the sharply declining mortality rate among mothers of newborn children during the past 32 years.

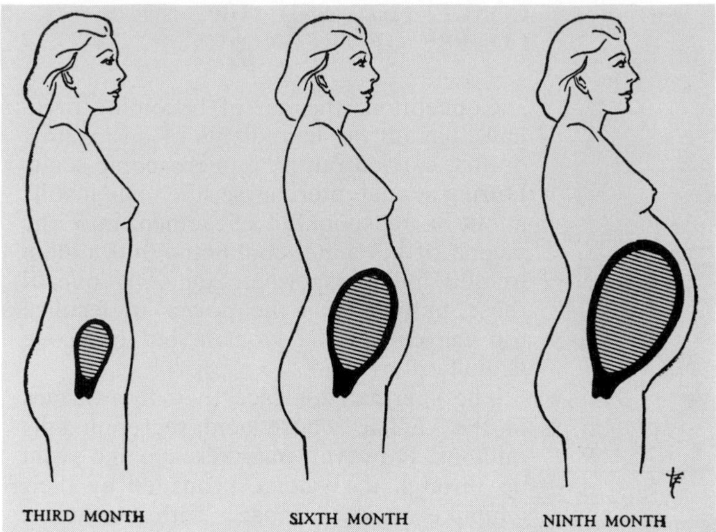

Figure 13–3. Pregnancy. Three stages, showing changes in the position and size of the uterus.

In one of these two tubes, an egg cell may be waiting if the female has ovulated. There is only a short period, no more than two days, when this egg cell, or *ovum,* is in the right place and in the right condition to be fertilized. Sperm can retain their potency for only about 48 hours within the woman's reproductive tract. But if all goes well, a sperm will reach the ovum and penetrate it; in that moment a new life is created.

George W. Corner, the well known embryologist, has said of this moment:

> The fertilization of an egg by a male sperm is one of the greatest wonders of nature. If this were a rare event, or if it occurred only in some distant land, our museums and universities would organize expeditions to witness it, and newspapers would record its outcome with enthusiasm.

The female egg is the largest of all human cells, and the male sperm, the smallest. But the sperm makes up in numbers what it lacks in size. A woman will produce only one egg each month, 300 to 500 in her lifetime, from puberty until ovulation ends about the time of the menopause. However, nature has provided adequate reserves for the female too: she is apparently born with a lifetime supply of immature eggs in her ovaries, as many as 400,000.

Once the head of the sperm has penetrated the egg, the tail, now unimportant, disappears. The vital material which is the father's contribution to the heredity of the offspring is in the forepart of the sperm. The moment a particular sperm has fertilized a particular egg, all the characteristics a child can inherit are determined. Whether the baby will be a blond or a brunet, or whether its eyes will be blue or brown, is settled. Whether it will be a boy or a girl is settled, too, because the sex is determined by whether a sperm with an X or a Y chromosome fertilizes the ovum. Shortly after the egg and sperm unite and the chromosome number is complete, the fertilized egg will divide, first into 2 cells, then 4, 8, 16, 32, and so on, building up a mass of cells and, eventually, differentiated tissues and organs, until nine months later, a baby composed of about 26 trillion cells (26,000,000,000,000) is ready to be born.

MULTIPLE BIRTHS

Sometimes, at the very first division, the two cells separate and go their independent ways, each developing into a baby. Because the original two cells were identical, these babies are identical twins and must be of the same sex. Occasionally two or more eggs mature and are released simultaneously into the fallopian tube, to be fertilized by two or more spermatozoa. These also develop independently, but into fraternal, or nonidentical twins. These twins may be of the same or opposite sex, depending on which type of sperm fertilized the eggs, and they are no more alike than any other brother-brother,

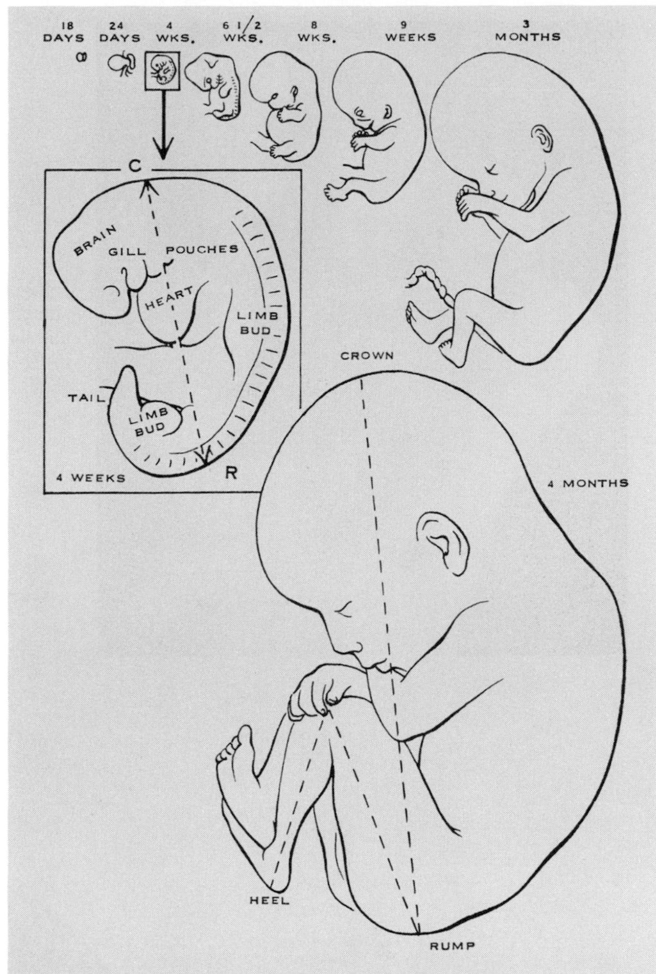

Figure 13–4. The development of body form. (From Martin, P. C., and Vincent, E. L.: *Human Development*. New York, Ronald Press, 1960.)

sister-sister, or brother-sister pair. About one birth in 80 in the United States produces twins, and 20 to 25 per cent of these are identical. This means that there are 1½ million pairs of twins, of which more than ⅓ million are identical.

Triplets occur about once in every 6000 to 7000 births: they can be identical, completely different, or a pair of identical twins from one egg, and a fraternal twin from another. Once in about 500,000 births, quadruplets develop.

The Dionne quintuplets, born in 1934, represented a rare event in medical history, that occurs once in every 50 to 60 million pregnancies. The birth of quintuplets is believed to have happened not more than 60 times in the last 500 years, and in all cases the babies died soon after birth. All five of the Dionne quintuplets survived and grew to adulthood.

DEVELOPMENT OF THE EMBRYO

Soon after the moment of fertilization, the egg cell begins to divide. Five to ten days later, the tiny embryo travels to the wall of the uterus, where it settles. A cover forms over it so that it is attached to the wall of the uterus in a protected, completely enclosed pocket, and at this stage it begins to grow rapidly.

Tests for Pregnancy

The best known sign of pregnancy is a missed menstrual period. However, menstruation is sometimes delayed or absent for reasons other than pregnancy, and in rare instances women menstruate for several months after conception.

Frequently the first clue to pregnancy

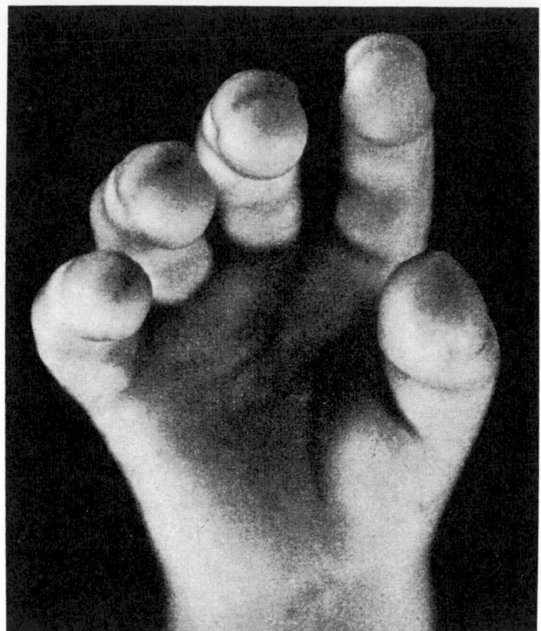

Figure 13–5. Hand plate and fingers in an attitude similar to that in shaking hands. Embryo approximately 46.5 mm. (From Blechschmidt: *The Stages of Human Development Before Birth.* Philadelphia, W. B. Saunders Co., 1961.)

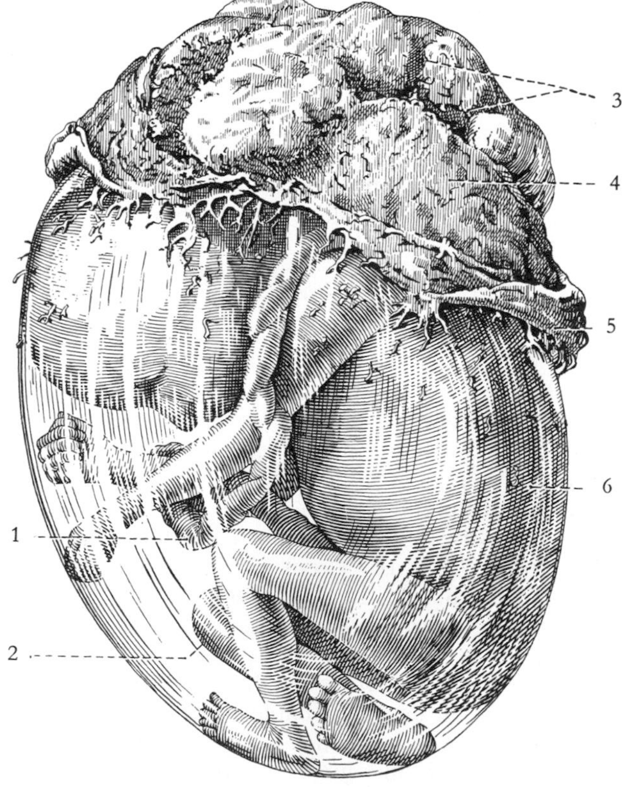

Figure 13–6. Fetus with its membranes (approximately 21 cm. crown-rump length). (From Blechschmidt: *The Stages of Human Development Before Birth.* Philadelphia, W. B. Saunders Co., 1961.)

comes when the breasts enlarge, the nipples become fuller or pigmented, and tiny new blood vessels form on the breasts. This may cause sensations of tingling and fullness. An experienced doctor can tell a great deal by examining the breasts.

At about the tenth week, his examination will enable him to detect pregnancy with a fair degree of accuracy. By pressing the abdomen in the proper place he can feel the slight enlargement caused by the swollen uterus. The tissues at the entrance to the vagina have a bluish hue, and if the fingers are inserted into the vagina, the cervix, or mouth of the womb, can be felt, definitely softer than it was in the nonpregnant state.

At the middle of the fourth or the beginning of the fifth month, x-ray will reveal the baby's bones; its movements can be felt, and its heart beat detected.

A very reliable laboratory test is the A-Z, or Aschheim-Zondek, test, named after the two German doctors who developed it. In this test, a small amount of urine voided by a woman in the morning is injected into a mouse or rabbit. If the woman is pregnant, changes will take place in the animal's ovaries. A similar, more recently devised test is carried out on a particular type of toad. If the woman is pregnant, the toad will put out a large number of spermatozoa within a few hours. This is faster and usually less expensive than those in which a mouse or rabbit must be sacrificed. However, it is also less reliable: false results are obtained at certain times of the year when the toad is insensitive to the hormones excreted in the urine. Also, tranquilizers, and perhaps other drugs, affect the results.

Prenatal Care and Activities

Until only a generation ago, many women had their babies with the help of only a female relative or a midwife. When they started using physicians, they would choose the doctor they wanted to handle the confinement, and that was usually the last the doctor and the patient saw of one another until the baby arrived. Unless something went wrong, a woman would not visit the doctor during her pregnancy.

One of the chief reasons things seldom go wrong today is that the doctor sees the patient frequently from the earliest stage of her pregnancy. *He knows her physical condition and can detect even the slightest indication of a complication.* This, together with his knowledge of how to handle such problems, accounts for the present safety and ease of pregnancy and childbirth. Even during a normal, uncomplicated pregnancy, a doctor's advice is invaluable to the mother. He supervises her diet, the amount and kind of activity she can engage in, and many other aspects of her day-to-day life. In addition, he can alleviate most of the discomforts that might otherwise plague a pregnant woman.

In general, the obstetrician is preferable to the general practitioner because of his specialization and greater experience. However, the choice is sometimes determined by what is available. The obstetric specialist is more likely to have his practice in larger communities. In small cities and rural areas, the general practitioner frequently handles prenatal care and deliveries as well as all other medical problems.

There is little the pregnant woman needs to do specifically for her baby. Taking care of herself is the best way to look out for him. Her thoughts, activities or dietary cravings will not alter his mental or physical characteristics. And visiting museums or attending concerts will not increase the chance of her having an artistic or musical child. Similarly, a craving, fright or emotional experience during pregnancy will not mark a child in any way. The little boy next door did *not* get his buck teeth because his mother was frightened by a horse, and the mole on his sister's back is *not* due to his mother's having had a craving for strawberries. The baby is growing in a protected, warm, comfortable, buoyant fluid, and is probably safer than he will ever again be in life.

Mothers worry a good deal about bumping their abdomens and endangering their babies' development. It is amazing how much direct abdominal pressure the baby and pregnant mother can tolerate without ill effects.

Louis F. Middlebrook, Director of the Department of Obstetrics and Gynecology of the Hartford, Connecticut, General Hospital, has described several unusual examples of this: a woman in her seventh month of pregnancy was in a severe automobile accident during which she was thrown from the car for a distance of 20 feet, and landed on a curb, striking her head and pregnant abdomen. She was taken to the hospital in critical condition, and hovered between life and death because of a severe head injury. Eventually, she made a complete recovery, and had a normal baby at full term. Another of Middlebrook's patients attended a costume ball, where she met a playful friend, disguised as a baseball player. Not knowing she was pregnant, and thinking she had stuffed a pillow under her clothing, he swung at her abdomen with a baseball bat! Nevertheless, she, too, had a normal and uneventful delivery.[1]

Pregnant women today have been freed from most of the onerous restrictions placed on them by their fears (and sometimes by their physicians) a generation or two ago. Today, she can dress attractively and comfortably during her nine months of waiting. The only rule is that her clothing should not be too tight or uncomfortable.

There are no restrictions on showering or bathing, although tub baths may present a danger from falls. Neither cigarettes nor alcohol – in moderation – is forbidden, and sexual intercourse is generally not discouraged until the last few weeks.

Pregnancy, instead of being a boring time full of real or imaginary indispositions, can be a time during which a woman may develop new skills or catch up on those she had to abandon after marriage because she was too busy. Sewing, painting, playing a musical instrument, experimenting with new recipes are all ideal during these nine months. Many women wish to continue working during pregnancy, and with her physician's permission the expectant mother may certainly do so. She will find in most places of employment, especially if she was on the payroll before she became pregnant, that there is no opposition to her continuing

[1]Middlebrook, L.F.: *Amicus Curiae,* November 1957.

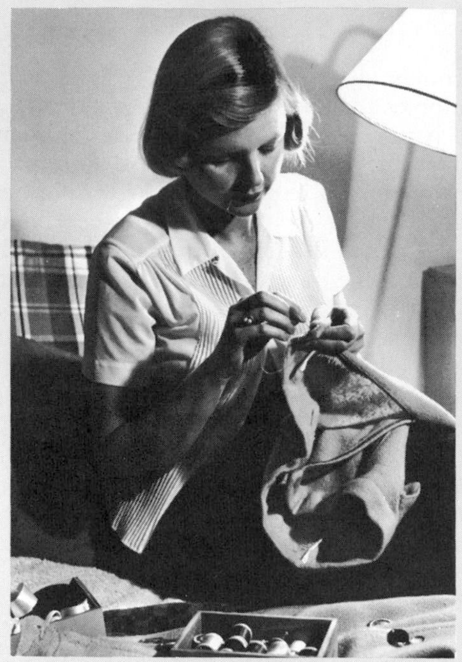

Sewing clothes for herself or the new baby is one of the rewarding activities with which the expectant mother can occupy herself without overtaxing her strength.

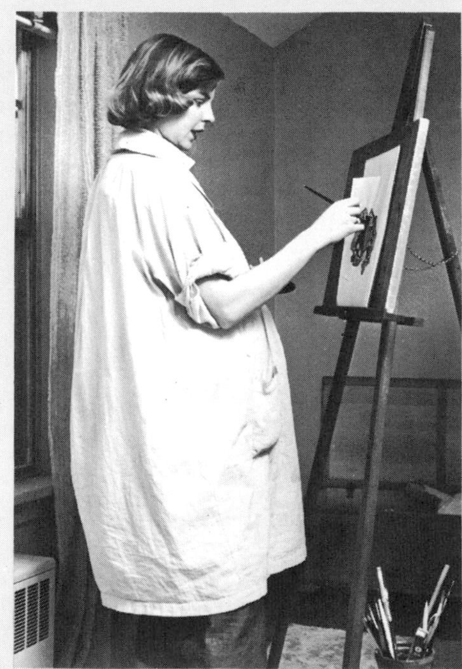

Pregnant women should keep themselves busy. Many find that pregnancy gives them time for hobbies, like painting, for which they were too busy before.

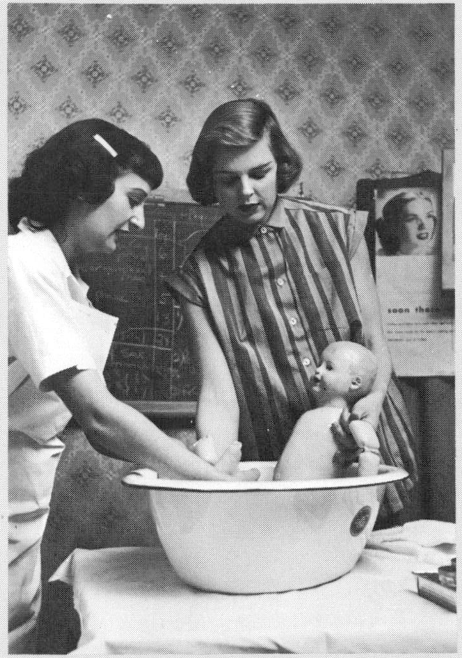

During pregnancy, the future mother should prepare to care for her child by learning from qualified people to perform such tasks as bathing the baby.

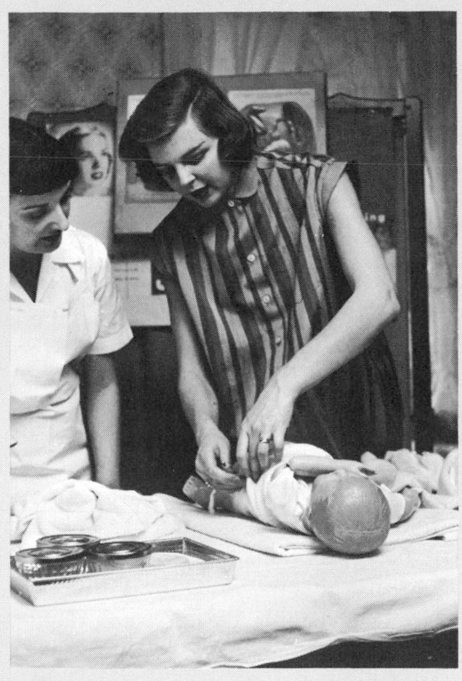

Changing the baby's diaper is a task that a mother performs frequently. It is advisable that she should know how to do it before the baby is born.

work, perhaps as far as the sixth or seventh month.

Discomforts and Dangers During Pregnancy

Pregnancy is a perfectly normal process, and a woman's body has been beautifully designed to incubate a baby and support its growth from the time it is a single, fertilized cell until the child is ready to be born.

The majority of women feel extremely well when they are pregnant. Many drive and take long motor trips, and engage in even quite strenuous sports. However, a woman's body is bound to undergo profound changes during this period. The center of gravity shifts—with the concentration of weight in the abdominal area—and this may cause more fatigue than usual, and some discomfort because of pressure on other organs. However, many obstetricians feel that most discomforts of pregnancy have their origin in old wives' tales. According to Howard P. Taylor, a Cleveland obstetrician, the widespread belief that *morning sickness* is natural and inevitable actually accounts for its developing in many cases. Friends and relatives enter into the plot, encouraging the pregnant woman to suffer from the classic symptoms of nausea and vomiting as soon as possible, so that she can feel miserable and "truly pregnant."

Infectious Diseases. Any serious disease or complication of pregnancy and childbirth is dangerous to the baby and the mother. However, there is one disease, *German measles,* which scarcely disturbs the mother but can seriously affect the unborn child, especially if the infection develops during the first three months of pregnancy. From 25 to 50 per cent of babies whose mothers had German measles early in pregnancy are born with an abnormality, such as cataracts, deaf-mutism, heart disease or mental retardation. *It is very desirable for girl children to be exposed to German measles* because contracting the disease usually provides a lifelong protection against reinfection.

The venereal diseases, syphilis and gonorrhea, are also very dangerous to

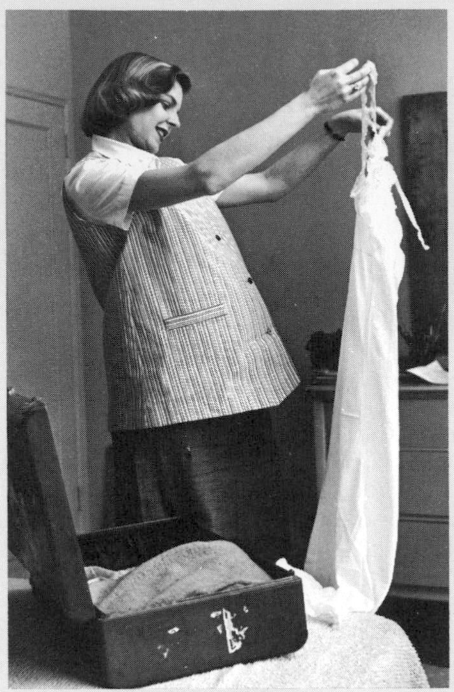

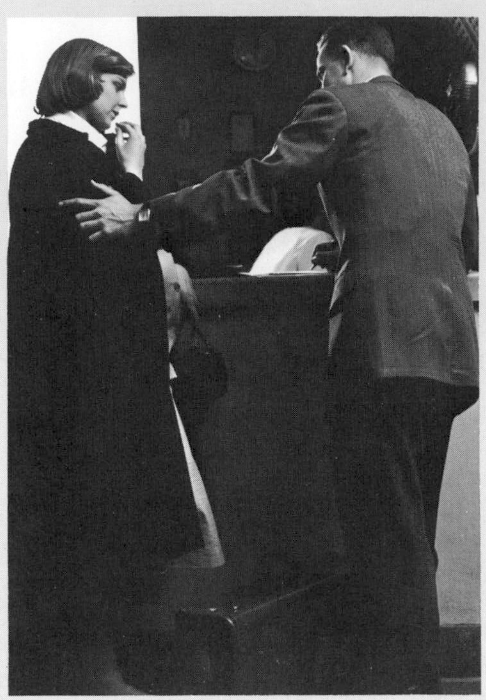

The expectant mother's two last tasks are packing the clothing she will need in the hospital after delivering her baby, left, and arriving at the hospital. It is important that she should not wait too long after labor begins before leaving for the hospital so that she has time to check in comfortably.

the baby. Unless they are treated while the disease is in its earliest stages, nearly half the women with syphilis deliver stillborn or infected babies. The babies that do survive are apt to be physically or mentally defective. *Gonorrhea* is less hazardous to the unborn child, but inflicts its damage when the baby is actually being born, while it is passing through the birth canal. If the germs responsible for gonorrhea get into the infant's eyes, they may cause blindness. The routine use of silver nitrate in the eyes of all newborn babies has prevented this disaster in most hospitals and home deliveries.

Studies made by Mila E. Rindge of the Connecticut Department of Health indicate that pregnant women are more susceptible to *polio* than nonpregnant women of the same age. This makes adequate vaccination against polio doubly imperative before pregnancy—and doubly advantageous, because the immunity against polio is also passed on to the unborn child. The higher the level of protection given prospective mothers, the greater and longer lasting is the protection for their infants.

The Rh Factor. Newborn babies face a risk if the mother happens to be Rh-negative and the father Rh-positive. A certain substance is present in the blood of about 85 per cent of all white people, and they are called Rh-positive; the 15 per cent who lack it are Rh-negative. (The percentage differs in dark-skinned races.) No problems result unless the mother is Rh-negative and the father Rh-positive. Even then, the first or second child will probably experience no difficulties. After that, a real danger exists in a large percentage of cases, unless there is very careful medical supervision.

This is what happens. The baby of such parents has a 50 per cent chance of being Rh-positive, like his father. If he is, the mother reacts to the Rh substance in her baby's blood by producing *antibodies*. With each new child, she produces more of these antibodies, and they remain in her blood. When the concentration of antibodies becomes high enough, they destroy the blood cells of the baby, and he may be born with a severe, even fatal, anemia.

The danger to the child is greatly minimized if the doctor has typed the mother's blood. If she is Rh-negative, the father's blood type must also be determined. The doctor then must be prepared to give the baby a transfusion that may save its life and fully restore it to health. In these transfusions, the baby's blood is almost completely replaced with Rh-negative blood.

Major Dangers During Pregnancy

In a very small proportion of births, serious complications which affect the mother may develop. Until recent years, these often progressed rapidly, and many mothers died during pregnancy. The tremendous improvements in prenatal care and deliveries have reduced the number of deaths to a very small figure, only about 3.4 in 10,000 live births. The poisonous condition known as *toxemia* of pregnancy is responsible for one-fourth of these deaths. Its cause is not known, but rapid recognition and treatment of the early signs usually prevent the high blood pressure and other very serious symptoms from developing later.

Other dangerous conditions which can occur during pregnancy or delivery of the child are hemorrhage, infection (sepsis), abortion and ectopic pregnancy.

Spontaneous abortion occurs in a small percentage of women, and they lose their babies during the first 16 weeks of pregnancy, either because of some abnormality in the baby, or some condition in the mother which prevents her from carrying her baby for the full nine months. (The loss of the baby after the sixteenth week of pregnancy is called a miscarriage.)

In ectopic pregnancy, the fertilized ovum burrows into the fallopian tube instead of the womb. Since the tube is too small to support the baby's growth, the fetus is apt to burst through after it has reached a certain size, rupturing the fallopian tube at the same time.

Puerperal or childbed fever, which develops after the delivery of the child, has declined tremendously since the days of Ignaz Semmelweiss, who died in 1865. Less than a hundred years ago, puerperal fever would sweep through a hospital ward, killing almost all the new mothers present. Dr. Semmelweiss discovered that this disease was due to an infection the doctor himself carried from

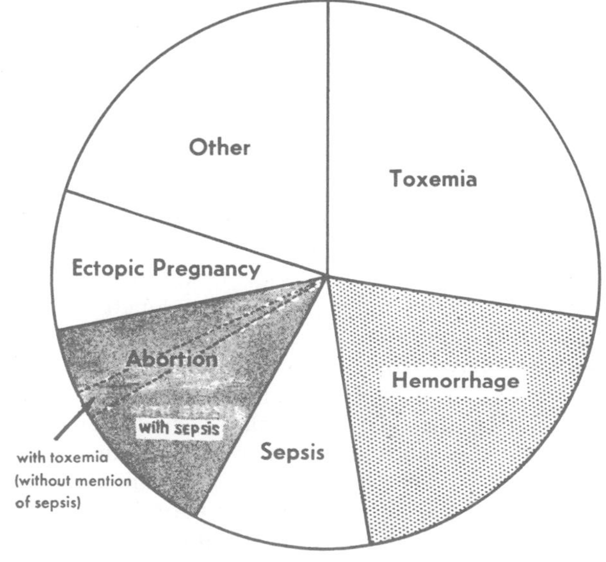

Figure 13–7. Causes of maternal mortality in the United States. (From the Health Information Foundation.)

the dissection room or from a woman who already had the disease. Oliver Wendell Holmes, the American author-physician, came to a similar conclusion at about the same time Semmelweiss made his great, though much opposed, discovery.

Today we know that puerperal fever is a streptococcal infection of the lining of the uterus, which spreads throughout the body. Because babies are delivered under strictly aseptic (bacteria-free) conditions today, puerperal fever has been practically eliminated. If, by any chance, it does develop, it is promptly treated with sulfa drugs or antibiotics, and usually responds very quickly.

A high proportion of these maternal deaths, especially from hemorrhage and toxemia, will be prevented by adequate prenatal care, better obstetric management and the prevention and control of infections. Deaths from ectopic pregnancy, which account for 8 per cent of the maternal mortality, can usually be prevented by early diagnosis and prompt surgery. A major part of the responsibility, however, rests with the pregnant woman herself. She must learn the importance of seeking prenatal care early, of observing good health and nutritional habits during pregnancy, and of cooperating completely with her physician. Community responsibility in this area involves the provision of adequate prenatal clinics and hospital and nursing facilities, especially in low-income areas.

BIRTH OF THE CHILD

The average pregnancy lasts 280 days in the human, but this gestation period varies tremendously from species to species. It is 11 days in the opossum and nearly 2 years in the elephant.

In humans, the gestation period also varies, probably influenced by the length of the mother's menstrual cycle. Most doctors agree that a baby will almost never live if it is born earlier than 196 days after the last menstrual period; a pregnancy extending for much more than 300 days is rare. The *average* pregnancy lasts 280 days, and the day the baby will be born is approximated by adding seven days to the date of the last menstrual period, and then counting back three months. For example, if the last menstrual period was November 16, the approximate day of delivery would be August 23.

The Three Stages of Labor

Several events indicate that labor is about to begin: a small amount of blood-tinged mucus may be passed; the "bag of waters" which encloses the baby may rupture, and water will either gush from the vagina, or leak out slowly; or labor pains will start.

The first stage of labor is the *dilation period*. The womb, which holds the baby, is like a large rubber bottle with a very small neck, about a half-inch long and almost closed. In order for birth to take place, the mouth of the bottle must be stretched to a diameter of about four inches to make room for the passage of the baby.

The walls of the womb are essentially a powerful set of muscles, and, at a certain time, for reasons unknown, these muscles begin to contract and force the baby downward. Gradually the mouth of the womb, the cervix, is stretched until there is room for the baby to pass through.

The labor pains are actually due to the intense contractions of the uterine muscles, fairly far apart at first and lasting for only a short time but closer together, more intense, and of longer duration as labor progresses.

When the cervix is fully dilated, or expanded, the second stage, the *expulsion period,* begins. The baby must now be pushed out through this narrow and resistant birth canal, and the mother achieves this by holding her breath, and pressing down to exert as much force as she can, augmenting the wavelike contractions of the uterine muscles.

The third and final stage of labor follows the birth of the baby, and is merely the *expulsion* of the *placenta* (or afterbirth), that remarkable tissue which nourished the baby throughout the pregnancy.

In an amazingly short time, nature returns the tissues to their original state, and soon the desirably slim figure is

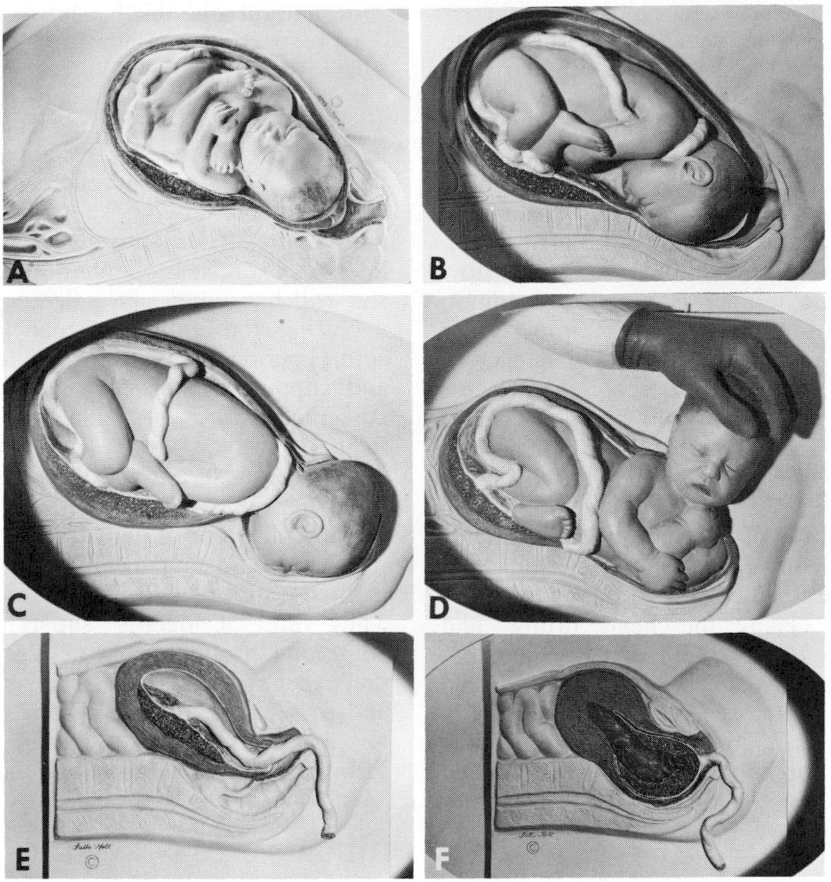

Figure 13–8. **A,** Early first stage of labor. Baby's head is engaged, the cervix is dilated 2 cm. and the membranes are intact. **B,** Late first stage of labor. The cervix is almost completely dilated (9 cm.), and the membranes are still intact. **C,** Early second stage of labor. Membranes have ruptured and the baby's head distends the perineal floor (bulging). **D,** Late second stage. The head is born, the shoulders have rotated and are ready to be delivered, and in a few seconds the rest of the baby's body will slip out. **E,** Early third stage. The placenta is separating from the uterine wall. **F,** Late third stage. The placenta is being expressed through the cervix and vaginal canal. (Photographed at the Museum of Science and Industry, Chicago.)

restored. Shortly after the baby is born, the uterus becomes tightly contracted, and involutes to its normal size. Breast-feeding the baby speeds up this process, and special exercises the doctor prescribes strengthen the abdominal muscles, which have become stretched and flabby.

Home Versus Hospital

Some of our mothers and most of our grandmothers had their babies at home, but today more than 95 per cent of women in the United States go to hospitals for their deliveries. Ninety-nine times out of a hundred everything goes smoothly during childbirth, but there is always that hundredth time, with complications. Physicians feel that obstetrical patients can be better cared for in a hospital where everything that could possibly be needed is available—special anesthetics, transfusions, oxygen tanks, good nursing care, and adequate rest.

Anesthesia and Instruments

Today, most doctors sanction the use of some form of anesthetic, or analgesic, or both, during childbirth. Analgesics, which are merely pain-relievers, are often used during the first stage of labor to help the mother relax between pains. Anesthetics are generally employed during the second stage, when the baby is actually being born. If the anesthetic is carefully chosen and administered by a skilled anesthetist, the risk to the mother or child is minimal.

In some instances it is necessary to hasten delivery before the head has appeared at the opening of the birth canal. For example, the journey may be slow because the mother is in poor condition and cannot expel the baby properly, or the baby may appear to be in danger of dying if it is not born quickly. The doctor will then reach into the birth canal and draw the baby out with *high forceps*. This instrument consists of two blades which are inserted separately into the vagina and the birth canal. When the doctor feels the baby's head between them, he clamps the handles of the forceps together. He then clasps the head firmly, and carefully extracts the baby in a manner simulating normal labor. An experienced obstetrician almost never injures a baby in this procedure, and because he does not use high forceps unless it is absolutely necessary, this instrument is a boon rather than a source of danger.

NATURAL CHILDBIRTH

Whether or not a woman admits it, she can hardly fail to give some thought to the question of the pain connected with having a child. How bad will it be? From what some women have told her, it must be unimaginably terrible, yet many mothers say they didn't feel a thing. Still others describe it as unpleasant but perfectly bearable. The truth lies somewhere in the middle, and there is no doubt that fear and tension aggravate pain, especially labor pains, and that they are far less intense if the patient can relax.

An English doctor, the late Grantly Dick Read, worked out the method called natural childbirth, or "childbirth without fear." Women in primitive countries usually have their babies with little difficulty. They may stop working in the fields to have a baby, and almost immediately return to their tasks. Why, he reasoned, shouldn't civilized women do just as well?

In natural childbirth, the doctor helps the prospective mother, from the earliest stages of her pregnancy, *emotionally* and *physically*. The emotional preparation attempts to rid the mother of her fears by telling her exactly what happens during her pregnancy and at each stage of the delivery, and how to keep the pain at a minimum. The physical preparation involves exercises to limber up the muscles she will use when she delivers her baby.

During the entire pregnancy and the actual period of labor, she has the help and support of her doctor and his staff. Anesthetics are available if she wants them. However, nearly half the patients do not request an anesthetic during the labor period, and some require it only at the final moment of delivery.

Women who have had their babies by this method are usually very enthusiastic. They find it deeply satisfying to be conscious throughout the delivery, to know the exact moment they have given birth, and to see and touch the baby the instant he is born. Without doubt, it is an incomparably beautiful experience.

THE ROOMING-IN SYSTEM

Chiefly for their own convenience, hospitals usually keep all babies in one large nursery. After the mother's flow of milk has been established, her baby is brought to her every three or four hours for a feeding. Unfortunately, some babies are hungry before that time, and may cry for quite a while before they are fed.

In the rooming-in system, the baby shares his mother's room, from a day or two after he is born until they leave the hospital together. The crib is arranged so that she can reach her baby without getting out of bed. She helps to care for him, changes and dresses him, feeds and comforts him, and in general learns to understand him. The only visitor permitted is her husband, and he, too, comes to feel at home with the baby.

The act of birth is probably a shocking experience for a child. Having lived comfortably in his mother's womb for nine months, he is suddenly on his own, forced to adapt to a great many new stimuli in a strange world. He is exposed to light, air, drafts, hunger, pain, and many other new sensations. The rooming-in system, which a number of hospitals have now established, makes this transition considerably easier for him.

CESAREAN BIRTHS

If, for some reason, the baby cannot be born through the vagina—because the mother is ill, or her pelvic structure too small—the doctor can perform an operation to remove it through the abdomen. This is called a cesarean delivery.

Many doctors prefer to deliver subsequent babies this way if a woman has had one baby by cesarean section, but it is possible for her to have other babies normally in some cases. The chief danger lies in that the wound from the first incision may open during a subsequent hard labor.

Although the cesarean operation is quite safe, it is still a major surgical procedure and is more hazardous than normal delivery. Few doctors perform it without a very good reason.

INFANT MORTALITY

The death of babies either during pregnancy or childbirth has declined steadily over the years, and we can anticipate even fewer deaths as improved care during pregnancy and delivery become available to wider segments of the population. In 1930, nearly 70 babies died for every 1000 live births in the nation as a whole, but by 1963 this figure was 18, not including stillbirths.

The use of hospitals and skilled obstetricians for confinement, specific medicines for infections, and wider extension of prenatal and postnatal care are responsible for the tremendous reduction in infant mortality in recent years. More and more babies will be saved in coming years when we learn how to reduce the number of premature births: approximately 60 per cent of infant deaths occur in premature babies who weigh less than 5.5 pounds at birth, although only 6 to 7 per cent of the babies born are this small.

Many factors affect the chances of the embryo or fetus[2] of surviving and being born alive. Genetic defects in the original germ cells or an abnormal environment in the uterus (such as disease of the mother), hormonal imbalance, or radiation may be incompatible with development and survival of the baby.

Even if development has progressed normally, the period of labor and delivery is critical for the baby. The major complications are cutting off its oxygen supply—

[2]*Embryo* is the term applied when the baby is in the very early stages of development, and *fetus*, for the later stages.

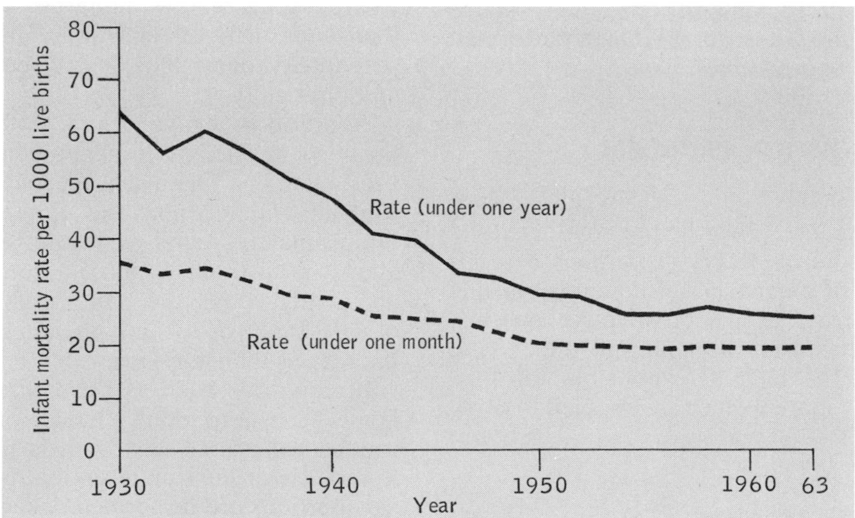

Figure 13–9. These curves show the leveling off in infant mortality rates in recent years, after the sharp declines of the preceding three decades.

by pressure or kinking of the umbilical cord—and traumatizing its head.

After birth the chief cause of death is prematurity. A baby who weighs less than 5.5 pounds is considered premature, and needs special nursing care to help it survive. A very large reduction in the deaths of premature babies weighing more than 1000 grams (2.2 pounds) has been achieved at the outstanding maternity hospitals. For example, at the Chicago Lying-in Hospital, approximately 90 per cent of premature babies weighing between 1000 and 2500 grams (2.2 to 5.5 pounds) survived in 1956 as compared with only 72 per cent in 1935. (At this hospital the death rate of newborn babies larger than 5.5 pounds has remained at the very low level of less than 5 per 1000 live births for the past 25 years). However, not more than 3 or 4 per cent of babies who weigh under 2.2 pounds can survive because they haven't reached a stage of development advanced enough to permit them to live in an artificial environment.

Other conditions which can be fatal for the infant shortly after birth are congenital malformations, respiratory diseases such as pneumonia and influenza, and intestinal infections such as diarrhea and enteritis.

Recent advances in medicine have made it possible to detect phenylketonuria (PKU) at birth. This disease causes mental retardation in about 4 persons in 100,000, but it can be avoided if detected shortly after birth. In view of this, many states now require a test for PKU be performed on all newborn babies.

THE ABORTION PROBLEM

Spontaneous abortion or miscarriage due to causes which the mother-to-be cannot control occurs in perhaps 8 to 10 per cent of pregnancies, frequently causing great sorrow in the prospective parents. Gradually we are beginning to understand some of the factors responsible for this, and many more women are enabled to carry their babies to term.

Therapeutic Abortions

A certain number of abortions must be *induced* for medical reasons in situations where carrying a baby to term might be hazardous, possibly fatal, to the mother. This might be the case when there is a serious disease, such as diabetes, advanced kidney disease, tuberculosis, and even certain mental illnesses.

In the United States, abortion for any other than medical reasons is considered illegal and is known as a *criminal abortion*. The number of such abortions is unknown, because a licensed physician is unlikely to see the patient unless there are serious medical complications. However, it has been estimated at anywhere from 200,000 to 1,200,000 a year. Compared to this figure, the number of therapeutic legal abortions is very small.

Most of the illegal abortions are performed on married women who either want no children or feel they already have a big enough family. A large number, however, must be attributed to pregnancies due to premarital sexual relations. According to a recent report by the Kinsey Institute, the girl or woman who engages in sexual experiences before marriage has one chance in five of becoming pregnant. Relatively few illegitimate children are born, and the rest must therefore be aborted in one way or another.

Ninety per cent of abortions are either self-induced or result from surgical intervention of some sort, generally by unlicensed, disqualified physicians and out-and-out quacks, at costs ranging anywhere from a few hundred dollars to thousands. Illegal abortions are always potentially hazardous, both emotionally and physically.

Abortion is legalized and performed by qualified physicians in a number of countries, including Denmark, Iceland, Sweden, Finland, Japan, and the Soviet Union. Unfortunately, many women have repeated abortions in these countries, because they apparently come to depend on this instead of birth control to limit their fertility and the size of their families.

In countries such as the United States, however, where only a small percentage can be performed legally, it is potentially a very hazardous undertaking. Many illegal abortions are performed under extremely unhygienic conditions. It is difficult to know how many deaths actually result, because they are generally hushed, but periodically we learn of them from hospitals or newspaper dispatches. Many undoubtedly go unrecorded, and other causes are reported on the death certificates. However, at least 17 per cent of the women reported by the Kinsey Institute to have had abortions reported some physical complications, half of them mild, and the remainder potentially very serious, including blood poisoning, peritonitis or other infections, long hospital stays, invalidism and almost fatal illness.

Questions

1. Do you think it is a healthy sign for our society that families are getting larger?
2. Describe the process of conception, implantation of the fertilized egg, and the early stages of development.
3. How do multiple births, identical and nonidentical, occur?
4. What are some of the tests for pregnancy, and what do they depend on?
5. If a woman feels completely well during her pregnancy, do you think she can manage without a physician until the time of her delivery? Discuss some of the advantages of prenatal care.
6. What are the effects of the following on pregnancy or on the development of the child: German measles; gonorrhea; the Rh factor?
7. What are the advantages of home versus hospital delivery? Do you know of any disadvantages?
8. Many doctors have little enthusiasm for natural childbirth and the rooming-in system. Do you think this is simply conservatism or that all their objections are rational?
9. What are the major causes of infant mortality and how could they be prevented or reduced?
10. How long does the mature ovum remain viable for conception? What is the life span of the male sperm after it arrives in a woman's reproduction organs?
11. Considering the answers to the preceding questions, how many days during the woman's menstrual cycle is she likely to become pregnant?
12. Examine the statistical probability of multiple births. Then estimate the possibility of sextuple births.
13. What is the size of the embryo at one month? Describe in gross terms the growth of the embryo and fetus, month by month, for the full term of pregnancy.
14. Speculate why so many restrictions were placed on pregnant women in the past. Do you think there are still some restrictions that might safely be lifted?
15. If you were an employer, how would you feel about having a pregnant woman at work until very late in her term?
16. Hospital delivery of babies is now practically universally accepted. However, what limitations or objections do you see to this system?
17. As a woman, would you prefer natural childbirth, with the option of being conscious throughout? As a man, would you want this for your wife?

Topics for Discussion

Superstitions concerning pregnancy.

Conquest of childbed fever.

Ectopic pregnancy.

Desirability of nursing versus bottle-feeding a baby.

The "fad" of a husband's presence in the delivery room.

Reasons for legalizing abortion in the United States.

Pressures in the path of legal abortion.

Reasons for the growing number of books of advice on pregnancy and child care.

Problems of a couple's adjustment to the first child.

Degree of a husband's responsibility for active care of a newborn child.

Desirability and need for government-sponsored aid for pregnant women and new mothers.

Problems of pregnancy and the need of further medical research.

Reading Suggestions

Discoveries on the Trail of Life's Beginnings, J. D. Ratcliff. Today's Health, March 1957. Clear, lucid discussion and excellent photographs of the fertilization process.

Fundamentals of Human Reproduction, E. L. Potter. McGraw-Hill, New York, 1948. This book discusses the important features of pregnancy intelligently and simply, and contains good drawings and photographs.

Pregnancy, Birth and Abortion, The Kinsey Institute. Harper & Bros., New York, 1959. An interesting presentation of the abortion problem, the result of surveys by the Kinsey Institute. It is digested in McCall's Magazine, March 1958, p. 34.

Primer for Pregnancy, Eve Stanton Featheringill. Simon & Schuster, New York, 1951. An informal and practical guide for the expectant mother.

Natural Child Spacing, M. Edward Davis. Hanover House, Garden City, N.Y., 1953. Describes in detail the body temperature method of contraception for planned parenthood.

Pregnancy and Birth, Alan F. Guttmacher. Signet Books, New York, 1962 (paperback). A well known obstetrician discusses pregnancy and birth in a clear manner, answering many of the questions pregnant women and new mothers are likely to ask.

Wisdom with Children, I. Newton Kugelmass. John Day, New York, 1965. The problems associated with bringing up baby discussed in this book are not new, but some of the detailed and insightful remarks and advice are. Substantial medical information is also included.

Baby and Child Care, Benjamin Spock. Pocket Books, New York, 1965 (paperback). A Bible on child care in millions of homes, Dr. Spock's work is well thought of by pediatricians, as well as by mothers. A clearly presented guide to most aspects of child-rearing.

The Gesell Institute's Child Behavior, Frances L. Ilg and Louise Bates Ames. Dell Publishing Co., New York, 1963. A guide to child behavior by members of the famous team of the Gesell Institute. Considers many problems and situations from birth to age 10.

Infant and Child in the Culture of Today, Arnold Gesell and Frances L. Ilg. Harper, New York, 1943. Now updated, this has become a standard work on child behavior, which is considered chronologically.

The First 5 Years of Life, Arnold Gesell, Frances L. Ilg, and others. Harper, New York, 1940. A detailed chronology, concentrating on the earliest years of life.

Hormones in Human Reproduction, G. W. Corner. Atheneum, New York (paperback). Dr. Corner clarifies the complex role of hormones in influencing physiological development and in regulating the reproductive cycle.

Expectant Motherhood, Nicholson J. Eastman. 4th Ed., Little, Brown and Co., Boston, 1963. An authoritative guidebook through pregnancy, by an obstetrician and gynecologist.

The Stages of Human Development before Birth, E. Blechschmidt. W. B. Saunders, Philadelphia, 1961. A technical text on embryology, profusely illustrated. Informative even for the undergraduate student.

Genetics Is Easy, Philip Goldstein. 2nd Ed., Viking Press, New York, 1961. A popular presentation of a difficult subject.

The Genetic Code, Isaac Asimov. Orion Press, New York, 1963; Also New American Library, paperback. A scientist-writer presents the elements of genetics in an unusually clear style.

Childbirth Without Fear, Grantly Dick Read. 2nd Ed., Harper, New York, 1953; Also Dell Publishing Co., New York, 1962 (paperback). The British physician who advocated natural childbirth describes in detail the emotional and physical preparation necessary. This book and its successors have influenced many women to undertake childbirth with little or no anesthesia.

Pregnancy, Birth and Abortion, Paul H. Gebhard, Wardell B. Pomeroy, Clyde E. Martin, and Cornelia V. Christenson, W. B. Saunders, Philadelphia, 1958.

Nine Months to Go, Robert M. Mitchell and Ted Klein. Lippincott, Philadelphia, 1960; Also Dell Publishing Co., New York, 1962 (paperback).

Abortion in the United States, Mary S. Calderone, ed. Hoeber-Harper, New York, 1958.

Reducing the Hazards of Being Born, Allan C. Barnes. Harper's Magazine, January 1964, p. 31. A professor of obstetrics tells what can be done to reduce the hazards of being born.

The Doctor Is a Detective. Today's Health, Sept. 1964, p. 31. A description of the physician's search for hidden birth defects in the newborn baby.

Abortion. Today's Health, April 1965, p. 24. A psychiatrist discusses the problem of abortion from several standpoints.

SECTION SIX

UNDERSTANDING DISEASE

14

THE NATURE OF DISEASE

A healthy body is a guest-chamber for the soul; a sick body is a prison.

BACON, *The Advancement of Learning*

If one has a *disease,* his body, or some important part of it, is not functioning normally. There are many kinds of diseases as might be anticipated from the great variety of causes: *infectious agents,* such as bacteria or viruses; *deficiency* of some essential vitamin or other nutrient; and *metabolic* derangements which develop when certain cells and tissues, such as the endocrine glands, show abnormal activities. The origin might also be *genetic* or *hereditary; psychosomatic; neoplastic* or *cancerous.*

Why certain diseases such as cancer, schizophrenia and high blood pressure develop is still a mystery, but when they are fully understood, they too will be shown to have definite causation. There is always cause and effect in illness, and never a supernatural origin.

Fortunately, many potentially serious illnesses give warning symptoms of some kind, and the most important ones are the following:

Fever. The mouth temperature of the average person is normally 98.6° Fahrenheit, and the rectal temperature, 99.6° F. An elevation in temperature may indicate a mild or serious disease or infection.

Pain. All of us occasionally suffer headaches and other fleeting, mild aches and pains, which rarely require medical advice unless they become chronic. But any new or unusually acute pain should be discussed with a physician.

Loss of Weight. Anyone who loses weight on an adequate, non-reducing diet is suffering from an illness of some kind.

Shortness of Breath. This may indicate obesity or too sedentary a life, but it may also represent the first sign of a potentially serious illness, such as heart trouble or anemia.

Bleeding. Bleeding without obvious cause is usually nature's warning that there

MAN BUILDS HIS RESISTANCE TO DISEASE

Highlights in the Development of Immunity

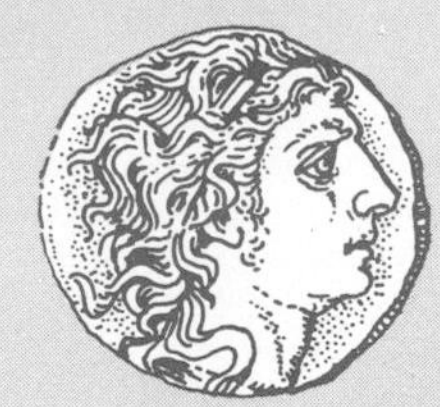

BUILDING THE BODY'S resistance to harmful agents is an old principle. Mithridates, king of ancient Pontus, regularly took small doses of poisons to accustom his system to poisons that could be used in attempts on his life.

VARIOLATION, a form of inoculation for smallpox, was known to most Oriental people for centuries. It was introduced to England about 1715. In 1718 Lady Mary Wortley Montagu had her three-year-old son inoculated in Turkey.

OPPOSITION TO VARIOLATION ran high at first. In 1721 Zabdiel Boylston inoculated 244 people during an epidemic of smallpox in Boston and was threatened with hanging. But in 1768 Catherine the Great of Russia was inoculated by Thomas Dimsdale, her English doctor. He was rewarded with a fee of about $50,000, plus $10,000 for traveling expenses, a life pension of about $2,500 a year, and the rank of baron of her empire.

PREVENTIVE INOCULATION based on scientific principles was introduced by Edward Jenner, an English country doctor. In 1796 he performed the first vaccination against smallpox on eight-year-old James Phipps. Lack of understanding often made Jenner's method the subject of crude caricature.

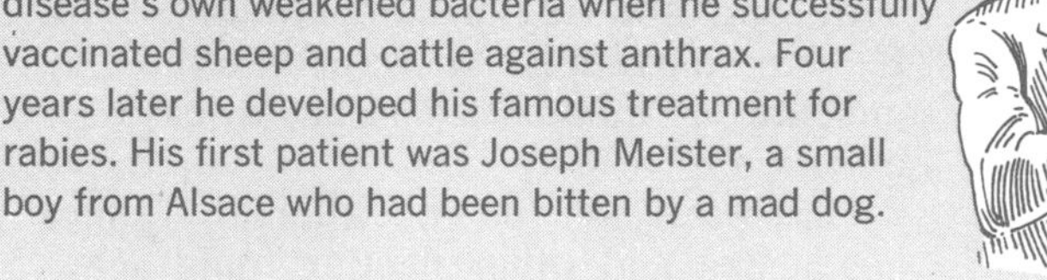

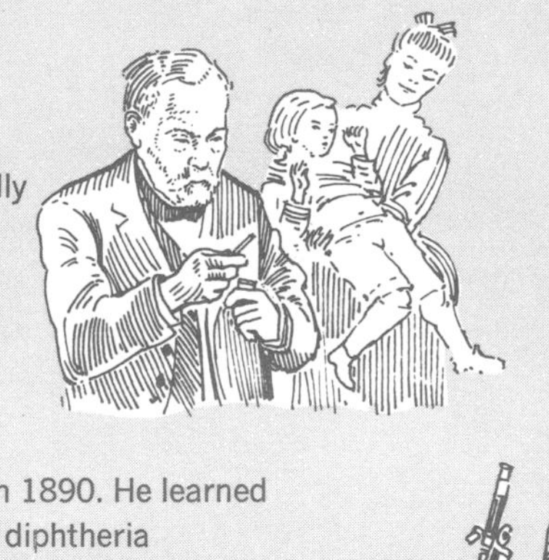

LOUIS PASTEUR, in 1881, proved the possibility of preventing disease through the injection of the disease's own weakened bacteria when he successfully vaccinated sheep and cattle against anthrax. Four years later he developed his famous treatment for rabies. His first patient was Joseph Meister, a small boy from Alsace who had been bitten by a mad dog.

ANTITOXINS were discovered by Emil von Behring in 1890. He learned that serums, made from animals immunized against diphtheria and tetanus, could immunize man from those dreaded diseases.

DR. JONAS SALK tested his vaccine against poliomyelitis in 1954 on nearly 2 million children in the United States and found it effective against the three types of virus that cause infantile paralysis. Today men like Dr. Salk continue to develop vaccines and serums to combat those diseases that remain unconquered.

is trouble somewhere, and every effort should be made to find the explanation.

INFECTIOUS DISEASES: TRANSMISSION, PREVENTION AND CURE

A century ago, tuberculosis (which was called *consumption*) was thought to be due to an inherited "weakness of the constitution." Doctors did not even recognize its contagious nature. It was believed that leprosy could be contracted simply by touching a leper's clothes, and that malaria came from breathing night air with its dangerous miasmas or vapors (malaria actually means "bad air"). A plague of locusts was blamed for diphtheria epidemics, and dysentery was attributed to becoming overheated.

Today we understand the causes of many infectious diseases, how they are transmitted, and how many of them can be prevented or cured. Tremendous progress has been made in this field following the proof by the French chemist, Louis Pasteur, in 1865, that bacteria are responsible for disease.

Microorganisms and Parasites

There are six types of infecting organisms which can cause a multitude of diseases: *bacteria, viruses, rickettsiae, fungi, protozoa, and parasitic worms.*

Bacteria are tiny forms of life visible

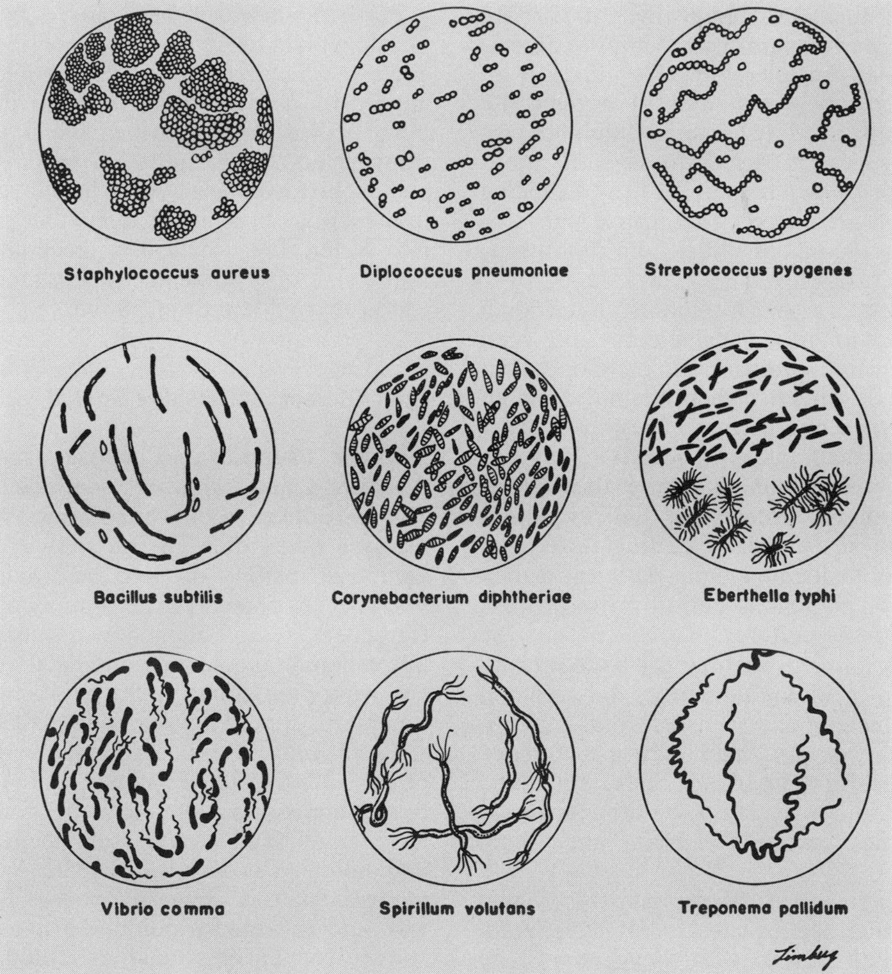

Figure 14–1. Types of bacteria. **Upper row,** Spherical forms (cocci); **middle row,** rod forms (bacilli); **lower row,** spiral forms. (From Villee: *Biology*. 4th Ed., Philadelphia, W. B. Saunders Co., 1962.)

only under a microscope. If all the millions of people in the city of New York were reduced to the size of bacteria, they would fit very comfortably into a drop of water.

Among themselves, the sizes, shapes, and habits of bacteria differ one from another. Many swim about, others remain still. Some bacteria are individualists, preferring to go it alone. The streptococci form chains like strings of beads, whereas the staphylococci found in boils live in clusters, like a bunch of grapes.

Rod shaped bacteria cause diphtheria, typhoid fever, tuberculosis, and leprosy, and syphilis is due to invasion by the corkscrew spirochete.

Bacteria are all around us, but, luckily, most of them are more beneficial than harmful to mankind. They are so skillful in destroying dead matter that we can consider them our most efficient garbage disposal department. Life without bacteria would not be possible. The growth of certain plants on which all animal life depends is aided by bacteria which convert atmospheric nitrogen into organic foodstuffs. Yet how pleasant our lives would be without the bacteria that cause tuberculosis, pneumonia, syphilis, and diphtheria, to name just a few.

Viruses are much smaller even than bacteria, so tiny they cannot be seen through an ordinary microscope but require the much higher magnification of the electron microscope. They are harder to study than bacteria because they are extremely fussy about where they grow. Only with the greatest of difficulty have scientists succeeded in getting viruses to multiply outside an animal body; now they are grown in animal cells by the process called "tissue culture."

Viruses are responsible for a great many diseases, including influenza, the common cold, chickenpox, measles and mumps. Moreover, most of them show a preference for a specific part of the body: smallpox, measles, and warts affect the skin, and polio and rabies invade the brain and spinal cord.

Rickettsiae are microorganisms which are smaller than bacteria, but sufficiently larger than viruses that they can just be seen with an ordinary microscope. Typhus fever, transmitted by a louse bite, and Rocky Mountain spotted fever, due to a tick bite, are both rickettsial diseases.

Fungi are present in nature in a tremendous variety of forms and kinds. They are related to mushrooms, but are very much smaller. The green mold which forms on stale bread is an example of a perfectly harmless fungus. Fortunately, only a few fungi are responsible for more or less serious human disease, such as ringworm of the scalp or nails, certain skin diseases such as athlete's foot, histoplasmosis (a lung condition), and coccidioidomycosis.

Protozoa are microscopic organisms which may be 50 times as large as bacteria, but are still visible only under a microscope. Important diseases caused by protozoa are malaria, amebic dysentery, and African sleeping sickness.

Parasitic diseases are caused by organisms which must pass part of their life cycle in animals. They include trichinosis, caused by a small roundworm in infected pork; hookworm; tapeworm, which may be transmitted by infected beef, pork or fish; and schistosomiasis, a tropical disease in which a snail discharges the parasite into water. The smallest of these parasites is the size of a pinhead, while a tapeworm can grow to a length of 30 feet.

How Microorganisms Are Spread

Many bacteria and viruses thrive in moisture, and *spitting, coughing* and *sneezing* keep them circulating. Motion pictures taken of a sneeze show that it is composed of tiny droplets, and that when you sneeze, you can expel a spray of liquid for several feet. This is how diseases such as the common cold, pneumonia, tuberculosis, whooping cough, influenza, and many others are spread.

Food and water are responsible for other infections. Typhoid and amebic dysentery organisms may be found in food, milk and water that have been contaminated in any way by feces. Moses recognized this several thousand years ago, and invented a combined sword-and-shovel so that his soldiers could cover their excrement. Later Aristotle advised

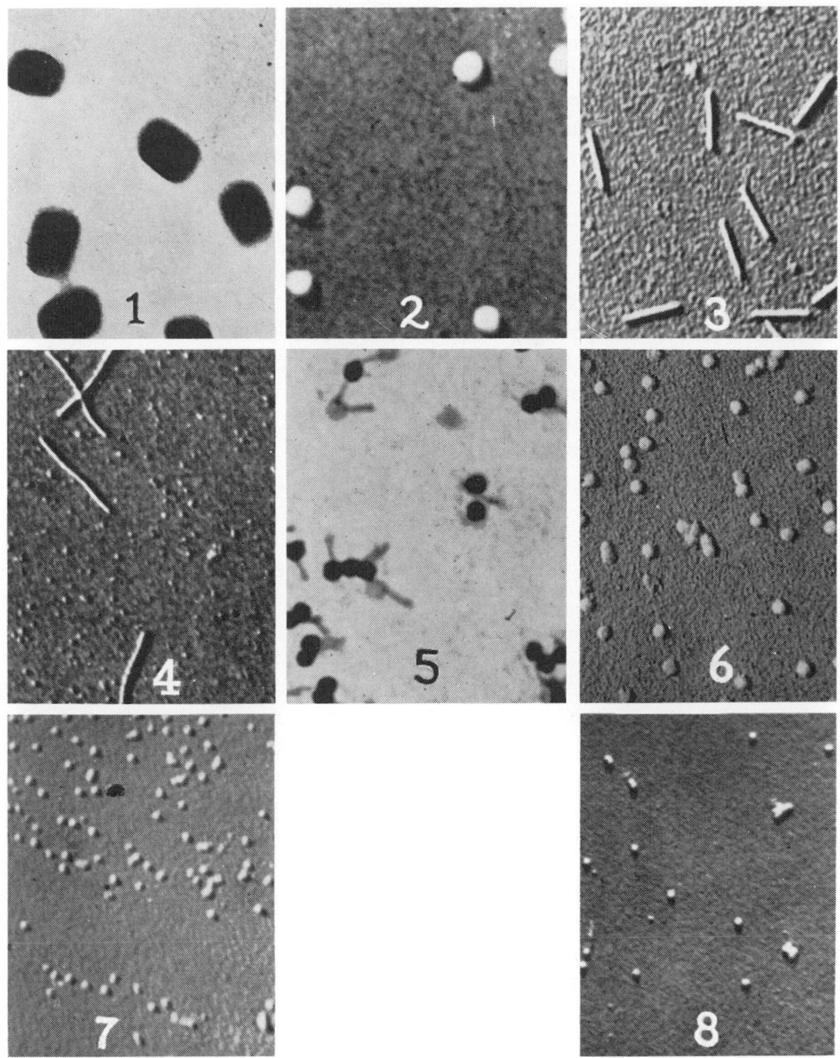

Figure 14–2. Electron micrographs of a variety of viruses. **1,** Vaccinia virus (used in vaccinating for smallpox). **2,** Influenza virus. **3,** Tobacco mosiac virus. **4,** Potato mosaic virus. **5,** Bacteriophages. **6,** Shope papilloma virus. **7,** Southern bean mosiac virus. **8,** Tomato bushy stunt virus. (Courtesy of Dr. C. A. Knight.)

Alexander the Great, during his campaign, to "Boil your water and bury your dung."

It is to prevent such contamination that you wash your hands after going to the toilet and before eating, and keep food protected from flies carrying bacteria. Contamination can be spread even by a person who is not ill, as in the case of typhoid carriers. One of the most famous of these was a cook, to become known as Typhoid Mary, who went from job to job spreading infection to more than 100 victims before doctors learned that she was a carrier.

The tremendous reduction in diseases spread by water and milk must be attributed to the greatly improved sanitation which public health measures have brought about: chlorination of water, pasteurization of milk, and sanitary sewage disposal. Proper canning and preservation of food, as well as care in its handling, are also important factors.

The story is told of an Army physician overseas who was responsible for the water supply in each new area. One day, he asked the sergeant in charge what was being done against contamination.

"Well, sir," said the sergeant, "first we boil it."

"And then?"

"Then we filter it."

The doctor nodded approvingly.

"And then," the sergeant went on, "just to be on the safe side, we drink beer."

More than 80 animal diseases can be communicated to man. *Incompletely cooked* pork may cause trichinosis, one of the commonest of these diseases. Raw fish and beef may contain tapeworms. Brucellosis, also called undulant fever, is a very debilitating illness which can be acquired from pork, beef, and unpasteurized milk or milk products such as cheese and ice cream.

Insect bites can be a source of infection because insects carry microorganisms either in the mouth or excrement. An insect bite makes a tiny break in the skin, like the puncture of a hypodermic needle. *Tick fever* (Rocky Mountain spotted fever) is similar to European typhus fever and is transmitted by the bite of ticks. In Mexico and the southern United States, a type more closely related to European typhus is transmitted by lice, ticks and mites living on rats. *Malaria* and *yellow fever* are carried by the *Anopheles* mosquitoes. Most of the United States is now free of malaria, but it has not yet been eliminated in all parts of the South.

Animal bites or scratches are responsible for several diseases, of which the most serious is *rabies*. This disease is most commonly spread by mad dogs, but other warm-blooded animals, including cats, foxes, wolves, skunks and bears can also carry it. The most recently discovered vector, or carrier, for rabies in the United States is the bat, and U.S. Public Health Service physicians have shown that bats in as many as 15 states carry this virus. Fortunately, we now have a safe and highly effective new vaccine for preventing this potentially fatal disease in individuals who have been bitten by rabid animals.

All *cuts, wounds* and *scratches* are potential entrances for infections, and should be thoroughly scrubbed with soap and water. The most serious danger is tetanus (lockjaw) and the tetanus bacillus is widespread. It has been found in the soil and wherever there are farm animals, as well as in the dust of city streets. Deep puncture wounds—by a nail, wood slivers, or other sharp object—are particularly hazardous. Fortunately, we can immunize against this organism, or can administer tetanus antitoxin as an emergency measure in someone who has not been immunized. The fatality rate from untreated cases of this disease may go as high as 50 per cent.

How Infectious Agents Produce Disease

One or even a few bacteria by themselves do not amount to very much. Because they multiply at such a prodigious rate, however, they can become dangerous. In the right environment, some bacteria can reproduce every 20 minutes. At this rate, as Claude A. Villee has calculated, "If there were plenty of food and nothing to interfere, one bacterium could give rise to about 500,000 bacteria within six hours. After 24 hours, the resulting mass of bacteria would weigh 4,000,000 pounds and in less than a week this single bacterium could give rise to a mass of bacteria the size of the earth. . . . Fortunately for all other forms of life, bacteria cannot reproduce at this rate for a very long time, for they soon are checked by a lack of food or by the accumulation of waste products.[1]

Nevertheless, hours after infection by certain bacteria, there is enough multiplication to give rise to characteristic symptoms. If bacteria did nothing but reproduce in the body they might still be dangerous because they could use up essential nutrients, and even block the blood vessels leading to certain tissues. But they do far more than this: many of them exert very destructive effects on tissues, and produce powerful and extremely poisonous toxins, most of which adversely affect specific tissues or organ systems. For example, diphtheria toxin can damage the heart muscle, and botulinus toxin specifically affects nerves.

Body Defenses Against Infectious Disease

Less than 100 years ago every fifth child died before reaching his first birth-

[1]Villee, C. A.: *Biology,* W. B. Saunders Co., Philadelphia, 1957.

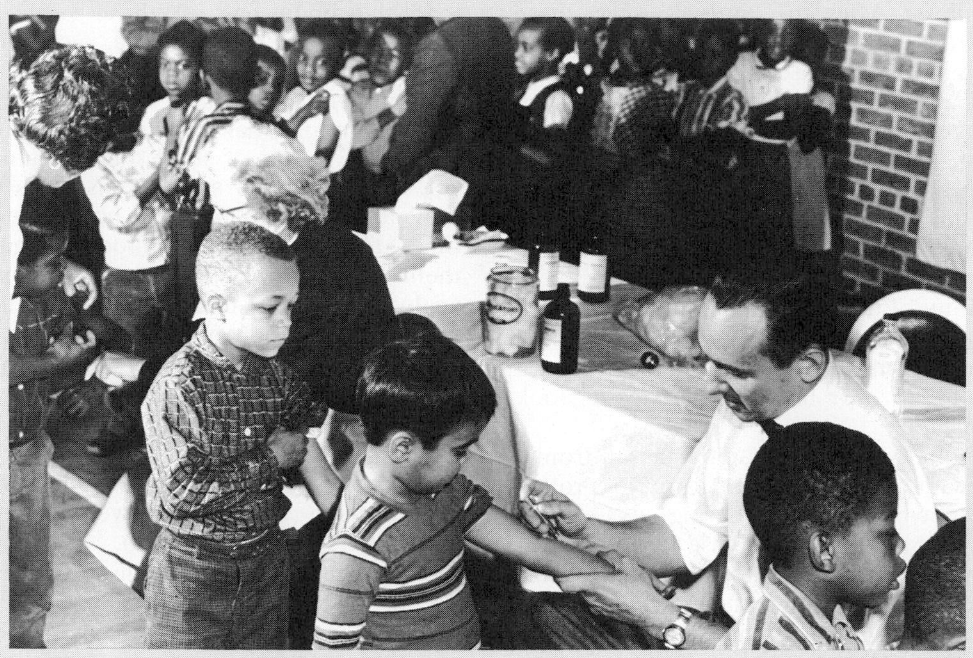

These children are receiving the Mantoux skin test for tuberculosis. Tuberculin, a sterile fluid with traces of tuberculosis bacteria, is injected into the skin. The reaction to the injection on the skin will tell the doctor if tuberculosis germs are, or have been, in the body.

day and almost as many more before the age of two, the majority succumbing to dysentery and childhood diseases. Epidemics of diphtheria have been reported which killed every child under 12 in a given area, and plagues of smallpox, yellow fever, and other diseases often decimated the population. Until doctors understood that bacteria and viruses were responsible, there was little they could do to prevent these fatal diseases.

Fortunately, our bodies are not completely helpless against harmful microorganisms. The *skin, mucous membranes* and *lining of the digestive tract* offer considerable resistance to invasion as long as they are unbroken. A scratch or wound in the skin will, of course, permit bacteria to enter. The *acid in the stomach* kills many bacteria that enter the gastrointestinal system. In addition, the *tiny hairs in the nose* act as filters to keep harmful organisms out, and secretions such as *tears* can kill these invaders or wash them away.

If microorganisms do enter, another defensive mechanism develops: the *leukocytes* (white blood cells) rush to the site of invasion to attack and devour the bacteria, and the body speeds up its synthesis of leukocytes. This is what happens during an *inflammation,* such as a boil. The pus contains innumerable bacteria engulfed and being destroyed by the white corpuscles. Severe bacterial infections can evoke a very marked increase in the number of circulating white blood cells. In appendicitis, for example, the leukocyte count may double.

Fever, too, has its beneficial aspects: many microorganisms are unable to proliferate at temperatures much above normal.

The body has another, even more powerful, weapon. It manufactures *antibodies* or *antitoxins* which counteract the infectious agents, and render their toxins harmless. After the battle is over, these substances may remain in the body and prevent the disease from gaining a foothold again. This is what happens when you recover from measles, chicken pox, mumps, polio, or any of the other diseases which people usually suffer from only once. You become immune to subsequent attacks because you have developed an *acquired immunity*.

Many of us are immune to polio, as well as to other serious infections, because we once had an attack that was so mild we didn't realize we had it, or perhaps mistook it for flu.

Enough antibodies can be passed from a pregnant mother to her baby to protect the newborn infant during its critical first few months. Otherwise it would have no resistance at all to the innumerable infectious organisms it encounters. Animals raised from birth in completely germ-free environment, in special equipment devised by James A. Reyniers of Notre Dame University, die very rapidly of overwhelming infections when they are brought into a nonsterile environment, because they have no antibodies against disease.

Natural immunity is the term used when people are immune to a disease without ever having had it, even in a mild form. This seems to be acquired on an hereditary basis, and is passed along to each generation. The reduced severity of certain infections which were originally highly contagious and serious—such as syphilis when it was first introduced into Europe—is probably due partly to inheritance and possibly to a change in the virulence of the infecting organism. Populations which have never been exposed to relatively mild diseases may develop acute and fatal illnesses when they first come into contact with them. This happened when measles was first experienced by the American Indians and South Sea Islanders.

Many immunities are *partial* or *temporary,* and do not protect an individual completely during his lifetime. The common cold, for example, confers immunity for only a very short time, and we can develop another cold just a few weeks after recovering from the previous one.

If the body has all these protective mechanisms against disease, you might wonder why we need vaccinations and why, if there is a threat of tetanus infection, tetanus antitoxin has to be used. The reason is that the toxins of some microorganisms act so rapidly and are so poisonous that they take effect *before* the body has had time to synthesize antibodies against them. We can develop immune antibodies against polio and suffer no ill effects if we are exposed to only a mild infection. But a massive invasion by very virulent polio viruses may permanently paralyze and even cause death because we cannot make the antibodies fast enough. However, if we have been vaccinated against the disease long enough in advance, we can resist even a very serious infection.

Vaccinations and Antitoxins. The practice of vaccination actually stemmed from observations that recovery from smallpox prevents it from recurring. Long before Jenner discovered vaccination, the people of the Far East had been *inoculating* against smallpox for centuries: this was done by infecting a minute wound with pus taken from a smallpox sore. A person inoculated in this way would usually develop a mild case of smallpox which could confer lifetime immunity.

In Massachusetts, Cotton Mather came upon an account of inoculation practiced in Turkey,[2] and spoke of it to a few physician friends. When smallpox appeared in epidemic proportions in Boston in 1721, Dr. Zabdiel Boylston inoculated his only son against it on June 27, 1721—the first person in the New World to submit to this operation. Dr. Boylston was mobbed by indignant citizens, and Cotton Mather had a bomb thrown into his window.

Despite fierce opposition at first, inoculation against smallpox was gradually extended, and prevented many fatal cases. The chief danger in this method was that the person who was inoculated did develop true smallpox, even though it

[2] Haggard, A. W.: *Devils, Drugs and Doctors,* Harper & Bros., New York, 1929.

was only a mild attack, but other persons in contact with him could develop as severe and fatal a case of smallpox as from the usual active cases of the disease.

Really safe vaccination was introduced in 1798 by Dr. Edward Jenner, of Gloucestershire, England, making use of the well known fact that in the countryside where he lived dairymaids who contracted cowpox from the cows they milked did not develop smallpox. In a cautious and scientific manner, Dr. Jenner collected data on this phenomenon for 18 years before he performed his first vaccination on a country boy, using matter from the arms of a milkmaid who had acquired cowpox. Two months later, he inoculated the boy with pus from a true case of smallpox, but the boy did not contract the disease.

Dr. Jenner's remarkable discovery met the usual opposition, but eventually became the established method for protection against smallpox. Today we have effective vaccines against a wide variety of microorganisms:

Bacterial diseases: diphtheria, whooping cough (also called pertussis), tetanus, typhoid fever and cholera.
Virus diseases: polio, rabies, influenza, smallpox, psittacosis (parrot fever), yellow fever, and measles.
Rickettsiae: typhus, Rocky Mountain spotted fever, Q fever.
Fungi: Histoplasmosis.

A great deal of research is being directed toward preparing effective vaccines against diseases for which we still have no protection.

Inoculation with an effective vaccine produces *active immunity,* and the patient does not have to suffer from the disease. The same basic principle is involved as in the *acquired immunity* which follows a bout of the illness. In both cases our cells synthesize *antibodies* in response to the *antigen,* or foreign protein, of the microorganism, whether it be a bacterium, virus or rickettsia. Vaccines contain strong enough antigens to stimulate the body to form antibodies against them, but not so strong as to bring on the symptoms of the disease. The toxicity of the antigen is reduced in various ways—treating the bacterial cell products with chemical agents, heat, or by drying; injecting only a minute amount of the bacterial toxin; weakening or attenuating the microorganisms by passing them through repeated cultures in the test tube until they become less toxic; and using less virulent strains of the organisms, which are nevertheless capable of evoking antibody formation. Preparations of viruses for use in vaccines are cultivated in chick or duck embryos, or in mammalian cells, such as kidney tissue, by tissue culture techniques. Killed or weakened preparations of the purified viruses are then used to prepare vaccines.

Sometimes an individual is exposed to a disease against which he has not been immunized, and the physician wishes to reduce the severity of infection, or prevent it altogether. This calls for either *passive immunization* or the use of specific *antitoxins*. Before the Salk polio vaccine was perfected, passive immunization was sometimes used for protection: the portion of blood (in blood banks) containing antibodies against various diseases was concentrated and injected into someone who had been exposed to polio. Because this so-called gamma globulin fraction of blood contains antibodies against polio, it affords a certain degree of protection. This technique is still used in measles and some other diseases. Unfortunately the immunity from these passive antibodies lasts only a few weeks.

Antitoxins against specific microorganisms are considerably more effective, and their use is essential, for example, when there is the threat of tetanus in an individual who has sustained a severe wound or cut and has not been previously vaccinated against tetanus. To prepare tetanus antitoxin, the tetanus toxin is injected into an animal; after the animal has had time to produce antitoxin against the tetanus toxin, the blood is removed, and the antitoxin concentrated. When this is injected into a human patient, it combines with and neutralizes the threatening tetanus toxin in his blood stream, and may be lifesaving.

The best method for the prevention of

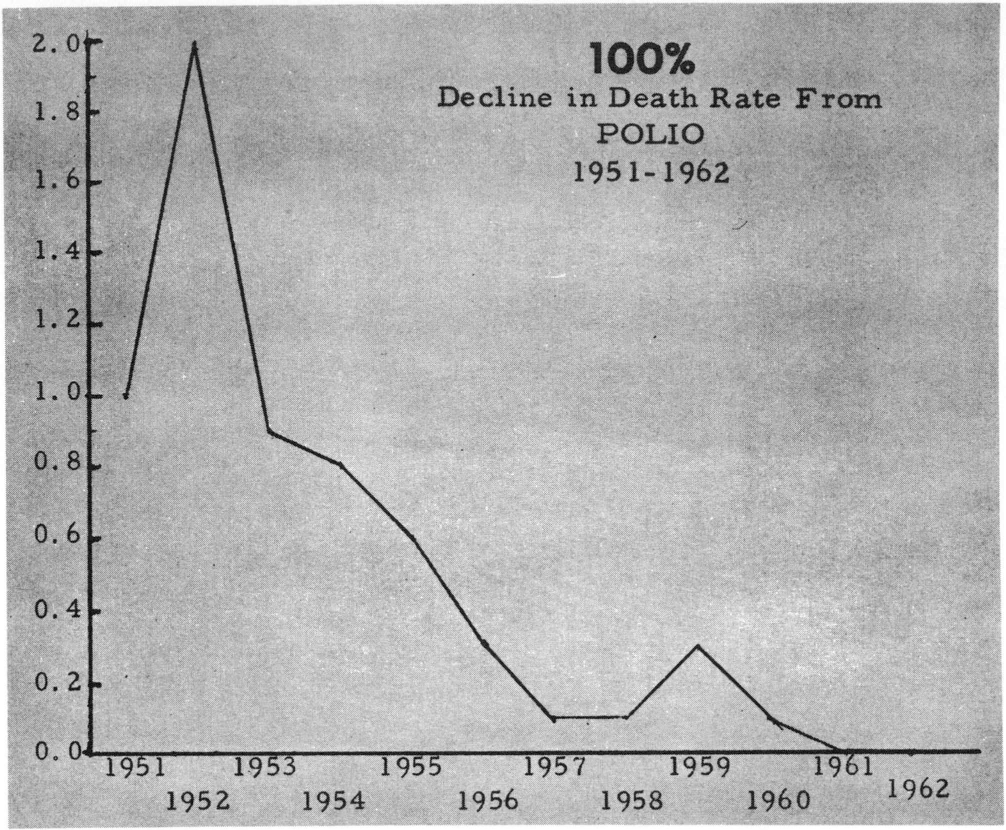

Figure 14–3. Decline in death rate from poliomyelitis. (From *Facts on the Major Killing and Crippling Diseases in the United States Today*. The National Health Education Committee, Inc., 1964.)

any infectious disease is vaccination. Unfortunately, scientists have not succeeded in preparing vaccines against all the serious communicable illnesses that affect mankind, but we can now protect against some of the most dangerous. In many communities, vaccination against diphtheria, whooping cough, smallpox and polio is compulsory, and *no intelligent person should subject himself to the hazards of any disease for which we have safeguards.* College students are in an age group which is very susceptible to polio, and polio vaccination should be a must for everyone in this age category. Tetanus vaccination would also be desirable. Travel in certain areas of the United States or in foreign countries requires vaccinations against special hazards that might be encountered, such as typhoid fever, Rocky Mountain spotted fever, tetanus, and even cholera and typhus.

Therapeutic Agents for the Infectious Diseases

In 1911, Paul Ehrlich announced the synthesis of *salvarsan,* an arsenic compound which could be used safely and successfully in the treatment of syphilis. It was also called "606," because it represented the 606th compound he had made in an effort to cure this disease. Since that time, and particularly in the years after 1935 when sulfanilamide was first used successfully by Gerhard Domagk in otherwise fatal bacterial infections such as streptococcal "blood poisoning," countless compounds have been synthesized by chemists in an effort to find specific curative agents for disease. The search has led to many remarkable substances, including drugs like *isoniazid,* which speeds up recovery from tuberculosis, and *chloroquine,* for the cure of malaria.

The accidental isolation of penicillin by Alexander Fleming from a mold which contaminated his bacterial cultures opened up the whole new field of *antibiotics*. These are the chemicals, synthesized by molds and certain other microorganisms, which have the ability to combat virulent bacteria. They have proved to be invaluable in the treatment of many bacterial and some rickettsial diseases, and an intensive search is being made at the present time throughout the world, in fields and forests, on land and in the sea, for organisms which can synthesize newer and better antibiotics.

Today, in addition to penicillin, we have a long list of effective compounds including streptomycin, Aureomycin, chloramphenicol, kanamycin, and erythromycin. Some are safer than others, with fewer and less dangerous side reactions; some affect a narrow, and others, a wide span of bacteria; and certain ones suffer from the disadvantage that sooner or later bacteria become resistant to them, and the antibiotics become ineffective. But, fortunately, we are constantly adding new ones to our armamentarium, and, to some extent at least, we can side-step the problem of resistance. So far, few really effective antivirus agents have been either synthesized or found to occur in nature, so that our chief weapons against virus diseases at the present time are vaccines and immune sera.

Even with the limitations of modern-day medical science, we can be grateful that we are living in the second half of the twentieth century instead of one hundred years ago when many diseases that today can easily be prevented or cured would then have meant death or disability.

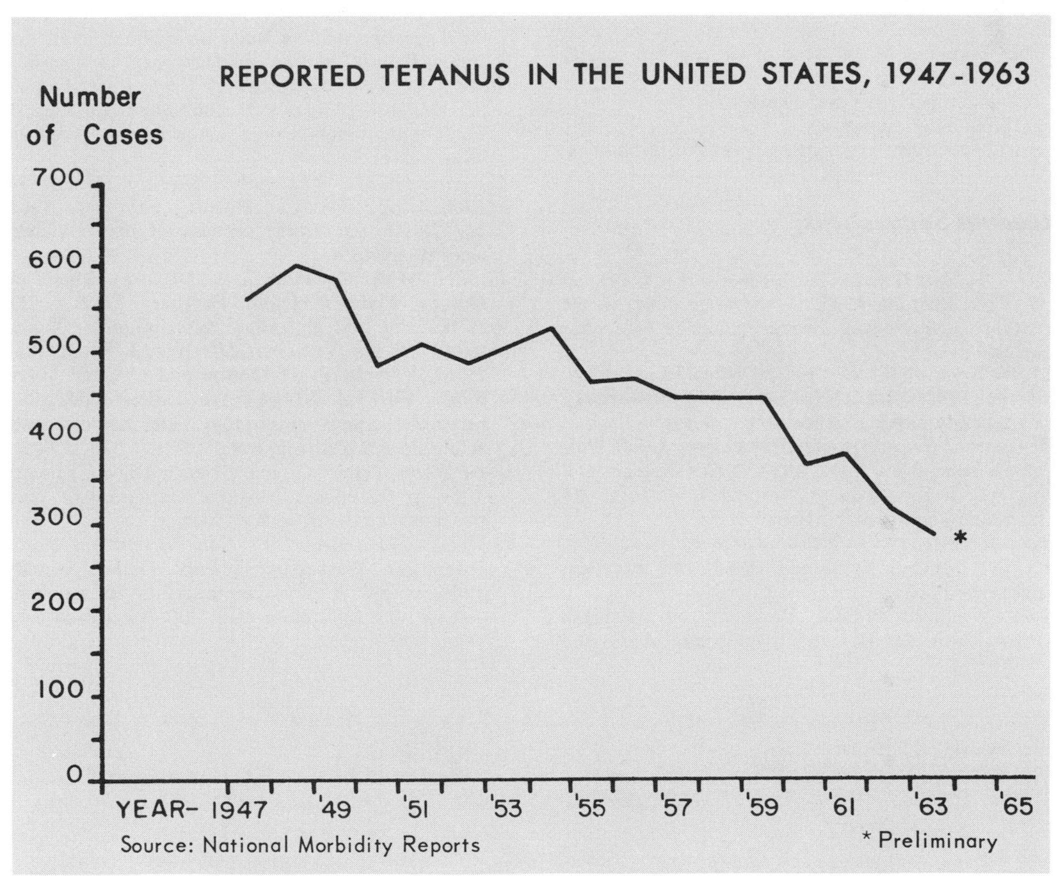

Figure 14–4. The number of tetanus cases reported in the United States from 1947 to 1963. (From *Morbidity and Mortality*. U.S. Department of Health, Education and Welfare, Public Health Service, June 12, 1964.)

Questions

1. Define disease. Give some general categories.
2. What are the common warning symptoms of disease?
3. Differentiate the following infectious agents, and give an example of a disease caused by each: bacterium, virus, rickettsia, fungus, protozoon, and parasitic worm.
4. What diseases could be spread by sneezing? food and water? insect bites? animal bites? raw fish and pork?
5. How do the white blood cells protect against bacterial invasion?
6. What is the difference between an *antigen, antitoxin, antibody?*
7. How does *passive* immunization differ from *active* immunization? Which is more effective?
8. What is the fundamental difference between smallpox vaccination and most other types of vaccination?
9. What are antibiotics? How were they discovered?
10. For what discoveries will Gerhard Domagk and Alexander Fleming be remembered?

Topics for Discussion

The "Typhoid Mary" type of carrier: can society isolate them?

The distemper virus and measles.

ECHO and adenoviruses.

Broad-spectrum and narrow-spectrum antibiotics.

Reading Suggestions

Rats, Lice and History, Hans Zinsser. Little, Brown & Co., Boston, 1935. A vivid account of the author's experiences during epidemics of typhus fever.

Science Book of Wonder Drugs, Donald G. Cooley. Pocket Books, Inc., New York, 1954 (paperback). By a highly expert science writer.

The Eternal Search, Richard Mathison. G. P. Putnam's Sons, New York, 1958. Man's diseases and his search for medicines throughout history. An interesting and readable book.

Communicable and Infectious Diseases, F. H. Top. C. V. Mosby, St. Louis, 1965. An excellent reference book.

Virus, Wolfhard Weidel. University of Michigan Press, Ann Arbor, 1965 (paperback). A revised book describing the origin, nature and control of viruses. Well written and witty.

Microbiology for Nurses, Martin Frobisher et al. W. B. Saunders, Philadelphia, 1964. A well-written and illustrated textbook. An excellent source book for the college student interested in microbiology.

The March of Medicine, H. S. Glasscheib. Macdonald Press, London, 1963. An interesting account of the history of medicine. Well illustrated.

The Book of Health, R. Lee Clark and Russell W. Cumley, eds. Van Nostrand, Princeton, N.J., 1962. An extraordinarily readable account of practically every human disease. Two hundred and fifty-five contributors tell what every family should know about health and disease.

Microbe Hunters, Paul de Kruif. Harcourt, Brace & Company, New York, 1954 (paperback). A fascinating introduction to the history of microbiology. An old but excellent book.

Eleven Blue Men, Berton Roueché. Berkley Publishing Corp., New York, 1953 (paperback). A collection of interesting stories about a variety of human diseases. Beautifully written and thrilling.

Curiosities of Medicine, Berton Roueché, ed. Berkley Publishing Corp., New York, 1964 (paperback). A fascinating collection of articles that provide a greater appreciation for the nature of medicine. Many of the articles are indisputably classics: John Snow on cholera, William Beaumont on digestion, William Budd on typhoid fever, and Peter Panum on the epidemiology of measles.

Have You Kept Your Immunity Up to Date? Donald A. Dukelow. Today's Health, April 1964, p. 7. Each student should read this article and heed the advice given.

Cowpox: Man's "Friendly" Disease, Frank H. Richardson. Today's Health, February 1964, p. 12. An interesting account of man's victory against smallpox.

Viruses: Molecules that Cause Disease, Donald G. Cooley. Today's Health, February 1962, p. 23. A readable and up-to-date description of viruses.

Viruses and the Nature of Life, W. M. Stanley and E. G. Valems. E. P. Dutton and Co., Inc., New York, 1961. A Nobel Prize Laureate describes research findings in virology. The book is both scientific and philosophical.

1964 Baby, Daniel Cohen. Science Digest, January 1964, p. 12. An informative discussion of what the future holds for today's baby.

Tetanus: The Disease We Can Prevent But Don't, Joseph D. Wassersug. Science Digest, January 1964, p. 85. A physican describes an agonizing disease that kills more than 400 Americans each year.

15

ENDOCRINE DISORDERS

. . . it is instructive to know that stress stimulates our glands to make hormones which can induce a kind of drunkenness. Without knowing this, no one would ever think of checking his conduct as carefully during stress as he does at a cocktail party. Yet he should.

HANS SELYE
The Stress of Life

When the only living species on earth was a microscopic single-celled organism, this creature still had to carry out many activities to survive; but since everything happened in a single cell, the processes could be regulated fairly easily. At this stage of evolution life was relatively simple. But as more complicated systems developed, culminating in the very complex figure of man himself, with many organs and tissues, and with a mind and conscious and unconscious activities, a multitude of controls had to be evolved to maintain stability. One type of control is exercised by the glands of internal secretion, the *endocrine glands*.

The endocrine glands determine what "metabolic tune" is to be played, how loud or soft, how vigorous or quiet. They set the rate, the mood, and the harmony among the organs and tissues of the body. Indeed, the endocrine glands have often been compared with an orchestra of which the *pituitary* gland is the conductor. All the other endocrine glands, although extremely important, play harmoniously under the direction of the leader.

The term *gland* is given to any part of the body that produces a secretion. The two types of glands are the *exocrine* and the *endocrine*. Exocrine glands are usually called glands of external secretion. Examples are the *salivary glands,* which pour saliva into the mouth, and the breast or *mammary* glands, which produce milk. Exocrine glands also secrete the digestive juices of the stomach and bile. Whereas the glands of external secretion send their products through a duct or tube, the secretions which endocrine glands produce go directly into the blood stream.

The substances these glands create are chemical in nature and are called *hormones*. In many cases, their exact chemical composition has been discovered by scientists, who can even create a few of them in the laboratory. A number of hormones have been extracted in pure form from the glands, which is a great advantage in using them medically.

We have learned much about what the various hormones do and about what happens to the body when a certain gland fails to function properly, creating too much or too little of its secretion. Although our knowledge of this subject is still incomplete, some of the most remarkable and dramatic treatments in medicine are possible because of advances in endocrinology.

THE FAMILY OF ENDOCRINE GLANDS

The endocrine glands include:

The *pituitary.*

The *thyroid.*

The *parathyroids,* which are actually four small glands attached to the thyroid.

The *islets of Langerhans,* tiny cells forming "islands" in the pancreas.

The *adrenal glands,* one above each kidney.

The *gonads* or *sex glands,* consisting of the testes in men and the ovaries in women.

In addition, there are the *pineal* gland, in the upper, back part of the brain, and the *thymus* gland, which is found below the thyroid in young people and which later atrophies. Very little is known as yet about these glands, although they are believed to belong to the endocrine family. Recent evidence indicates that the thymus gland may play a role in the development of immunity to disease.

The hormones which these glands send through the blood to the various parts of the body act like messengers. (The word *hormone* derives from a Greek word meaning "to excite" or "to stir up.") They don't actually initiate processes, but rather they catalyze certain activities, encouraging or discouraging them. They exert their influence on such fundamental processes as growth, reproduction and sex. How great a part they play in our mental and emotional states is not yet fully understood. However, it is known that some glandular disturbances cause mental conditions or personality changes, and that these disappear with treatment.

The endocrine glands form an *interdependent* system. In that respect they are like a family: what happens to one can affect them all. For example, the removal of one gland often alters the functioning of all the others. Similarly, an increase in the functioning of one will change the others. That is one reason why it is *extremely dangerous to dose one's self with hormones, glandular tissue or extract,* or whatever it may be called, for the purpose of reducing, getting rid of excess hair, developing the breasts, becoming more virile, or for any other reason.

The Pituitary Gland

The most important function of the pituitary is the part it plays in stimulating, regulating and coordinating the functions of the other endocrine glands. It is rightfully called the "master gland."

This gland is located at the base of the brain. Imagine a line drawn through your head from ear to ear and another line going backward from between your eyes. The pituitary gland lies at the spot where these two lines cross. It is about the size of a pea, and consists of an anterior lobe, an intermediate part and a posterior lobe.

One hormone of the pituitary gland has a powerful effect on growth of the body in general. Another controls the adrenal glands; this is the adrenocorticotrophic hormone, popularly known as ACTH. Pituitary hormones regulate the thyroid and stimulate the development of the ovaries and testes, making sexual development and reproduction possible. Still another hormone stimulates milk production by the breasts.

Too little pituitary secretion causes certain types of *dwarfism,* while too much makes the body grow to gigantic proportions. Pituitary tumors may press on the optic nerves and cause some loss of vision and headaches. *Acromegaly,* in which the bones, particularly those of the face and hands and feet, increase in size, results from an overactive pituitary gland.

Underactivity, or pituitary insufficiency,

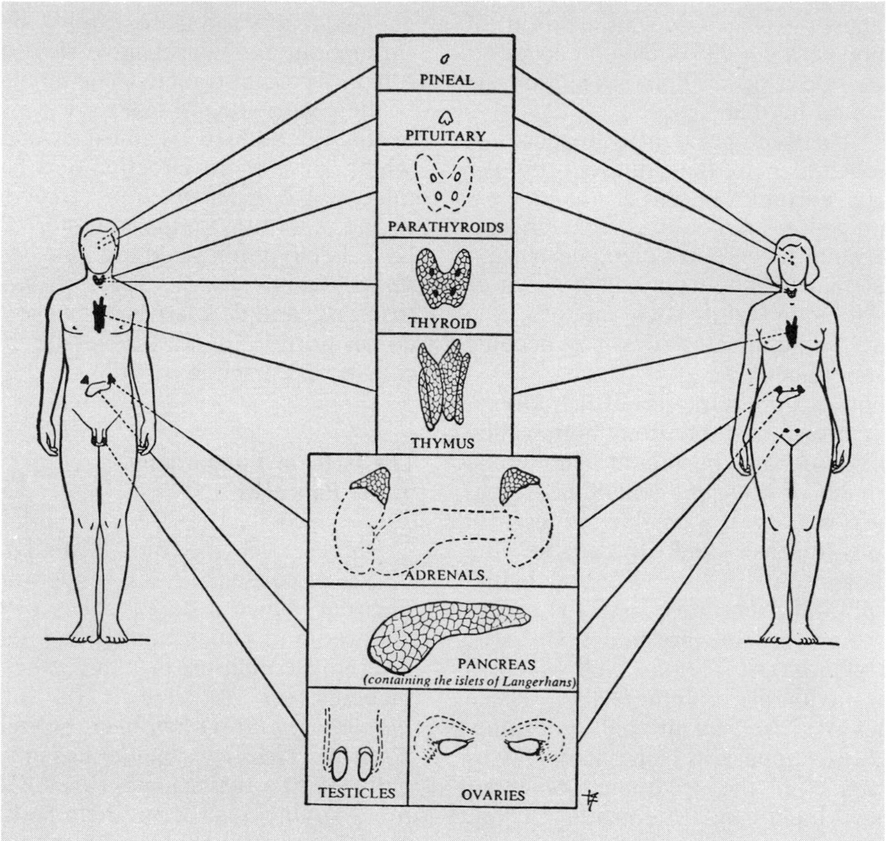

Figure 15–1. Location of the endocrine glands.

may produce a condition called *Frölich's syndrome*. Children so affected are excessively fat and underdeveloped sexually, although mentally bright. If given pituitary extract in time, they will become normal and will be spared unhappy lives.

If the pituitary secretion decreases after puberty, fat may accumulate around certain portions of the body, particularly the hips.

When the posterior portion of the pituitary fails to function properly, excessive urination results. The output of urine may amount to as much as 30 quarts a day. This rare malady is called *diabetes insipidus,* not to be confused with the more common diabetes mellitus.

The Adrenal Glands

Each adrenal gland is divided into two parts: the *cortex* or outer portion, and the *medulla,* the central section. The cortex and the medulla produce quite different hormones.

The medulla secretes the hormone *epinephrine,* more commonly called *adrenaline.* The output of this hormone is immediately stepped up when you become angry, fearful or excited. This quickly makes the heart beat faster and produces chemical changes that prepare the body for action. You have undoubtedly observed the effects of adrenaline when you were angry or alarmed, for it makes you feel tense and on edge; or perhaps you have said, "I was so scared (or angry) that I did things I couldn't possibly have been able to do normally."

The three main functions of the adrenal *cortex* and of its various steroid hormones are:

1. To control the salt and water content of the body.

2. To control sugar and protein metabolism, acting exactly opposite to insulin. In some tumors of the adrenal cortex,

where there is excessive production of its hormones, a condition called *Cushing's syndrome* develops. This condition is accompanied by diabetes.

3. The cortex appears also to secrete a hormone similar to that put out by the testes. In certain tumors of the cortex, females develop marked masculine characteristics, such as a deep voice and hair on the face; menstruation may slow down or cease. In men with such tumors, the secondary sex characteristics may become more pronounced.

Atrophy or underfunction of the adrenal cortex causes a rare condition called *Addison's disease*. The recent commercial development of *cortisone* and other steroid hormones makes it possible to control Addison's disease and to enable the afflicted person to lead a normal life.

The pituitary hormone, ACTH, stimulates secretion of hormones by the adrenal glands. ACTH, as well as cortisone, is available commercially. These hormones are used in adrenal underfunction and also appear to bring about favorable results in the treatment of other diseases, including rheumatic fever, arthritis, asthma, hay fever, bursitis and skin and eye disorders. The reason for these remarkable effects is not yet clearly understood. People with these diseases do not appear to be deficient in adrenal hormones, yet adding to their normal secretion brings about striking improvement in some cases.

An epoch-making discovery in medicine was the successful treatment of patients with rheumatoid arthritis by cortisone. The first reports of this were made by Philip Hench and his associates at the Mayo Clinic in Rochester, Minnesota, about 1948, and their work stimulated a search for other and better, synthetic steroid derivatives. Because this hormone was originally obtained from animal adrenal glands, salvaged at the slaughter houses, the amounts available were very limited. An intensive search was initiated for better natural sources. Curiously, the Mexican yam, a kind of sweet potato, proved to contain a steroid which could be used in the synthesis of many other derivatives.

Since Hench's first report, organic chemists at various research laboratories throughout the world have devised many other steroid hormones. The chief purpose of their work was to make greater amounts available, and to synthesize compounds which were more effective and had fewer undesirable side reactions than had cortisone. The most important steroids which have been synthesized are *hydrocortisone, fluorohydrocortisone, prednisone, prednisolone,* and derivatives of these in which some portion of the molecule has been transposed or altered.

The Islets of Langerhans in the Pancreas

Diabetes is the most familiar of the diseases caused by an endocrine gland disorder. Once a major cause of death in children and young adults, and a seriously disabling condition in many older people, diabetes (or, to give it its full name, *diabetes mellitus*) has been brought under control. This was made possible in the early 1920's when insulin was discovered by a young Canadian doctor, Frederick G. Banting, assisted by Charles H. Best.

Many years ago, a scientist named Langerhans studied small clusters of cells that formed what he called "islets," scattered throughout the *pancreas*. (The pancreas is the flat organ situated below and behind the stomach; the pancreases of animals are the sweetbreads of our dinner menus.) Although the masses of cells which are now called the islets of Langerhans lie within the pancreas, their function is entirely different. The main part of the pancreas produces juices which enter the intestines and help in the digestion of proteins and fats.

The islets of Langerhans secrete the hormone called *insulin*. This enables the body to use (or burn) sugar and starch after it has been converted into glucose by the digestive juices. The body depends on glucose for heat and energy, and to help in the utilization of other foods.

When the islets of Langerhans fail to provide the insulin to "spark" this process, the sugar passes, unused, into the blood and is eliminated in the urine. The quantity of urine eliminated increases, causing the diabetic to be thirsty and drink more water, which in turn is quickly eliminated. Thus diabetes is due to the failure of the body to provide an essential hormone, insulin. It is not a contagious or infectious disease.

We do not know all the reasons why the islets of Langerhans sometimes fail to provide sufficient insulin. A disease of the pancreas can be responsible. There is a tendency for diabetes to run in families; certain ones of us may have less ability to produce insulin than others. Diabetes occurs most frequently in people who are overweight; the islets of Langerhans, trying to make enough insulin for the tremendous amount of sugar and starch fat people consume, may be simply unequal to the task. Another cause for diabetes is overproduction of hormones from the adrenal glands, which neutralize or antagonize the insulin. Derangement of pituitary gland function can also affect insulin activity.

(Diabetes is also discussed on p. 259.)

The Thyroid Gland

The thyroid gland is situated in front of the throat, below the Adam's apple and just above the breastbone. It is roughly U shaped, the ends of the U flaring out to a lobe about the size of the big toe.

This gland is extremely important in maintaining the all-round health of the body, because it regulates the rate at which the body uses oxygen taken in by breathing. It also controls the rate at which the various organs of the body function, and the speed with which the body uses food.

Too much thyroid secretion would speed up metabolism so that you would be overactive and nervous, your heart would palpitate, and you would be kept at so high a pitch you couldn't relax and sleep well. Too little thyroid output would make you drowsy, fatigued, and slow-moving. You might gain weight and develop coarse features and a thick, scaly skin.

The hormone of the thyroid gland, *thyroxine,* has many important functions. It regulates the metabolic rate. It also influences growth, temperature sensitivity, intellectual development, and, directly or indirectly, the proper functioning and coordination of many other tissues. Among these are the brain, the cardiovascular system, the blood-forming system and the reproductive organs.

Myxedema. Myxedema is caused by an underactive thyroid. A person suffering with this condition is sluggish physically and mentally. He cannot stand the cold. Sometimes his tongue is so large and thick that it sticks out of his mouth. Treatment usually brings marked improvement.

Cretinism. Cretinism develops if a child is born without a thyroid gland, or if the gland degenerates. Unless the disease is detected early, the child remains physically and mentally undeveloped. However, if thyroid therapy can be started on very young infants, growth may be normal, and a marked improvement in mental status can be achieved. Women who tend to have cretinous babies can be given thyroid hormone during pregnancy to prevent this.

This disease occasionally occurs even if the mothers are on a normal diet, because of poorly functioning thyroid glands. However, mostly it is found—or was found, until its cause was recognized—in the so-called "goiter belts" of the world. These are the places where the soil and water, and foods grown in these areas, are dangerously low in *iodine.* This is true in certain parts of the Alps and the Himalayas, as well as in our own Great Lakes region and the valley of the St. Lawrence. Adding iodine to ordinary salt can prevent this so-called *endemic* cretinism.

Simple Goiter. The thyroid gland needs iodine in order to function properly, and to manufacture the normal quantity of *thyroxine.* In an effort to compensate for iodine deficiency, the gland becomes enlarged. As the swelling continues, a noticeable lump appears in the throat. This swelling or goiter may be large enough to interfere with breathing or swallowing. Girls and women are more likely to develop goiters than are boys and men. The hormone of the thyroid gland contains about 65 per cent iodine, but the amount of iodine needed in food to avoid goiter is very small. The amount of *iodized* table salt we use in meals is sufficient, even in areas where the soil is completely lacking in natural iodine. Consuming iodine sometimes makes a simple goiter subside. If not, surgical removal is necessary.

It is especially important for expectant mothers who live in such regions as the Rocky Mountain states, the Great Lakes basin, or the upper Mississippi River Valley, where the soil is lacking in iodine, to use iodized salt. Insufficient iodine in the diet may cause a pregnant woman to produce a child with thyroid deficiency. In extreme cases, cretinism results.

Hyperthyroidism. A more serious type of goiter develops when the thyroid manufactures *too much* hormone. (*Hyper* means too much.) People with hyperthyroidism are nervous and irritable and suffer from insomnia. Heat makes them extremely uncomfortable, so that they frequently sleep with the covers thrown off, even in cool weather. The excess secretion also produces an overactive heart, manifesting itself in palpitation (which is sometimes mistaken for a true cardiac condition). Another symptom of this disease is loss of weight—as much as twenty pounds or even more—in spite of increased hunger.

Other names for hyperthyroidism are thyrotoxicosis and Graves' disease. Hyperthyroidism is sometimes called *exophthalmic goiter* because many patients have protruding eyes, causing them to look continually startled.

For many years the only treatment was surgery. About 90 per cent of the gland was removed, and most patients were cured. Today, radioactive iodine can be employed to cut down the gland's activity. Like ordinary iodine, radioactive iodine is taken up by the thyroid, and the radiation given off within the gland suppresses its functioning. A medicine called propylthiouracil may also be used in treatment, either by itself or in preparation for surgery.

Any enlargement or lump in the throat should be examined by a physician. One of the tests employed to determine the activity of the thyroid gland is the *basal metab-*

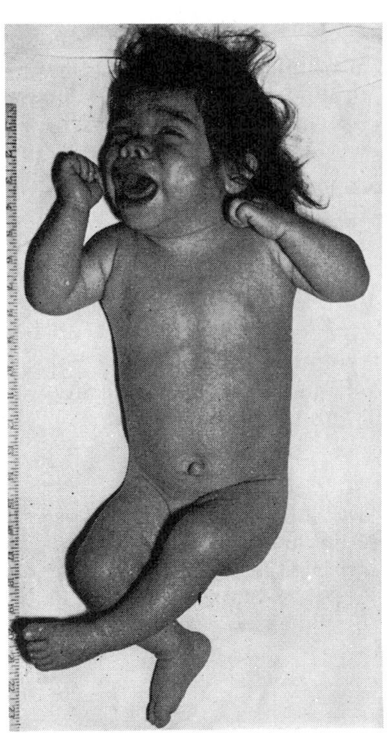

A

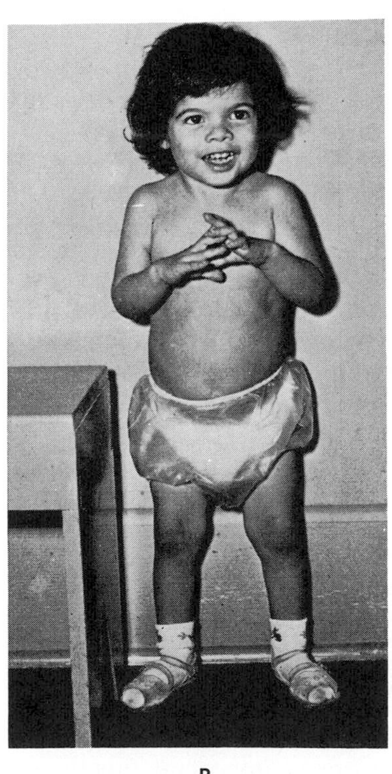

B

Figure 15–2. **A,** Cretin, aged 3 years, 10 months. No previous treatment with thyroid hormone had been administered. **B,** The same child after 14 months of optimum continuous treatment with desiccated thyroid. (From Williams, B. H. and Cramm, C. J. *The Medical Clinics of North America,* July, 1955.)

olism test, which records the amount of oxygen you use. In hyperthyroidism this is increased, and in myxedema the absorption of oxygen during breathing decreases. Another laboratory test for thyroid disorders utilizes radioactive iodine as a *tracer*. The severity of the disease can be determined by the amount of iodine taken up by the thyroid gland: an overactive gland will use up more iodine, an underactive one, less.

The Parathyroid Glands

These tiny glands, about the size of a very small pea and usually found in clusters of four, are embedded near the base of the thyroid. They control the excretion in urine of the bone minerals, calcium and phosphorus.

The parathyroid glands are so much smaller than the thyroid that in the past they were sometimes accidentally removed with the thyroid when it had to be taken out surgically. The significance and location of the parathyroids are well known today, and there is little danger of their accidental removal.

In *parathyroid deficiency* the calcium regulation is disturbed and the muscles are subject to spasms *(tetany)*. In severe cases, convulsions and death may result. The administration of the parathyroid hormone, or certain synthetically manufactured compounds with similar actions, or a potent vitamin D preparation, will keep the calcium output normal and stop the spasms. *Parathyroid tumors* cause *hyperparathyroidism*. When this occurs, there is generalized depletion of calcium, with loss of bone mineral, and sometimes kidney stones form.

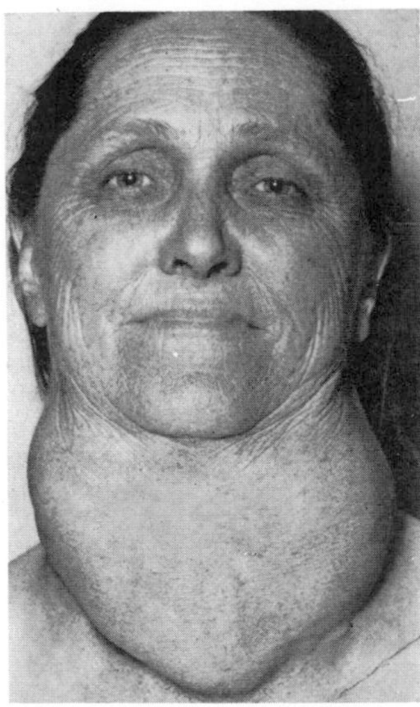

Figure 15–3. Large multinodular goiter. Gradual enlargement since childhood. (From Crile: *Practical Aspects of Thyroid Disease*.)

The Sex Glands (Gonads)[1]

The gonads (from the Greek word *gonē*, meaning *seed*) consist of the *testes* in men and the *ovaries* in women. Besides producing *sperm* and *ova*, the sex glands make the hormones which are responsible for the special characteristics of the male and female.

Human beings have always been aware of the outward physical difference between men and women, but understanding the cause of these differences has been a slow process. The discovery of the gonads and isolation of their hormones have gradually removed much of the mystery from sexual differentiation.

At an early stage of development, the embryo possesses rudimentary male and female sex organs. However, normally only one or the other matures and the sex of the child is determined. In rare cases, both, or parts of both the male and female sex glands may develop. Such an individual is a *hermaphrodite* and will need surgery to determine the sex.

Advances in Endocrinology

Remarkable advances have been made in recent years in *endocrinology*, the branch of science which deals with the endocrine glands and their hormones. Today, with the use of purified natural hormones, and in some cases, even better *synthetic* hormones, we can treat diseases which were once fatal. There have even been implantations of glands in individuals

[1]Reproduction is discussed in Chapters 10 and 11.

in whom the glands were lacking from birth or became diseased. For example, parathyroid glands have now been successfully transplanted.

Perhaps the many problems involved in transplanting glands or tissues of any kind from one individual to another will some day be solved. If—and when—this happens, we shall think nothing of transplanting thyroids, adrenals, ovaries and all the other glands. But that millennium has not yet come.

When iodine achieved its apparently miraculous effects in the residents of the goiter belts, a tremendous wave of enthusiasm—and hysteria—struck the world. Glands, wonderful glands, could do anything. The fountain of eternal youth was just around the corner, in the form of transplanted monkey glands. Articles, books, and even plays were written dealing with this new way of staying young and virile forever. These claims soon proved to be unfounded, and the monkey gland craze went the way of other fads.

Questions

1. What is a *hormone*? Give at least three examples of hormones, telling what function each one plays.
2. Differentiate between *exocrine* and *endocrine* glands, and give an example of each.
3. Why is the pituitary gland called the "conductor" of the endocrine gland orchestra?
4. Why is self-dosage with hormones so dangerous?
5. What causes dwarfs and giants? cretins?
6. What is the chief role of the parathyroid glands?
7. How does the *basal metabolism* test indicate thyroid gland activity?
8. What are the gonads? Contrast the endocrine and sexual functions of the male and female gonads.
9. What causes "sterility" in the male and the female?
10. Compare the adrenal medulla and cortex.

Topics for Discussion

Thyroid gland and temperature sensitivity.
Diabetes insipidus.
The discovery of insulin.

Reading Suggestions

General Endocrinology, C. Donnell Turner. 3rd Ed., W. B. Saunders Co., Philadelphia, 1960. Endocrinology in its biologic aspects.

The Thymus Hormone, R. H. Levey. Scientific American, July 1964, p. 66. A new role of the thymus gland is described.

The Story of Insulin, G. A. Wrenshall, Indiana University Press, Bloomington, 1962. A vivid description of triumphant discovery of insulin and its historical use. Also discussed are the most up-to-date ideas on diabetes mellitus and its management. A highly readable book.

Structure and Function In Man, Stanley W. Jacob and Clarice A. Francone, W. B. Saunders, Philadelphia, 1965. A basic textbook in integrated anatomy and physiology. It contains a very up-to-date and well illustrated chapter on the endocrine system.

The Wonderful Human Body, American Medical Association, 1961. Contains an excellent description of the endocrine system. Well illustrated.

The Stress of Life, Hans Selye. McGraw-Hill, New York, 1956. An informative discussion of the role of the endocrines in normal living.

The Hormone Quest, Albert Q. Maisel, Random House, New York, 1965. A review of the exciting research being conducted with hormones. An up-to-date and readable book.

Our Hormones and How They Work, Sarah R. Reidman, Collier Books, New York, 1962 (paperback). The study of hormones written for the layman.

The Chemicals of Life: Enzymes, Vitamins, Hormones. New American Library, New York, 1962 (paperback). An interesting discussion of the chemistry of life. Very readable.

A Modern Pilgrim's Progress for Diabetics, Garfield G. Duncan. W. B. Saunders Co., Philadelphia, 1956.

Hormones: Your Body's Chemical Rousers, Donald G. Cooley. Today's Health, November 1962, p. 28, and December 1962, p. 28. A two part article describing the production and action of hormones. The articles are comprehensive, scientific, readable, and very well illustrated.

The Parathyroid Hormone, Howard Rasmussen. Scientific American, April 1961, p. 56. An up-to-date account of current knowledge regarding this hormone.

Function of the Human Body, Arthur C. Guyton. W. B. Saunders, Philadelphia, 1964. A very readable college level physiology book.

How We Discovered Insulin, Charles H. Best. Reader's Digest, March 1964, p. 47. One of the participants in the discovery of insulin gives a firsthand account of the experience.

16

SOME COMMON "NUISANCE AILMENTS"

Very often we are bothered by ailments which, though not really serious, may still be annoying enough to interfere with our comfort and happiness, and even be temporarily incapacitating. Sinusitis, acne, fungus infections, premenstrual pain and tension, and many other conditions have already been discussed in previous sections.

In this chapter, five such "nuisance ailments," which are bothersome to many people, are described: *headaches,* the *common cold, allergies, constipation,* and *varicose veins.*

HEADACHES

Probably more people suffer from headaches than from any other medical condition, and the proof is that $350 million a year – 10 per cent of the cost of all drugs and medicines – goes into headache remedies. A survey made by Henry Ogden of the Louisiana State University School of Medicine showed that headaches were common problems with more than 60 per cent of the population, and the rate among college students, especially medical students, exceeded 80 per cent. According to Dr. Ogden, more women experienced headaches than men, 71 per cent compared with 50 per cent of the males interviewed. Age was also found to be a definite factor, and the percentage of headaches dropped steadily over the decades, with only about 28 per cent of people over 60 complaining of these distressing symptoms.[1]

Defective vision and *eyestrain* are common causes of headaches, and countless people suffer needlessly without

[1]*Drug and Cosmetic Industry,* October (1956).

realizing that eyeglasses, good lighting and better reading and television habits would bring relief. Headaches can also be triggered by *anxieties* and *tensions,* as well as by hunger, lack of sleep, too much drinking or smoking, overexertion, or even eating ice cream too fast. *Sinusitis, colds, hay fever,* and other *allergies* may be accompanied by headaches; and in *measles, influenza, polio, meningitis,* and many other infectious diseases, headache may be the first symptom. *Anemia, disorders of the intestinal tract,* and *constipation* may bring headaches on, too.

You certainly don't have to visit a doctor every time you have a headache, because it will often respond to aspirin or some other simple pain reliever, and will frequently disappear spontaneously when the cause is eliminated. However, if headaches are accompanied by other disturbing symptoms, if they seem to be increasing in severity or frequency, and if they persist when there isn't any obvious cause for them, a medical consultation is certainly in order.

A great many ordinary headaches are classified as *tension* or "nervous" headaches, because they are simply the expression of some emotional stress. One group of physicians studying over 500 such patients discovered that they responded rapidly to a *placebo,*[2] which was described to them as a new headache cure. This does not mean that the patients were not in true pain, but it does suggest that the headache had a psychosomatic origin, since it could be alleviated by the doctor's solicitude or the completely inert pill—or both combined.

Whether the tension which causes headaches comes from the nature and pace of daily life or from the emotions of the individual—or both—the result is the same. The solution is to reduce the tensions, or to relieve the pain.

If aspirin, or some other safe pain reliever, does not work, try to relax by resting in a quiet place. Some people find that gentle massaging of the neck muscles relieves a headache; others massage the entire scalp quite vigorously. Application of an ice bag to the head for from 5 to 10 minutes may also prove beneficial.

Migraine is a special form which is sometimes called a "sick headache," because it is often associated with nausea and vomiting. Its cause is unknown, but it does appear to be related to an individual's psychological makeup. It is found most frequently in certain personality types, especially tense, "perfectionist" individuals, and an attack may follow some emotional disturbance. In women, episodes of migraine often coincide with the menstrual period, and nearly three times as many women as men suffer from these headaches. Also, there seems to be a family tendency toward migraine.

A typical attack starts with changes in vision—a flickering before the eyes, flashes of light, or a blacking out of part of the visual field. Migraine headaches generally are located either in the right or left part of the head, and scarcely ever involve the entire head. They may be almost intolerably painful and nauseating, and the pain is not relieved by aspirin. However, other medicines, especially those containing *ergotamine,* have been used successfully, both to prevent the headaches and to relieve them.

Individuals who suffer from migraine sometimes experience strange hallucinations, ranging from blurred vision and distorted images to bizarre bodily sensations. Some patients say they feel that their bodies are "ballooning out" and swelling to unnatural proportions, or that their heads are floating above the neck. Others describe sensations of "shrinking to about one foot high," or stretching to twice normal height. Possibly these hallucinations were the inspiration for *Alice in Wonderland* by Lewis Carroll, who was himself a severe migraine sufferer.

Headaches are probably an ancient disease of man. Archeologists working in prehistoric burial sites have dug up skulls into which openings have been chiseled out, or *trephined.* They believe these skulls might have come from patients who suffered headaches or other troubles ascribed to evil spirits pounding the insides

[2]This is a pill that contains no medicine but merely sugar or some other inactive substance.

of their heads. The artificial "hole-in-the-head" was to let the devils out. An easier and safer treatment for many headaches, both the tension and migraine types, might be to follow the "Nine Commandments for Headache Patients," which a physician interested in the emotional aspects of this problem has recommended:

This is not a perfect world. Families and friends have many foibles. Perfection is rarely attained, so be satisfied with less.

Tolerance makes understanding the other fellow easier. It sets an attainable standard.

Do not be a slave to the clock. Work at your own pace; do as much as you can. Trying to meet too many deadlines only creates tension.

You cannot please everybody, so stop trying. Popularity comes by giving your friends and family a chance to love you for yourself, not for your best performance.

Be efficient but not to the extent that perfection becomes a burden.

Speak up if you want to. You cannot please everybody; honesty and directness break down barriers and make friendships easier.

Approve of yourself. You are as good as the next fellow. If you are given a compliment, take it and make use of it.

Stop being so critical of your negative feelings. Everyone is ambivalent at times, so do not worry so much about loving and hating.

Stop feeling guilty. We are all human and we all make errors. Give a little and you will get a lot, *maybe even reduction of that pain in your head.*

THE COMMON COLD

It's called the common cold because at least 40 million Americans suffer from it not once but several times each year. We spend millions of dollars on aspirins, antihistamines, and innumerable other medicines in the hope of relieving some of the distress it causes, but a much greater cost is the 150 million work days lost each year to the common cold and associated viruses.

"Three days coming, three days with you, and three days going" is still a fairly accurate description of the course of a cold. First there is the brief "dry" stage when the nose feels prickly and there is a tickling sensation in the throat. Then the eyes begin to water, and this is followed by sneezing, a "running" nose, cough and sore throat, and possibly some fever. After a few days, the secretions become thicker and the cold starts to dry up.

In themselves, colds are little more than an annoying nuisance, and even so famous a physician as Sir William Osler, felt that "the only way to treat colds is with contempt." However, colds *do* warrant care because they can pave the way for potentially serious respiratory infections.

Cause and Prevention

Colds are caused by a virus to which the body is particularly susceptible when its resistance is lowered. It is, unfortunately, an extremely contagious virus, readily transmitted by close contact, particularly kissing, and by handling contaminated objects such as handkerchiefs. But the *chief* method of transmission is a cough or a sneeze; photographs taken by highspeed cameras show a cloud of particles spread approximately three feet in front of the person who sneezes. Because most of these particles could be caught by covering the sneeze or cough with a tissue, many colds could be prevented from spreading by this simple precaution.

Chilling lowers the body's resistance to colds, and forgetting your rubbers on damp days or a warm coat in cold weather can increase the number of colds you contract and transmit to others. Change into warm, dry clothes as soon as you can when you become wet or chilly.

Taking vitamins won't prevent or cure a cold, but it still pays to eat a well balanced diet because people in good physical condition are better able to resist some of the complications which follow colds.

You will have some *immunity* after a cold, but it is so brief you can't count on it. Therefore, the preventive measures should be used routinely.

How to Treat an Ordinary Cold

If you possibly can, go to bed as soon as you feel that you are coming down with a cold. You should stay away from other people anyway, in order not to spread your cold, so why not go to bed where you, too, will be better off? Keep warm until you are past the "runny" stage, and drink plenty of liquids. You can eat moderately of

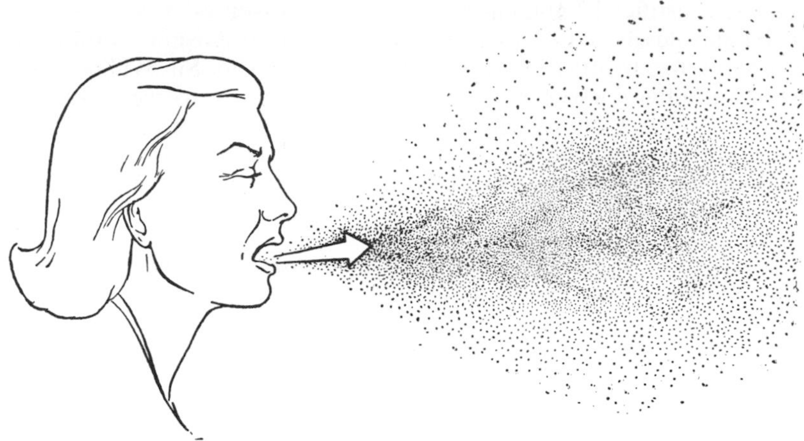

Figure 16–1. How microorganisms are spread by a sneeze.

anything that appeals to you. Be careful about blowing your nose too hard because you might force infection into the sinuses and ears. If your nose is badly stopped up, *ask your doctor* what kind of drops to use. Don't use nose drops or inhalers just because your friends or advertisements recommend them. They can do more harm than good. And don't waste your money on medicines that promise to "relieve the symptoms of a cold." Plain aspirin (or buffered aspirin, if the ordinary preparation upsets your stomach) brings the quickest and safest relief.

Protect People Around You. Smother your coughs and sneezes in tissues, and put the tissues into a paper bag so that they can be disposed of without contaminating anyone else.

Be Sure to Call a Doctor if:

1. You have a fever that lasts more than two or three days, or goes above 103° F.
2. You have a severe headache that doesn't respond to aspirin.
3. You have chills, severe cough, chest pains, blood-stained or rusty-looking sputum.
4. Your back, neck, or any other bones ache; you "ache all over"; you have an earache.
5. Your cold symptoms don't clear up. (You may actually be suffering from hay fever or some other allergy.)

What About Cold Vaccines?

Cold vaccines have been used for a number of years, but their prophylactic value is uncertain. One study with college students reported that cold vaccines were of no more value than injected sterile water. It is interesting to note, however, that sterile water reduced colds by 61 per cent—an obvious psychological effect.

Dr. John H. Dingle of Western Reserve University Medical School has aptly described the current status of the cold vaccine:[3]

> . . . Before any virus associated with respiratory illness is incorporated in a vaccine for general use in our population, it should be clearly demonstrated that: the virus caused the disease in question, the disease is followed by immunity, the virus can be grown in sufficient quantity to prepare a vaccine effective in the stimulation of antibodies, there is a positive correlation between the presence of antibodies and resistance to infection, and finally, the incidence of illness caused by the virus is sufficiently great to warrant attempts to immunize on a mass or a broad scale. At the present time these criteria can be met only in the case of the adenoviruses producing acute respiratory disease in military populations. There is no apparent justification for the use of even adenovirus vaccine on a mass scale in civilian populations at the present time.

[3]Dingle, J.H.: *American Journal of Public Health, 50*:293, 1960.

ALLERGIES

If you suffer from allergies in any form, you don't have to be told how miserable they can make you. And you are only one of millions. It is estimated that allergy is the third most prevalent illness in the United States, responsible for a major disease in one out of every 10 individuals, and affecting, in some degree or other, perhaps as many as *one out of every two people*. Neither infants nor octogenarians are spared, and although allergies are more common in early childhood, you can develop an allergy at any time in your life. Fortunately, they are not contagious.

The costs of allergic diseases in income loss and in discomfort are tremendous. Twenty-five million working days are lost each year because of hay fever and asthma alone, and occupational skin diseases cost industry over 100 million dollars. A large proportion of absenteeism from work and from school both must be blamed on allergic diseases.

You are not born with an allergy, but you may inherit the tendency to develop one or several. Geneticists report that if one parent is allergic, one-third of the children will show some allergy before they reach the age of ten. If both parents are allergic, about two thirds of the children will have similar tendencies, usually more severe, and manifest by the age of six.

However, you don't have to inherit the tendency in order to develop an allergy. Given the right conditions, almost anybody can become allergic to something, and the severity of the illness may range from a mildly annoying skin irritation or sniffles, to complete invalidism, to death.

The important allergic diseases are *asthma* and *chronic bronchitis,* which can be major disabling conditions, *hay fever, hives, eczema and contact dermatitis, gastrointestinal disturbances,* and certain types of *headaches*.

Causes of Allergies

An allergy is an abnormal sensitivity of the body to a foreign substance which is otherwise essentially harmless. The reaction may develop after eating, breathing, touching, or inhaling the offending material. *Antigen* or *allergen* is the name given to the substance which provokes the allergy, and the protein which the body synthesizes to combat it is called the specific *antibody*. If a person has once been exposed to a substance to which he is sensitive, the process is called *sensitization*.

All of us are constantly surrounded—while we eat, drink, work, play, study, and sleep—by chemicals or other agents which are allergens to some people. But not everybody reacts. For reasons still not understood, some individuals become sensitive to certain antigens.

The number of substances which have been reported to cause allergic reactions is enormous.

Things you breathe include pollens from grasses, flowers, and trees; dusts, such as house or insect dust; animal dander—the skin or hair shed by dogs, cats, rabbits, and other animals; particles from feathers; cosmetics; insecticide sprays; tobacco dust; and many chemicals.

Foods most frequently responsible are eggs, milk, wheat, fish, nuts, peas, beans, chocolate, strawberries, and other fruits.

You may also become allergic because of certain *things you touch,* referred to medically as *contactants*. Among these are wool or nylon, poison ivy, nail polish, hair dyes, permanent waving solutions, newspapers, certain plants, detergents, and flowers. You can even become allergic to money—to the metal in a nickel or the dye on a check.

Allergic *injectants* are substances which cause reactions when they *penetrate the skin*. These include insect stings: bee, ant, spider, or wasp; vaccinations or serum injections; medicines which are injected; and animal bites. Penicillin is responsible for many allergic reactions. If you are sensitive to it, you may even react to milk from a cow which has been treated with penicillin for some infection.

Bacterial allergy or *autosensitization* is the term applied when individuals are sensitized to bacteria present in their own bodies. A person who has experienced numerous infections of the sinuses, nose, throat, tonsils and adenoids may become sensitized to the infecting microorganisms.

Repeated respiratory infections are often attributed to this cause.

Surprisingly, even *physical conditions,* such as heat, cold, sunshine, changes in barometric pressure, humidity, and hot or cold drinks can cause true allergic symptoms. Hives may occur in cold-sensitive individuals after a swim in cold water, or after a cold shower. Bright sunlight causes rashes in some people.

The relation of the emotions to allergic reactions is a complicated one, but is particularly important in asthma and hives. Hives are actually called *angioneurotic* edema. It is unlikely that the emotions *cause* allergies, but they may represent a triggering mechanism which can precipitate an attack if the stage is already set.

Common Forms of Allergy

Hay Fever. Seasonal hay fever is the most common type. If it occurs in the early spring, it is usually due to tree pollens, and, in the summer, to the pollens of grasses. Ragweed pollen is generally the offender in the very common fall allergies. In some sections of the country pollens are present throughout most of the year, and the exact dates for seasonal allergies will vary.

Perennial hay fever can occur at any time of the year, because it is generally due to house dust, animal hair, feathers, and other substances, including *foods,* that we are constantly exposed to.

Common names for year-round hay fever are *allergic* or *vasomotor rhinitis;* many so-called "colds" are really perennial hay fever attacks.

Hay fever symptoms usually center in the nose, eyes and face—tickling, stuffiness, a watery discharge, and itching of the eyes and face.

If you suffer from this condition, *be sure to see a doctor,* because it can become far more than just a nuisance. It may lead to sinusitis or even to asthma (see p. 224).

Treatment varies according to the allergen responsible. In some cases the offending object can be avoided—for example, getting rid of a cat or dog will eliminate the allergy if it is due to this animal's dander, or parting with that "sable" coat which is actually made of rabbit fur, a common allergen. Spend your vacation at the seashore if pollens in the country are responsible. If you cannot escape from an area abounding in pollens to which you are allergic, an air conditioner with a good filter unit may mean the difference between misery and comfort. In addition, your physician may be able to immunize you against attacks: these injections contain minute amounts of the sensitizing pollen, and provoke the response of an antibody which may protect you. However, they must be given in ample time if you suffer from seasonal allergy. It is usually too late if you delay until the attacks have begun.

No medicine will cure hay fever—or any other allergy—but many substances available today afford tremendous relief. Among the newer treatments are the *antihistaminics,* so-called because they combat histamine release in the body. This chemical is thought to be responsible for some of the unpleasant allergic reactions. Cortisone and other steroid compounds are also helpful in some cases.

The medicines are administered in various forms—pills, capsules, sprays, eye drops, injections, or suppositories. Sniffing hydrocortisone powder was found to give tremendous relief to a group of ragweed hay fever sufferers. However, it is not wise to use any medications except under a doctor's supervision, because some of them produce undesirable side effects. Drowsiness is one of the commonest side effects of the antihistaminics, and they may be dangerous in driving or hazardous occupations.

Hives, or Urticaria. This disease is a form of allergy, in which there is a swelling, due to leakage of body fluids. It is not a true skin allergy, although the hives frequently appear on the skin as wheals or welts. Actually, they are very commonly *internal,* and foods, medicines, infections, and emotional disturbances may bring them on. The itching or burning they produce may be extremely uncomfortable.

Giant hives *(angioneurotic edema)* may appear on the lips, tongue, throat, eyes, and other parts of the body. Because an attack in the throat may interfere seriously with breathing, a person subject to hives should discuss *emergency* treatment with his physician in advance, and not wait

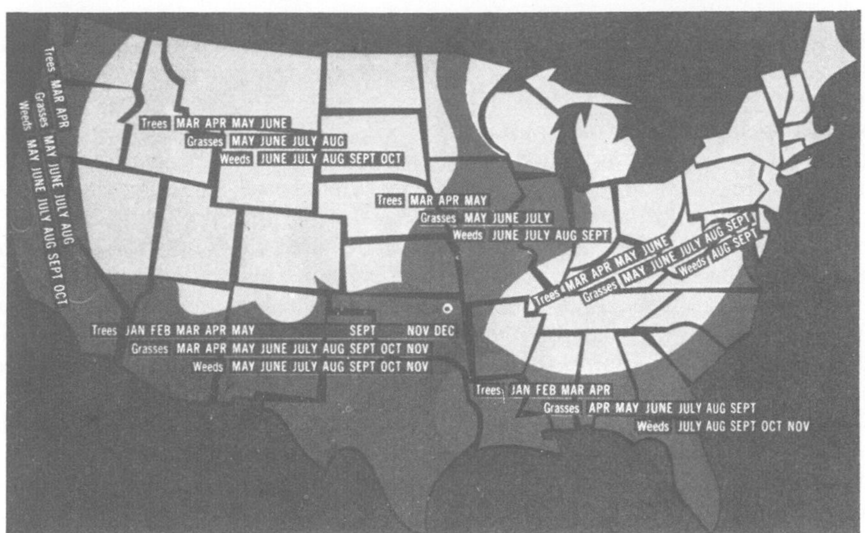

Figure 16–2. Maximum pollen dispersal. (From *Pfizer Spectrum,* May 15, 1958.)

until a potentially fatal attack occurs.

Eczema. This term means many things to many people. One of the greatest recent advances in dermatology has been the differentiation of various types of eczema, making the development of effective treatments possible.

A rough, red, itching rash appears in this disease, which soon turns into scaly, "weeping," crusted patches of skin. These are often located around the elbow and the back of the knee, but may cover practically the entire surface of the body, including the face. The physical discomfort and emotional suffering from the unsightliness of this disease can cause great distress.

Not all cases of eczema are of allergic origin, but this is the commonest factor. *Allergic eczemas* may result from foods, medicines or substances which are inhaled. *Contact eczema,* essentially the same as contact dermatitis, means that the condition is caused by something touching the skin, and this embraces a wide variety of

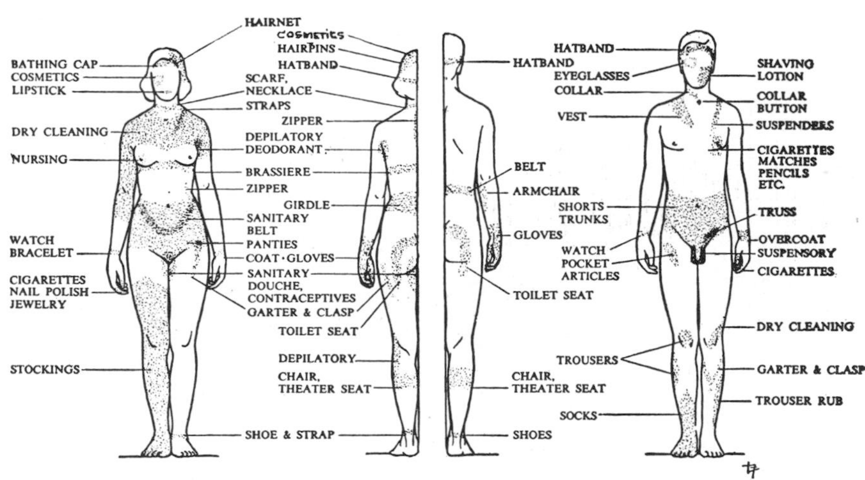

Figure 16–3. Dermatitis. Areas and causes of dermatitis due to allergy or irritation.

substances. The hands are usually hardest hit; "housewives' eczema," for example, frequently results from sensitivity to a detergent, and can be prevented by washing with "soapless" skin cleaners, or employing rubber gloves whenever soaps and detergents must be used.

Contact Dermatitis. Skin reactions such as reddening, itching, blisters, or watery discharge can be caused by direct contact between sensitizing agents and the skin. They can also result from allergens that are absorbed via the nose, mouth or from injection. Sometimes, the rash is limited to one area, but it may be very widespread, and accompanied by sneezing or other nasal symptoms.

The most common contact dermatitis is poison ivy, but the complete list of causative agents is almost endless, and includes industrial oils, medicines, cosmetics, perfumes, soaps, mouthwashes, clothing made of various materials or treated with certain preservatives, and dyes.

The tests used for determining sensitivity to allergens are the patch, scratch and injection methods; a complete screening for skin sensitivity may require a large number of tests.

Poison ivy (and the closely related *poison oak* and *sumac*) are responsible for an acute contact dermatitis which causes an enormous amount of misery. There are close to a half million cases every summer, and about 60 to 80 per cent of adults tested react to an oily extract of the plant.

Poison ivy grows in the form of climbing vines, shrubs which trail on the ground, and erect shrubbery, flourishing abundantly in town as well as country. The leaves are one to four inches long, green and glossy in summer and russet or red in fall, and the fruit is grayish and waxy, resembling mistletoe. Although poison ivy assumes many forms and displays seasonal color changes, one constant characteristic makes it easy to recognize: *the leaves always grow in clusters of three,* one at the end of the stalk, and two opposite each other. *"Leaflets three, let it be!"*

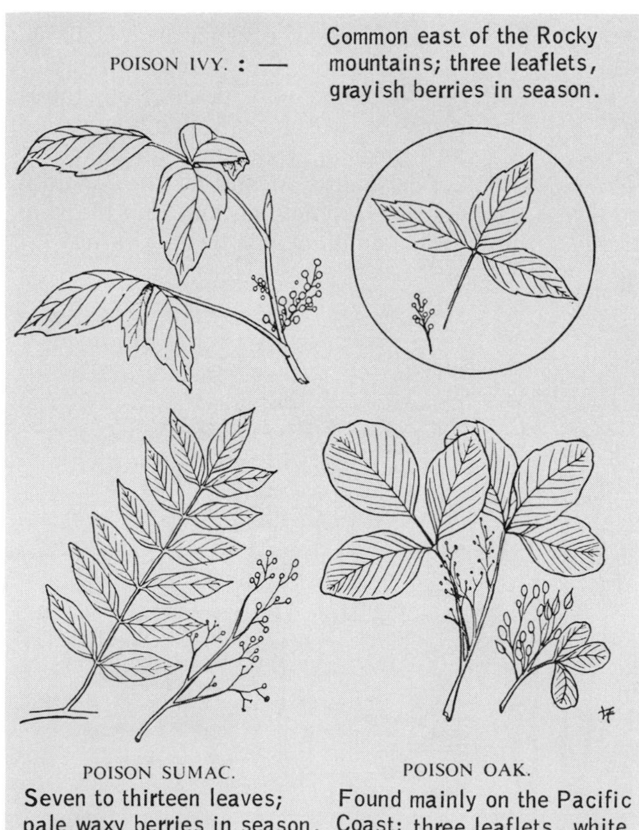

Figure 16–4. Leaves and fruit of poison ivy, poison sumac, and poison oak.

Most cases of poison ivy are due to direct contact with the plant, but even clothing, garden tools and pets may be contaminated with sufficient oil to cause irritation. Some people are so reactive that they develop an acute dermatitis after exposure to the smoke of plants which are being destroyed by fire.

The first symptom is an itching or burning sensation, followed by a rash, swelling and small or large blisters, sometimes so painful that they are incapacitating. Symptoms may develop anytime from a few hours to seven days after contact.

If you know you are sensitive to poison ivy, wash your skin thoroughly with yellow laundry soap as soon as possible after handling it. An acute reaction may require a doctor's help to relieve discomfort and guard against secondary infections until the attack subsides. Stubborn cases may be due to repeated contact with contaminated clothing. Any suspected garments should be washed or dry cleaned.

Soothing baths or compresses and the use of sedatives help relieve some of the discomfort, but until cortisone and other steroid hormones became available, no medication was consistently effective. The use of corticosteroids has revolutionized the treatment of dermatitis due to poison ivy, oak and sumac.

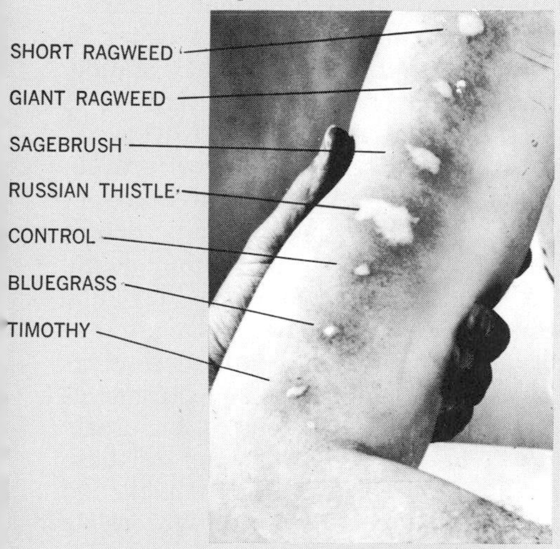

The results of a scratch test. In this case, the patient has reacted positively to Russian thistle and to sagebrush and short ragweed. The control and the other tests show no reaction.

The best way to *prevent* poison ivy is to *eliminate the plants* wherever they are found, preferably by uprooting them. Unfortunately, an attack of poison ivy does not confer immunity. It merely warns you that you are sensitive and must avoid it. Attempts to protect sensitive individuals by inoculating against poison ivy have not been uniformly successful, although some physicians feel that several newly developed preparations reduce the severity of subsequent attacks. Robert J. Langs of the Albert Einstein College of Medicine in New York has reported that a "poison-ivy pill' can provide season-long immunity against both poison ivy and oak.[4]

Skin Eruptions from Sensitivity to Medicines. Allergic reactions are so universal that it is not surprising to find many people acutely sensitive to certain *medicines*. Individuals who tend to have marked allergic reactions in general should inform their physicians, especially if a new medication is being prescribed.

This is one of the reasons penicillin is not an unmixed blessing. According to a three-year nation-wide survey of 800 hospitals and more than 1600 physicians made by Henry Welch and his associates of the Food and Drug Administration in Washington, penicillin causes more reactions and deaths than any other antibiotic. The greatest danger comes when this medication is injected intramuscularly; the allergic conditions which develop include urticaria, angioneurotic edema, reddening or a definite rash. In a very small proportion of patients, a fatal reaction occurs.

To avoid such hazards, sensitive patients should be identified by having them take scratch tests with penicillin before injecting what might prove to be dangerous amounts. If a reaction does occur, a penicillin-destroying enzyme, called *penicillinase*, can be administered, and it may overcome the troublesome and dangerous effects of penicillin.

[4]*Medical Science*, July 25, 1958, and January 10, 1959.

Streptomycin occasionally causes a mild allergy which subsides fairly quickly, but tetracycline, erythromycin, and other broad-spectrum antibiotics, which cure a large number of bacterial infections, rarely induce allergic responses.

About 5 per cent of patients who take the sulfonamide compounds also develop skin eruptions. Other causes are the metals used as therapeutic agents, such as gold, arsenic, and mercury; isoniazid and para-aminosalicylic acid, which are employed in the treatment of tuberculosis; and even the familiar sedatives, phenobarbital and related barbiturates. In most cases, the skin allergy disappears as soon as the medication is stopped, so that there are rarely any serious consequences.

Injection of tetanus antitoxin and other serums may also be hazardous in this respect, and allergic patients should first receive a small test dose to determine their sensitivity.

Allergic Reactions of the Digestive System. Although allergic reactions to foods usually cause hay fever and skin reactions, there are some that involve the digestive system, and produce nausea, vomiting and dizziness. Gastrointestinal allergies may show up anywhere from the mouth to the rectal area, and common reactions are canker sores in the mouth and hives in the intestinal tract.

Allergic Headaches. These are fairly common, and even attacks of acute migraine may be sparked by allergy to a food or inhalant.

Sensitivity or Anaphylactic Shock. An individual may show no reaction to a particular allergen the first time he is exposed. But the second time, since he has become highly sensitized, he may go into a condition of shock which may even be fatal. Such reactions have been reported from bee, wasp and other insect stings, animal bites or scratches, serum injections and certain drugs, such as penicillin.

If a severe reaction does occur, special emergency measures may be lifesaving: injection of antihistaminic drugs or epinephrine solution (the same as the adrenaline we secrete from our adrenal glands); and the use of corticosteroid hormones. If the individual knows that he is very sensitive to a particular allergen, he should have a physician attempt careful immunization to prevent a more serious reaction. Fortunately for the survival of the human race, fatal reactions of this type are extremely rare.

CONSTIPATION

About 24 hours after a meal is eaten, the undigested residue has passed into the *sigmoid* region of the colon, just above the rectum, waiting for ejection as fecal matter. It is retained in the colon until a valvelike structure at this junction opens. The rectum is endowed with a very efficient network of nerves which transmits a sense of fulness to the brain, and the valve will open in response to a message from the headquarters in the brain.

This fairly complicated process doesn't always function perfectly. In some individuals, the bowel may be sluggish, and the fecal mass moves too slowly, or the sensitivity of the rectal nerve system may be diminished. *Hemorrhoids* (piles) and *anal fissures* also interfere with normal, painless bowel movements, and may cause constipation.

However, most people actually suffer from *imaginary* constipation, which has been called "the great American disease." Bowel movements simply don't occur as often as most persons think they should. But there is no law of nature that states that if the bowel isn't emptied every 24 hours, serious consequences will result. The interval may be 36 hours, 48 hours, or even longer. Unfortunately many people become extremely concerned if they do not have a bowel movement every day, and immediately conclude they are dangerously constipated. They begin dosing themselves with all kinds of laxatives and purgatives to correct the situation, and often create a very vicious cycle, because these medicines may irritate the bowel and actually cause constipation. We waste millions of dollars a year on patent medicines and other "cures" for a condition which is nonexistent.

Our modern mode of living, with its strains and stresses and sedentary habits, helps promote self-induced constipation. In some primitive languages, there is no such word as constipation, and no need for it because the condition doesn't exist. It can be prevented by a proper diet, adequate fluids, some exercise daily, relaxed living, regular habits of elimination and *not worrying about your bowels.*

Walter Alvarez gives this good advice on the treatment of constipation.[5]

> Not all constipated persons can or should be treated the same way. Some need not even be treated at all. To illustrate: years ago a healthy young woman, a teacher of physical education, consulted me in regard to a bowel which she was accustomed to empty once a week with the help of an enema. When I found that this delay in defecation did not cause her any distress, I asked her why she was wasting her time and money in my office. Her answer was that she hadn't wanted to come, but her mother and sisters and family doctor were constantly upbraiding her for her neglect of her bowels that finally she had given in. Amused, I wrote her out the following certificate: *To whom it may concern: Miss Blank is to be permitted to let her bowels go unopened as long as she pleases.*

If you do need a cathartic, use the mild ones like petrolatum and agar, aromatic cascara sagrada, or milk of magnesia. But *never* take any cathartic if there is fever, nausea, pain or general feeling of illness associated with the constipation. It can cause fatal consequences if the condition is caused by appendicitis.

Constipation *can* be *organic,* that is, due to actual physical change in some organ, such as a tumor which is obstructing the intestines, a stricture which narrows them, or some other disease process. That is why it is important to *consult a doctor* if constipation comes on fairly suddenly, without obvious cause.

VARICOSE VEINS

Varicose veins are knotlike, twisting enlargements of the veins, usually just below the skin of the legs. They are the result of a breakdown of the valves found at regular intervals in the veins. It is through these valves that the blood flows back to the heart, after having been pumped to the extremities through the arteries. These valves divide the veins into sections, each valve forming a floor to support the blood above it. When a valve is faulty or degenerates, it cannot support the blood. When several valves in a surface vein break down, the weight of the column of blood becomes sufficient to distend the vein.

Varicose veins are estimated to affect one out of every two women and one out of every four men over 40 years of age. Here four-legged animals have an advantage over us. The dog and horse, for example, never develop varicose veins.

This condition is seen most frequently in people whose work requires them to stand or sit upright for long periods. The tendency to develop weak valves runs in families. Increase in the internal or back pressure of the blood in the veins is also a strain on the valves. This can be caused by heavy lifting or pregnancy. Varicose veins may also occur as a sequel to phlebitis—an inflammation of the veins that may damage the valves. Also, there may be a connection between the endocrine glands and the valves, which tend to degenerate with age.

In addition to being unsightly, varicose veins may result in some symptoms, generally in the form of dull, nagging aches and pains. The ankles may swell. The enlarged vein can become the site of an infection, and since the resistance of the surrounding tissue has decreased, a bruise or injury can become serious. The resulting varicose ulcers are not easy to clear up, especially in elderly people or diabetics; they may not yield to medication and require surgery, including skin grafting.

The most serious consequence of varicose veins is the possible formation of an embolus—a circulating blood clot. It is possible for a blood clot to form in a distended vein. If such a clot returns to the heart and is pumped to the lungs, the results can be very serious.

In mild cases, varicose veins can be handled adequately by such measures as: eliminating tight shoes and tight garters that restrict the circulation, and elevating the feet at intervals and walking about occasionally instead of standing still for long periods. Sometimes wearing an elastic stocking or bandage for even part of the day will support a varicose vein and

[5]Alvarez, W.: *How to Help Your Doctor Help You,* Dell Publishing Co., New York, 1955.

prevent it from becoming more distended.

In severe cases, or with individuals to whom appearance is especially important, varicose veins can and should be eliminated. There are two ways in which this can be done. One method is surgical; the distended veins can be cut out, or else ligated (tied off). Afterward, the blood will flow through other veins. The other method is medical; a fluid is injected into the varicose vein, causing it to harden, after which the blood can no longer flow through it and will flow through other veins. The technique for injecting veins has been steadily improved during the one hundred years since it was first attempted, and this procedure is now perfectly safe in experienced hands. It is far simpler and quicker than surgery, and it does not require the patient to be hospitalized or to stay away from work. The discomfort is slight, and unless there are a great many varicose veins or the patient is extremely nervous, one appointment is usually sufficient. (However, very large veins or other considerations may make the surgical treatment the better one.)

The varicose veins of old people can safely be injected, or those of pregnant women if they would otherwise suffer pain for some months before childbirth. It should not be done in those rare cases in which an infection of the blood vessels has injured the deep veins, because this would interfere with the circulation in the leg. Of course, eliminating one or more varicose veins will not prevent other valves from breaking down and other varicose veins from developing. People who have to work in certain occupations, or who have a marked tendency toward faulty valves in the veins, are apt to have to contend repeatedly with this condition.

Questions

1. What is a "nuisance disease?"
2. Name some important causes of headaches. How would you cure a "tension" headache?
3. Describe an attack of migraine headache.
4. What are the chief dangers from the common cold? Do you think it is the sign of a strong person, a "Spartan," not to "give in to a cold?" Or might this reaction not actually be a sign of some weakness and suppressed fear of more serious illness?
5. Why do you think colds are so common and have been so resistant to medication?
6. Define the terms "allergy" and "allergen."
7. What are the most important types of allergic reactions?
8. Give an example of the following allergens: inhalant; food; contactant; injectant.
9. What hereditary factors are involved in the development of allergies?
10. Explain why constipation is sometimes considered a psychosomatic disease.
11. What are varicose veins? What can be done to prevent this condition? How is it treated?

Topics for Discussion

Emotions and allergy.
Antihistaminics.
The action of penicillinase.

Reading Suggestions

Your Allergy and You, Kay Kempton Haydock. Henry Holt & Co., New York, 1958. A practical book, written in clear language for the lay reader, describing causes, symptoms and treatment for allergic conditions.

Poison Ivy, Patricia Jenkins. Today's Health, June 1958. How it is caused and what to do about it.

Constipation, Harper & Bros., New York, 1952. What the patient needs to know about the causes, symptoms and treatment.

Help for the Headache Prone, Joseph D. Wassersug. Parents Magazine, April 1964, p. 139. A noted internist discusses the many causes of headache. An excellent article.

More Cold Viruses, D. D. Rutstein. Scientific American, March 1962, p. 70. An informative article for the advanced student.

What Science Has Learned About Varicose Veins, Noah D. Fabricant. Today's Health, April 1963, p. 35. An authoritative and up-to-date account of knowledge regarding the treatment of varicose veins.

They're Closing in on the Common Cold, J. D. Ratcliff. Today's Health, October 1961, p. 48. An interesting account of medical advances against the common cold.

America's Laxative Addicts, J. D. Ratcliff. Today's Health, November 1962, p. 52. The author tells why the indiscriminate use of laxatives is foolish and sometimes dangerous.

Headache—Our Most Common Malady, Theodore Berland. Today's Health, February 1965, p. 20. An authoritative and up-to-date discussion of a common complaint.

Sore Throat Can Be Serious, Theodore Berland. Today's Health, January 1965, p. 26. The "sore throat" is discussed as a symptom of a variety of diseases.

Uncommon Knowledge of the Common Cold, Robert Mines. Science Digest, January 1963, p. 18. A discussion of what recent research has shown about the common cold.

17

THE DISABLING DISEASES

In this section we restrict ourselves to those diabling diseases which constitute major hazards for students of college age or which are of the greatest importance to the nation in terms of numbers afflicted. The illnesses of infectious origin included are *poliomyelitis, infectious mononucleosis, infectious hepatitis, influenza,* and *venereal diseases. Epilepsy, multiple sclerosis, cerebral palsy, blindness,* and *deafness* involve the brain or central nervous system. The following conditions affecting muscles, joints and bones are discussed: *muscular dystrophy, myasthenia gravis,* and *hernias; arthritis, gout, backache,* and *bursitis; osteomyelitis* and *osteoporosis. Anemias* are also described, as well as three diseases with a strong psychosomatic component—*asthma, ulcerative colitis,* and *peptic ulcer.*

POLIOMYELITIS (INFANTILE PARALYSIS)

Polio has ranked high among the disabling diseases. However, this affliction, which first appeared in epidemic form in Sweden in 1887, which affected 27,000 people in the United States in 1916 and claimed 6000 lives, and which struck Franklin D. Roosevelt in 1921, is now preventable. For this accomplishment we are deeply indebted to many scientists. (See Table 17–1). Generally, polio is a mild virus infection of the intestinal tract, and most people who have been infected either show no symptoms or develop only a minor illness. In a small percentage of cases, however, it spreads to the central nervous system and may cause paralysis by destroying or weakening

Table 17–1. Chronology of the victory over polio

Year	*Scientist*	*His Contribution*
1789	Michael Underwood British physician	Dr. Underwood was the first to recognize polio.
1798	Edward Jenner British physician	*Discovery of immunity:* Dr. Jenner produced immunity to smallpox in 8 year old James Phipps by injecting him with material taken from a milk-maid suffering with cowpox.
1840	Jacob Heine German physician	Dr. Heine presented the first systematic description of polio.
1880's	Louis Pasteur French scientist	Demonstrated that infections were caused by tiny organisms (germs). Demonstrated that organisms kept in a suitable culture could be modified and made less lethal. Developed vaccines for rabies and anthrax.
1908	Karl Landsteiner Austrian physician (later worked in U.S.)	Dr. Landsteiner was the first to transmit polio to a monkey. This made it easier to study the disease.
1949	Dr. John F. Enders Harvard University physician	Dr. Enders and his associates found a way of culturing the polio virus on monkey kidney cells kept alive in test tubes. He and his associates received the Nobel Prize for discovery of this method to grow polio virus in quantities large enough for use in vaccines.
1955	Dr. Jonas E. Salk University of Pittsburgh physician	Developed a vaccine consisting of chemically killed viruses. It was licensed for use in the United States on April 12, 1955.
1961 1962	Dr. Albert Sabin University of Cincinnati physician	Developed three oral polio vaccines consisting of live viruses. Type I was licensed for sale in the United States on August 17, 1961; Type II on October 10, 1961; and Type III on March 27, 1962.

the nerve cells that control muscles. Most commonly, it affects the arms and legs, but it can also paralyze the muscles concerned in breathing and swallowing. *Polio does not affect the mind.*

Young children are the most frequent victims, but it can attack people of all ages. Except for women in the childbearing period, more males develop polio and the mortality is greater than among females. For example, between 1950 and 1954, there were 46 per cent more deaths among men, and 22 per cent more in 1955–1956. The highest incidence of the disease is in the spring and summer.

At least three types of polio virus have already been successfully crystallized and, like many other viruses, these are well defined chemical compounds called *nucleoproteins*. There are paralytic and nonparalytic polio viruses, but the majority of people who develop the disease do not suffer from paralysis or weakened muscles. Of those whose muscles are weakened, many are never paralyzed; and of those whose muscles are paralyzed more than half recover without serious aftereffects. However, polio *can* cause permanent paralysis, and it *can* be fatal.

Polio viruses have been found in the nose and mouth and also in the excreta, and are present not only in polio patients, but also in individuals who do not appear to have the disease. This explains why polio can be spread by patients who are actually suffering from the disease, as well as by those who have mild, often undiagnosed cases, and even by carriers who are not ill but carry the virus about in their bodies. Objects which have been contaminated by patients or carriers can also transmit polio.

Many people have apparently been infected with polio virus in so mild a form that the disease passed unrecognized, but the exposure was still sufficient to leave them with a permanent immunity. This is perhaps the reason most of the victims are children and young adults, who have had too little exposure to develop immunity.

Early symptoms of polio include fever, headache, vomiting, fretfulness, drowsiness, sore throat, change in bowel habits, stiffness, and pain in the back and neck. These do not necessarily mean polio, but they should not be ignored.

Treatment

During its acute stages, polio should be treated in a hospital, preferably one specializing in this disease. An iron lung or respirator may be needed if the muscles of breathing become paralyzed. Skilled care is often essential to prevent muscles from becoming permanently weakened.

If paralysis of the arms or legs occurs, rehabilitation will be necessary. Remarkable success has been achieved by the proper techniques, and patients who would otherwise be crippled have been restored to activity.

In some cases, reconstructive surgery can be performed to give better use of the impaired limbs.

So far, no chemical or antibiotic has been discovered which can cure polio.

Prevention

Two effective vaccines against polio are now available and widely used in the United States—the Salk vaccine, developed by Jonas E. Salk of the University of Pittsburgh, and the Sabin oral polio vaccine, developed by Albert Sabin of the University of Cincinnati.

The Salk vaccine consists of three chemically killed polioviruses mixed into a single vaccine. When injected, this vaccine produces disease-fighting antibodies, which prevent the polioviruses from getting into the central nervous system and causing polio. Most people can gain immunity to paralytic polio from four properly spaced injections. The vaccine appears to be completely safe.

The Sabin oral vaccine is made from attenuated live viruses for all three types of polio. Actually, it consists of three vaccines, one for each type of polio. The vaccine is usually dropped on a sugar cube or made into a sweet tasting liquid.

Regarding the oral vaccine, the United States Public Health Service states:

> A characteristic of the oral vaccine is that it prevents the intestinal tract from harboring polioviruses. Theoretically, when enough people take the oral vaccine in a concentrated period of time, these disease-producing viruses will die out of the community because they can find no human host. For this reason, and because it is easy to administer quickly to large numbers of persons in a short space of time, oral vaccine is particularly suitable for the control of epidemics.

It is recommended that Type I vaccine be given, followed six weeks later by Type III, and six weeks later by Type II. A fourth dose containing all three types is recommended for infants; it should be given six weeks after Type II. The vaccine is completely safe.

The reduction in polio following development of the Salk vaccine in 1955 and the Sabin vaccine in 1961–1962 may be seen in Table 17–2.

About the polio era, John Wilson has written that:[1]

> Soon, unless something very surprising happens, the polio drama will be over. As disease cycles go, it was a surprisingly short one. In the epidemic form with which we have been concerned, it is an affair concerning no more than fifty years of so. Epidemic polio was the disease of affluence. It attacked advanced twentieth-century society, and was conquered by that society. Viewed from one angle, the story is a breath-taking demonstration of the power of modern science and technology.

Scientific victory over disease, however, is not enough; all of us must participate and keep a strong safeguard against polio.

[1]Wilson, J.R.: *Margin of Safety,* Doubleday & Co., Garden City, N.Y., 1963.

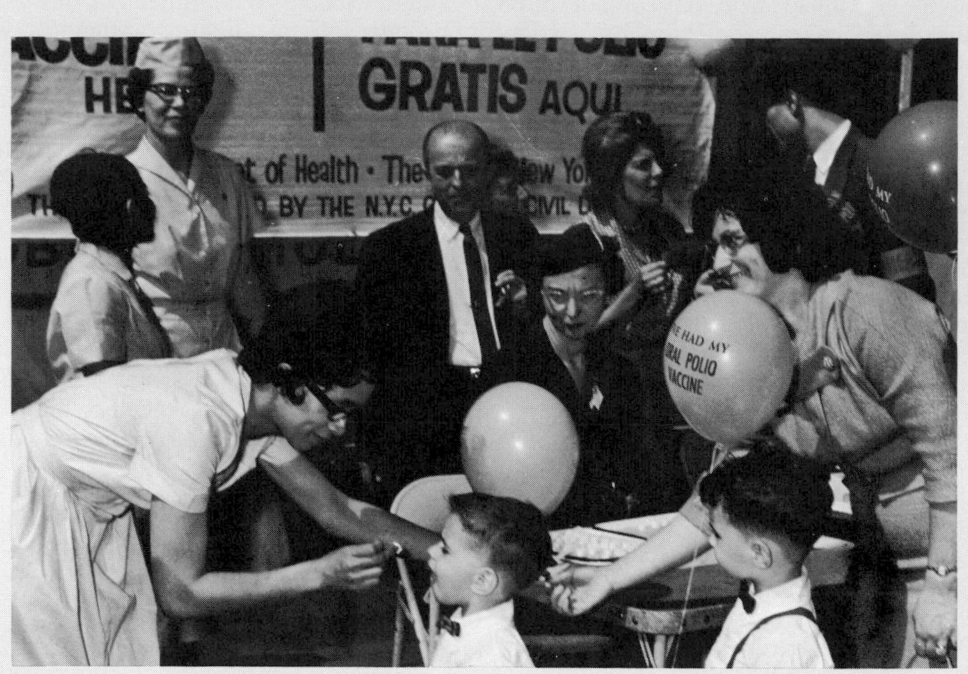

Children receiving Sabin oral polio vaccine. As part of a nationwide campaign to prevent poliomyelitis, many communities throughout the country provided Salk and Sabin vaccines to children and adults.

Table 17–2. Poliomyelitis cases reported in the United States from 1952 through 1965*

Year	*Total*	*Paralytic*	*Nonparalytic*	*Unspecified*
1952	52,879	21,269	12,802	23,808
1953	35,592	15,648	12,144	7800
1954	38,476	18,308	13,221	6947
1955	28,985	13,850	12,453	2682
1956	15,140	7911	6555	674
1957	5485	2499	2826	160
1958	5787	3697	1941	149
1959	8425	6289	2045	91
1960	3190	2525	626	39
1961	1312	988	305	19
1962	886	707	125	54
1963	445	381	46	18
1964	113	89	13	11
1965	52	38	10	4

*From U. S. Public Health Service, Department of Health, Education and Welfare

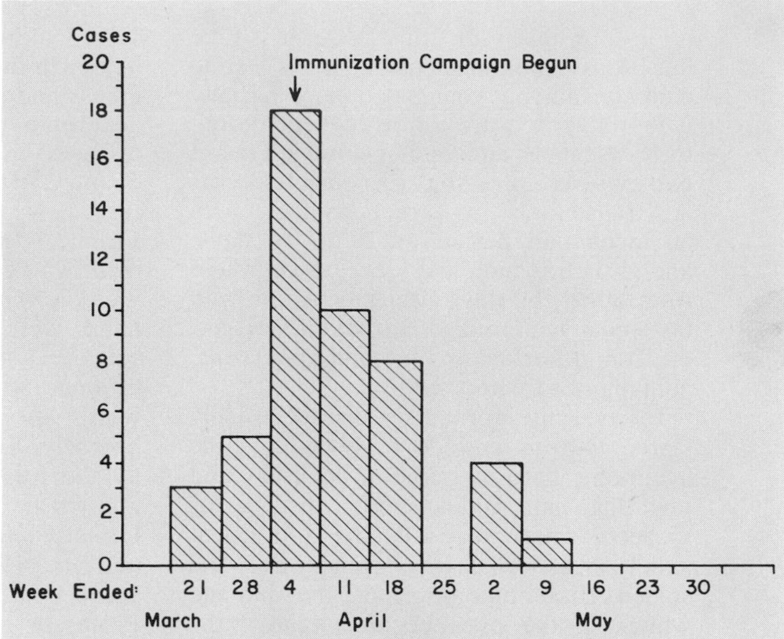

INTERNATIONAL NOTES

Figure 17-1. Poliomyelitis cases by date of report, Bahamas, 1964. (From *Morbidity and Mortality.* U.S. Department of Health, Education and Welfare, Public Health Service, July 24, 1964.)

This means that everyone should be immunized, and babies should get a full course of vaccine by the time they are one year old.

INFECTIOUS MONONUCLEOSIS

Infectious mononucleosis is also called "the kissing disease" or "students' disease" because young people between the ages of 15 and 30 appear to be the most susceptible. It is apparently caused by a virus, although the specific virus has never been isolated and the disease has not been transmitted experimentally from man to man, or from man to animals. Spread of the disease does not occur as in the common cold—through coughing, sneezing or even ordinary conversation with an infected person—but only by very close contact, such as kissing. This is why experts in the field feel that "precisely the age group most interested in osculation" provides the bulk of infectious mononucleosis patients.

The symptoms of this infection are fever, sore throat, swelling of lymph glands in the neck, weakness and fatigue. In addition, there may be jaundice, if the liver becomes involved, and a skin rash. *Any time you suffer from this combination of symptoms and have felt constantly tired for a prolonged period of time, you should consult a doctor, because if you do have infectious mononucleosis, rest is extremely important.*

There is no specific medication for infectious mononucleosis, and antibiotics and other medicines do not influence its course. However, some physicians feel that antibiotics are desirable because they decrease the danger of secondary infections by other organisms. The standard treatment includes ice packs to reduce the pain of swollen glands, soothing gargles for the sore throat, a good diet and *complete rest.* Usually, this illness clears up within a few weeks, but it may leave the patient weak and easily fatigued for months thereafter. Because liver damage sometimes occurs, adequate rest is a *must* in this disease to prevent this potentially serious complication.

INFECTIOUS HEPATITIS

A virus localizing in the liver and producing signs and symptoms of liver damage is responsible for this disease. Like infectious mononucleosis, it is quite common among young people, especially if they live in army camps, college dormitories, schools and similar groups. One of two viruses may be responsible: virus A, transmitted by direct contact, with an incubation period of 20 to 40 days; and virus B, which may develop anywhere from 60 to 160 days after inoculation with inadequately sterilized needles or syringes, or from transfusion of blood or plasma, contaminated with the virus.

In its acute form, the disease usually starts with an episode of fever, and the symptoms are weakness, nausea and vomiting, pain and a sudden distaste for tobacco. There may also be a transient skin rash, as well as a very tender liver and spleen. If jaundice develops, the skin and whites of the eyes become yellow, the urine is much darker than normal, and the stools are light in color. However, sometimes the disease is so mild that few or none of these symptoms appear.

After a week or so of jaundice, recovery usually sets in and the jaundice gradually subsides. As in the case of infectious mononucleosis, there is no specific therapy, and bed rest and diet are considered of greatest importance. Antibiotics and corticosteroid hormones may be helpful, but the most important feature of treatment is rest and diet to *protect the patient against the development of a chronic, prolonged form of the disease, and especially from serious and permanent liver damage.*

INFLUENZA

Because influenza, usually called "the flu," often resembles a common cold, many people fail to take it seriously. This is a grave mistake, because pneumonia may go hand in hand with influenza. During the epidemic of 1918, approximately 20 million people lost their lives from this combination of diseases. The chief danger is to the very oldest and the very youngest age groups, to cardiac patients and pregnant women.

Influenza probably is a very old disease and was accurately described as early as 1510, although it was not known as influenza at that time. It created so much illness and so many problems that nationalist pride made nations insist that the disease had originated in some other country. In Tolstoi's *War and Peace,* this new and fashionable illness from France is discussed by a group of noblemen, who call it "grippe," from the French word, *gripper.* The French, on the other hand, were certain it came from Russian soil, and they insisted that the name, *gripper,* was derived from the Russian word *khripet,* which means to speak hoarsely. The Germans, less polite, called it "the Russian pest," and in Italy, it was known as "the German disease." In the United States, the same tendency persisted, and the 1918 epidemic was called "the Spanish flu." According to David Rutstein, Professor of Preventive Medicine at Harvard, influenza is the only disease in modern times which still causes world-wide epidemics.[2]

Influenza is caused by a virus and its symptoms include fever, sore throat, cough, a runny nose, chills and aches, especially in the head, back, and legs. Like a cold, it is spread from one person to another, most commonly by coughing and sneezing the virus into the air, and is so contagious that once it appears in a community, health authorities are seldom able to prevent it from becoming an epidemic. Fortunately, these epidemics usually last no longer than a month, and we do have vaccines now against some of the flu viruses.

Even when there are no complications and the fever and other symptoms last only a few days, influenza tends to leave people as weak and generally disabled as though they had gone through a long siege of illness.

Temporary immunity does follow the flu, but there are a number of different strains of the influenza virus, and *having had one kind doesn't keep you from catching another.* Within the past 10 years, at least 18 types of viruses responsible for upper respiratory tract infections have been isolated, and ten of these occur

[2]Rutstein, D.D.: The influenza epidemic, *Harper's,* August 1957.

commonly. That is why vaccination does not afford protection against all varieties of flu.

Treatment

The best way to get well quickly and avoid dangerous or disabling complications is to give yourself all possible odds in your fight against this virus. Go to bed if you have any symptoms of a cold or the flu, or even if you just don't feel well when there is influenza about. If it turns out to be nothing, think of your "wasted" day as well-spent insurance.

Don't overtreat yourself with nose drops, sprays or antihistamines. If you have any aches and pains or a fever, call the doctor, and let him prescribe the medication you need. Although the sulfa drugs and antibiotics will not cure your flu, they are valuable in guarding against pneumonia and other diseases for which influenza paves the way. Eat a bland diet and drink plenty of fluids. Stay in bed as long as your doctor tells you to, even if your symptoms have disappeared, and don't be surprised if you continue to feel fatigued for several weeks.

Prevention

Avoid crowds and unnecessary contact with other people, get sufficient rest, and don't allow yourself to become overtired or chilled when you know that influenza is on the increase. Keep as far away as possible from people who don't smother their coughs and sneezes in tissues, and be especially careful about contact with anyone who is coming down with the "sniffles." Regard every cold as potential influenza, and remember that it is most contagious during the early stages.

Effective vaccines against flu can be prepared from killed viruses which have been grown in the chick embryo. The chief problem is that so many varieties produce influenza and that the vaccine must be able to act against any offending virus. Fortunately, most widespread epidemics are caused by one—or only a few—strains, and it is possible to prepare multivaccines, effective against several viruses. Two injections of vaccine must be administered at intervals of approximately six weeks to provide the necessary immunity, and if you are planning to be vaccinated, have it done in the early fall, because it takes time to establish immunity; the peak season for flu is from January to March.

VENEREAL DISEASES

The term *venereal disease* connotes sex and sin today, but historically the name derives from Venus, the Roman goddess

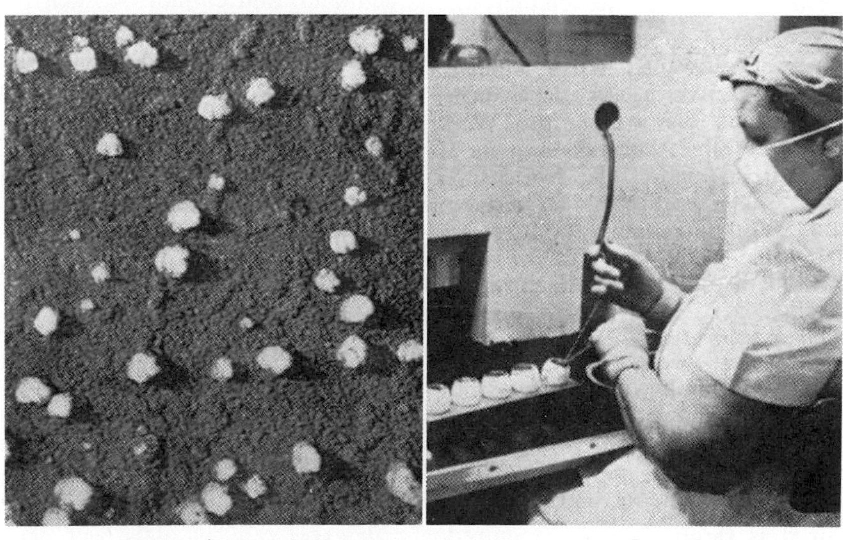

Figure 17–2. **A,** Influenza virus (enlarged 115,000 times). **B,** Growing influenza virus in eggs.

of love. Throughout the Roman Empire, there were temples devoted to Venus; she was also worshipped in Phoenicia as *Astarte,* and as *Aphrodite* in Greece. At the Temple of Venus in Corinth during the first century A.D., there were a thousand famous and beautiful prostitutes, who attracted visitors from the entire eastern Mediterranean area. No opprobrium was attached to the word prostitute, and the money these handmaidens of Venus received for their favors was used to support the temple. It was actually considered a meritorious act for *all* women to spend a day, a week, or even longer periods at the temple, offering themselves to the visitors, and giving the money they received to the temple. The Greeks, in addition, established a form of *civic prostitution* as a means of obtaining revenue. In many parts of the ancient world, the custom of *hospitality prostitution* provided the more notable travelers and visitors with women from the household—female servants, and even wives and daughters.

It is easy to understand how rapidly venereal disease could spread from this ancient, and at that time, honorable profession. There was little effort to stop it, except among the Hebrews who, according to the Old Testament, warned against the harlot, and attempted to stamp out the worship of Astarte.

Medical historians believe that gonorrhea and venereal sores, such as chancroid, are described on the clay tablets and papyri and in the writings of Greek and Roman writers of ancient times. Assyrian tablets as far back as 900 B.C. clearly describe gonorrhea. Syphilis is supposed to have been brought to the Old World from the Western Hemisphere by Christopher Columbus's sailors. However, it is possible that many illnesses and skin lesions diagnosed as leprosy in Biblical times may actually have been syphilis.

Syphilis—also called "the pox," "siff," and "bad blood"—is caused by a spiral-shaped organism, *Spirochaeta pallida,* or *Treponema pallidum.* It is generally transmitted through sexual contact, although infection can occur through kissing, but it is rarely, if ever, acquired from contact with toilet seats.

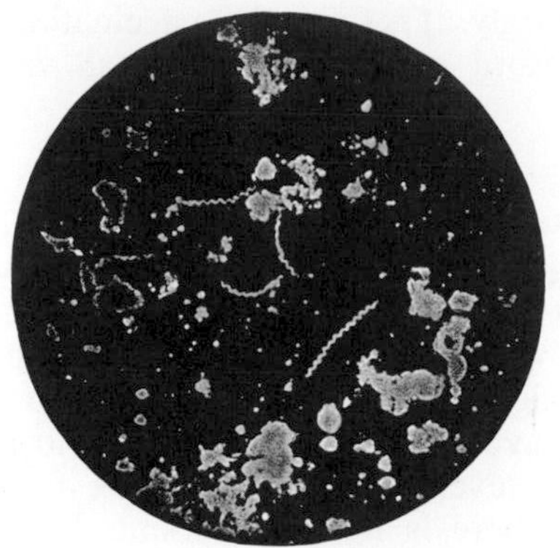

Figure 17-3. *Treponema pallidum* (darkfield preparation × 1000). (From Davidsohn and Wells: *Clinical Diagnosis by Laboratory Methods.* 13th Ed., Philadelphia, W. B. Saunders Co., 1962.)

After the syphilis microorganisms have entered the body, they are silent for a period of from 10 days to as long as three months. The first sign of their presence is a *chancre,*[3] which resembles a pimple, blister, or open sore, and it usually appears on the sex organs but may be on the lips or fingers. In men the chancre is generally on the penis, although it sometimes forms on the adjacent skin or on the thighs; in women it is often concealed in the genitalia, and cannot be seen or felt. Not all people infected with syphilis develop chancres, and unfortunately, the Wassermann and other blood tests for syphilis usually fail to detect the disease at this early stage.

If a chancre does develop, even competent physicians cannot always tell whether it is syphilitic until they study material from it under the microscope, and actually detect the characteristic spirochete of syphilis. *Any* sore on the sex organs should be examined immediately by a physician. If it isn't caused by syphilis, a great deal of needless worry will be avoided. If it is syphilis, treatment can be started at once with the assurance of a prompt cure.

The chancre heals of its own accord,

[3]Pronounced *shan'ker.*

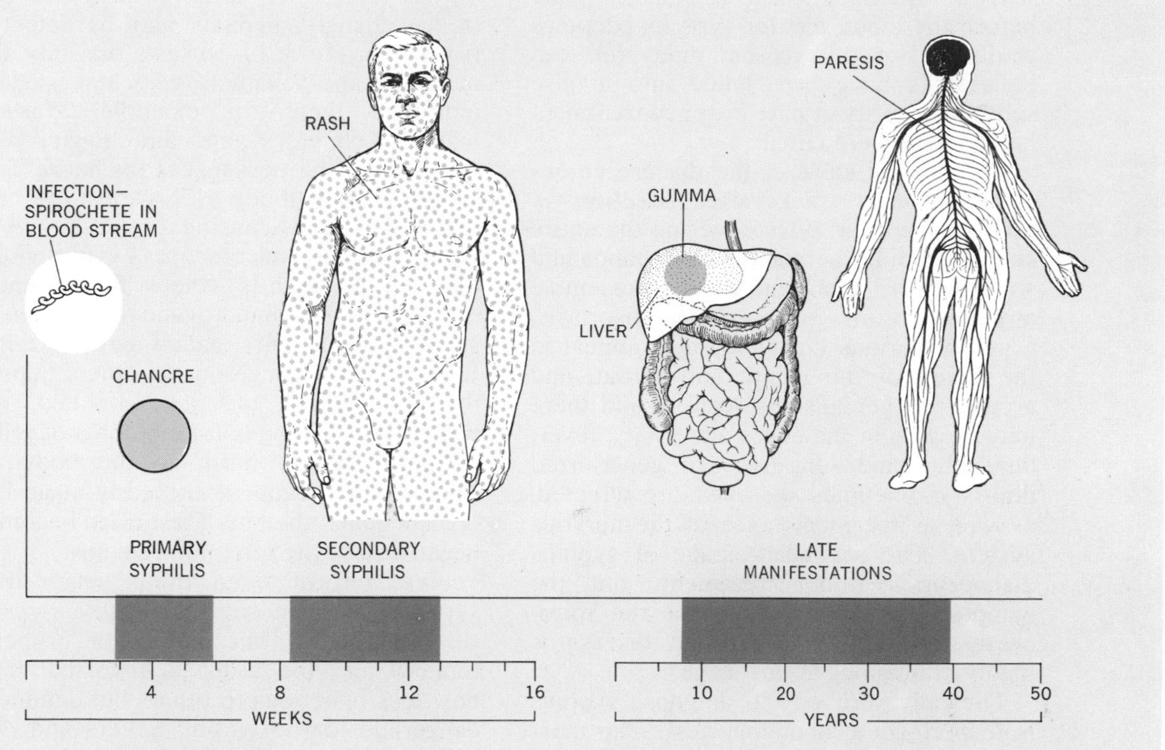

Chart at base of diagram represents typical course of untreated syphilis. Chancre usually appears within a few weeks of exposure, although it may not be noticed. Secondary symptoms can include fever, bald patches, and other symptoms, as well as a rash, beginning 1-12 months after exposure. Syphilis is not cured when the symptoms disappear. Such late manifestations as gumma of the liver and nervous system damage can ensue up to 40 years later.

Table 17-3. Reported venereal disease cases[1,2] and rates per 100,000[3] by calendar year—United States, 1954-63

Calendar year	Syphilis: Primary and Secondary		Early Latent		Late & Late Latent		Congenital		All stages[4] of Syphilis		Gonorrhea		Chancroid		Granuloma Inguinale		Lymph Granuloma Venereum	
	Cases	Rates	Cases	Rates	Cases	Rates	Cases	Rates	Cases	Rates	Cases	Rates	Cases	Rates	Cases	Rates	Cases	Rates
1954	7,147	4.5	23,861	15.1	89,123	56.5	6,676	4.2	130,697	82.9	242,050	153.5	3,003	1.9	618	.4	875	.6
1955	6,454	4.0	20,054	12.5	86,526	53.8	5,354	3.3	122,392	76.2	236,197	147.0	2,649	1.7	498	.3	762	.5
1956	6,395	3.9	19,813	12.0	95,168	57.6	5,498	3.3	130,314	78.9	224,683	136.0	2,138	1.3	357	.2	500	.3
1957	6,581	3.9	17,818	10.6	91,378	54.3	5,321	3.2	123,888	73.6	214,872	127.6	1,637	1.0	348	.2	448	.3
1958	7,184	4.2	16,569	9.7	83,129	48.5	4,901	2.9	114,053	66.5	232,818	135.8	1,603	.9	314	.2	435	.3
1959	9 799	5.6	17,025	9.8	86,740	49.7	5,130	2.9	120,824	69.2	240,254	137.6	1,537	.9	265	.2	604	.3
1960	16,145	9.1	18,017	10.1	81,798	45.9	4,416	2.5	122,538	68.8	258,933	145.3	1,680	.9	296	.2	835	.5
1961	19,851	11.0	19,486	10.8	79,304	43.8	4,163	2.3	124,658	68.8	264,158	145.8	1,438	.8	241	.1	787	.4
1962	21,067	11.5	19,585	10.7	79,533	43.3	4,070	2.2	126,245	68.7	263,714	143.5	1,344	.7	207	.1	590	.3
1963	22,251	11.9	18,235	9.8	78,076	41.9	4,031	2.2	124,137	66.5	278,289	149.2	1,220	.7	173	.1	586	.3

[1] Alaska and Hawaii included after 1955.
[2] Civilian cases only. Known military cases excluded.
[3] Civilian population only.
[4] Includes "stage not stated."

*From *Morbidity and Mortality*. U.S. Department of Health, Education and Welfare, Public Health Service, 1964.

without treatment, and is usually gone before the blood test for syphilis becomes positive. For this reason, many infected individuals have been lulled into a false sense of security or have dropped treatment before they were cured.

The second stage of the disease comes on about nine weeks after infection. A rash may appear, often covering the entire skin, including the palms of the hands and soles of the feet, and it can resemble anything from measles to psoriasis. Sores of various kinds may also appear in the lining of the mouth and throat, and around the genitals and rectum, and there may be pain in the bones and joints, fever, headache, and sensations of generalized illness. Sometimes the eyes are affected, as well as the membranes of the nervous system. The secondary stage of syphilis disappears without treatment, but the symptoms may return because the spirochetes are still present. The disease is highly contagious at this stage.

The only sure way to diagnose syphilis is to perform a laboratory test. The most satisfactory test for the first stage of syphilis is the examination of material from the chancre to see if it contains spirochetes. Two to three weeks after the disappearance of the chancre, syphilis may be detected from a variety of blood tests that take the names of the scientists who first used or improved them—for example, Wassermann, Kolmer, Kahn, and Eagle. The most promising new test is the fluorescent treponemal antibody (FTA) test. In this test the syphilis-causing organism, when viewed with a microscope by ultraviolet light, glows with a yellow fluorescence.

The *primary* (chancre) and the *secondary* stages together are called *early syphilis* and are more dangerous to others than to the person who has it. Untreated, the disease may continue for a number of years without obvious harm to the body. If treatment is begun in the early stage but is inadequate, the blood test often becomes negative, but the infection remains.

Five, ten or even more years after syphilis has been contracted, *late syphilis* develops (if it has not been properly treated) and the order is reversed: it is now less infectious to others but definitely dangerous to the victim. Severe and disabling diseases of the bones and joints, the skin or the internal organs are not uncommon in late syphilis, because the

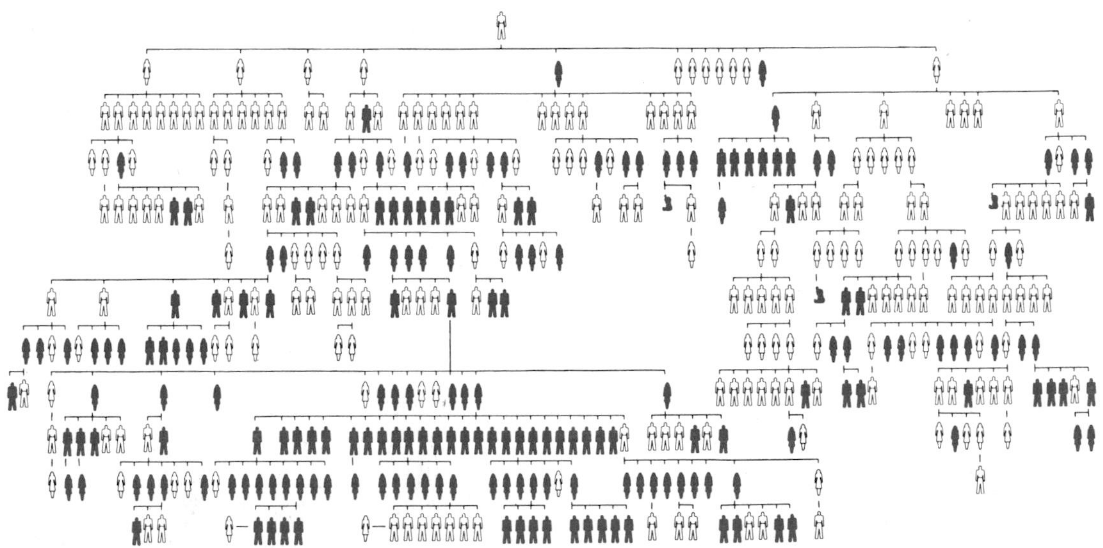

Figure 17–4. Persons involved in a typical syphilis epidemic. White figures represent adults; blue figures represent persons under 20; small blue figures represent infants. (Courtesy of U.S. Public Health Service Task Force on Eradication of Syphilis, 1962.)

unchecked spirochetes can invade any cell of the body. The most serious conditions result if the heart and nervous system are affected.

Syphilis can attack the heart itself, the aortic valve, and the aorta (the main blood vessel leaving the heart), and it can cause very disabling cardiac disease. Involvement of the nervous system often leads to the condition called *tabes dorsalis* or *locomotor ataxia,* in which the sensation of position is lost. An individual so affected doesn't know where his legs are and loses his balance in the dark. Extensive invasion of the nervous system causes *paresis* which leads to prolonged insanity and eventually to death.

An especially tragic form of this disease is *congenital syphilis,* in which the spirochetes are transmitted from the mother to the unborn infant. This may happen even when there is no visible sign of illness in the mother. Babies infected *in utero* may be born dead or be seriously handicapped later because of blindness, deafness, or other deformities. *All* pregnant women owe it to their children to have a routine blood test for syphilis in the early months of pregnancy. Early diagnosis and therapy prevent infection of the unborn child.

With the discovery and widespread use of penicillin, the *treatment* of syphilis became a relatively simple matter. Before modern methods of rapid treatment, when arsenic and mercury compounds were the only medications available, it was usually necessary for the patients to take them for a year and a half. Today, syphilis can be completely cured in a week or two with three injections of penicillin. A single injection of penicillin (1,200,000 or 2,400,000 units), given 30 hours before or after exposure, will *prevent* infection, and other antibiotics can be used in individuals who are penicillin-sensitive.

The reported cases of primary and secondary syphilis in the United States decreased between 1950 and 1956, but since 1957 there has been a threefold increase in the incidence. For 1963, the rate for primary and secondary syphilis was 11.9 cases per 100,000 population; the corresponding death rate was 1.6 per 100,000 (see Table 17–3).

Gonorrhea is our most widespread venereal disease, but is less dreaded than syphilis because, ordinarily, it is less dangerous. However, *gonorrhea can become serious,* and is a cause of sterility in men as well as women, and of many disorders of the reproductive organs. It can lead to painful arthritis and destruction of the joints, and can even cause death if the organisms enter the blood and lodge in the heart valves. If the bacteria get into the eyes, blindness may result, and most states now require doctors to use a disinfectant in the eyes of newborn babies. This has practically eliminated blindness due to gonorrheal infection during passage through the birth canal.

This disease is caused by the gonococcal organism, *Neisseria gonorrhoeae,* which attacks the genital organs of men and women. The common slang terms for gonorrhea are "clap" and "dose." It is almost always contracted by sexual intercourse, and *not* by kissing or from toilet seats. Vaginal infections in little girls and eye infections in children and adults are the exceptions, and they can develop from nonsexual transmission of the gonococcus.

The first symptoms of gonorrhea usually appear five to seven days after exposure.

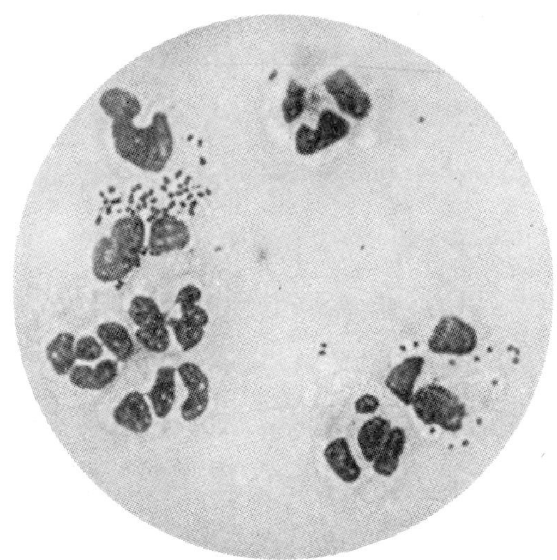

Figure 17–5. *Neisseria gonorrhoeae.* (gonococcus). (Courtesy *Therapeutic Notes*; Parke, Davis.)

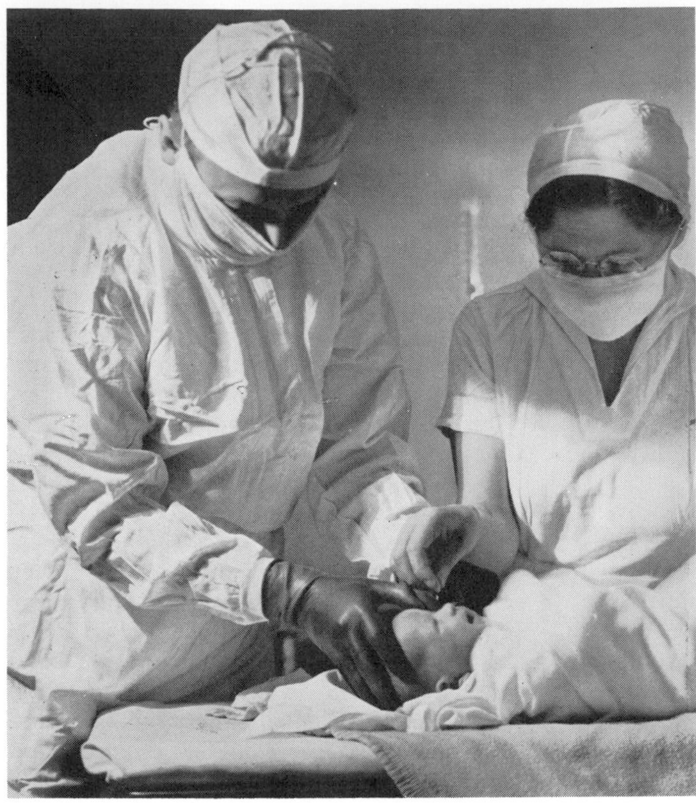

Figure 17–6. Physician and nurse placing silver nitrate solution in eyes of infant shortly after birth to prevent gonorrheal ophthalmia. The solution is contained in a wax ampule to be crushed between the fingers of the nurse. Note the caps, gowns, gloves, and other equipment used to assure asepsis so necessary during the puerperium. (Courtesy of National Society for the Prevention of Blindness.)

In men there is a whitish discharge from the penis or a burning sensation during urination. Women may develop pain in the lower abdomen with or without a period of burning urination or a whitish vaginal discharge. Because organisms other than those responsible for gonorrhea may cause similar symptoms, a precise diagnosis of gonorrhea can be made only by microscopic examination. This requires a reputable physician, hospital clinic, or venereal disease detection center. Although gonorrhea and syphilis are caused by two different microorganisms, it is possible to contract both diseases at the same time.

Until recently, the treatment of gonorrhea was very simple and rapid, because the organism was highly sensitive to antibiotics. Most cases responded to a single injection of penicillin, only 300,000 to 600,000 units, and very refractory cases could be cured by several injections. Despite the extensive use of this antibiotic, the number of cases in the United States has increased steadily since 1957. However, when these figures are corrected for population increases, a slight decrease in rate is observed. The incidence for 1963 was 149.2 cases per 100,000 population. However, an Army physician, Ernst Epstein, reported recently that penicillin failed to cure gonorrhea in 20 per cent of the soldiers treated at a camp in Inchon, Korea. Similar findings have been made by other physicians in both the United States and Great Britain, indicating an increasing prevalence of penicillin-resistant strains of the gonococcus. Fortunately, other antibiotics are still effective against these strains.

In addition to syphilis and gonorrhea, there are three other less common types of venereal disease—*chancroid, lymphogranuloma venereum,* and *granuloma inguinale*. Symptoms of these diseases are sores on the genital organs, swellings or lumps in the groin, or sores around the groin and the anus.

An attack of syphilis or gonorrhea does not produce immunity to these diseases, which means that even if an individual has been cured once, he is vulnerable to repeated attacks of both diseases. *The surest way to prevent venereal disease is to avoid contact with infected persons.* Unfortunately, these infections are not confined to prostitutes and promiscuous men, and it is impossible to tell from a person's appearance, social status or wealth whether he or she is infected.

According to a report by the United Nations Secretariat for the Social Commission of the Economic and Social Council, the *part-time* prostitute has become as great a problem to the world as the professional.[4] In some areas of Europe and North America, "the good-time girl has become a competitor and the trend is apparently toward a decreasing demand for prostitution. Because of this ... the professional prostitute is no longer the main source of venereal disease."

In 1957, 6581 cases of primary and secondary syphilis were reported in the United States. From this all-time low value, there has been an increase to 22,251 cases reported in 1963. However, it is estimated that only 10 per cent of the cases of infectious syphilis treated by private physicians are reported. Consequently, the 1963 total was probably closer to 100,000 cases. Of these cases, 43 per cent were among persons less than 25 years of age.

Venereal diseases will be eliminated completely when we recognize that they breed on fear, shame and ignorance. Today, this fear is absolutely groundless, nor is there any need for shame. From the doctor's viewpoint, syphilis and gonorrhea are preventable and curable illnesses, not a moral punishment for sin. "It is not a divine moral purpose, or a satanic punitive ingenuity that connects syphilis with genital activities, but a mere biological accident, no more significant in the last analysis than the fact that potatoes grow in sandy loam."[5] Understanding this fact will prevent innocently infected people from sneaking off to quacks and "doctors for men" because they are ashamed to face a reputable physician.

[4]*New York Times,* April 1, 1959.

[5]Stokes, J.H., Beerman, H., and Ingraham, N.R., Jr.: *Modern Clinical Syphilology,* 3rd Ed., W. B. Saunders Co., Philadelphia, 1944.

EPILEPSY

In recent years the public has adopted a sensible, frank and open attitude toward many illnesses, including tuberculosis and venereal disease. However, for some reason, a "hush-hush" policy still prevails when it comes to epilepsy.

At least 1 of every 200 Americans has epilepsy in mild or severe form, making it as common a disease as tuberculosis and diabetes, and four times more frequent than polio. Epilepsy afflicts 200,000 to 300,000 young people under 20, and the incidence is greatest in children under five.

In the past, people who suffered from epilepsy were shunned, because they were regarded as insane, or, at least, peculiar. Consequently they had to endure not only the disease but humiliation and a sense of inferiority which made them feel lonely and set apart.

That so many cases of epilepsy were concealed actually hampered research, but starting about 1937, largely through the outstanding work of Tracy Putnam, H. Houston Merritt, and W. G. Lennox, we have made great progress in understanding and treating this disease. We know now that epileptics are *not* inferior people, and that it is *not* a kind of insanity; only a small percentage of affected people suffer brain damage and deterioration. Nor are they particularly superior, even though a number of exceptional people have had epilepsy, including Socrates, Julius Caesar, Napoleon, Paganini, Peter the Great, Lord Byron, Dostoevsky, Flaubert, and many others. Tony Lazzeri, the great Yankee second baseman of the Babe Ruth era was an epileptic, but this fact was never revealed until after his death. The old myth that the fits and convulsions of epilepsy must be due to invasion by a witch or demon died very slowly.

Symptoms

The word epilepsy means a seizure, often called a "fit," and is specifically applied to a certain type of seizure characterized by loss of consciousness and involuntary convulsive movements.

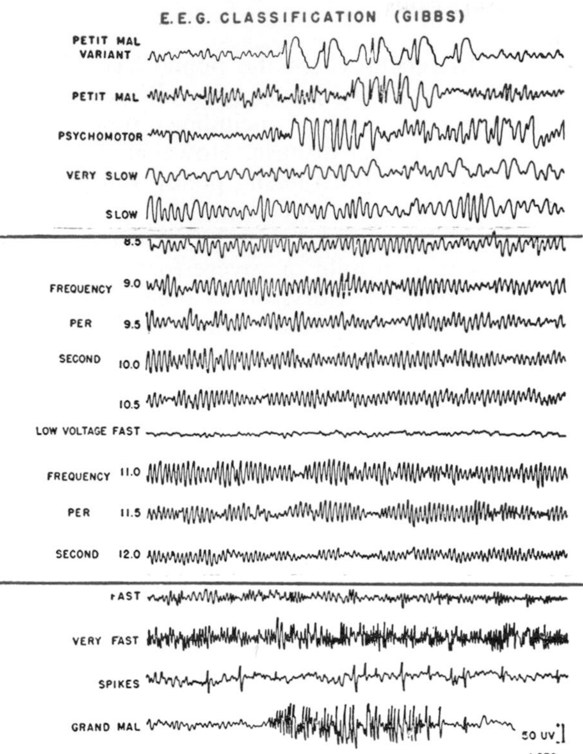

Figure 17–7. Normal and epileptic electroencephalograph records. The upper five and the lower four are considered abnormal. A paroxysmal record (i.e., petit mal, psychomotor, or grand mal) is 33 times as common in epileptics as in controls; it is considered extremely abnormal and strongly suggestive of epilepsy. Very slow or very fast records are 20 times as common in epileptics as in controls; they are therefore considered abnormal and suggestive of epilepsy or a related disorder. Incidence determined on adults. (Courtesy of F. A. Gibbs.)

In minor seizures, or *petit mal,* the loss of consciousness is momentary. There may be a twitching about the eyes or mouth, but the epileptic remains seated or standing, and appears to have experienced little more than a lapse of attention or a moment of absent-mindedness. However, in major seizures, *grand mal,* the victim falls to the floor unconscious, often foaming at the mouth, biting, and shaking his limbs violently. The observer may mistake it for fainting, blacking out, or even a stroke, although the convulsive movements should indicate that it is an attack of epilepsy. Fortunately, people with epilepsy frequently experience a warning (the *aura*) before a major attack occurs and this enables them to lie down and avoid falls.

The seizure is due to a temporary disturbance of the brain impulses, an abnormal electrical discharge comparable to static on your radio. Medically, it is known as *cerebral dysrhythmia,* meaning a disturbance of the brain's normal rhythm.

Fainting spells, fleeting unconsciousness, convulsions, or fits of any kind may be due to epilepsy, but they may also result from other diseases. To establish a definite diagnosis, special tests are necessary, such as an electroencephalograph (the brain-wave pattern is very distinctive in epilepsy), x-rays of the skull, and air injections into the ventricles of the brain which permit special x-rays to be taken.

Cause and Treatment

Ordinary epilepsy, the most common type, also called *genuine* or *idiopathic epilepsy* (which means that the cause is unknown) usually begins early in life. It is not directly inherited, although a predisposition or tendency towards it may run in families. Several very effective medicines, including phenobarbital, Dilantin, and Tridione, are now available to prevent or greatly reduce the number of seizures.

Acquired epilepsy, also called *symptomatic epilepsy,* may be the result of a brain tumor or other injury which irritates the brain and sets off the abnormal electrical discharge. Removing the tumor or repairing the injury frequently cures the symptoms.

More than 90 per cent of epilepsy sufferers can now expect to lead normal lives with modern medical and surgical treatments. However, complete therapy must also include education and reassurance of the patient—as well as of the general public—to remove the stigma which is attached to this disease. Even today, residual ancient fears and superstitions continue to handicap the epileptic, no matter how well-controlled his disease is and how normal a life he leads. A successful small businessman, honorably discharged from the U.S. Air Force after four years of active duty, wrote anonymously of some of the problems he faces as an epileptic:

> Many U.S. laws are attempting to breed me out of existence. In some of them . . . I am separated only by a comma from habitual criminals and imbeciles. In 14 states the law refuses me the right to marry; in four states I can be surgically sterilized against my wishes; and seven states require that a doctor report me to the state capital if I go to him for treatment. In six states I can marry only if I submit to sterilization or am too old to have children. . . . In Michigan my wife may be sent to jail for as much as five years and be fined $1,000 for marrying me. . . . In ten states, to get a job I may be forced to waive my rights under Workmen's Compensation, and, if I am injured, receive reduced aid or none at all. And if I were foreign born seeking admission to the U.S., I would be lumped with the feeble-minded, the insane, the alcoholics, the lepers, the prostitutes and the paupers, and denied entry under Federal immigration laws. . . . Actually I could live normally only if I became a liar.[6]

MULTIPLE SCLEROSIS

Multiple sclerosis is second in incidence only to epilepsy as a disease of the nervous system, and is far more widespread than infantile paralysis. It is not so well known to the public as polio because it strikes far less dramatically, being an insidious, chronic disease of long duration. Periods of improvement alternate with periods of symptoms, but, at its worst, it can be an almost completely disabling disease. Tragically, most of its victims are young adults, and in two thirds of the patients symptoms first appear between the ages of 20 and 40.

In this disease, hardened patches due to inflammation are scattered throughout the brain and spinal cord, interfering with the activity of nerves in the affected areas. Why these patches become inflamed and hardened is still unknown. Bacteria or viruses have been suggested, but not yet definitely established, as causative agents. Heredity is apparently not an important component in the disease, for it often develops in one identical twin and not in the other, and multiple sclerosis in three generations of a single family is rare. The greatest number of cases seems to be found in cold climates, such as northern Europe.

Symptoms and Effects

Because the location, extent and duration of disability vary tremendously from one patient to another and even in the same patient at different times, it is difficult to describe a typical case. However, the most common symptoms include:

Marked tremor or shaking of the limbs, interfering with fine movements such as sewing or writing, and often making the patient extremely weak. Speech may also become slow and monotonous.

Unsteadiness of stiffness in walking, and inability to maintain balance.

Visual difficulties: the patient may "see double" or lose part of the visual field. For example, he may be unable to see toward the upper left with either eye.

Rigidity or paralysis, which may occur in any part of the body.

Treatment

Treatment consists mainly of good general care to keep up the body's health and resistance to disease, and, when necessary, expert nursing care, because multiple sclerosis is apt to grow worse following an illness. *Physiotherapy,* including massage and exercise, helps prevent the affected muscles from becoming unnecessarily weakened or paralyzed. Emotional disturbances may aggravate the disease and sufferers from this prolonged malady are apt to become very depressed. For this

[6]*My Illness Makes Me Untouchable* (as told to Evan Hill). Coronet, March 1958, p. 132.

reason, *psychotherapy* and mood-elevating drugs may be helpful.

Patients with multiple sclerosis can, and often do, lead long and useful lives. The average duration of the disease is about 25 years, but cases continuing for 60 years have been reported, marked by many periods of spontaneous improvement.

CEREBRAL PALSY

Cerebral palsy is one of the most common disabilities in the United States, affecting about 550,000 people—one-third of whom are under 21 years of age. Each year, about 10,000 babies are born with cerebral palsy—one every 53 minutes. This is one of the saddest of the disabling illnesses because it strikes at infants, many of whom are treated for the rest of their lives as though they were helpless mental and physical cripples. This is particularly tragic because, in the great majority of cases, skilled rehabilitation can be very helpful for victims of cerebral palsy.

This disease results from damage to certain areas of the brain, and was for many years attributed to birth injuries, caused by the use of forceps. Now we realize that the difficulty is initiated far more frequently during the developmental stage, *before* the baby is born, and sometimes it occurs after birth.

About two of every six children born with cerebral palsy will be feebleminded, and the remainder will be of normal mentality, but show greater or less physical impairment. This disease affects the nerves which control the muscles. As a result there may be *spastic* paralysis, with stiffness and acute difficulty in muscular movements, causing a scissors-like gait; *tremors* and jerky motions of the limbs and head, often accompanied by bizarre grimaces; and *poor coordination*. There may also be sight or hearing defects.

The treatment of cerebral palsy varies according to the nature and extent of the brain injury. Muscular spasms can be partially relieved by certain medicines, and some deformities can be corrected by surgical means. However, *training* is

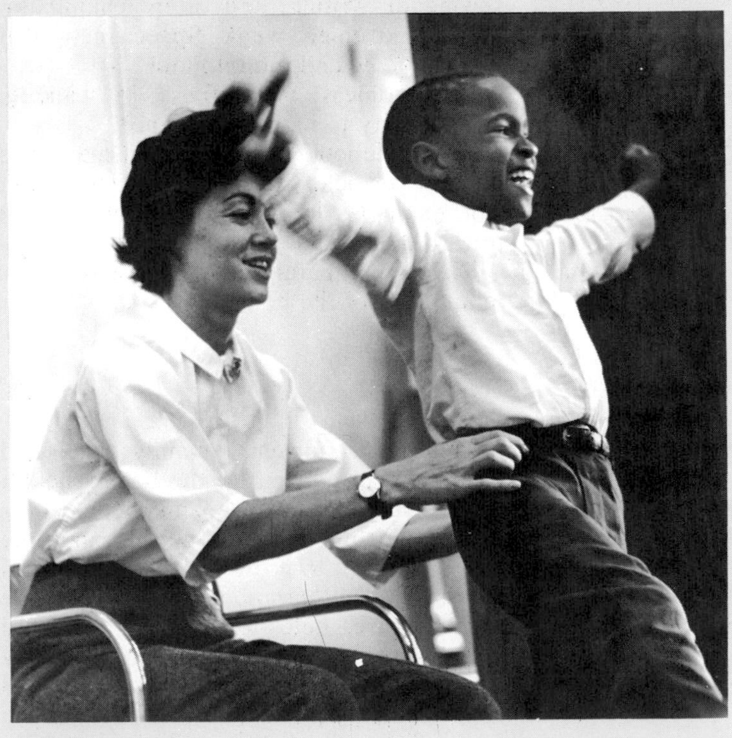

Physical therapy is a form of rehabilitation for patients recovering from diseases. This boy, whose walking was hampered by a disease affecting his legs, learns to walk again with help from a therapist.

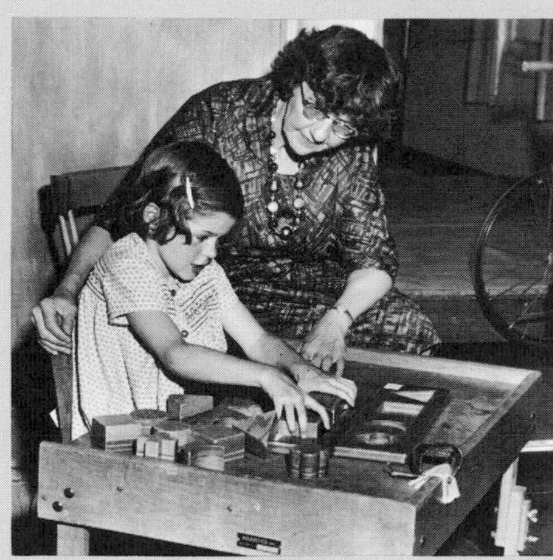

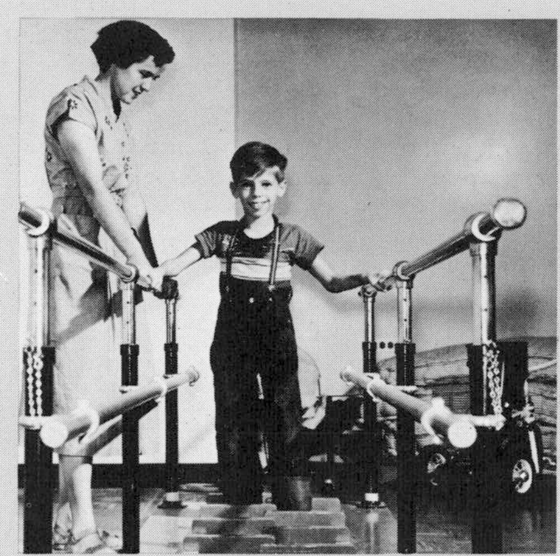

Most children with cerebral palsy benefit from occupational and physical therapy, which not only teaches them to control their muscles, but offers them an opportunity to play. The boy on the right is learning how to walk.

the real key to the conquest of this disease, and has made possible useful, normal lives for countless victims. The earlier such training begins, the less difficulty there is in overcoming the disabilities.

Indications of cerebral palsy are usually apparent to the parents or physician when the baby is only a few months old. Parents of such children need to learn how to help them walk, talk and do the many things which are so easy for the normal child and so difficult for one who can't control his muscles. Most large communities have special schools for such children—and to help the parents. Time, patience and knowledge can work miracles in cerebral palsy.

BLINDNESS AND OTHER SERIOUS VISUAL DISORDERS

Despite the best that modern medicine and surgery can do, there are still many people whose vision is severely and irreparably damaged or who are totally blind. The National Society for the Prevention of Blindness estimates that 400,000 people in the United States are either totally blind, or have enough visual impairment to prevent the conduct of normal activities. In about 16.7 per cent of the cases, prenatal and hereditary disorders are the cause; infectious diseases account for 5.3 per cent and accidents for 2.9 per cent. Glaucoma, cataracts, diabetes, and arteriosclerosis are also responsible for a significant number of cases, but in many instances the precise cause of blindness is not known.

As Franklin M. Foote has pointed out, to envisage the estimate of this many blind people in the United States, you have to imagine a city as large as Miami, Florida, or Omaha, Nebraska—in which every man, woman, and child is blind.

More than 27,000 persons lose their sight each year, and unless we develop more effective preventive measures, 3/4 million people now living will become blind before they die.

The cost of caring for the blind, in terms of education, braille and talking books, seeing-eye dogs, pensions, and other services, amounts to $150 million each year, according to the American Foundation for the Blind. If we also take into consideration industrial compensation, medical expenses and lost production, eye injuries cost industry more than $200 million a year. These expenditures are in contrast to the few million dollars

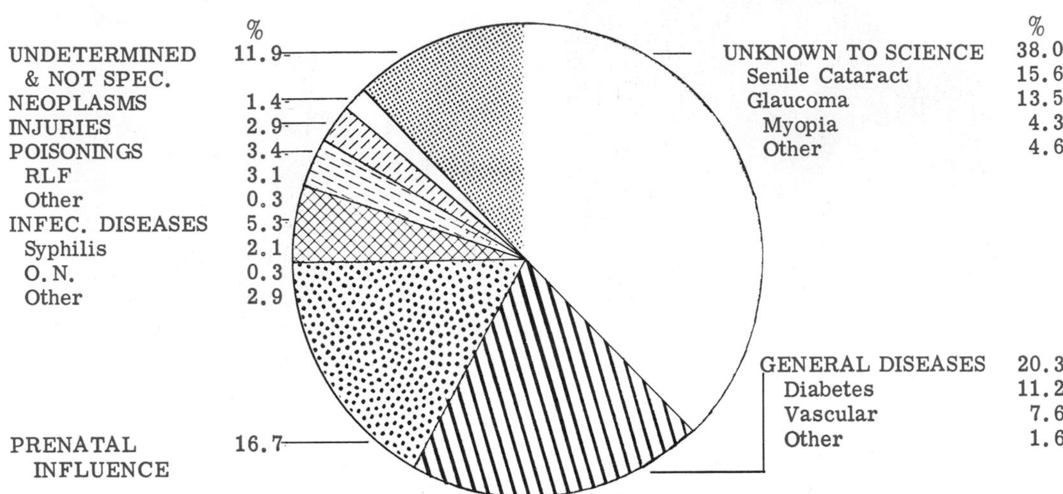

Figure 17–8. Causes of blindness in the United States. (From *Facts on the Major Killing and Crippling Diseases in the United States Today.* The National Health Education Committee, Inc., 1964.)

spent each year for research on this problem.[7]

Major Causes

Trachoma is an eye infection caused by a virus, which affects the membranes lining the lids and covering the eyeball, and in advanced cases may cause severe scarring and blindness. This disease is especially prevalent in areas of the world where poor nutrition and hygiene and crowded living conditions prevail, and where the climate is hot, dry, and dusty. Fortunately, the sulfonamides and antibiotics can keep trachoma under control, and prevent its dangerous progression.

Glaucoma is caused by an abnormal accumulation of fluid in the eyes, producing intraocular pressures which seriously impair vision. Normally, fluids flow freely into and out of the inner chamber of the eye, but in some individuals, for reasons unknown, this equilibrium is disturbed. Glaucoma is the result, and it afflicts about 800,000 people each year. One of every eight blind persons is a victim of this disease, and the tragedy is that, in most cases, their eyesight could have been saved by early diagnosis and treatment.

In the acute type of glaucoma, dimming of the vision may be sudden: the eyeball becomes painful, and the affected person feels quite ill. However, the insidious type doesn't cause pain, and injures the vision only very slowly. It sometimes makes itself known by the appearance of colored rings and halos about bright objects, or by the fact that the vision remains good in front, but dims on the side. Tranquilizers have been helpful in some cases of glaucoma, because the emotions have a profound influence on ocular pressure, but the commonest treatment is to use "miotics," eyedrops which relieve fluid accumulation in the eyeball.

Blindness is one of the complications of *diabetes* of long duration and, despite insulin therapy, occurs in about 6 per cent of people with diabetes.

[7]In 1963, the federal appropriation for research on blindness was $8½ million.

Cataracts

Cataracts are opaque areas which develop on the lens. This occurs chiefly in older individuals, and merely represents part of the aging process. When they are large enough, cataracts interfere seriously with vision, but, fortunately, almost all of them can be removed by surgery, which provides great relief for this condition.

Scarring or opacity of the cornea sometimes follows inflammations, ulcerations or injuries of various kinds, and, if extensive enough, it, too, may lead to blindness.

Transplants have been very successful in curing blindness due to scarred cornea. Unfortunately, of the approximately 400,000 blind people in this country, only about 15,000 are suitable for corneal transplants, because blindness in the remainder is from causes other than a scarred cornea.

Detached Retina

The retina, which is essentially an extension of the optic nerve which lines the interior of the eyeball, receives the light rays and transmits the impulses to the brain where they register as sight. Sometimes—after injury or inflammation—the retina becomes detached and separated from the eyeball. Retinal detachment can interfere seriously with vision and may eventually cause blindness. In about half the cases, surgical treatment can save the sight.

Prevention of Blindness

Preventive measures and research are largely responsible for a 70 per cent reduction in blindness caused by infectious disease in school children. The use of prophylactic eyedrops for every newborn child has practically eliminated blindness caused by gonorrhea, and health education and sulfa drug treatment have cured most of the trachoma in this country. A 60 per cent reduction in syphilis as a cause of blindness in children over the past 20 years has resulted from premarital and early pregnancy tests for syphilis, coupled with antibiotic therapy and widespread education about this disease.

Retrolental fibroplasia, a form of blindness which formerly occurred among premature babies, has become very rare since physicians stopped administering oxygen in high concentrations to these babies. About 8000 children and young people in this country can attribute their blindness to retrolental fibroplasia.

Eye safety programs, especially in industry, have reduced blindness due to injury about 30 per cent.

Early diagnosis and treatment of pathological eye conditions are the best method to prevent blindness, according to the National Society for the Prevention of Blindness. This organization has been conducting surveys in several communities with the help of ophthalmologists to detect previously undiagnosed, potentially serious eye conditions. A study in Baltimore, for example, showed that 50 per cent of the blindness found could have been prevented. The value of such surveys is indicated by the results obtained in Cleveland: in a survey involving 12,000 persons older than 40 years, 240 cases of glaucoma were found, or about 2 per cent. Only 23 of these 240 had previously been diagnosed as glaucoma.

Blindness actually appears to be increasing in the older age group, largely because there is a steady growth in the number of elderly people in the population. This makes health examinations for glaucoma and cataract, as well as for changes due to degenerative vascular diseases, even more important today, especially in individuals past middle age. Another important preventive measure against blindness is the use of protective lenses for industrial workers, and nonbreakable lenses for children.

DEAFNESS

Approximately one of every ten, or 18,500,000, people in the United States have some hearing impairment, and

225,000 cannot hear human speech. Even the best hearing aids can't help the auditory mechanism after it is completely destroyed.

Signs of Deafness

Impaired hearing may come on suddenly or gradually, and manifest itself in many ways. School children who appear listless and inattentive, mispronounce words, show voice or speech peculiarities, and in general do poorly at school, may be suffering from a simple and easily corrected hearing loss. A shocking number of school children have been called stubborn and irresponsible by their parents, or labeled subnormal in intelligence by their teachers simply because these children are deaf.

Many emotional problems can also be traced to hearing defects. A deaf person, child or grown-up, often avoids other people if he is unable to hear them and follow what is being said.

If you answer "yes" to the following questions, you are suffering some hearing loss and should see an ear specialist (otologist) *without delay:*

Do you frequently find yourself asking that words and phrases be repeated?

Does a faucet drip in the room without your hearing it?

Do you find that you don't hear well if your back is turned to a speaker?

Do you strain to hear, turn one ear or bend your head toward a speaker, or watch his lips intently?

Unfortunately, many hearing defects are not recognized until there is some permanent loss of hearing.

Causes of Deafness

Deafness results most commonly from disturbances in the sound-conducting mechanism of the middle ear, *conduction deafness;* from damage to the sound-perceiving apparatus in the inner ear; and from disease of the auditory nerve, leading to *nerve deafness.* Infections invading the middle ear may damage the ear bones, restrict their motion or fill up the area with pus. Perhaps the greatest single danger is secondary infections associated with the common cold, and these are blamed for as much as 40 per cent of all cases of impaired hearing. Diseased tonsils and adenoids and running ears, if neglected, may cause a temporary loss of hearing which can lead to some degree of permanent deafness.

Measles, mumps, scarlet fever, chicken-pox, whooping cough, and meningitis are responsible for many cases of deafness. Hearing should always be checked after these illnesses.

Sometimes accidents injure, perforate, or even destroy, the eardrum. Nerve deafness, perforated eardrum, and middle ear infections account for about half the deaf population.

A foreign object or wax hardening in the ear and covering the eardrum, infections after swimming and a sharp blow on the ear are also hazardous. The cauliflower ears, shambling gait, and stupid incoherence of prize fighters who have been bruised in contest after contest are the outward signs of damage to both the brain and hearing mechanism from repeated blows.

Industrial noises and high-intensity sound of any kind should either be reduced to a minimum, or protective devices employed to prevent deafness. Noise affects the hearing by destroying the small hair cells in the inner ear. Once this mechanism has been damaged, hearing loss becomes permanent. If the defect is great, even amplification of sound by a hearing aid is ineffective. The noise around jet planes, for example, is so intense that exposure for even a few minutes can cause temporary hearing loss, with some permanent residual damage. Earplugs, earmuffs, or helmets may be slightly uncomfortable, but they afford important protection against the hazards of too much noise, and should always be worn by individuals working in excessively noisy areas or exposed to high-intensity sounds.

Hereditary and congenital defects are responsible for a small percentage of deafness. Deafness "runs" in certain families because of hereditary defects in the development of some portion of the hearing mechanism, such as the nerve or the tiny bones of the midear.

Otosclerosis, which means "hardening of the ear," is a slowly progressive type of deafness caused by new bone formation and a gradual fixing or immobilization of the hammer, anvil, and stirrup bones in the middle ear.

Prevention and Treatment of Deafness. Much deafness can be prevented by recognizing the potential seriousness of generalized diseases or of specific infections involving the ears.

Certain types can be corrected or greatly helped by one of the many varieties of hearing aids available today.

Lip reading is enormously beneficial to deaf people, and it is especially important that young children who are deaf become skillful in this technique as soon as possible.

Fluid accumulation in the ear may cause a mild, easily corrected type of deafness. Also, hearing impairments due to overgrowth of lymphoid tissue—which often accompanies inflamed adenoids and tonsils—can be taken care of by minor surgery. If deafness is due to otosclerosis, the operation called *fenestration* is often very successful. As the name suggests, this means "making a new opening, or window" in the hardened bone overlying the inner ear. The eardrum is then placed over the new opening, so that sound waves can be transmitted through it.

MUSCULAR DYSTROPHY AND MYASTHENIA GRAVIS

In polio and similar diseases which affect the brain and nerves, the muscles are useless and waste away because the *nerves* which control them die. In contrast to these, *muscular dystrophy* and *myasthenia gravis* cause severe disabilities by affecting the muscles directly.

Muscular dystrophy is a particularly distressing disease because it strikes at children and teen-agers, weakening and gradually shriveling the muscles away. Three males for every female suffer from this condition, and hereditary influences have been demonstrated in about 80 per cent of the cases. Very important muscles can be affected, and as the illness progresses, it may incapacitate the patient so completely that he cannot stand or sit. However, there are several forms of muscular dystrophy and not all lead to total incapacitation.

A less severe variety appears between the ages of 10 and 20, which involves the muscles of the face and shoulders, but may also affect the leg or trunk muscles. Patients with this form of muscular dystrophy usually live out their years, and the fortunate ones suffer minimal disability.

There is no really specific therapy for muscular dystrophy, and we do not even know what causes it. However, intensive research on the cause and cure is in progress, and perhaps this will lead to hopeful developments in the near future.

In *myasthenia gravis,* there appears to be a chemical defect at the site where nerves and muscles interact. As a result, the muscles don't function properly, and people with this condition tire very quickly and have extreme muscle weakness. Usually their strength returns after rest, and they tend to feel strongest in the morning and most fatigued at night. The muscles most frequently affected are those of the face, eyelids, larynx, and throat, and often a patient can detect the onset of myasthenia gravis by the fact that his eyelids droop or he has difficulty in swallowing. The muscles of the trunk and extremities are less frequently involved.

This disease usually begins between the ages of 20 and 50, and affects more females than males. There is no true paralysis of muscles, and in most cases myasthenia gravis is a chronic illness, often with long periods of remission and only minor symptoms. *Neostigmine* and other medications, as well as surgical treatment, bring relief to a large number of patients.

HERNIAS

Hernia is the medical term for a rupture. It is not actually a tear, but a weak spot that develops in the bands of muscle tissue of the abdominal wall, permitting the intestines to bulge through and form a soft lump.

There are various types of hernias, and they occur more frequently in men

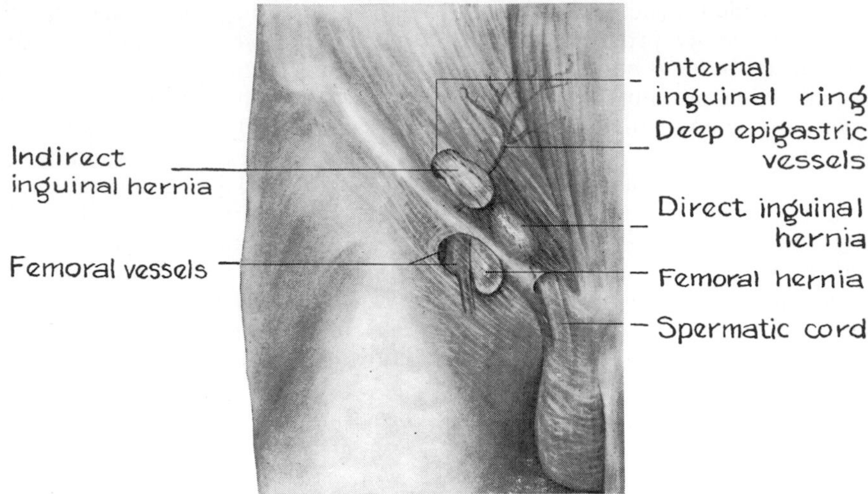

Figure 17–9. Hernias. Diagrammatic projection of the sites of origin of a femoral hernia and a direct and an indirect inguinal hernia. (From Dunphy and Botsford: *Physical Examination of the Surgical Patient.* 3rd Ed., Philadelphia, W. B. Saunders Co., 1964.)

than women, but they may develop even in children. *Inguinal* hernias in the male groin are the most common. This is where the spermatic cord passes to the testicles, and is the weakest spot in the male's abdominal wall because in some male infants, the wall does not shut tightly around the cord. In later years, constant straining or excessively heavy lifting may force the weakened wall to give way, suddenly or gradually. At first inguinal hernias may cause little pain and be scarcely noticeable, but before long the bulge may become bigger than a hen's egg, and sometimes extends into the scrotum.

In women, *femoral* hernias develop most frequently, on the upper thigh just below the groin. *Umbilical hernias,* in which the navel protrudes, are the most common in children. A similar condition sometimes results from surgical operations if the scar does not heal properly and the newly closed tissue is not strong enough to prevent intestinal bulging. Coughing, sneezing, or straining during defecation may aggravate the pain and protrusion of the hernia.

Anyone with this condition should seek medical care, instead of wearing a truss. It can and should be corrected by relatively minor surgical procedures. Not only are hernias unsightly and inconvenient, they can also become dangerous if a loop of intestine becomes "strangled" in the bulge, and its blood supply is cut off. This necessitates an emergency surgical procedure.

Hernias can be prevented by following certain sensible rules in lifting and carrying heavy loads:

1. Start doing heavy muscular work gradually, to adjust your muscles to the increased strain.
2. When lifting heavy weights, face the object, with your feet close to it and spread about 12 inches apart. If you are picking something up from the floor, keep your knees bent and rise slowly, using leg rather than back muscles.
3. Carry loads on your shoulders instead of your hips whenever you can.
4. Don't reach too high for heavy packages. Use a stool.

ARTHRITIS, GOUT, BACKACHE AND BURSITIS

More than 12,000,000 persons in the United States are suffering from arthritis and related rheumatic diseases, according to a recent report. New victims are added at the rate of 250,000 a year. Of the total suffering from arthritis, 624,000 are unable to work, and 3 million are limited in their activities.[8]

Of every 100 patients who consult a doctor because of "rheumatism," about 40 have rheumatoid arthritis; 30, osteoarthritis; 15, muscular rheumatism, neuritis, and sciatica. The remainder probably are suffering from gout, rheumatic fever, and other miscellaneous forms of rheumatic disease.

Women seem much more susceptible than men to arthritic diseases: for every man who is stricken, there are two or three women. This can create serious psychological and economic problems for the family, because it strikes such a high percentage of wives and mothers.

The term arthritis is widely misused and is frequently applied to vague aches in almost any part of the body. You cannot have arthritis in the middle of the thigh, for example, because there is not any joint there. However, you could develop it in the joints at the knees, wrists, elbows, fingers, toes, hips, shoulders, neck, and even between the bones of the spine. But a pain in the joint is not necessarily due to arthritis; it might arise in the ligament, tendon, muscle, or bursa.

Symptoms of arthritis are pain, swelling, stiffness, and deformity in one or more joints. An attack may be set off or aggravated by any one of many factors, including exposure to cold and dampness; infection of the teeth, tonsils or some other part of the body; injury to a joint or constant strain upon it; attempting physical labor that is too hard for one's age or strength; constant fatigue; and great nervous tension. However, the underlying cause of many cases of arthritis is unknown.

The three commonest types are *infectious* arthritis, *osteoarthritis,* and *rheumatoid* arthritis; the latter two are most prevalent.

Infectious arthritis is due to a bacterial infection inside a joint, originating either from the blood stream or from a wound that damages the joint. For example, in gonorrhea the microorganisms are often carried from the infected genital organs to the joints *via* the blood stream. Tuberculosis and brucellosis (undulant fever) sometimes have the same effect. Because the organisms involved are killed by antibiotics, treatment of infectious arthritis is very successful with penicillin and related medicines, but it must be started promptly.

Osteoarthritis rarely develops before the age of 40, but it is fairly common in people past this age. It appears to be due to wear and tear of the joint tissues and the formation of bony bumps at the joints which interfere with ordinary movements. The pain and disablement are usually minor.

The most serious variety is *rheumatoid* arthritis, common among young adults and usually starting before the age of 40. Individuals with mild cases need not fear that joint deformities are inevitable, but they should be under the regular care of a physician to make sure the disease does not progress. Acute attacks of rheumatoid arthritis can produce permanent changes in the joints, which leave them stiff and deformed. In this respect, it differs from an attack of *rheumatic fever,* in which the joints always return to normal after recovery. However, like severe rheumatic fever, rheumatoid arthritis can produce many symptoms, such as a rundown feeling, poor appetite, anemia, fever, and pleurisy.

The cause of this disease is not definitely known, but some experts believe that it may be caused by an allergy to the streptococcal bacteria. The most serious complication is such extreme stiffening of the joints, including the fingers, that they cannot be bent or unbent. People who suffer repeated attacks over a number of years may be forced to curtail their activities seriously.

Perhaps more than any other disease, arthritis has been a lucrative field for quacks and medical fakers peddling special diets, radioactive waters, alfalfa tea, "guaranteed-to-cure" copper bracelets for the afflicted joint, blackstrap molasses, special "lubricating" cocktails of cod liver oil in orange juice, "conjure bags," and "health belts." All these so-called treatments are both useless and dangerous, because they prevent or delay the arthritic patient in seeking real medical aid.

[8]*Facts on the Major Killing and Crippling Diseases in the United States Today,* The National Health Education Committee, 1964.

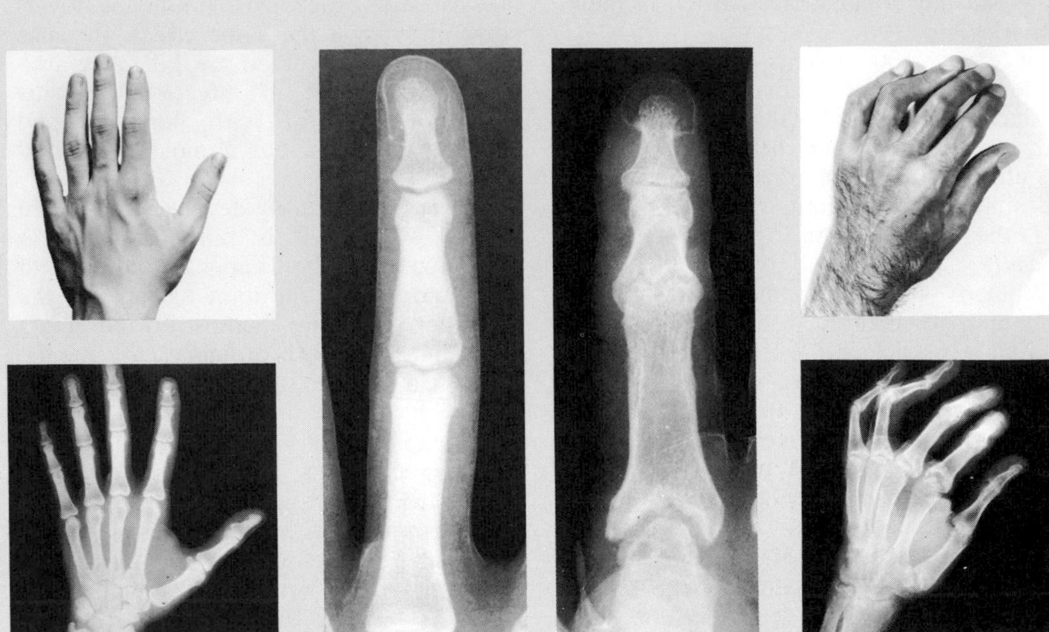

When arthritis affects the hands, it may be difficult to move the fingers. In the X-ray photographs, the normal hand (left) has room for the joint to move freely. The arthritic joint (right) is "locked" with bone and scar tissue.

Mild attacks of rheumatoid arthritis are treated by adequate physical and emotional rest, applications of heat to the affected joint, and aspirin or related preparations for pain relief. ACTH and the steroid hormones or other medications may be required for more severe cases. If the joints have become so stiffened that they can't be moved, reconstructive surgery often affords relief. Unfortunately, there is no cure for this disease, but because there is often a large psychosomatic component, psychotherapy may be very helpful.

Another form of arthritis, called *spondylitis,* is limited almost entirely to the spine, and may produce a stiff, fused vertebral column.

Children are rarely afflicted with crippling arthritis but they occasionally develop a very severe form called *Still's disease*.

Gout is a generalized disease in which excessive quantities of uric acid accumulate in the blood, tissues and urine. Like the severest forms of arthritis, it may affect the joints and even destroy them, and, in addition, it can injure the kidneys. The first indication of a gouty condition is often an attack of extremely severe pain, frequently in the big toe. About 400,000 people suffer from this illness, and 96 per cent of them are men. Unfortunately there are so many jokes about gout and high living that many people don't realize that it can progress into a very disabling disease of the joints, kidneys, or both. Because good dietary and medical treatments are available today, these complications can be prevented.

Two other ailments of the joint structure which can be extremely disabling unless treated properly are *backache* and *bursitis*. The backbone, or spine, is a column made up of many small bones which are held together by ligaments. Between the layers of bone lie cartilage disks which act as cushions. (Cartilage is the firm material which shapes the ears and nose.) Through this spinal column of bones runs a tube which holds the spinal cord, and from it extend many of the main nerves of the body. Because the bones and disks are loosely strung together, the backbone is very flexible and permits bending and a variety of other movements.

Backaches may result from many causes—a slipped disk, sacroiliac strain, sciatic neuritis, and arthritis—but incorrect posture is one of the commonest causes. When you were a small child in school, your teacher probably *made* you stand up straight, but as you grew older you might have forgotten this good advice and found it much easier to slump over a desk, or developed the habit of stooping. Unfortunately, if your back is thrown out of shape by poor posture or strained from carrying too much weight, the bones, ligaments, nerves and muscles are either pressed too close together or stretched too far apart, and may cause pain in either case.

If you are healthy otherwise and still develop backaches, check the following:

1. *Your mattress may be soft* and sagging and may make your spine curve too much when you sleep. A strong plywood bedboard between the spring and mattress will correct this.

2. *It may be only your posture that is wrong.* A good test of posture is to stand with your back against the wall, your weight resting evenly on your feet. Your shoulder blades and buttocks should touch the wall. If only your shoulders touch, you are round shouldered; if only the middle of your back touches, your spine is curved too much. If you stand up straight, you will find that, automatically, your abdomen is also held in, a good way to prevent sagging abdominal muscles.

3. *You may be carrying too heavy a load on one side.* This tends to curve your spine either to the right or left, and strain the back muscles and ligaments.

4. *Your work habits may be wrong.* When you sit at a typewriter, or desk, don't slump, but try to sit upright. If you must do a lot of bending, make sure you take time out at regular intervals to stretch and straighten up.

5. *Watch out for drafts.* Try to avoid

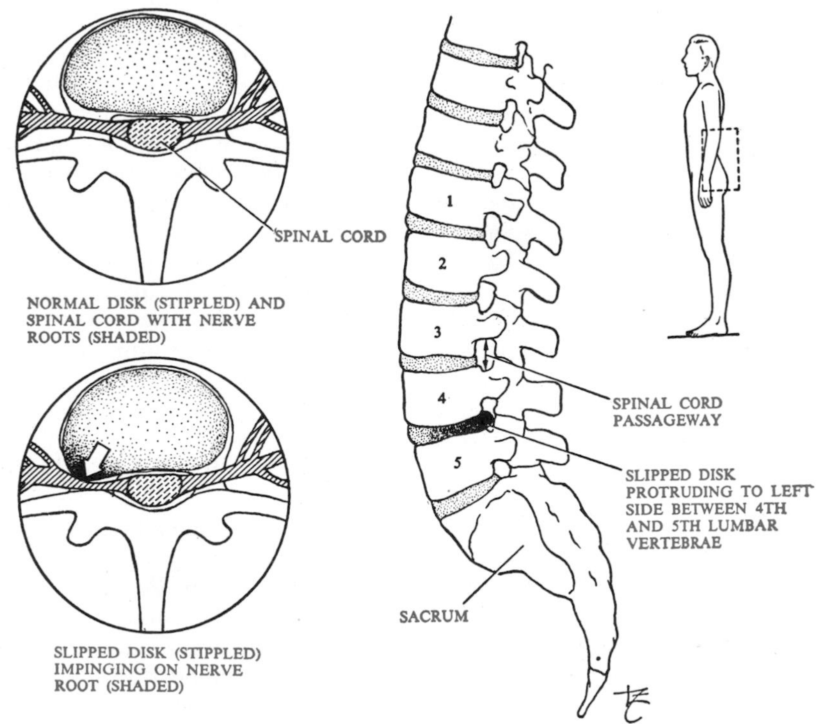

Figure 17–10. Slipped intervertebral disk. **Left,** Cross sections of vertebra and disk as viewed from above. **Right,** Lower spine as viewed from left side; nerve roots are omitted.

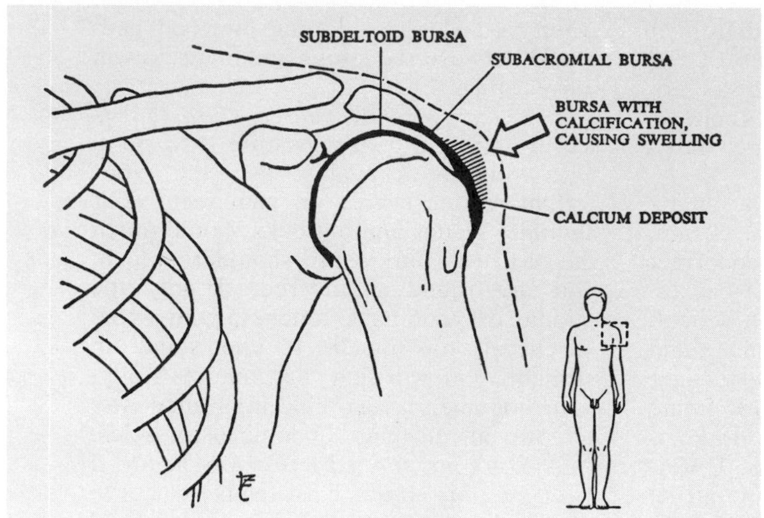

Figure 17–11. Bursitis with calcification.

sitting with your back exposed to drafts from hallways, open doors or windows.

6. In women, backaches are often associated with the *menstrual period,* or abnormality in the position of the pelvic organs.

If none of these factors is responsible for your backache, go to your doctor for a checkup. He may find that you have a dislocation, most commonly a sacroiliac strain or slipped disk. Occasionally the disks slip out of place from between the bones, or even rupture. When this happens, they may press on the nerve roots emerging from the spinal cord and cause considerable pain and disability. Surgery may be required to correct this.

Bursitis: Our joints would creak and wear out if we didn't have an efficient "oiling system" in the smooth surfaces inside the joints and the bursae around them. However, bursae sometimes become inflamed and even accumulate calcium deposits around them, setting off the extremely painful condition called bursitis.

This may appear in an acute or chronic form. The acute form comes on suddenly, often after chilling or exposure to a draft, or from excessive use of a joint as in typing, piano playing or athletics. Most commonly it affects the shoulder, but almost any joint in the body can be involved in bursitis. Sometimes nature will heal the acutely painful attack by rupturing and draining the inflamed area if the joint is rested in a sling or the patient goes to bed. Pain-relieving medications, moist heat, and especially, cortisone and related medicines often afford relief from the pain. If these do not help, a skilled doctor can frequently insert a needle into the inflamed area and draw out the fluid and calcium salts. At the same time he may puncture the bursa in several places to prevent recurrence.

Chronic bursitis, with persisting pain and limitation of motion around a joint, sometimes follows the acute attack. If rest, heat and the proper medicines don't relieve it, surgery may be necessary to remove the calcium deposits or free the area of chronic inflammation. "Tennis elbow," "typist's shoulder," and "housemaid's knee" are common forms of chronic bursitis.

DISABLING BONE CONDITIONS

The major bone afflictions are *infections, dislocations,* and *fractures.*

Acute osteomyelitis is a bone infection caused by the same staphylococci and streptococci that are responsible for boils and blood poisoning. It affects children and young adults most frequently, generally striking the long bones of the arms and legs, and usually causes severe pain and fever. An acute attack is a serious emergency, demanding immediate medical care. Fortunately, prompt treatment with antibiotics such as penicillin is generally effective, although in some cases drainage of the infected area by surgery is also required.

If antibiotic therapy is not effective, *chronic osteomyelitis* may develop and pus continue to drain from the infected area for long periods of time. Modern medications have brought about a great decrease in this terribly disabling bone disease.

Tuberculosis can affect almost any bone in the body, as well as the hip and other joints. Most of you have seen individuals with disabling hunchback, which is caused by the erosive action of tuberculosis on the bones of the spine. This is called *Pott's disease,* and is caused by drinking *unpasteurized* milk from tuberculous cows. There is no better argument for pasteurization of all milk and milk products than this guarantee that tuberculosis bacteria cannot be ingested.

ANEMIA

Anemia literally means "without blood," and indicates that there are fewer red blood cells than normal, or that they contain too little hemoglobin to transport adequate amounts of oxygen from the lungs to the tissues of the body. The symptoms of *mild* anemias are usually rather vague, often little more than lack of pep and a greater tendency to fatigue, but the decrease in effective blood cells can easily be detected by a physician with standard laboratory tests. *Severe* anemia is often recognized by the unusual pallor of the palms of the hands, fingernails, or the inner part of the eyelid, the conjunctiva. In addition, a truly severe anemia can cause shortness of breath on exertion, and many other symptoms—pounding of the heart, a rapid pulse, loss of appetite, severe headaches and dizziness, and even fainting spells. A person usually knows he is sick if he has a severe anemia.

There are many and varied causes for ordinary anemias. The important are severe loss of blood, either from the massive hemorrhage of a wound or a slow chronic loss, as in a stomach ulcer; dietary deficiency of the iron, copper, and cobalt which are needed for hemoglobin synthesis; destruction, or *hemolysis,* of red blood cells; and impairment of the bone marrow where red cells are synthesized. *Pernicious*

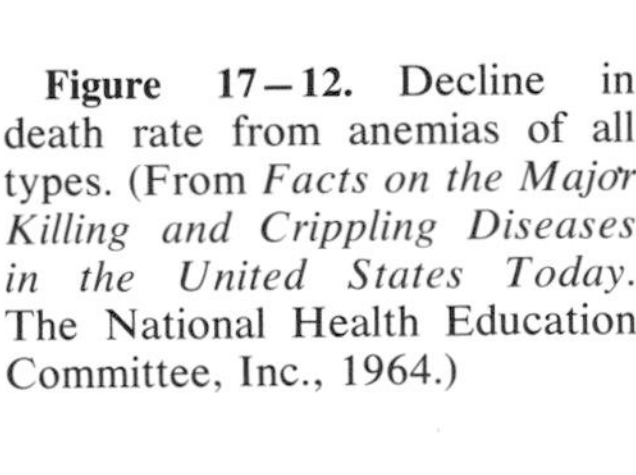

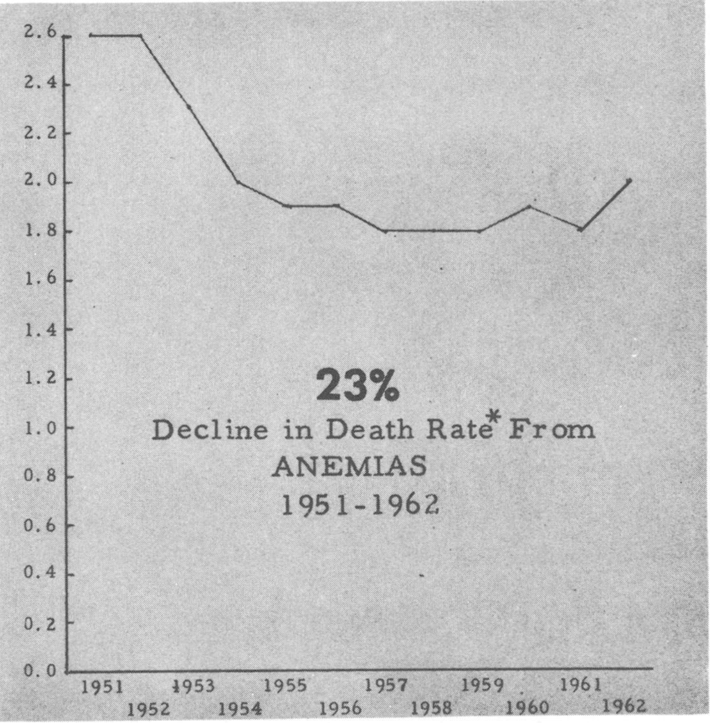

Figure 17–12. Decline in death rate from anemias of all types. (From *Facts on the Major Killing and Crippling Diseases in the United States Today.* The National Health Education Committee, Inc., 1964.)

anemia is a special variety, and there are also certain hereditary types, such as Cooley's anemia and sickle-cell anemia.

Rh incompatibility and mismatched blood transfusions are the commonest causes of red cell destruction. However, certain chemicals and medicines, and illnesses such as malaria and widespread cancer may also be responsible.

Any disease process which affects the activity of the bone marrow where red cells are manufactured can also lead to anemia. This can happen if cancer crowds out the blood-producing marrow or if it is destroyed or depressed by radioactive or other toxic chemical materials.

In *pernicious* anemia, the body is unable to make red cells because it lacks a substance in the stomach which is necessary for the absorption of vitamin B_{12} (cyanocobalamine). This vitamin is essential for the synthesis of certain elements of the red cell. For many years before vitamin B_{12} was known, pernicious anemia was treated successfully with concentrated liver extract. Today we know that the effectiveness of the liver is due to its vitamin B_{12} content, and we can now replace it with injections of the purified vitamin. Pernicious anemia can't be cured, but it can now be kept under control and the symptoms alleviated except in patients with serious complications and advanced central nervous system damage.

ASTHMA, ULCERATIVE COLITIS AND PEPTIC ULCER

These three diseases seem to have a strong psychosomatic component and are aggravated by emotional tensions. Asthma can be a problem at any age, ulcerative colitis very commonly affects students of college age, whereas ulcers are usually confined to a somewhat older group in the population.

Asthma is a chronic disease of the bronchial tubes which lead from the windpipe (or *trachea*) into the lungs. Ordinarily these tubes don't offer any resistance to the entrance or exit of air, and we aren't even conscious of the fact that we continually inhale and exhale at the rate of about 16 times a minute. In asthmatic attacks, however, the bronchial tubes tend to close down and the patient begins to wheeze, struggling for air. If the attack is severe, the sufferer seems almost to be suffocating, and uses all his strength just trying to breathe. Frequent and prolonged attacks can permanently damage the lung tissue and put a strain on the heart. Fortunately the average case of asthma is mild and more of a recurrent nuisance than a threat to health.

One type of bronchial asthma is definitely of allergic origin. An individual may have hay fever and asthma simultaneously during the ragweed season, or he may experience attacks of asthma only at this time. Other pollens, as well as house dust—a very common offender—animal fur or feathers, face powder, and certain foods may also be responsible. A person suffering from asthma may therefore have to be tested with a great many substances to discover the responsible allergen. In some cases he can be successfully immunized against it and protected from future attacks. A laboratory worker eventually tracked down the cause of his asthma: he could handle any animals except rabbits, but when he touched them or even cleaned their cages, he developed a typical attack. In his case, the cure was obvious: a change of jobs.

Often asthma is associated with bacterial infection of the sinuses, throat and nose, and improves rapidly when the infection clears up.

In some individuals, nervous tension is the only apparent cause and there is a tremendous improvement in the disease when the emotional problems are solved. Even cases of asthma of allergic origin may become worse if the patient is emotionally disturbed or tense. It is interesting that this was known as far back as Hippocrates, who recognized that anger and hostility often precipitated acute attacks. For some patients, emotional storms are far more dangerous than dust storms.

Epinephrine (adrenaline), one of the hormones produced by the adrenal gland, has been used for many years in the relief of asthmatic attacks, and recently even more effective medicines have become available—the antihistaminics, ACTH, cortisone, and related steroids.

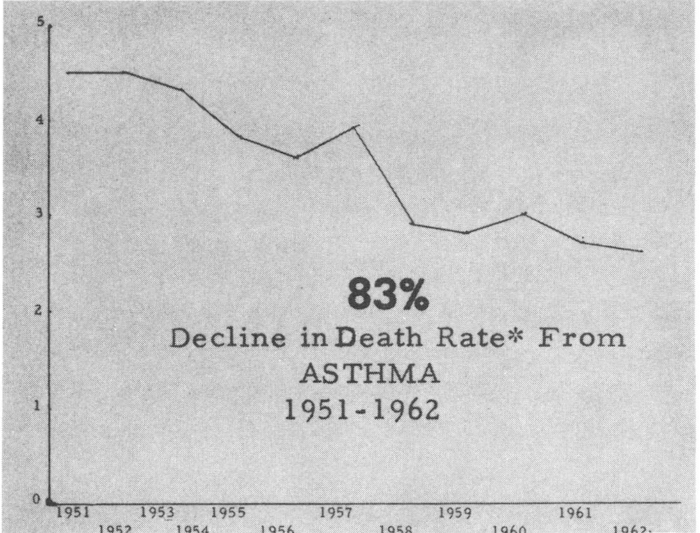

Figure 17–13. Decline in death rate from asthma. (From *Facts on the Major Killing and Crippling Diseases in the United States Today*. The National Health Education Committee, Inc., 1964.)

Ulcerative colitis is a potentially serious disease which can be very disabling. The most common symptom is severe diarrhea, with as many as 15 to 20 watery bowel movements a day, often containing blood. Weakness and loss of weight are usually associated with this condition. Careful medical examination and tests are required for diagnosis, including x-rays of the large intestine after it is filled with barium, and examination of the rectum and colon with a *proctoscope* or *sigmoidoscope* through which the lining of the bowel can be seen. Marked reddening and, sometimes, actual ulcers or sores are observed. Today, prompt medical treatment can prevent the disabling effects of this disease, which otherwise often make its victims miserable. Rest, special dietary treatment and psychotherapy, and in advanced cases, even surgical intervention may be required.

The word *ulcer* simply means a sore, or irritated area, and a *peptic ulcer* is a sore in the stomach or the duodenum, that part of the intestines which connects with the stomach.

This condition is extremely common, and appears to be on the increase. According to some estimates there are approximately 10 million cases in this country alone, responsible for an inestimable amount of distress and disability. It is more common in men than in women, the ratio in the United States being about 3.5 to 1, and may occur at any age, although it is rarely seen in children under ten. Business executives and other people who work under very high tension appear to be particularly susceptible to peptic ulcer, and ulcers have become a very prominent disease of our times. This is undoubtedly due to the relationship between ulcers and worry or anxiety. For example, it was found that cases of peptic ulcer increased among the troops during wartime, especially those who were in combat zones.

The cause of ulcers is not fully understood, but it is definitely associated with the presence of an excessive amount of the highly acid gastric juice, which the stomach secretes for digestion. In people with ulcers, there is excessive secretion, not only after eating, but also between meals and at night during sleep. Because worry and anxiety can increase the secretion, ulcers are considered to be a *psychosomatic disease*. Very severe ulcers can be produced in monkeys by subjecting them to alternate periods of anxiety and rest.

The most common *symptoms* are *pain* and *discomfort* in the upper abdomen, usually a few hours after meals or in the middle of the night. These so-called "hunger pains" generally subside after eating, drinking milk or taking bicarbonate of soda. There may also be nausea and vomiting.

Bleeding: Untreated peptic ulcer may produce a slow seepage of blood, which is

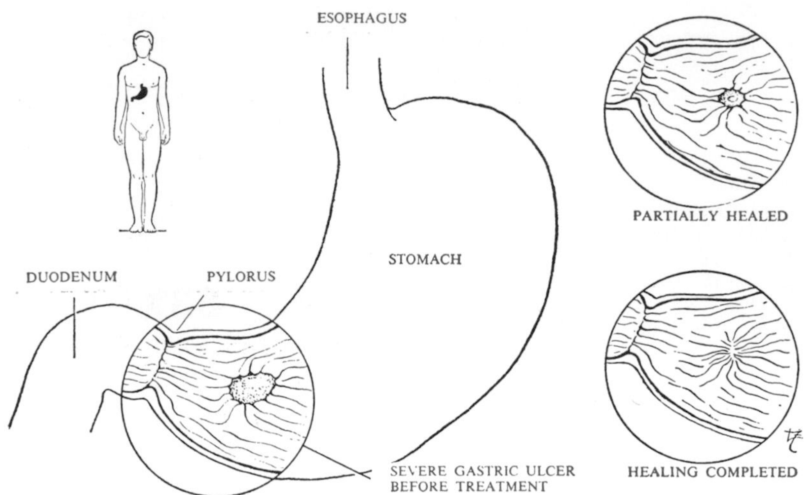

Figure 17–14. Severe gastric ulcer, before and after healing.

vomited or passed through the bowel in black, tarry stools. However, if a sizeable blood vessel is eroded, there may be a massive hemorrhage.

The ulcer may also *perforate* and break through the wall of the stomach or duodenum. This is an emergency situation and requires immediate surgery to repair the perforation, and prevent peritonitis or other serious infection.

Diagnosis of ulcers involves tests on the stomach acid, after passing a tube through the mouth or esophagus and taking a sample of the stomach contents. X-rays of the stomach and duodenum, and sometimes a *gastroscopic* examination in which the doctor looks into the stomach with an instrument resembling a flexible periscope are also very helpful.

The *treatment* and *cure* of ulcers require a carefully planned, soothing diet, "antacid" medicines which can neutralize some of the stomach's acid, reduction of worries and emotional tension, and in certain cases, surgery.

Questions

1. Many diseases are much more common than polio. Why has it been so feared? What is the recommended vaccination schedule for polio, and why is it stressed that all people under 40 should be vaccinated?
2. Describe the symptoms of infectious mononucleosis and the method of transmission.
3. What are the two important ways in which infectious hepatitis is transmitted? What symptoms should make you suspect this disease?
4. Compare colds and influenza. What are the chief dangers in both?
5. Compare syphilis and gonorrhea in the following respects: microorganism responsible; mode of transmission; signs of the disease; method of treatment; hazards and end results.
6. What is the cause of epilepsy and how is it treated? How do you think we could overcome the stigma attached to this disease so that the well-controlled epileptic could lead a normal life?
7. Discuss the major causes of blindness and methods of prevention.
8. Review the process of hearing (Chapter 6) and show how different types of deafness could develop.
9. Differentiate arthritis, bursitis and gout. What are the commonest types of arthritis?
10. What are the causes of most backaches and how can they be relieved?

Topics for Discussion

Live polio virus vaccine.
Eye banks for corneal transplants.
Education of the deaf.

Reading Suggestions

Born That Way, Earl R. Carlson. John Day Co., New York, 1941. This is the very moving autobiography of a physician who was born with cerebral palsy.

Margin of Safety, John Rowan Wilson. Doubleday & Co., Inc., Garden City, N.Y., 1963. A very interesting account of our victory over polio and the development of the Salk and Sabin vaccines. The student interested in a research career or in the philosophy of science will find this a most informative book. It is as much a discussion of scientists as it is of their work. Very well written.

Nervousness, Indigestion, and Pain, Walter C. Alvarez. Collier Books, New York, 1962, paperback. In the author's words, it is a book written "in simple speech in order to help those many persons with nervousness, indigestion, and pain who would like to learn more about their personal problems of illness than their physicians have time to teach." A good book by a well known physician.

Slipped Discs, Kenneth C. Hutchin. ARC Books, Inc., New York, 1964, Paperback. A physician discusses the vertebral column and problems associated with it. A timely book for the many Americans who suffer low back pain. Written for laymen.

Venereology For Nurses, A textbook of the Sexually Transmitted Diseases, R. D. Catterall. Charles C Thomas, Springfield, Illinois, 1964. A timely book that describes the major venereal diseases. It contains a complete glossary covering the language of venereology and is readable by the college student.

A History of Syphilis, Charles Clayton Dennie. Charles C Thomas, Springfield, Illinois, 1962. An interesting account of the disease of syphilis from the time that Schaudinn and Hoffmann discovered *Treponema pallidum* to the present day.

The Great Epidemic, A. A. Hoehling. Little, Brown & Co., Boston, 1961. The story of "Spanish Influenza"—a killer that slew millions and then disappeared. A very readable account of one of the worst plagues in history.

Teen-Agers and Venereal Disease, U.S. Public Health Service, 1961. A sociological study of 600 teen-agers in New York City social hygiene clinics.

What Doctors are Learning About Arthritis, Joseph J. Bunim and Howard G. Earl. Today's Health, August 1964, p. 38. A report of recent research by the clinical director of National Institute of Arthritis and Metabolic Diseases, the National Institutes of Health.

What Most People Don't Know About Epilepsy, Shirley M. Linde, Today's Health, July 1964, p. 38. Thirteen important questions about epilepsy are discussed in detail.

Crippler of Young Adults, Russell N. DeJong. Today's Health, November 1964, p. 36. A report on recent advances against multiple sclerosis.

Gonorrhea: Present Knowledge, Research and Control Efforts, James D. Thayer and M. Brittain Moore, Jr., Medical Clinics of North America, May 1964. An authoritative discussion of gonorrhea today and tomorrow.

18

THE DEADLY PAIR

For all of us, the most precious element we have is time. But time runs out too soon for millions because of a health enemy that takes more lives than all other diseases combined—heart disease.

TYRONE POWER *in a special film for the American Heart Association shortly before his own sudden and fatal heart attack.*

Today it is virtually impossible to pick up a newspaper or magazine, whether it be popular or scientific, that does not deal in some way with either cancer or heart and circulatory disease. Why are we so preoccupied with these diseases? The answer is a simple one: collectively, these untamed killers snuff out the lives of well over a million of our citizens each year. Heart disease is responsible for an estimated 849,000 deaths annually. Cancer strikes an estimated 540,000 persons each year and claims the lives of 284,000.

HEART DISEASE AND OTHER CARDIOVASCULAR CONDITIONS

Sixty years ago, pneumonia, tuberculosis, intestinal diarrhea, and other infections were the leading killers. However, with the control of these diseases, another killer has taken over the number one spot—heart disease.

This is due at least in part to the years that have been added to our lives. People who might formerly have died of pneumonia or some other infectious illness while they were in their forties, now survive to be 65 or more; and heart disease is more common in the older age group. Heart disease is compared with other leading causes of death in Table 18–1.

Symptoms of Heart Disease

There are certain general symptoms that *suggest,* but do not *prove* there is something wrong with the heart. But they are sufficiently important to warrant medical examination. Only a doctor (or in special

Table 18–1. Leading causes of death

Cause of Death	1964	1963	1962	1961	1960	1959	1958	1957	1956	1955
All Causes—Crude	745.9	741.4	690.7	688.0	671.2	665.3	662.4	656.8	617.0	620.4
—Adjusted† ...	740.6	759.8	739.1	747.9	756.7	763.2	779.3	777.8	765.8	772.7
Tuberculosis—all forms .	3.9	5.0	4.9	5.1	5.4	5.7	6.7	6.7	7.1	7.9
Communicable diseases of childhood	0.1	0.1	0.1	0.1	0.1	0.1	0.2	0.1	0.2	0.3
Acute poliomyelitis	‡	‡	‡	‡	0.1	0.2	0.1	0.1	0.3	0.6
Malignant neoplasms ...	162.1	160.1	148.7	148.3	142.4	141.9	139.8	136.1	128.7	128.2
Diabetes mellitus	17.8	17.2	15.5	15.4	15.2	14.7	15.2	15.2	14.9	14.7
Diseases of the cardio-vascular-renal system	394.1	391.9	367.9	368.7	357.1	355.5	352.0	348.6	328.6	327.7
Vascular lesions, central nervous system.	71.1	71.2	66.2	67.0	66.5	67.7	66.5	66.5	63.4	63.9
Diseases of heart	292.7	289.9	274.6	273.8	263.9	261.5	260.4	256.2	240.9	239.3
Chronic rheumatic heart disease ...	10.3	11.6	10.7	11.3	10.6	10.8	11.4	11.6	11.5	12.0
Arteriosclerotic and degenerative heart disease	243.2	237.8	224.6	221.5	211.9	207.9	206.5	200.5	187.4	185.0
Hypertension with heart disease	25.2	26.8	26.9	28.5	29.3	30.6	31.5	33.6	33.4	34.0
Other diseases of heart	14.0	13.7	12.3	12.5	12.1	12.2	10.9	10.5	8.6	8.3
Nephritis and nephrosis	5.6	6.0	5.8	6.4	6.7	7.1	7.4	8.2	7.6	8.3
Pneumonia	18.5	20.6	17.2	17.0	19.7	17.7	18.9	17.4	13.3	13.2
Influenza	0.4	1.9	0.9	0.6	1.8	0.8	1.4	2.6	0.7	0.9
Cirrhosis of liver	13.7	13.2	12.6	12.2	11.8	11.1	11.3	11.0	10.6	9.9
Complications of pregnancy, childbirth	0.6	0.5	0.8	0.6	0.6	0.8	0.8	0.9	0.9	1.0
Suicide	6.8	6.9	6.5	6.3	6.1	6.5	6.1	5.7	5.6	6.1
Homicide	3.3	2.9	2.9	3.1	2.8	2.8	2.9	2.9	2.4	2.5
Accidents—total	37.8	35.3	33.9	32.9	32.4	33.1	34.2	34.9	35.6	35.1
Motor vehicle	17.8	16.0	15.2	14.3	14.0	14.6	14.8	15.3	15.7	15.3
Home	7.4	6.9	6.6	6.6	6.5	6.5	6.2	6.5	6.5	6.5
Occupational (civilian)	1.9	1.9	1.9	1.6	2.2	2.2	2.4	2.7	2.7	2.6
All other causes	86.8	85.8	78.8	77.7	75.7	74.4	72.8	74.6	68.1	72.3

cases, a cardiologist, or heart specialist) can decide how significant they are, and he may find it necessary to take an *electrocardiogram,* which records the activity of the heart.

1. *Dyspnea (shortness of breath) on exertion.* Almost everyone becomes short of breath or even gasps for air after rushing to catch a bus or climbing a number of stairs. Breathlessness is also apt to occur, to a slight extent, as people get older, especially if they are overweight. But when ordinary activities which formerly caused no difficulty suddenly bring on shortness of breath, it *may* suggest heart disease.

2. *Nocturnal dyspnea* (shortness of breath at night) means awakening from sleep with a choking sensation or a feeling of suffocation.

3. *Edema* (swelling) of the ankles may result from numerous relatively harmless conditions like varicose veins and premenstrual water retention, but it may also indicate poor circulation because of heart disease.

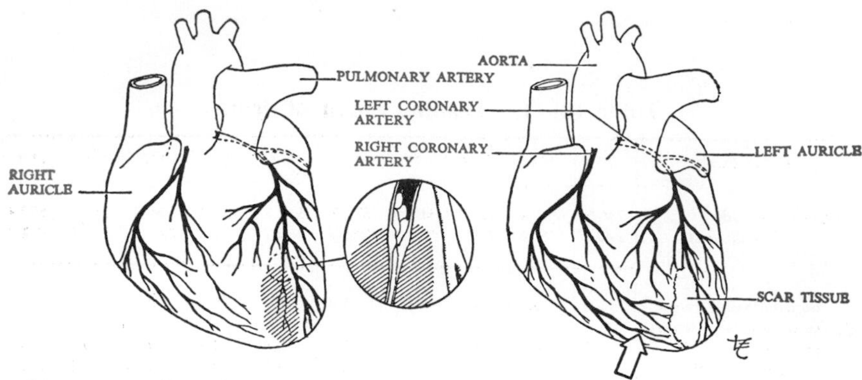

Figure 18–1. Coronary thrombosis. **Left,** At time of attack. The flow of blood through part of the left coronary artery is blocked *(shown in inset),* cutting off the circulation in the shaded area. **Right,** Recovery from attack. Scar tissue has built up. Blood vessels of the right coronary artery *(indicated by arrow)* now supply the affected area.

4. *Angina pectoris* means pain over the heart or in the middle of the chest, and has been described as feeling as if a rock had been placed on the chest or over the heart. However, it is important to remember that not all distress in this area originates in the heart. It may be only a gas pain or indigestion!

5. *Other symptoms* may be dizziness, fainting spells, blue lips, attacks resembling asthma, extreme fatigue, palpitation (fluttering of the heart), even coughing up blood, or a persistent cough.

Coronary disease refers to some abnormality in the coronary arteries, the vital blood vessels of the heart itself. This may be caused by *arteriosclerosis,* or hardening of the coronary arteries, which impairs the heart by damaging the arteries supplying blood to the heart muscle. It does this by narrowing their diameter, making it difficult for the blood to flow through, and by causing irregularities in the otherwise smooth lining of the arteries. When the flow of blood is slowed down and the heart muscle receives too little blood, brief attacks of *angina pectoris* may result. In addition, blood is apt to stagnate in the narrowed blood vessels and form clots.

If such a clot forms within a coronary artery and blocks off the blood supply to part of the heart muscle, it will cause a *heart attack* (the medical term is "coronary thrombosis" or "coronary occlusion"). This may either injure or destroy part of the heart muscle. Heart attacks resulting from blood clots are usually characterized by severe and prolonged pain, and may require extended periods of hospitalization until adequate recovery and repair of the damaged heart muscle has set in.

Years ago it was felt that such an attack, if not immediately fatal, would lead to death within a few years. Now we know this is not true, for there are numerous cases on record of complete recovery after coronary thrombosis. Usually some symptoms remain but these can be controlled by cooperation on the patient's part in his schedule of activities and by special medicines prescribed by the doctor. A useful technique for patients who have a tendency to form clots in vital blood vessels is to administer one of the numerous anticoagulant drugs which prolong the clotting time of blood, and prevent any more dangerous clots from forming.

An interesting research lead in this field centers about the use of certain chemicals—the enzymes, or biological catalysts—which can dissolve blood clots when they are injected into the body. They can't cure an already damaged heart muscle, but they may prevent further damage.

What Causes Heart Attacks?

Hardening of the arteries, usually accompanied by *obesity,* which imposes an

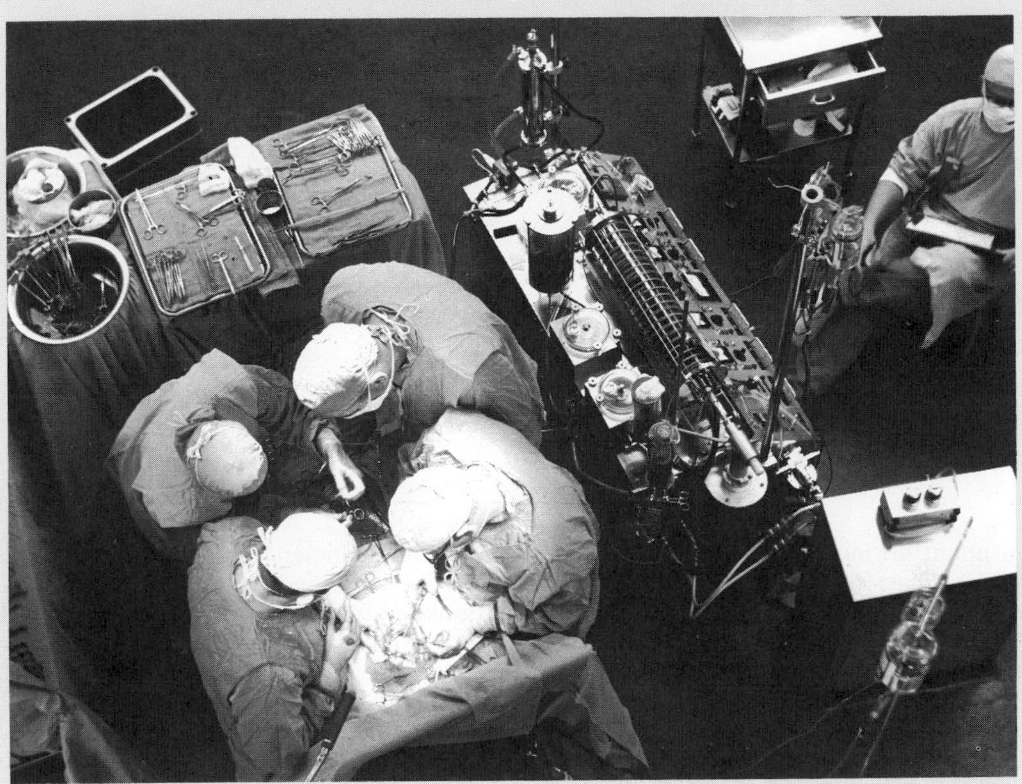

Surgeons perform open-heart surgery in a modern hospital operating theater. Behind them at right is a heart-lung machine, which temporarily takes over the functions of the heart and lungs.

extra strain on the heart, *physical inactivity* and *emotional strains* are probably the major causes of heart attacks. Two predisposing conditions are *high blood pressure* and *diabetes*. *Hereditary factors* and the *endocrines* are also involved. Physical inactivity is probably a major contributing factor, both in encouraging obesity and in reducing the healthy tone of all muscles, including the heart muscles. Since antiquity, the best candidates for heart disease have been the physically lazy, overfed members of the higher economic classes, who suffer from "loafer's heart".

According to a study made by J. N. Morris among British workers, death from coronary heart disease among hairdressers, clerks, and others engaged in relatively light work is almost twice as high as in agricultural and industrial laborers.[1] It's also interesting that in some of the Scandinavian countries, where the bicycle and not the automobile is the standard method of transport, the death rate from heart disease is considerably lower than in the United States. This is true even though the fat consumption—and therefore the possibility of obesity and arteriosclerosis—is nearly the same as ours.

The dangers of exertion and physical activity in people who suffer from coronary disease have apparently been exaggerated. Dr. Paul D. White, who was called in as a

[1]Raab, W.: *Archives of Internal Medicine*, February 1958.

At left, the plastic ball is lowered, and blood enters the ventricle. Right, pressure resulting from the contraction of the ventricle forces the ball to rise, which seals the auricle and stops the flow of blood.

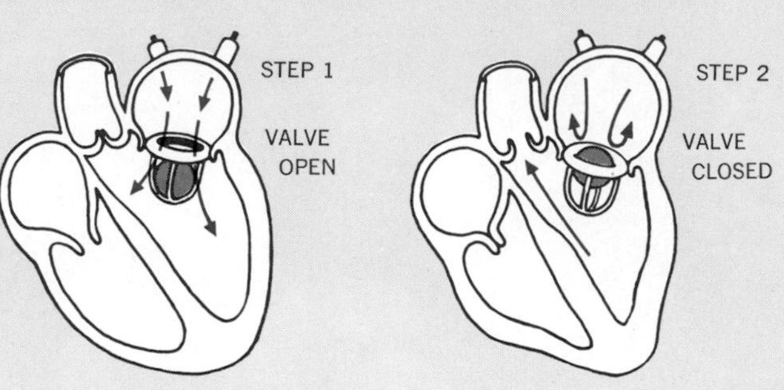

OPERATION OF THE SYNTHETIC MITRAL VALVE

consultant during former President Eisenhower's heart attack, feels very strongly that a reasonable amount of exercise is not only desirable, but essential for maintenance of good health. He prescribes golfing, walking and gardening in moderation as sensible activities even for cardiac patients. Many doctors believe that severe exertion is *not* a major factor in precipitating heart attacks. For example, Dr. Arthur M. Master of the Mount Sinai Hospital in New York studied the type of activity 1603 patients were engaged in when they suffered coronary occlusions: 440 of these attacks occurred when the patients were at rest, 412 during mild activity, 367 during sleep, 212 while walking, 142 during moderate activity, and only 30 (2 per cent) during unusual or strenuous exertion.[2]

The role of the emotions in heart attacks is a very real one, although sometimes difficult to assess. However, many physicians feel that the occupational stress, the speed at which a man has to work and the nervous tension he suffers are important factors. Dr. Stewart Wolf, of the University of Oklahoma, who is very interested in psychosomatic disease, described the coronary attack-prone individual as "a man who is highly competitive in his attitudes, if not in his behavior, concerned with self-sufficiency and with doing things on his own and usually the hard way. Looking for new worlds to conquer, he takes less than the usual satisfaction between chores." The "coronary" candidate finds life a long, uphill struggle; he never quite gets to the top to rest and enjoy the satisfactions of achievement.

Although coronary thrombosis is usually explained as a secondary complication of arteriosclerosis, it has been observed in persons with perfectly normal arteries. In

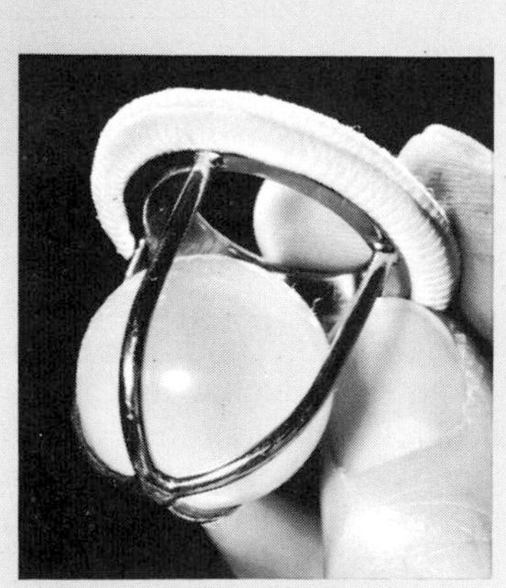

A plastic ball valve, which can replace either the mitral valve of the heart, as shown above, or the aortic valve.

[2]Annual Meeting, American College of Chest Physicians, 1958.

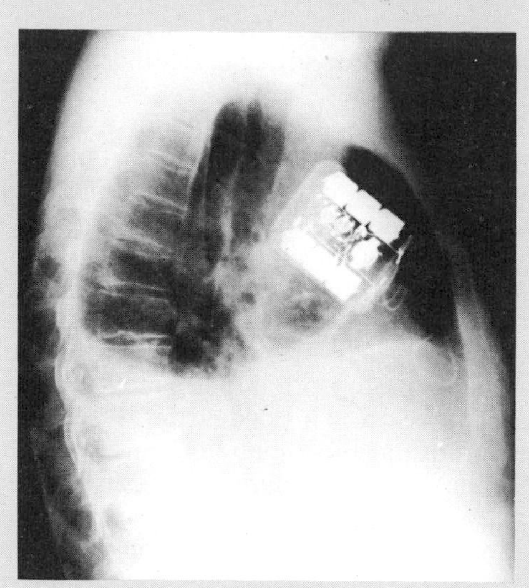

The electronic artificial pacemaker is seen in an X-ray photograph, above, in position near the heart. New models are placed in the flanks so that batteries can be replaced more easily. Below are a pacemaker, the wires that lead to the heart, and the electrodes that are connected to the heart muscle. At bottom, the battery-powered electronic circuit in the pacemaker. A book of matches beside it shows its small size.

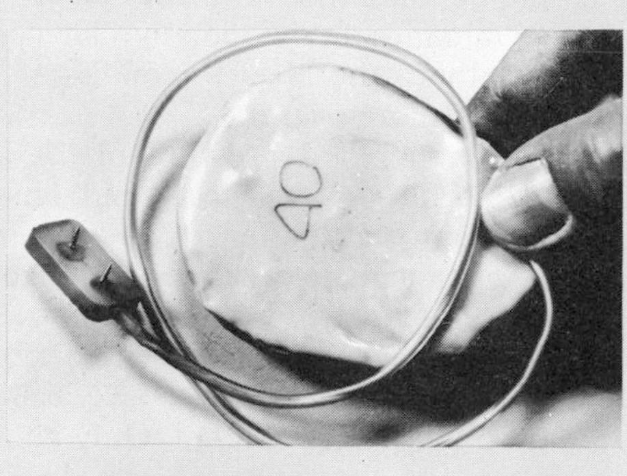

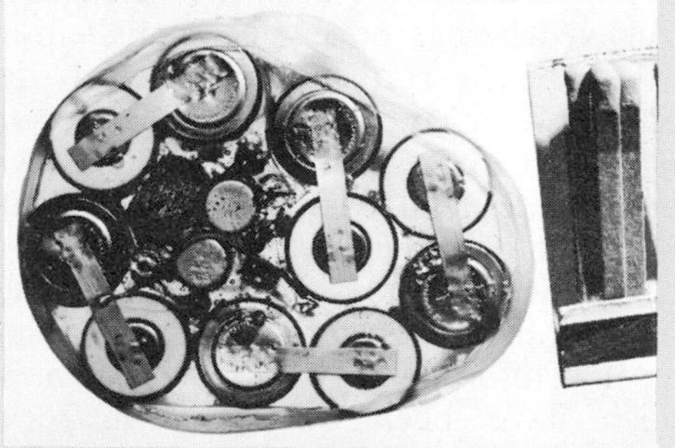

such cases, a defect in the clotting mechanism is implicated. It has, in fact, been suggested for several years that increased coagulability of the blood may be a factor in thrombosis.

In this connection, Dr. Meyer W. Friedman and his associates of San Francisco have shown that chemical changes which might be the prelude to clot formation and coronary occlusion—such as the accelerated clotting time of blood—occur at periods of great emotional stress.[3]

In contrast to this, a study reported in *Circulation Research*[4] indicated that when chickens were forced to exercise by walking four miles a week, their blood clotted more slowly than when they were caged. Likewise, in a study[5] of medical students in England, a meal high in fat was found to accelerate the clotting time, whereas exercise reversed this effect. Moreover, Keys and his associates[6] have found the clotting times of people engaged in active occupations to be significantly longer than those of individuals employed in sedentary type jobs.

Sex and race differences in coronary disease may be very striking. Between the ages of 35 and 44, the death rate among white American males is nearly seven times that of females. But a recent study[7] indicates that women living under the same psychological strain as men have the same incidence rate of heart disease as men. In this regard, it is interesting to note that the death rate of colored males is only 1.5 times that of colored females, and it varies little with age.

That the female sex hormones may be of some value in preventing heart disease is suggested from some interesting research by a group of physicians at the University of Southern California Medical School, led by Dr. Jessie Marmorsten. In this study, a group of female patients (many of them over 70) who had suffered

[3]American Heart Association Meeting, San Francisco, 1958.

[4]Warnock, N. H., *et al.*: *Circulation Research, 5*: 478, 1957.

[5]McDonald, G. A., and Fullerton, H. W.: *Lancet, 2*: 600, 1958.

[6]Keys, A., and Buzina, R.: *Circulation, 14*:479 (abstract), 1956.

[7]Friedman, M.: *Progress in Cardiovascular Disease, 15*:419, 1962.

heart attacks were given minute amounts of female sex hormones regularly; in a similar group of control patients who did not receive the hormone, there were more than twice as many deaths from subsequent heart attacks, or worsening of the disease, than in the group taking hormones.

Hypertension (High Blood Pressure)

As a nation we have become "high blood pressure conscious" in recent years. This is not an unmixed blessing because along with valuable information, a good deal of misinformation has been absorbed, and many essentially healthy people worry needlessly about this disease. High blood pressure may actually be a very mild condition.

The Cause of Hypertension. When the heart pumps blood into the arteries in order to distribute it throughout the body, the blood presses against the walls of these strong, elastic tubes. The pressure is highest when the blood is being forced ahead by the pump (the *systolic* pressure) and lowest between beats (the *diastolic* pressure); and these two pressures are measured by a doctor when he puts a blood pressure cuff around the arm. In normal children, the systolic pressure is from 75 to 100 mm. of mercury; young adults range from 100 to 120, and older people, from 120 to 140. For college age students, the diastolic pressure normally ranges from 70 to 90, the average being 80.

Sometimes, because of illness, emotional tension or for unknown reasons, the walls of the arteries constrict, narrowing the space through which the blood must flow. When this happens, greater force must be exerted by the heart to push the blood through the arteries. This increased pressure is called *high blood pressure* or *hypertension.*

In about 80 per cent of the cases, the cause can't be determined, and these are called "essential," "idiopathic," or "primary" hypertension. Most of the remaining 20 per cent can be traced to Bright's disease or other kidney ailments, tumors of the adrenal gland, *coarctation* of the *aorta* (a congenital narrowing of the main artery), and narrowing of one or more arteries in a kidney. Some of these can be cured by modern surgical techniques.

In many cases, an *apparent* high blood pressure is caused by an emotional disturbance. Nervousness and strain during a medical examination, for example, can cause the blood pressure to rise, but this is only temporary and should cause no concern. Repressed anger and other emotional tensions can also produce a marked increase in blood pressure, and if this happens too often, permanent damage might develop. This would be *true* hypertension of psychosomatic origin.

If the blood pressure stays consistently high, a diagnosis of hypertension is made. However, the doctor does not judge the severity of the disease by the height of the blood pressure alone. He also observes the condition of the small blood vessels in the retina with an instrument called an *ophthalmoscope.* (Because the retina is transparent, it is the best place to study small blood vessels). Electrocardiograms or x-rays also indicate whether the heart has been damaged or enlarged by having to work against the high pressure, and tests on the kidneys provide information about their condition. On the basis of these examinations, the doctor can conclude whether the heart condition is mild, moderate or severe.

Because high blood pressure places an increased strain on the heart and blood vessels, patients may suffer from symptoms such as headache, weakness, fatigue, or shortness of breath. However, contrary to popular opinion, people who die from high blood pressure are not usually killed by a stroke (shock, apoplexy). Only about 15 per cent of these deaths are due to strokes, whereas 65 per cent of them are caused by heart disease. Relatively few people die of their high blood pressure, in comparison with the number who continue to lead useful lives, with little restriction of activities.

Treatment. Even in severe cases, considerable relief and a longer life span can be afforded by various treatments which have been developed in recent years.[8] Several medicines now available,

[8]Palmer, R. S.: *American Practitioner and Digest of Treatment, 8*:33, 1957.

including *chlorothiazide* and *reserpine* (a remedy used in India for centuries), help reduce the blood pressure or relieve its symptoms and prevent complications. In some cases, salt intake is restricted and a reducing diet may also be prescribed, because obesity apparently increases the tendency to high blood pressure.

Psychotherapy is frequently helpful if severe emotional strain is a contributory factor, and, when all other measures fail, a surgical procedure called *sympathectomy,* which involves severing certain nerves deep in the back, may bring relief.

Ordinary forms of hypertension occasionally develop into the so-called *malignant* form. If this happens, the destructive action of the high blood pressure on the blood vessels of the body is speeded up, and unless the condition is checked promptly, it may prove fatal in a matter of months or a few years. The blood vessels of the retina, kidney, heart and brain are hardest hit in malignant hypertension.

Arteriosclerosis (Hardening of the Arteries)

Arteriosclerosis is frequently—but not always—present along with hypertension, and the greatest damage occurs if both diseases exist simultaneously. Arteriosclerosis causes a narrowing of the coronary arteries which supply blood to the heart muscle, and hypertension injures the heart by making it work against pressure. If the heart muscle is already handicapped by an inadequate supply of blood, it becomes endangered to an even greater degree when forced to do the extra work required in high blood pressure.

A great deal of scientific research is being directed toward the cause and cure of arteriosclerosis. To date, however, only theories exist as to what the cause of this disease might be. The most accepted theory is that arteriosclerosis results from the deposition of lipids (fats and fatlike materials) into the walls of the arteries. This theory stems from the facts that lipids are found in excess in nearly all arterial plaques, that excess ingestion of this type food has produced arteriosclerosis in many animals, and that people with high lipid levels seem to have a higher incidence of coronary artery diseases. It is obvious, therefore, even to the opponents of this theory that blood lipids are more than innocent bystanders in this pathologic process.

Yet, a number of questions are not explained by this theory. Why, for example, are the coronary arteries more susceptible than other arteries of comparable size? Why is the American female, who eats the same diet as her husband and who has the same concentration of lipids in her blood, relatively immune to this disease? It is unlikely, some research scientists believe, that this protection is afforded by sex hormones, and as Dr. M. Friedman and his associates have noted:[9]

> . . . it would seem strange indeed that the white American female should derive a protective influence against clinical coronary artery disease from a hormone that so singularly fails to offer a similar reputed protection to the American Negress, the Italian female, or the Mexican female.

These and other questions add to the complexity of the problem, which now seems to have many facets.

In connection with this theory, it has been repeatedly observed that persons suffering from coronary artery disease have difficulty in clearing fat from their blood.[10, 11] For example, after the normal person eats a high-fat meal, the concentration of lipids in his blood increases for three or four hours and thereafter are rapidly cleared. On the other hand, the patient suffering from coronary artery disease may have an elevated concentration of fat in his blood for 12 or more hours after the meal. Moreover, the peak concentration is frequently observed to correspond with attacks of angina pectoris.

One apparently beneficial effect of physical exercise is related to its ability to accelerate the clearing time of fat from the blood. In a study[12] recently reported in a British medical journal, a group of 40 young men were randomly divided into two groups. Both groups ate a high-fat

---

[9]Friedman, M.: *Progress in Cardiovascular Diseases, 15*:419, 1962.

[10]Stutman, L. J. *et al.: American Journal of Medical Science, 5*:242, 1961.

[11]Barritt, D. W.: *British Medical Journal, 2*:640, 1956.

[12]Esko, A. N. *et al.: Lancet, 1*:1151, 1962.

meal, whereupon the first group went on a two hour march while the second group remained at rest. After comparison, the group that exercised had cleared the fat from their blood at a much faster rate. On the basis of this finding, the investigators suggested that the favorable correlation observed between physical activity and the incidence of occlusive heart disease depends on a reduction of the concentration of lipids in the blood after meals.

In another study,[13] it was found that exercise promotes the release of an enzyme (lipoprotein lipase) capable of accelerating lipid metabolism, and it was suggested that this might be the mechanism by which physical activity results in the rapid clearance of lipids.

Another theory concerning the etiology of arteriosclerosis is the *fibrin deposit theory*. This theory suggests that small amounts of a sticky protein substance called fibrin are deposited on the walls of arteries and later are incorporated into the walls. Fibrin is actually the final product in the blood coagulation process, and it is thought by many that fibrin is constantly being formed and broken down in the blood stream. At any rate, evidence is rapidly accumulating to implicate fibrin deposition as a factor in arteriosclerosis. The most convincing of this evidence comes from a study[14] in which fibrin was tagged with radioactive I_{131} and traced in the circulation. It was, indeed, found to be deposited on the walls of the arteries and later was incorporated into a mural thrombus (a clot attached to the wall of an artery). More recently this process has been observed with the electron microscope.[15]

In connection with this theory, it is significant to note that the human body has a system especially suited for the destruction of fibrin—the fibrinolytic system. The potency of this system is very great: suitably activated, this fibrinolytic mechanism can destroy all the fibrin the body is capable of forming. A good example of this is the Russian practice of using for transfusions the blood obtained from persons having died a traumatic death. The trauma experienced in such cases constitutes a stimulus capable of maximally activating the fibrinolytic system and rendering the blood incapable of clotting.

According to another study,[16] physical exercise has a favorable effect on this clot-dissolving system. In this research, ten young men were observed while working on a treadmill. Their fibrinolytic activity was found to increase in direct proportion to the amount and intensity of work performed. It was further demonstrated that during exercise a chemical was produced or released that activated the fibrinolytic system. This activator usually disappeared within an hour after exercise.

It appears, therefore, that if the fibrin deposit theory of arteriosclerosis is tenable, then exercise can play an important role in the reduction of coronary artery disease. Moreover, because the effects of exercise on fibrinolytic activity are both transient and proportional to the amount of work performed, a daily work-out seems to be advisable.

The Diet and Heart Disease

Those persons who fall into the "high risk" category for developing coronary artery sclerosis usually show elevations of both cholesterol and triglycerides (neutral fat) in their blood serum. Physicians have no absolutely certain method of reducing the cholesterol and triglycerides to normal, but they attempt to do so by prescribing a low-calorie diet with relatively low-fat content. Also, some doctors believe that the coronary-prone individual should favor unsaturated over saturated fatty acids in his diet to reduce the serum cholesterol level. The unsaturated fatty acids are abundant in plant and seed oils; the saturated fatty acids are high in beef and milk fats. Fish, poultry, vegetables, and margarine are recommended by enthusiasts for this regimen. Some medical research workers oppose this type of diet, especially when it contains very large

[13]Cantone, A.: *The Journal of Sports Medicine and Physical Fitness, 4*:32, 1964.

[14]Page, I. H. (ed.): *Connective Tissue, Thrombosis and Atherosclerosis* (Proceedings of a Conference Held at Princeton, New Jersey, 1958), Academic Press, New York, 1959, p. 26.

[15]*Medical Tribune,* June 1964.

[16]Ogston, D., and Fullerton, H. W.: *Lancet, 2*: 730, 1961.

quantities of unsaturated fats, because it may lead to increases in body weight, and as reported by Dr. A. L. Tappel, a biochemist at the University of California, it may accelerate the aging process.

However, we do know that eating too much fatty food causes overweight, and obesity is a definite menace to health. It is like carrying around a heavy knapsack; the added poundage puts an extra strain on the heart, making it work that much harder to pump blood. It is a well known fact that thin people have a longer life expectancy than obese ones, and all doctors agree that after the age of 35 it is better to be slightly underweight than overweight. Thanks to the dictates of fashion, the doctor can usually persuade women to reduce; but too many men, especially as they advance toward middle age, get careless in their eating habits and begin to develop a paunch. Since men in general have a shorter life expectancy than women and more coronary-artery disease, the fat man is deliberately encouraging his own demise.

Smoking and Coronary Heart Disease

Epidemiologic studies have been remarkably consistent in demonstrating a significant relationship between cigarette smoking and increased death rate from coronary heart disease. There is little dissenting evidence. The 1964 Surgeon General's report states:

> Male cigarette smokers have a higher death rate from coronary artery disease than non-smoking males. . . . It is also more prudent to assume that the established association between cigarette smoking and coronary disease has causative meaning than to suspend judgment until no uncertainty remains.

This topic is discussed more fully in Chapter 22.

Strokes

The brain has a tremendous need for a constant oxygen supply, and this relatively small organ uses about 20 per cent of all the oxygen the body consumes. If denied its oxygen quota for a very short time, actually a matter of minutes, brain tissue will die. When the blood supply to the brain, or even a significant portion of it, is cut off, the severe oxygen deprivation which results can cause a *stroke,* also called *apoplexy* and, in some sections of the country, a "shock." This is almost always a disease of older people, and the average age of stroke victims is 64.

The four major causes of strokes are *blood clots, hemorrhage, tumor,* or *blood vessel spasm* in the brain, and the commonest cause is a blood clot. It may form in a blood vessel of the brain itself which has been damaged by arteriosclerosis, or may break off from a clot which has developed in the heart or elsewhere and travel to the brain.

A stroke can also follow *hemorrhage* through a weakened blood vessel, the diseased spot ballooning out like a defective area in the inner tube of a tire. Other causes are *pressure* on vital brain tissue or arteries by clots or *brain tumors,* and *spasm,* or constriction, of the muscular walls of the blood vessels.

The words stroke and apoplexy have an ominous sound to most people, and it is true that they can be serious and even fatal. Major strokes can lead to prolonged and crippling illnesses, often involving loss of sensation in certain parts of the body, disturbances of speech, vision or memory, and loss of locomotion. It is estimated that there are 2 million paralyzed and bedridden stroke victims in the United States today, many of whom could be at least partially rehabilitated with proper care and attention. On the other hand,

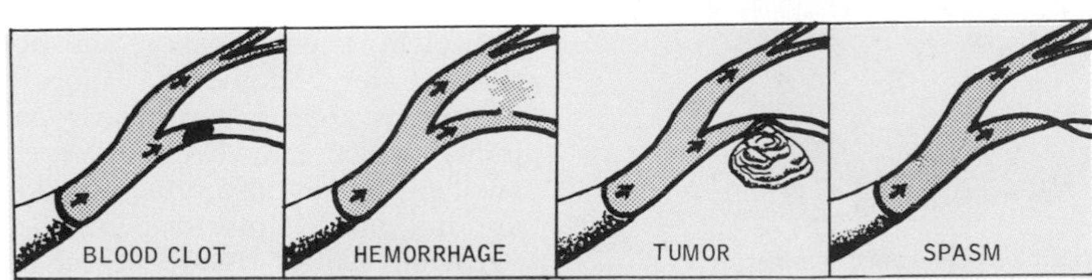

Figure 18–2. Major causes of strokes.

HARDENING OF THE ARTERIES

The Progress of Atherosclerosis

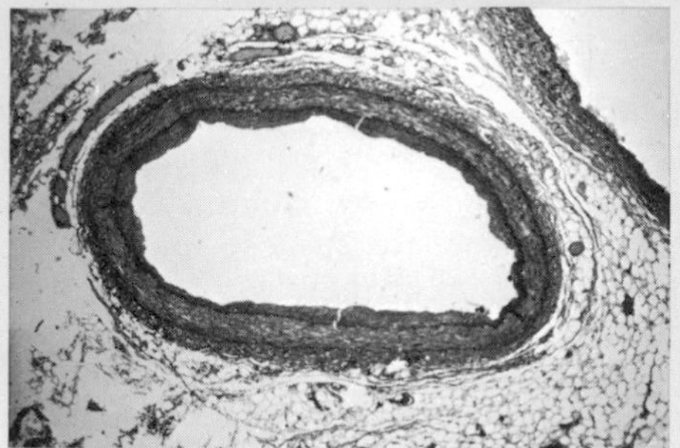

Cross section of a normal artery

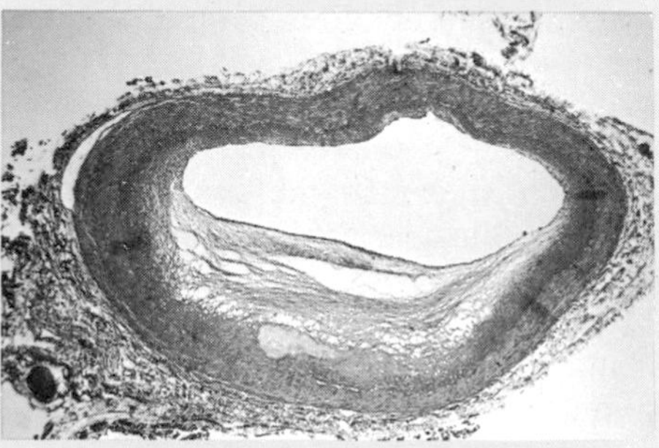

Fatty deposits form on the inner lining

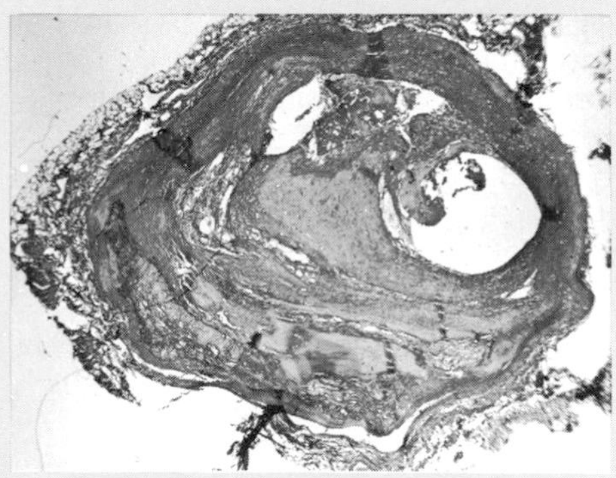

Channel narrows as fat deposit increases

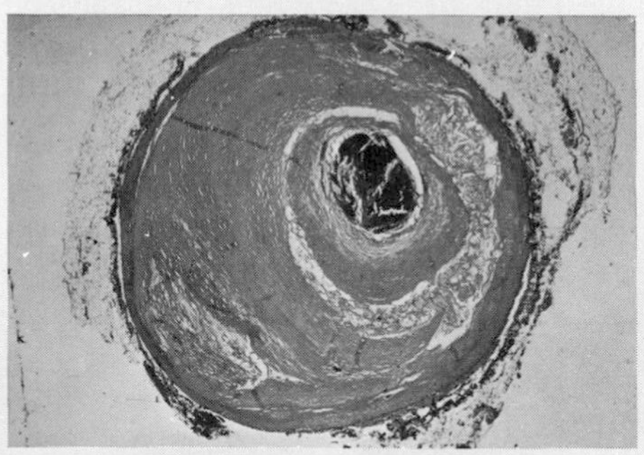

Blood clot blocks narrowed channel

many strokes are so mild that they produce no, or few, lasting effects.

Fortunately, some initial strokes may now be prevented by reduction of high blood pressure or preventive therapy in arteriosclerosis-prone persons. The person who is fortunate enough to have recovered from one is forewarned that he should maintain a normal weight and take advantage of what we do know about preventing arteriosclerosis and high blood pressure. It's encouraging to realize that a severe stroke does not necessarily mean the end of a productive life. Louis Pasteur experienced such a stroke when he was only 45, yet he lived another 27 years, during which period he made many of his most celebrated discoveries in the field of medicine.

Rheumatic Fever

Rheumatic fever is the delayed result of a streptococcal infection such as a "strep" sore throat, scarlet fever, tonsillitis, or middle-ear infection. The initial attack of the disease usually occurs in childhood and may affect many parts of the body, the most important being the heart. If rheumatic heart disease does develop, it sometimes injures the heart muscle and its valves. This creates a serious mechanical hindrance to adequate pumping of the blood: the valves may leak or their openings may shrink until they are too narrow to permit blood to flow through properly.

Children and young adults are the commonest victims, but often heart symptoms from early rheumatic fever don't show up until years later. Many adults experience their first symptoms after they reach middle age.

Rheumatic fever is sometimes difficult for a doctor to diagnose because the early signs are rather vague and are characteristic of many other diseases—fatigue, loss of weight, anemia, pallor, and poor appetite. Later, however, more definite symptoms appear, particularly pain in the joints, which may even become red and swollen. It may also attack tendons which are not near joints, causing the familiar "growing pains." Blood vessel damage in children with rheumatic fever may first show up in frequent nosebleeds, because they have weakened blood vessels in the nose. At least 50 per cent of the people who have chronic, long-standing rheumatic heart disease which is discovered when they are grown, never knew they had rheumatic fever as children. Careful questioning by doctors sometimes reveals merely repeated nosebleeds or "growing pains."

The key to prevention of this disease is *early recognition of streptococcal infections and intensive treatment with penicillin.* Later, penicillin or one of the sulfonamides may be used to prevent subsequent attacks.[17] Many physicians recommend that penicillin be given regularly to children who have had rheumatic fever until they reach adulthood.

Bacterial Endocarditis

Many bacteria, including one called the "green," or *viridans,* streptococcus can be found in the nose and throat of perfectly healthy people. Unfortunately, these bacteria sometimes invade the blood stream after a tooth extraction or operation involving the mouth, nose or throat, or even the intestines. If these virulent streptococci reach heart valves that are already damaged by rheumatic fever or congenital heart disease, they may lodge there and cause *bacterial endocarditis.* This is the reason anyone with such heart damage should consult his doctor about preventive measures before even minor operations like tooth extractions. We are fortunate that these microorganisms yield to penicillin, and rheumatic fever no longer has the completely fatal outcome it once had.

Syphilis

This disease affects the circulatory system, most often by injuring the aorta, the main artery leading from the heart. It is especially dangerous when it weakens and scars the aortic heart valve which separates this great blood vessel from the heart itself. If this happens, the valve may leak, permitting blood to pour backward instead of forward from the heart.

[17] *Prevention of Rheumatic Fever and Bacterial Endocarditis,* American Heart Assoc., Committee on Prevention of Rheumatic Fever and Bacterial Endocarditis. *Circulation, 15*:154, 1957.

Congenital Heart Disease

Defects of the heart and circulatory system are prominent among the abnormalities present at birth in a small percentage of babies. In the "blue baby," for example, the blood doesn't flow properly from the heart to the lungs. Many of these conditions are immediately obvious at birth, but some congenital abnormalities do not reveal themselves until much later in life. Great progress has been achieved in recent years in correcting or improving such heart conditions by newly devised surgical operations.

Kidney Diseases

Because they are closely related to the cardiovascular illnesses, several kidney diseases are usually included under the general grouping of *cardiovascular-renal* diseases. The chief reason for this is that hypertension and arteriosclerosis cause many of the deaths due to kidney disease by severely damaging the blood vessels of the kidneys, and preventing them from functioning properly, *Uremia,* or kidney failure, is the result.

The function of the kidneys is to remove waste products of the body, and they accomplish this with approximately 2 million highly selective filtering units. If these can't perform properly because of disease, the waste products accumulate, and if the kidneys fail completely, death results because no other tissue can carry out the excretory function. One healthy kidney is all we need, but a disease affecting both kidneys can be extremely serious.

In *glomerulonephritis,* commonly called *Bright's disease* or *nephritis,* the delicate membranes of the filtering units are injured, permitting blood cells and proteins to pass into the urine. An acute attack of this disease also affects the blood capillaries of the body, and water leaks out into the tissues, causing swelling and puffiness around the eyes and ankles, as well as other parts of the body. The heart may also be affected, but the kidneys suffer the major damage.

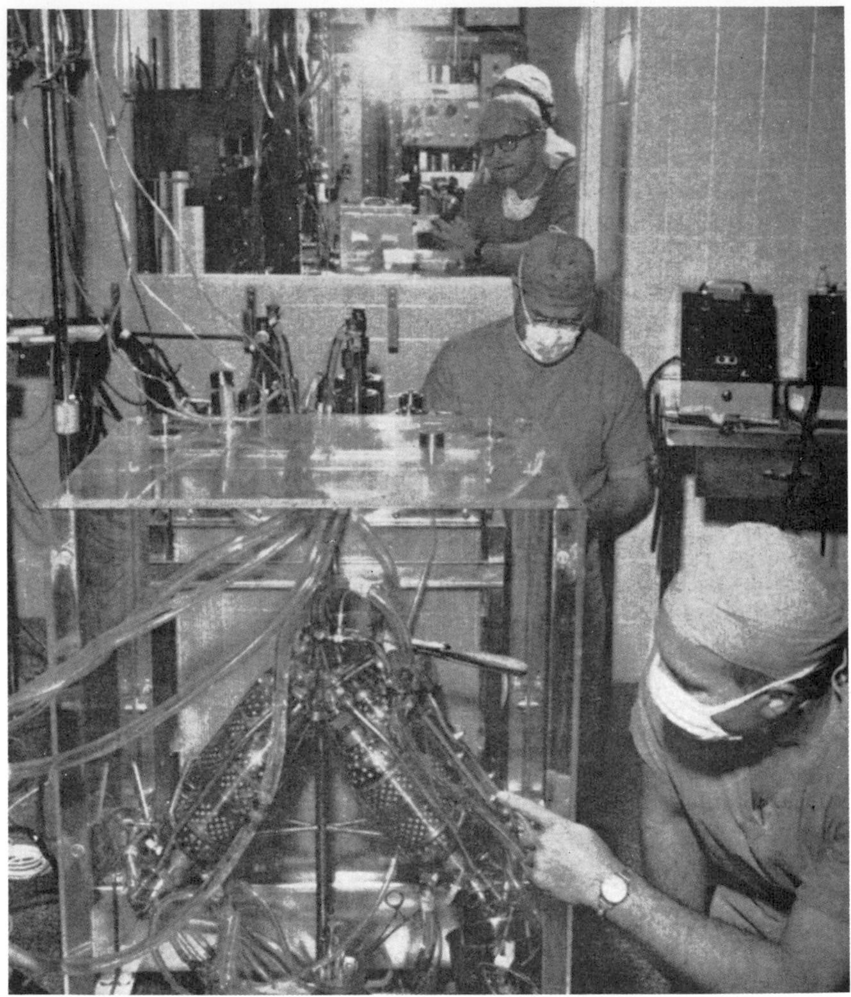

Figure 18–3. Open-heart surgery with the heart-lung machine. Surgeons check blood pumps on complicated heart-lung machine which takes over breathing and pulse for patient during open-heart surgery. Operator (outside, in background) is at control unit with cardiologist, who checks heart diagrams. (Courtesy of Globe Photos.)

Nephritis may follow shortly after a streptococcus infection of the throat, tonsils or sinuses because, in a small percentage of patients, the bacteria sensitize the kidney, in a manner not yet clearly understood. Only certain varieties of streptococci cause nephritis: scarlet fever *may* be responsible, but streptococcus infections of the skin, such as erysipelas, do not cause Bright's disease.

Fortunately, most patients recover completely and remain well the rest of their lives. However, some continue into the chronic stage and the kidneys are eventually damaged beyond repair. Even in such individuals, however, there may be many years of comfortable, productive living before the kidneys fail completely.

The prompt use of sulfa drugs and penicillin for all sore throats, tonsillitis, sinus infections and painful neck glands will *prevent* many cases of Bright's disease. Another precaution is to avoid chilling the feet and body for several weeks after recovering from such infections.

Nephrosis is a special form of nephritis which is characterized by a tremendous accumulation of edema fluid. The tissues under the skin and the abdominal cavity may hold quarts of this watery fluid because the affected kidneys have lost their ability to regulate body fluid balance. However, the kidneys are not usually badly damaged, and with modern medicines it is possible to ward off the deadly pneumococcus, streptococcus, and other bacteria which killed so many nephrosis victims in the past. Nature itself can cure the kidney lesion, if given enough time.

Pyelitis is an infection usually centering in the kidney pelvis, the small funnel-shaped reservoir which collects urine from the kidney. Common symptoms are back pains, fever and a burning sensation on urination. It usually responds readily to modern medicines, but if not treated promptly, pyelitis sometimes becomes chronic and develops into the more serious *pyelonephritis*. This may ultimately lead to destruction of the kidneys.

Uremia means, literally, "urine in the blood," and develops when the kidneys are so badly damaged that they can no longer purify the blood of urea and other waste products of the body's metabolic activities. In advanced uremia, even the breath has the ammoniacal odor of urine.

Temporary, transient uremias sometimes develop after blood transfusions of mismatched or infected blood, certain types of poisoning or in complications of pregnancy, and can usually be successfully treated, with no residual damage, by a number of methods. One of these is the so-called *artificial kidney,* a device through which the blood can be circulated and purified until the kidneys can again take over the job. This equipment is available in many leading hospitals and medical centers today.

When the kidneys are hopelessly and irreversibly damaged by disease, the artificial kidney is sometimes used at frequent intervals to prevent the accumulation of the uremic process. Another hope in such cases is to replace the diseased kidney with a normal human kidney from some other person. Research doctors are attempting to transplant human kidneys to open up a new life for many patients doomed to die of chronic, irreversible uremia.

NORMAL VERSUS ABNORMAL GROWTH: THE PROBLEM OF CANCER

The very word cancer is horrible to most people. Fear of this disease casts a shadow on lives cancer will never touch, and many who do develop it often become so terror-stricken they are unable to fight back. This is especially tragic because in many instances *a malignant cancer is curable if it is diagnosed soon enough.*

Cancer is one of the greatest killers for all age groups, and can affect almost any part of the body. Cancer seldom issues clear and obvious warnings, and there is no simple test that can definitely rule out all possibility of its presence or absence. It is sometimes a painful, lingering disease, and becomes emotionally and economically exhausting to both the patient and his family. Finally, we do not understand how it develops, and tend to feel helpless facing such a mysterious, dangerous adversary.

However, far too much attention has been devoted to this "enigma" of cancer. *We don't know everything there is to know about it, but we already know enough to prevent and cure many cases and to prolong even more lives.*

What Cancer Means

The tissues of our bodies grow by the division of cells, and the new cells are smaller, but otherwise exactly like the parent cells. They grow until they reach their normal size and have formed all the necessary organs and structures, but when the body reaches maturity, growth stops and the body settles down to the size it will maintain for the rest of its existence. A certain number of new cells are developing constantly to replace dead tissue and to repair damage. If you cut yourself, the wound heals by the formation of new tissue, but when a certain point is reached in this process, nature again cries halt.

It is still a mystery why normal cells divide only until they have produced the required amount of tissue and then stop. Nor do we understand why the process sometimes goes wild, and cells continue to multiply until there is too much tissue. A *tumor* is the lump or mass produced by such unchecked growth.

A *benign* tumor may be large or small, but it never *spreads* as does a malignant tumor. A *cancer*, also called a *neoplasm,* is a malignant tumor, a shapeless mass

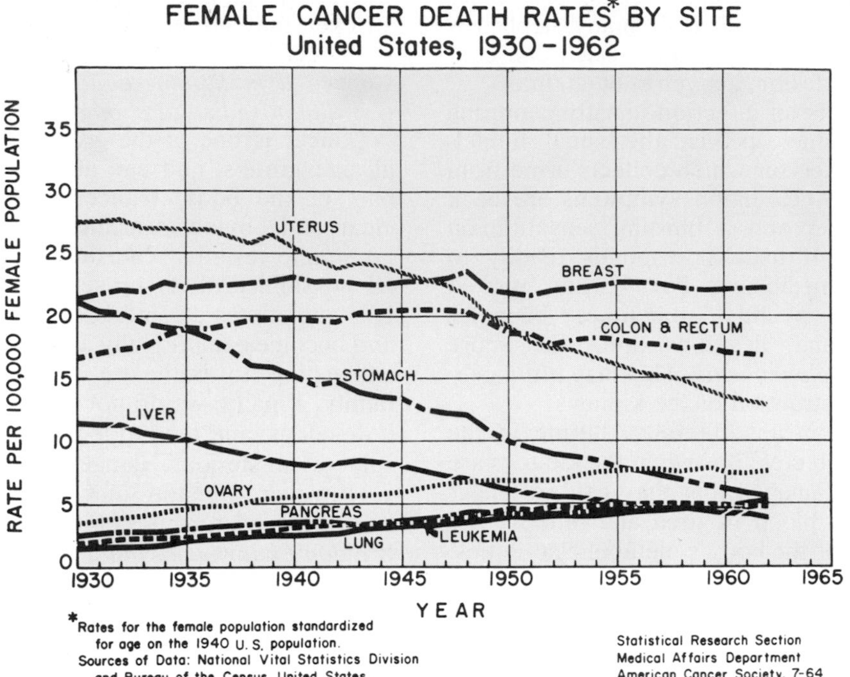

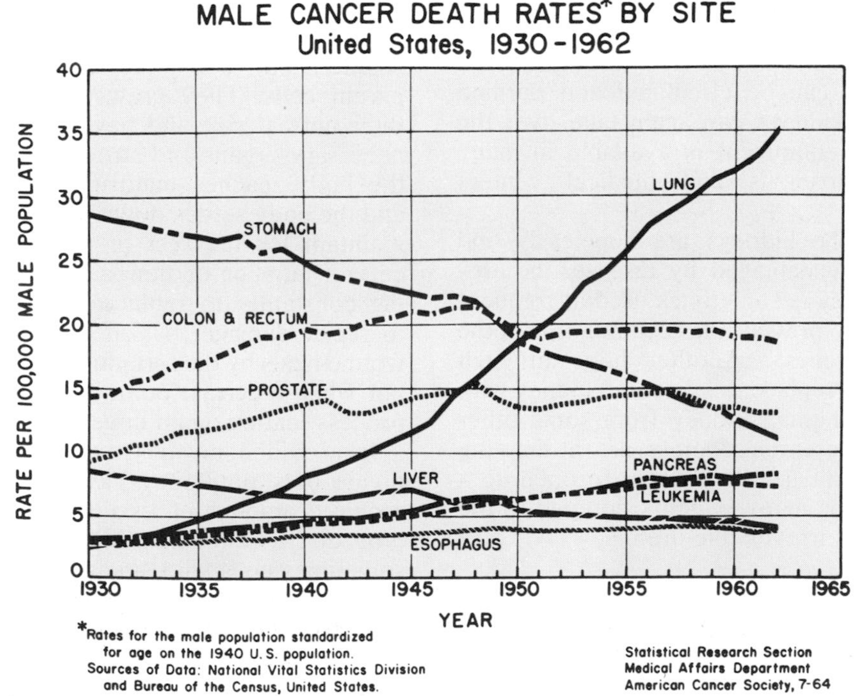

 Figure 18–4. Age-adjusted death rates per 100,000 population of selected sites of cancer in the United States from 1930 to 1962.

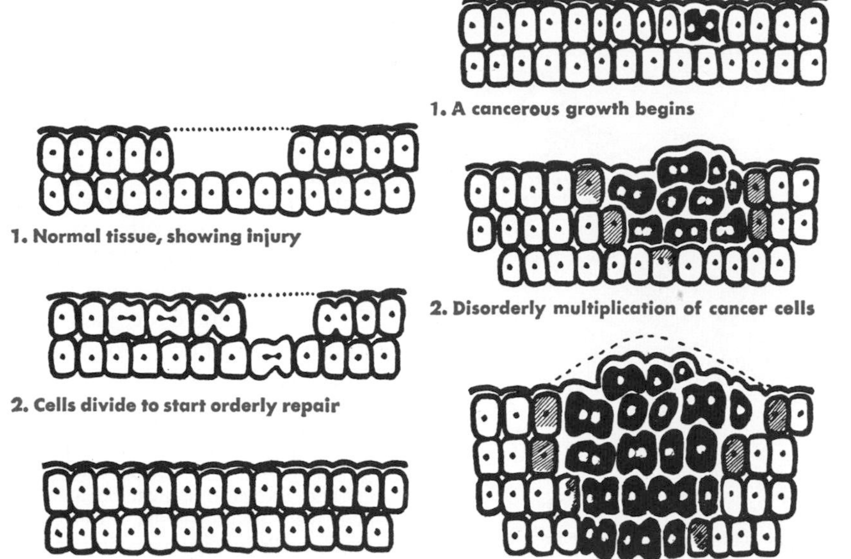

Figure 18–5. Normal and cancerous growth. (From American Cancer Society Bulletin: Who, What, Why, Where and When of Cancer? 1957.)

which continues to grow in a disorderly fashion, sometimes rapidly, sometimes slowly, and it *does not remain confined to a small area.* Unless it is checked, a cancer can spread until the enlarging tissue crowds and presses on other organs of the body, preventing them from carrying out their normal functions and robbing healthy cells of their food and blood supply.

Pieces of the malignant growth may break off and be carried by the blood or lymph fluid to some other part of the body, dividing and growing until they form *metastases.* Cancer can spread in this way from the kidney to the bones, or from the lungs to the brain. In this late stage, the disease becomes very difficult to cure, and can be compared to a fire which started in the basement and sends a spark up the stairway to the attic to set off another fire there.

Types of Cancer

There are two major groups of malignancies. *Sarcomas* usually affect the bones and muscles, and are apt to grow rapidly and be very destructive. Most neoplasms of the breast, stomach, womb, skin, and tongue are *carcinomas.*

Precancers are relatively harmless tissue changes which have a tendency to become cancerous. They include the thickened white patches (not ordinary canker sores) on the mouth and tongue called *leukoplakia;* some *moles;* any chronically *irritated spot* on the skin or on the mucous membranes of the mouth; *polyps,* such as those of the large intestine; and some forms of lymph-gland tumors.

Hodgkin's disease is a potentially serious illness which usually afflicts young people, causing a progressive enlargement of the lymphatic glands throughout the body. In most cases, it starts in the glands of the neck, groin, armpit, or even the chest or abdomen. There is some disagreement about whether this disease is a true cancer. However, because it can become widespread, invasive and destructive, and because it responds to treatment in the same way as cancer, it is usually classed as a malignancy.

In *leukemias,* the number of white blood corpuscles increases tremendously, sometimes reaching levels a hundred times normal. The term *acute* or *chronic* is used to describe leukemia, depending on how rapidly it develops. The acute form appears suddenly and usually progresses

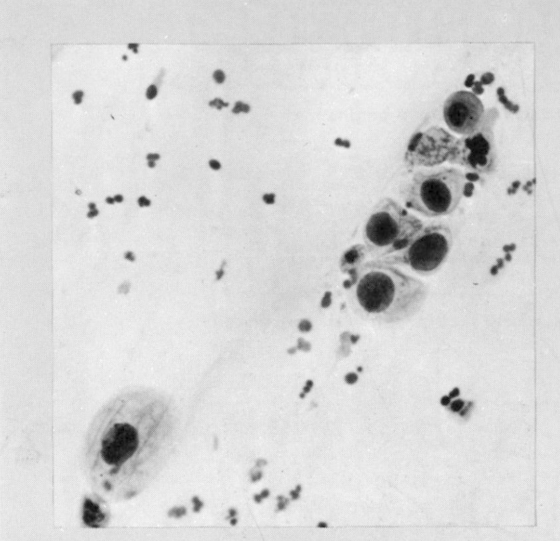

Pap Test: This is a photograph, magnified 900 times, of a Papanicolaou smear test, or Pap test, for cancer, as applied to a secretion from the vagina. The cluster of large cells at upper right have reacted positively by absorbing large amounts of stain, revealing cancer of the uterus. The test is a simple, painless procedure that can detect cancer at an early and curable stage.

so rapidly that often it is not even discovered until the disease is far advanced. This type is found most frequently in young children, whereas the chronic, slower form is more likely to develop after the age of 35. The most important types are *lymphocytic* leukemia, which involves the lymphocytes (the white cells originating in lymph nodes or spleen); *granulocytic* leukemia, an overgrowth of the white cells of the bone marrow, called granulocytes; and *monocytic* leukemia, in which the number of monocytes from connective tissue is increased enormously.

The Magnitude of the Cancer Problem

The American Cancer Society estimated that, in 1964, 290,000 persons died of cancer—that is, 795 persons a day or one every two minutes. Cancer strikes one out of every four Americans, two out of every three families, and is responsible for one out of every six deaths.

The death rate from cancer increased steadily from 1930 to 1950; since then it has leveled off. The date rate per 100,000 population was 112 in 1930, 120 in 1940, 125 in 1950, and 125 in 1960. Currently, there are about 540,000 new cancer cases diagnosed each year; 830,000 Americans annually receive medical care for cancer.

The future, however, is somewhat more encouraging. The American Cancer Society states:

> Of every six persons who get cancer today, two will be saved and four will die. Numbers 1 and 2 will be saved. Number 3 will die but might have been saved had proper treatment been received in time. Numbers 4, 5 and 6 will die of cancers which cannot yet be controlled; only the results of research can save these patients. This means that today half of those who get cancer could and should be saved—by early diagnosis and prompt treatment. Thus, the immediate goal of cancer control in the United States is the annual saving of 270,000 lives, or half of those who develop cancer each year.

How Cancer is Detected

Malignant growths cause different symptoms according to their location and state of development, but, unfortunately, pain is not usually one of the early warning symptoms. The *early danger signals are:*

1. Any lump or thickening, especially in the breast, lip or tongue.
2. Irregular or unexplained bleeding, such as blood in the urine or bowel movements; bloody discharge from the nipple or any body opening; unexplained vaginal bleeding or discharge, or any bleeding after the menopause.
3. A sore that does not heal, particularly around the mouth, tongue, or lips, or anywhere on the skin.
4. Noticeable changes in the color or size of a wart, mole, or birthmark.
5. Loss of appetite or continual indigestion.
6. Persistent hoarseness, cough, difficulty in swallowing, chest pains.
7. Marked change in normal elimination (bowel habits and urination).
8. Continued, unrelieved headaches, dizziness, disturbances of vision, nausea, and vomiting.

Table 18–2. Cancer status chart

SITE	ESTIMATED NEW CASES 1965	ESTIMATED DEATHS 1965	DANGER SIGNAL (WHEN LASTING LONGER THAN TWO WEEKS SEE YOUR DOCTOR)	SAFEGUARDS	COMMENT
BREAST	62,000	26,000	LUMP OR THICKENING IN THE BREAST.	ANNUAL CHECKUP. MONTHLY BREAST SELF-EXAMINATION.	THE LEADING CAUSE OF CANCER DEATH IN WOMEN.
COLON AND RECTUM	73,000	43,000	CHANGE IN BOWEL HABITS; BLEEDING.	ANNUAL CHECKUP, INCLUDING PROCTOSCOPY.	CONSIDERED A HIGHLY CURABLE DISEASE WHEN DIGITAL AND PROCTOSCOPIC EXAMINATIONS ARE INCLUDED IN ROUTINE CHECKUPS.
KIDNEY AND BLADDER	29,000	14,000	URINARY DIFFICULTY. BLEEDING — IN WHICH CASE CONSULT YOUR DOCTOR AT ONCE.	ANNUAL CHECKUP WITH URINALYSIS.	PROTECTIVE MEASURES FOR WORKERS IN HIGH-RISK INDUSTRIES ARE HELPING TO ELIMINATE ONE OF THE IMPORTANT CAUSES OF THESE CANCERS.
LUNG	52,000	47,000	PERSISTENT COUGH, OR LINGERING RESPIRATORY AILMENT.	PREVENTION: HEED FACTS ABOUT SMOKING. ANNUAL CHECKUP. CHEST X-RAY.	THE LEADING CAUSE OF CANCER DEATH AMONG MEN, THIS FORM OF CANCER IS LARGELY PREVENTABLE.
MOUTH, LARYNX AND PHARYNX	20,000	9,000	SORE THAT DOES NOT HEAL. DIFFICULTY IN SWALLOWING. HOARSENESS.	ANNUAL CHECKUP. INCLUDING LARYNX.	MANY MORE LIVES SHOULD BE SAVED BECAUSE THE MOUTH IS EASILY ACCESSIBLE TO VISUAL EXAMINATION BY PHYSICIANS AND DENTISTS.
PROSTATE	33,000	16,000	URINARY DIFFICULTY.	ANNUAL CHECKUP, INCLUDING PALPATION.	OCCURS MAINLY IN MEN OVER 60. THE DISEASE CAN BE DETECTED BY PALPATION AND URINALYSIS AT ANNUAL CHECKUP.
SKIN	80,000	4,000	SORE THAT DOES NOT HEAL, OR CHANGE IN WART OR MOLE.	ANNUAL CHECKUP. AVOIDANCE OF OVEREXPOSURE TO SUN.	SKIN CANCER IS READILY DETECTED BY OBSERVATION, AND DIAGNOSED BY SIMPLE BIOPSY.
STOMACH	21,000	18,000	INDIGESTION.	ANNUAL CHECKUP.	A 40% DECLINE IN MORTALITY IN 20 YEARS, FOR REASONS YET UNKNOWN.
UTERUS	44,000	14,000	UNUSUAL BLEEDING OR DISCHARGE	ANNUAL CHECKUP INCLUDING PELVIC EXAMINATION AND PAPANICOLAOU SMEAR.	UTERINE CANCER MORTALITY HAS DECLINED 50% DURING THE LAST 25 YEARS. WITH WIDER APPLICATION OF THE "PAP" SMEAR, MANY THOUSAND MORE LIVES CAN BE SAVED.
LEUKEMIA	17,000	14,000	LEUKEMIA IS A CANCER OF BLOOD-FORMING TISSUES AND IS CHARACTERIZED BY THE ABNORMAL PRODUCTION OF IMMATURE WHITE BLOOD CELLS. ACUTE LEUKEMIA STRIKES MAINLY CHILDREN AND IS TREATED BY DRUGS WHICH HAVE EXTENDED LIFE FROM A FEW MONTHS TO AS MUCH AS THREE YEARS. CHRONIC LEUKEMIA STRIKES USUALLY AFTER AGE 25 AND PROGRESSES LESS RAPIDLY.		
			CANCER EXPERTS BELIEVE THAT IF DRUGS OR VACCINES ARE FOUND WHICH CAN CURE OR PREVENT ANY CANCERS THEY WILL BE SUCCESSFUL FIRST FOR LEUKEMIA AND THE LYMPHOMAS.		
LYMPHOMAS	20.000	15,000	THESE DISEASES ARISE IN THE LYMPH SYSTEM AND INCLUDE HODGKIN'S AND LYMPHOSARCOMA. SOME PATIENTS WITH LYMPHATIC CANCERS CAN LEAD NORMAL LIVES FOR MANY YEARS.		

(From *1965 Cancer Facts and Figures,* American Cancer Society.)

None of the above signs necessarily means cancer, and very commonly they do not. But the only way to be sure is to have a thorough medical examination.

Many special techniques and instruments have been devised for cancer diagnosis to supplement the medical examination. X-ray photography is used to detect neoplasms of the lung and the gastrointestinal tract, and, with certain modifications, the kidneys and brain.

Special *endoscopic* instruments which work on the principle of a periscope have proved extremely valuable in studying the internal organs and locating small cancers in the early, curable stage. Essentially, these are tubes which can be inserted into the area to be studied, illuminating the tissue by a tiny bulb at the end.

A *biopsy* is *the* definite way of determining whether a growth is cancerous: a small portion of the suspected tissue is removed and examined under the microscope by a *pathologist,* a physician who specializes in concluding from the appearance of the organs and their cells whether they are normal or diseased. Biopsies of some tumors are taken through endoscopic examining instruments. For example, a growth in the rectum can be biopsied with the proctoscope and those in the lung with the bronchoscope. If the tumor is readily accessible, the procedure is very simple and is often performed in the doctor's office. In other cases, it may require surgery.

The Papanicolaou cell smear test has been described as one of the greatest diagnostic aids to cancer in the twentieth century. This is sometimes called the *cytologic* method (cytology is the study of cells). It is a relatively simple test, which depends on the fact that tissue fluids bathing cancerous areas carry away cells which have been shed by the cancer tissue. Microscopic examination of these cells on a glass slide is enough to reveal the presence of cancer, because when the cells are stained with special dyes, they usually show such bizarre structures that they can easily be differentiated from normal cells. Cytological techniques have been used very successfully in picking up cancers of the lung, stomach, breast and, particularly, the cervix, or mouth of the womb.

According to Seymour M. Farber, of the University of California, cytological studies of sputum are about 90 per cent effective in detecting unsuspected cases of lung carcinoma. Cancer of the uterus, the second largest cause of malignancy in women, can be demonstrated by the Papanicolaou cell smear when it is in its early, pre-invasive, *curable* stage. Theoretically this cancer is 100 per cent curable, but actually only about 40 per cent of the cases are cured because they are diagnosed too late.

A new technique in the diagnosis of breast cancer is mammography. Using this soft tissue x-ray procedure, physicians in a recent California survey of 1223 women detected eight cases of breast cancer in women who had been judged free of this type of cancer by conventional techniques.

Another promising technique in cancer detection is thermography. This method is based on the measurement of heat radiated from the surface of the body. Because normal and pathologic tissues emit different amounts of radiation, it is frequently possible to locate cancer cells by measurement of tissue temperature. A recent study by Dr. K. Lloyd Williams of London revealed a 1° C. rise in the temperature of the skin overlying breast cancers in 95 per cent of women previously known to have breast cancer.

It would be wonderful if there were a simple chemical blood test to detect cancer in any part of the body. Unfortunately, medical science has not yet advanced this far although the blood can be tested chemically for cancer of the prostate and for a rare bone marrow malignancy called *multiple myeloma.* Also, blood smears and counts help in the diagnosis of leukemia.

More recently, cancer of the cervix is being tested by mail. Women are furnished a soft plastic pipet to obtain samples of cervix cells. In turn, the pipets are mailed to a hospital for analysis.

Is Cancer Contagious?

Fortunately, human cancer does not appear to be contagious. It is therefore perfectly safe to visit, associate with, or care for anyone who is sick, or even dying, from cancer.

Causes of Cancer

Most diseases result from a single, specific cause: pneumonia is caused by either a virus or a particular bacterium; streptococcal sore throats are set off by the streptococcus organism; rickets is produced by vitamin D deficiency; characteristic disorders appear if there is underactivity or overactivity of endocrine organs. The situation is quite different with cancer, however, because many and quite varied conditions can contribute to its development.

Some of the known factors are chronic or prolonged irritation—by chemicals, friction, or heat—which may cause cancer in internal organs, body openings or on the skin. Repeated exposure to certain chemicals produces cancer in laboratory animals and in human beings, as well. One of the first recognized carcinogens (the scientific name for cancer-inciting agents) was isolated from chimney soot. It produces a characteristic neoplasm which was formerly very common in chimney sweeps in England.

It is a popular misconception that cancer can be caused by a blow to the breast or other parts of the body.

Certain warts or moles, especially if they are irritated, and chronic mouth sores caused by ill-fitting dental plates or jagged teeth sometimes become malignant.

Cancer of the lip can develop in smokers who habitually hold a hot pipe stem or cigar in one corner of their mouths.

Prolonged exposure to sunlight is the important factor in "sailor's skin," "farmer's skin," and other similar malignancies. However, these take many years to develop.

Radiation. Exposure to excessive amounts of radioactive chemicals and radiation is a very definite cause of malignancy. This (as well as genetic mutations), is one of the reasons for serious concern about the testing of atomic weapons and the dangers of atomic warfare.

In the early days of x-ray use for diagnostic purposes, the enormous hazards of this technique were not recognized. As a result, many physicians and x-ray technicians developed cancer because of excessive exposure to these dangerous rays. Even today, despite very careful shielding devices, radiologists have a shorter life span and more cancer than nonradiologists.[18]

Madame Curie, the world-famous scientist who discovered the radioactivity of radium, died of cancer. The use of radioactive paint to make luminous watch dials caused malignancies and the early death of many unsuspecting young workers in watch factories during the early years of this practice.

Data which have accumulated from Hiroshima and Nagasaki prove that survivors of the atomic explosions who were near the *center* of the blast have 12 times as much leukemia as survivors who were at the *periphery* of the blast area.

In recent years, many studies have been made on individuals who received large amounts of x-ray for the *treatment* of certain diseases. (For *diagnostic* x-rays, a much lower exposure to irradiation is needed than for *treatment,* or *therapeutic,* x-rays). As a result of these studies, *many physicians feel that x-rays should not be used in the treatment of any disease, unless the disease is of an essentially fatal nature, or all other treatment methods have failed.* This might be the case in the treatment of cancer, for example.

The reason for the concern about therapeutic x-rays is that *they appear to have actually caused cancer* in certain individuals.[19]

Radiological techniques are immeasurably valuable in medicine, and actually represent one of the greatest contributions to medical science. However, it is now generally accepted that radiation has a

[18]*American Journal of Medical Science, 220*: 282, 1950.

[19]Dameshek, W., and Gunz, F. A.: *Journal of the American Medical Association, 163*:838, 1957.

Table 18–3. Applying cancer statistics locally

SIZE OF COMMUNITY	ESTIMATED NO. CANCER CASES UNDER MEDICAL CARE IN 1965	ESTIMATED NO. WHO WILL DIE OF CANCER IN 1965	ESTIMATED NO. OF NEW CASES IN 1965	ESTIMATED NO. WHO WILL BE SAVED FROM CANCER IN 1965	ESTIMATED NO. WHO WILL EVENTUALLY DEVELOP CANCER	ESTIMATED NO. WHO WILL DIE OF CANCER IF PRESENT RATES CONTINUE
1,000	4	1	3	1	250	150
2,000	9	3	6	2	500	300
3,000	13	4	8	3	750	450
4,000	18	6	11	4	1,000	600
5,000	21	7	14	5	1,250	750
10,000	43	15	28	9	2,500	1,500
25,000	107	37	70	23	6,250	3,750
50,000	215	75	140	47	12,500	7,500
100,000	430	150	280	93	25,000	15,000
200,000	860	300	560	186	50,000	30,000
500,000	2,150	750	1,400	465	125,000	75,000

NOTE: The figures can only be the roughest approximation of actual data for your community. It is suggested that every effort be made to obtain actual data from a Registry source.

(From *1965 Cancer Facts and Figures,* American Cancer Society.)

cumulative biological effect, and greater precautions must be exercised in its use.[20]

Viruses. Evidence is increasing that leukemia and Hodgkin's disease may be caused by a virus, and that certain other cancers may also have a virus origin. However, most of the proof comes from studies with experimental animals. Wendell M. Stanley, Nobel Prize winner and head of the Virus Research Laboratory at the University of California, recently stated: "I believe the time has come when we should assume *that viruses are responsible for most, if not all, kinds of cancer, including cancer in man.*"

Stanley pointed out that we harbor a great many viruses in our bodies, and that some of them–like the one responsible for cold sores–may persist in a dormant form for years, or even a lifetime. Perhaps, again like the cold sore virus, they are activated by irritation, chemicals or some other condition, and flare up to generate a cancer. It will take many years of study and special kinds of experiments to determine whether Stanley's theory can be applied to the cancer problem generally, but it is a very challenging one.

Smoking and Lung Cancer[21]

Lung cancer is a continuously increasing threat to life. Today, the death rate from this disease is ten times what it was 30 years ago. In 1964, the number of deaths from lung cancer was estimated at 43,000 persons–37,000 men and 6000 women. It is the leading cause of male cancer deaths.

Is lung cancer related to smoking? The answer to this question is an unequivocal "yes." In fact, Dr. Alton Ochsner, an internationally known chest surgeon, states: "I am convinced that every heavy smoker will develop lung cancer–unless heart disease or some other disease claims him earlier." In addition, the 1964 report of the Surgeon General's Committee on Smoking supports his contention.

Heredity and Cancer

To investigate heredity as a cause of cancer, Dr. Bent Harvald and Dr. Mogens Hauge of the University of Copenhagen have made a study of identical twins. Among 1528 of these twins, who had identical genes, 164 cases of cancer developed. But in 143 of these cases, only one partner developed cancer. Moreover,

[20]Radiation as a cause of cancer is discussed in greater detail in Chapter 32.

[21]Smoking as a cause of lung cancer is discussed in greater detail in Chapter 22.

there were only eight cases in which both partners had the same type of cancer.

It would appear, therefore, that heredity does not play a significant role in the cause of cancer in human beings. Therefore, just because some member of your family has developed cancer, there is no reason to spend the rest of your life worrying about a similar fate.

The Treatment of Malignant Tumors

The aim of cancer treatment is the *complete* removal or destruction of all cancerous tissue. Once this has been accomplished, the malignant growth is gone just as surely as a fire that has been extinguished. In many cases, this can be done before it has caused any damage.

Surgical methods are of great importance: the surgeon cuts away some of the normal tissue as well, so that he can be certain of getting all the cancer cells, and if the malignancy is large or is internally located, this can be a major procedure.

Irradiation treatments, such as x-ray, radon, cobalt, and super voltage therapy, depend on the fact that the penetrating radiation damages tissue, especially if it is growing at a rapid rate. For this reason, cancer cells are more sensitive than normal ones, and are destroyed sooner.

Radioactive isotopes have been helpful in several malignant conditions: radioactive *iodine* is employed in the treatment of thyroid cancer, *phosphorus* in some diseases of the blood-forming organs, including leukemias, and *gold* for carcinoma of the womb and prostate.

Chemotherapy of cancer, which means treatment of the disease with hormones and other chemicals, has received a great deal of attention in recent years. At the present time, there is no medicine, chemical or drug which can *cure* cancer. However, certain substances are effective in *retarding* its growth and in prolonging life.

Some cancers respond to treatment with *hormones:* stilbestrol, a female hormone, is given for cancer of the prostate, and certain of the male hormones are used in treating breast malignancies.

Thyroid hormone has been employed to suppress the activity of cancerous fragments left in the thyroid after surgery.

Removal of the pituitary or the adrenal glands has slowed down the progress of cancers in certain areas. Also, hormones from the adrenal gland have prolonged life in leukemia patients.

About 70,000 chemical compounds have already been tested in experimental animals as anti-cancer agents, and some of these have been very successful in retarding malignant growths in humans. These range from poison gases—such as *nitrogen mustards* and related compounds—to antivitamins, antibiotics and special anticancer viruses. Just as in the case of irradiation, the rapidly growing cancer

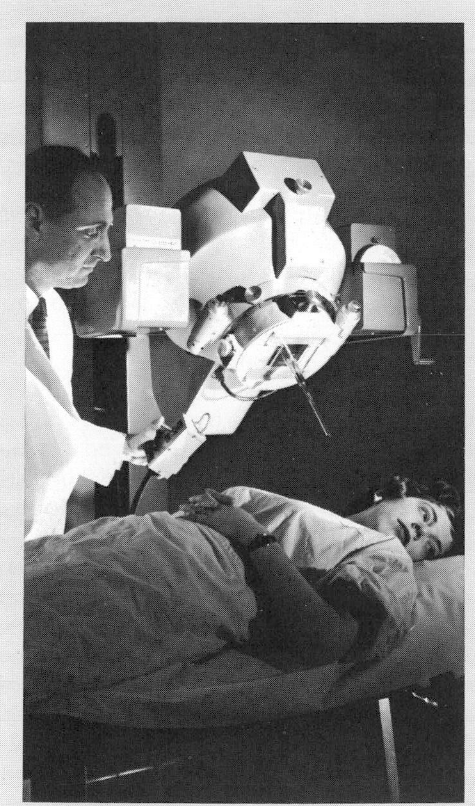

Radiation Therapy: A machine is being used to administer cobalt-ray treatment to a patient suffering from cancer. The rays are directed so that the diseased tissue only is affected.

Table 18–4. Man's progress against cancer

CATEGORY	1937	1964
Saved (alive five years after treatment)	Fewer than one-in-five	One-in-three
Uterine cancer	Chief cause of cancer death in women	Death rate cut 50%. Could be reduced much more
Lung cancer	Mounting: no hope of control	Still mounting: but upward of 75% could be prevented
Research support	Less than $1,000,000	More than $215,000,000
Cancer clinics and registries approved by American College of Surgeons	240 in USA and Canada	963 – plus expansion of teaching, research, treatment centers
State control measures	Seven states	All 50 states
Chemotherapy	Almost no research	Major research attack has produced 24 useful drugs
One-in-two patients could be saved today by early diagnosis and prompt treatment.		

(From *1965 Cancer Facts and Figures*, American Cancer Society.)

cell is more sensitive to many chemicals than normal, slow-growing tissue.

Even though none of the compounds so far discovered appears to cure cancer, some have prolonged life for many years. An enormous amount of time and money is being invested in research to find truly curative chemical substances which can selectively destroy malignant cells.

Many techniques for treating cancer are available today, sometimes even more effective when combined—for example, surgery and irradiation. They have effected a tremendous reduction in the loss of life from cancer, and are responsible for many added years of life. According to Dr. I. S. Ravdin, a president of the American Cancer Society, 44,000 cancer patients who would have died in 1953 were saved in 1963.

We can all help conquer cancer by observing several common-sense rules:

1. The most important is the regular physical checkup. Half of all cancers occur in parts of the body which the doctor can readily examine. The American Cancer Society estimates that 70,000 people in this country are saved every year by *early* treatment of cancer. Unfortunately, it also estimates that *another 90,000 could be saved*—but are not.

2. Learn the danger signals. If you have, or suspect you have, any of them, go to a reputable physician or clinic *at once.* Time is cancer's greatest ally.

3. Beware of "sure cures" for cancer. They are promised by quacks, either deliberate fakers or self-deceived crackpots. No matter what the "cure" consists of—ointments, salves, herbs, lotions, medicines, mysterious "rays," or vapors—it is a fraud and a menace to health. It not only takes the money needed for proper treatment, but also loses valuable, often critical, time which should be spent under a doctor's care. Only a reputable doctor or clinic can make proper use of surgery, x-ray, radium, and other reliable methods of curing or treating cancer.

Questions

1. What is the chief reason that coronary disease and cancer have become leading causes of death?
2. What are some factors that predispose to heart attacks?
3. What physical changes in the arteries force

the heart to pump blood at a higher blood pressure than normal? How do you think emotional disturbances could bring about a temporary hypertension? Could this be considered a psychosomatic disease?

4. List some of the possible values of exercise in the prevention of heart disease.

5. List the major causes of strokes, and show why they lead to strokes.

6. What is bacterial endocarditis, and what causes it?

7. Define glomerulonephritis, and indicate the cause and effects.

8. How does a benign tumor differ from a malignant one? What is the meaning of the word "metastasis"? Precancer?

9. List at least five danger signals which might be indicative of cancer.

10. How can cancers be detected with certainty?

11. Is human cancer a contagious disease?

12. Describe important methods for treating cancer.

Topics for Discussion

Cholesterol controversy.
Causes of arteriosclerosis.
Transplantation of the kidney.
The theory that viruses cause cancer.
Smoking and lung cancer.

Reading Suggestions

Death Be Not Proud, John Gunther. Harper & Bros., New York, 1949. A moving story by John Gunther of the development of a brain tumor in his teen-age son, which ultimately caused his death.

Cancer and Common Sense, George Crile, Jr. Viking Press, New York, 1955. A remarkably sensitive discussion of how this horrifying disease can be understood and accepted by the patient and the family. Written by a distinguished surgeon.

Heart Attack: New Hope, New Knowledge, New Life, Myron Prinzmetal and William Winter. Simon & Schuster, New York, 1965 (paperback). A leading cardiologist describes what happens to the human body when it experiences a coronary thrombosis. Diagnosis, treatment, and prevention are discussed for the layman.

Heart Disease and High Blood Pressure, Kenneth C. Hutchin. Arco Publishing Co., New York, 1964 (paperback). An easy-to-understand book for the layman, fully explains heart and circulatory problems.

Strokes: How They Occur and What Can Be Done About Them. Collier Books, New York, 1961 (paperback). Dr. Irvine H. Page and six other medical authorities discuss the causes and treatment of strokes. Very readable.

Your Heart: A Handbook for Laymen, H. M. Marvin. Doubleday, Garden City, 1960. An excellent book to aid the student in understanding his heart.

Report to the President: A National Program to Conquer Heart Disease, Cancer and Stroke, U.S. Government Printing Office, 1964. This report, prepared by the President's Commission on Heart Disease, Cancer and Stroke, represents the most up-to-date discussion of our current battle against these untamed killers.

Your Heart and Your Future, Alton Blakeslee and Jeremiah Stamler. Today's Health, July 1964, p. 23. A very interesting discussion of cardiovascular health. It is taken from the authors' more comprehensive book entitled *Your Heart Has Nine Lives,* Prentice-Hall, Englewood Cliffs, N. J., 1963.

Surgeons Now Replace Your Damaged Arteries, J. D. Ratcliff. Today's Health, May 1964, p. 58. An enlightening report of new techniques in surgery.

Hot-weather Target: Your Heart, Donald G. Cooley. Today's Health, July 1963, p. 21. An informative and authoritative article on how to cope with hot weather.

Message from Your Heart: the Electrocardiogram, John Lentz. Today's Health, June 1963, p. 26. An explanation of the electrocardiogram.

Hardening of the Arteries: Everybody's Disease, Irvine H. Page. Today's Health, October 1961, p. 28. A leading medical scientist describes arteriosclerosis in plain language.

When the Heart Stops, Paul W. Kearney. Today's Health, November 1960, p. 14. A description of the first-aid technique of artificial circulation.

High Blood Pressure: How Dangerous Is It?, Irvine H. Page. Today's Health, June 1960, p. 61. The author answers 15 questions about high blood pressure.

What You Should Know About Your Kidneys, Howard Earle. Today's Health, June 1961, p. 52. A famous doctor answers questions about the kidneys and explains how an artificial kidney works.

Science and Cancer, Michael B. Shimkin. U.S. Department of Health, Education and Welfare, 1964 (paperback). An excellent book addressed primarily to the reader outside the scientific community. A very readable account of cancer and the efforts of science and medicine to control it.

Normal Growth and Cancer, Grace Medes and Stanley P. Reimann. J. B. Lippincott, Philadelphia, 1963. A good survey of current knowledge in the field.

Cancer and Public Education, John Wakefield. Charles C Thomas, Springfield, Ill., 1963. The executive director of the Manchester (England) Committee on Cancer makes known the results of his vast experience and thoughts on cancer education.

Prostate Cancer: Needless Killer, J. D. Ratcliff. Reader's Digest, September 1963, p. 147. Male college students should read this informative article.

New Weapon Against Cancer, J. D. Ratcliff. Today's Health, July 1960, p. 50. Description of a modified use of the heart-lung machine in the treatment of cancer.

Breast Self-examination. National Cancer Institute, Superintendent of Documents, U. S. Government Printing Office, Washington, D. C. A well illustrated pamphlet on breast examination for cancer.

The Savage Cell, Pat McGrady. Basic Books, New York, 1964. The science editor of the American Cancer Society has written a comprehensive book about cancer that should be read by all college students. Vividly discussed are such related factors as environment, food, drugs, air pollution, occupation, tobacco, radiation, emotions, hormones, heredity, and many others. Written for the layman.

The student will find the following publications of the American Heart Association and the American Cancer Society very readable and enlightening.

Heart Disease Caused by Coronary Atherosclerosis.
Facts About Heart and Blood Vessel Diseases.
Questions and Answers About Heart and Blood Vessel Diseases.
If Your Child Has a Congenital Heart Defect.
101 Questions About Cancer.
Cancer Facts and Figures (annually).
Youth Looks at Cancer.
Facing the Facts About Cancer.

OTHER POTENTIAL KILLERS

These diseases are killers primarily because of our indifference or ignorance about them.

The tremendous advances in medicine since the turn of the century have added 22 years to our life span. To accomplish this feat, it was necessary to check a number of would-be-killers—for example, pneumonia, tuberculosis, diabetes, and appendicitis. We are able now to defend ourselves against several once dreaded diseases—but only if we utilize the knowledge that our painstaking scientists have accumulated. That many people ignore this knowledge each year is indicated by often senseless deaths.

To the list of senseless killers, we have added suicide and accidents. It is in our power to defend against these killers if only we will take the trouble to do so.

PNEUMONIA

Pneumonia is an infection of the lungs that partially solidifies the normally spongy tissues of this important organ. This is the reason the doctor hears a "solid" instead of a "hollow" sound when he taps the chest of a patient with pneumonia.

This disease is caused by either the *pneumococcus* or certain other *bacteria,* or by *viruses,* and both types are infectious. Most people carry the microorganisms in their throats all the time, but don't succumb to the disease unless the body is weakened and their resistance to infection becomes lowered. The time to be most on guard against pneumonia is a few days after an ordinary cold begins, and during and after an attack of influenza, whooping cough or measles. Overexposure to cold after intensive sweating and insufficient rest also create conditions favorable for pneumonia.

Lobar pneumonia is the term used if the disease affects the lobes of the lung,

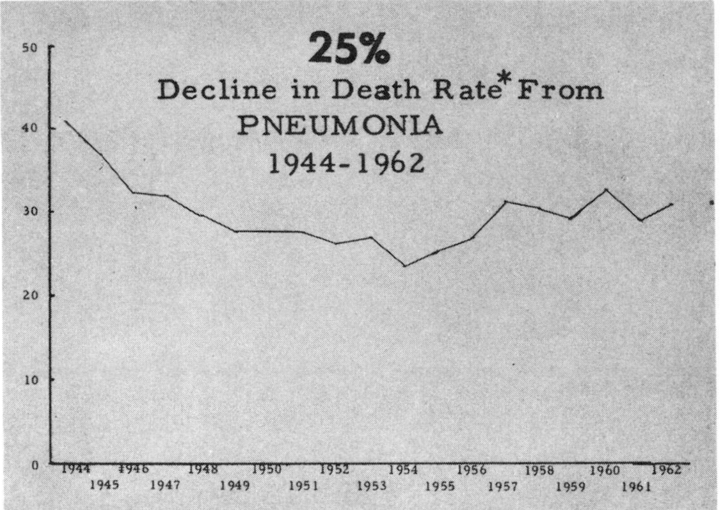

Figure 19–1. Decline in death rate from pneumonia. (From *Facts on the Major Killing and Crippling Diseases in the United States Today.* The National Health Education Committee, Inc., 1964.)

and when both lobes are affected, it is called *bilateral* or *double* pneumonia. *Bronchopneumonia* is localized in or around the bronchial tubes and is usually, but not necessarily, milder than lobar pneumonia.

The *symptoms* of this disease are a cough, sharp chest pains, blood-streaked sputum, and a high fever which is generally preceded by a chill. Anyone with these danger signals should get into bed immediately and remain there until the doctor arrives.

Bacterial pneumonia was one of the leading killers a generation ago, but today, thanks to penicillin and other antibiotics as well as the sulfa drugs, the danger to the patient's life has been practically eliminated if treatment is started in time. Miraculous as they are, these drugs are not effective if the disease process has made too much headway.

Virus pneumonia is also called *primary atypical pneumonia* because it was once far less common than the bacterial variety. But now that pneumonias due to bacteria are under control, the virus type has become quite prevalent. Fortunately, it is rarely fatal except in patients with advanced heart disease or other complicating illness. Antibiotics are also employed in the treatment of virus pneumonias, but with limited success.

When the mucous membranes of the *bronchi,* the tubes which lead from the windpipe to the lungs, are inflamed, the condition is called *bronchitis. Acute* bronchitis is often referred to as a chest cold, and is usually associated with an elevated temperature, chest pains, cough and loss of energy. *Chronic* bronchitis, with its characteristic dry cough and, sometimes, shortness of breath, may follow repeated attacks of acute bronchitis. People who live in damp and foggy areas tend to develop bronchial afflictions more often than those in dry climates. Bronchitis usually responds to good nursing care, rest and antibiotic therapy.

SUICIDE

Self-destruction ranks seventh among the causes of death in the United States for the entire population, and third for the 15 to 24 year age range, outranked only by accidents and cancer. More than 19,000 people are known to die each year by suicide, twice as many as by homicide; many more are saved from attempted suicide. The true figure is probably even higher than 19,000 because the moral and religious stigma attached to taking one's own life makes many families conceal the real cause of death.

Many countries have much higher rates than ours, which is 10.1 per 100,000 adults, but some are also considerably lower.

Nearly four times as many men commit suicide as women, but women attempt or threaten to do so more often. Firearms and explosives are the commonest way out for men, followed by hanging and poisons, whereas women most frequently choose poisons, very commonly barbiturates. The incidence for both sexes rises sharply with age, reaching its peak in men between the ages of 50 and 65, and in women, 40 to 55.

Although the incidence rate of suicide is lower among young people than adults, it has become sufficiently high to cause concern among parents, educators, and doctors. In fact, suicidal adolescents and children represent 3 per cent of all suicides.

Suicides are motivated by many complex factors, but one of the most important considerations is severe depression. Certainly not every depressed person commits or even thinks of suicide as an answer to his melancholy, but it is most frequent among depressed psychotic patients, and also occurs in other psychoses and serious neurotic illnesses. Sociological factors are also important: it is three times more common among whites than among Negroes, and greater among the economically well-off professional persons than among the nonprofessionals, and among white-collar workers as compared with laborers. An individual's integration with the world around him is also reflected in the suicide rate, and he is much less likely to attempt self-destruction if he has a deep, intimate relationship with other people than if he is isolated from truly meaningful relationships.[1] For example, suicide is more common among individuals who live alone or in boarding-houses, among the single, widowed, and divorced than the married, and among people in urban areas than rural areas. The rural rate is only half the urban rate.

Contrary to popular opinion, most suicides occur in the early morning, and not in the sad, dark hours of the night; on Monday and Tuesday, and not on the lonely weekends; in late spring and early summer, instead of on cold, depressing winter days. Perhaps the reason is the psychological weakness or inability to face a new day, a new week, a new season. The tensions of the premenstrual period also increase suicides at this time of the month.

The prevention of suicide is extremely difficult, but certain clues and premonitory symptoms can be very helpful. Chief among these are chronic insomnia, especially early morning awakening, loss of interest in customary activities and sexual drive, mental and physical sluggishness, and despondency to the point of despair.[2] If such symptoms become chronic or severe, the individual or his family should be alerted to the danger, and seek psychiatric help. The most critical period for such individuals is the first three months after an emotional crisis or after leaving a psychiatric hospital; almost half the suicides occur within this period. For this reason, physicians and the patient's family must be very alert during these months, even if the patient seems to be improving.

Our hope for the future is that the teaching of mental hygiene at an early age, the extension and greater use of guidance by teachers and religious leaders, and an increased awareness of danger signs by physicians and families will bring about a reduction of the suicide rates throughout the world.

TUBERCULOSIS

Tuberculosis is an ancient disease, yet it has serious implications for us, even in this second half of the twentieth century. Judging from bone changes seen in mummies which were buried before 2000 B.C., it apparently affected the early Egyptians. The Babylonians also referred to this disease and Hippocrates described "consumption" in some detail. The famous Greek physician, Galen, who practiced in the second century, wrote about the possibility of transmitting tuberculosis from one person to another.

There is evidence that more than half the human race contracts tuberculosis at some time during their lives; the lungs of

---

[1]Schneidman, E. S., and Farberow, N. L.: *Clues to Suicide*, Blakiston, McGraw-Hill, New York, 1957.

[2]Kavanaugh, P. R.: *Marquette Medical Review*, *22*:33, 1956.

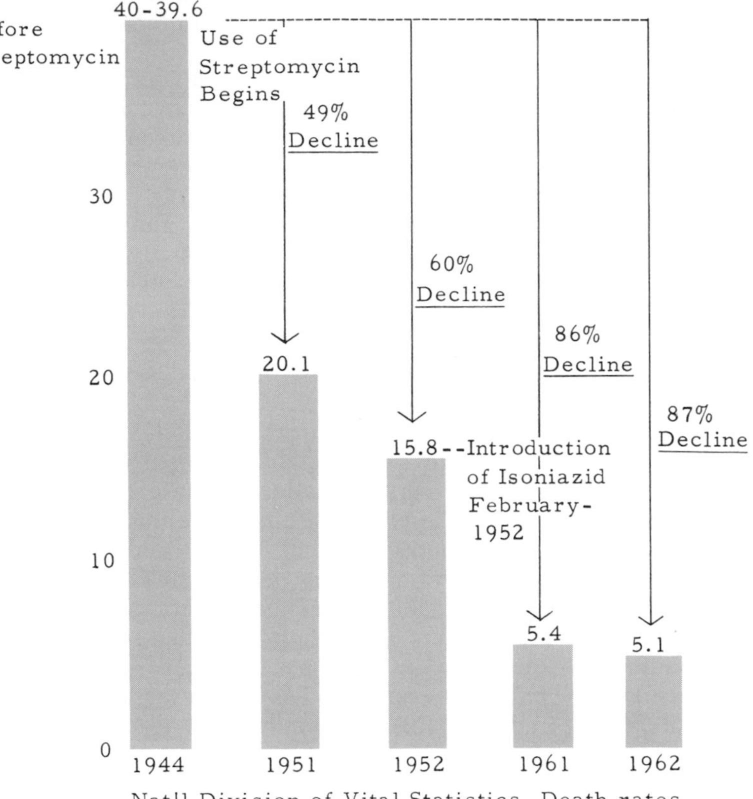

Figure 19–2. Decline in the tuberculosis death rate. (From *Facts on the Major Killing and Crippling Diseases in the United States Today.* The National Health Education Committee, Inc., 1964.)

many of us show old scars of tuberculosis even though we were never aware of the disease.

The microorganism responsible, the *tubercle bacillus,* was first isolated in 1882 by Robert Koch, who had wanted to be an explorer but became a village doctor instead. Actually, Koch became a splendid explorer—but in medicine, a far different field.

In the past 50 years, there has been a tremendous decline in deaths from tuberculosis. A survey made in 1857 in Massachusetts indicated that out of every 100,000 people 450 died of tuberculosis. By 1900, the national death rate in the United States was down to 194 per 100,000 population, still a sizeable figure, but by 1963, this figure had declined to the record low of 5.1 deaths per 100,000 population. Unfortunately, the *decline in death rates is not paralleled by a corresponding decrease in the number of new cases of this disease. It is still very much with us, because of a tremendous reservoir of undiagnosed and untreated cases, who are a constant threat and source of infection.* The National Tuberculosis Association estimates that there are about 250,000 active cases of tuberculosis in the United States, and that *100,000 of these are not known to health officials and are therefore not receiving treatment.* In addition, there are about 1,750,000 inactive cases—individuals who have had active tuberculosis at some time in their lives.

It is true that many tuberculosis sanitaria

Table 19–1. Death rate from tuberculosis*

Year	*Number*	*Rate per 100,000*
1963	9660	5.1
1962	9506	5.1
1961	9938	5.4
1960	10,866	6.1
1959	11,456	6.5
1958	12,361	7.1
1957	13,324	7.8
1956	14,061	8.4
1955	14,940	9.1
1954	16,392	10.2

*From Vital Statistics Report, U. S. Department of Health, Education and Welfare, March, 1963.

have closed down, and that fewer hospital beds are being occupied by tubercular patients. Still, the number of people receiving some hospitalization is now greater than ever. Fortunately, newer methods of therapy have cut down the length of the hospitalization period required.

The most striking change in tuberculosis incidence is the shift in death rates in various age groups. New cases continue to be reported in young people, but today the disease in this age group is much less likely to be fatal. This is certainly a tremendous advance because the decrease in deaths during the most productive years of life is a great social gain. However, statistics prove that we should abandon the once prevalent belief that tuberculosis is uncommon among old people. It is frequent, and it is serious. Some years ago a tuberculosis sanitarium resembled a college dormitory. Today, it is more like an old folks' home.

The economic distribution of tuberculosis has also changed decidedly. A few generations ago, it could be found in all classes. Today, it is associated primarily with low-income groups, and especially with unskilled laborers and their families, and the Negro in America carries a heavy tuberculosis load.

How Tuberculosis Is Contracted

Tubercle bacilli usually attack the lungs, although they may also invade the kidneys, lymph nodes, skin, larynx, bones, joints, intestines and even the male and female genitals. Only rarely is the heart, liver or brain involved. These microorganisms work more slowly than many other infectious agents, which gives us valuable time to fight the disease before it can do permanent damage. But although it takes a long time for tuberculosis to develop, it may take even longer to cure it.

A certain number of tuberculosis cases are caused by *unpasteurized* milk and other dairy products. However, tuberculosis of the *lungs* develops when bacteria in sputum are transferred to healthy people from the lungs of an infected person who coughs or sneezes without protection. It can also be spread by kissing or by using contaminated eating utensils. Some patients discharge the microorganisms in their stools, and pass them on to others if they are careless in their toilet habits. *But the chief method of spread is coughing, and the tubercle bacilli can live for months in dried sputum.*

When the microorganisms reach the lungs and begin to multiply there, the body rushes its defenses to the infected area and is almost always victorious in this first skirmish, killing some of the bacilli and walling off the remainder with tough scar tissue. Although the imprisoned organisms stay alive, they are rendered powerless and this first infection usually causes no symptoms.

A simple skin test, the *tuberculin test,* enables a physician to determine whether tubercle bacilli have entered the body. If this is positive, an x-ray should be taken to find out whether the bacteria are safely imprisoned or are active and causing disease.

Resistance

Resistance to tuberculosis depends primarily on two factors: the condition of the body and the extent of exposure. *Poor health* due to chronic fatigue, inade-

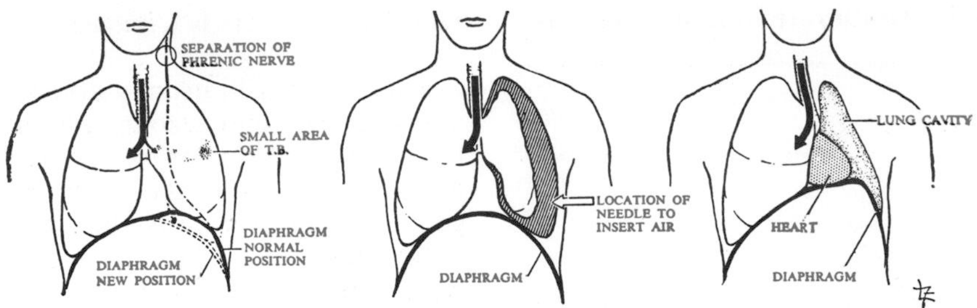

Figure 19–3. Surgical treatments for pulmonary tuberculosis. **Left,** The phrenic nerve is separated, immobilizing one side of the diaphragm. This helps keep the lung at rest while scar tissue forms. **Center,** Artificial pneumothorax. Air is periodically introduced into the lung cavity to collapse one lung and thus completely immobilize it temporarily. **Right,** Complete removal of lung. Tissue in process of filling the gap.

quate nutrition or other illness, and crowded, substandard living conditions can lower the body's defenses and permit the bacilli to gain a foothold. However, even a healthy person may not be able to withstand repeated exposure to the bacilli, or brief contact with overwhelming numbers. This might happen if a husband or wife didn't know the other had active tuberculosis, and even more often when a child is exposed to a tuberculous person, because children are particularly susceptible to this disease.

Symptoms of Tuberculosis

The symptoms most people associate with this infection—cough, fever, loss of weight, and hemorrhage from the lungs—rarely appear when the disease is in its early and easily curable stage. However, *loss of pep, poor appetite, loss of weight,* and *low-grade fever* may be early warning signals, and only an x-ray of the lungs can indicate whether these symptoms are actually due to tuberculosis or to some other illness.

Treatment and Cure

Years ago, everyone placed great faith in climate as a cure for tuberculosis. Today we realize that there is no magic in any particular climate or area of the country, and now every state and many large cities have excellent sanitoria. In recent years, new medicines have been developed for this disease, such as *streptomycin, PAS (para-aminosalicylate),* and *isoniazid.* Although these have proved to be very helpful, none of them is "the magic bullet," even when they are given in combination. However, their use has markedly reduced the period of hospitalization required for treatment.

Medication alone is not always enough and, in some cases, it must be supplemented with surgery or other methods of treatment. In *pneumothorax,* air is injected into the space around the affected lung to collapse the lung and aid healing by putting the infected area at rest. *Crushing the phrenic nerve,* which moves the diaphragm by carrying the electrical impulse to it from the brain, prevents the diaphragm—and therefore the lung, as well—from moving on the affected side of the chest.

In *thoracoplasty,* the lung is collapsed by cutting out portions of several ribs. The chest wall caves in and holds the affected lung firmly, like a splint, permitting the infected portion to rest. *Pneumonectomy* means surgical removal of part, or even all, of a lung, and is performed much more frequently and safely now that we have such excellent anti-bacterial drugs.

Tuberculosis of the lymph glands, kidneys, genitals and other tissues is treated in much the same way as lung tuberculosis, by rest and medicines.

Prevention of Tuberculosis

The major factors in prevention are keeping in good condition, avoiding unnecessary exposure to tubercle bacilli, and detecting the disease in its earliest stages. A burning match may go out by itself, but *it may also cause a fire*. Why not put it out when it can easily be extinguished?

Here are some important rules to follow:

1. Have a medical checkup every year, and be sure it includes a tuberculin test. Your doctor can decide if and when a chest x-ray is necessary.
2. See your physician if you have a cough, cold or bronchitis that doesn't clear up in two or three weeks, if you are constantly tired or listless, lose weight, have pains in your chest, "night sweats" or fever, or cough up blood or blood-streaked sputum.
3. Keep your resistance high by regular and sufficient rest, well balanced meals, and relaxation.
4. Use only pasteurized milk and milk products.
5. Keep a good distance from people who cough and fail to cover their mouths with handkerchiefs or tissues.
6. Wash your hands before meals or after you have touched anything which might be contaminated—for example, after riding in a bus, streetcar, or subway.
7. A checkup for tuberculosis should always precede marriage.
8. If you have a family history of tuberculosis, be sure to tell your physician and to be especially careful about observing these rules. Although tuberculosis is not inherited, it does appear more frequently in some families than in others.
9. If you have had close contact with someone who has developed tuberculosis, be sure to have a checkup immediately, and again in six months. But don't get panicky about it. Being exposed doesn't necessarily mean that you have been infected.

What About Vaccines For Tuberculosis?

The only vaccine we have available at the present time for this disease is the one called BCG (Bacillus Calmette Guérin, after its inventors), and, unfortunately, there are certain possible hazards in its use. The chief objection to BCG is that it interferes with tuberculin testing. However, the vaccine is being used in population groups exposed to a large number of people with tuberculosis. For example, many medical students and student nurses at medical schools and hospitals in Pennsylvania are being vaccinated with BCG if they show a negative reaction to tuberculin.

Since the beginning of this century, tuberculosis has dropped from number one to number fifteen in the list of killers. This has not happened by accident. Our knowledge of this disease should make it possible to remove it from the list entirely, to force this enemy into unconditional surrender.

DIABETES

The word *diabetes* comes from the Greek for *fountain,* and was used to describe this disease because excessive urination is such a characteristic symptom. *Mellitus* means *sweet* or *sugary,* and the scientific name for the disease is *diabetes mellitus,* describing the sugary urine.

In diabetes, there is a relative or absolute deficiency of *insulin,* and the body's ability to burn sugar or starches is impaired. Normally this hormone is produced in adequate amounts by the pancreas, but in the diabetic either too little insulin is produced or its effects are counteracted by over-activity in other glands.

No matter how much the untreated diabetic eats—and he is apt to eat a great deal—he is always hungry and thirsty, because without insulin, sugar cannot be utilized properly, and the body is deprived of an essential food. As a result, in untreated diabetes much of the sugar is excreted in the urine. However, it piles up faster in the blood than the body can eliminate it, and this reduces resistance to infection. Diabetic patients who are not taking insulin are also apt to feel weak, tired, and nauseated, and they may develop even more serious symptoms later.

Symptoms

Everyone should be alert for the following symptoms of diabetes:

1. Excessive thirst and urination (in children, bed wetting may be a sign).
2. Loss of weight, especially if there is increased consumption of food.
3. Decreased resistance to infection—often manifested in frequent boils and carbuncles.

Even in its early stages, diabetes can be detected by testing the urine and the blood for sugar. A complete physical examination should always include an analysis of the urine.

The Magnitude of the Diabetes Problem

Diabetes warrants careful consideration because it is a surprisingly widespread disease with potentially serious consequences. *One person in eighty of the general population is diabetic,* according to several surveys which have been made; and among students of college age, about one in a hundred.[3] Unfortunately, only about half the community's diabetics have been diagnosed, and the remainder don't know they have the disease.

Every year 65,000 additional people are added to the roster of diabetics, part of the group of nearly 5 million potential diabetics. One person in four of the general population is a carrier, a nondiabetic individual who can transmit the tendency to diabetes to his or her offspring.

A survey made by H. L. C. Wilkerson and L. P. Krall covering 71 per cent of the population in a New England town revealed three hidden diabetics for every four persons known to have the disease.[4] Similar studies by other investigators have

[3] Reinberg, M. H., Greenley, P. O., and Littlefield, M. S.: *Journal of the American Medical Association, 148*:1177, 1952.

[4] *Journal of the American Medical Association, 152*:1322, 1953.

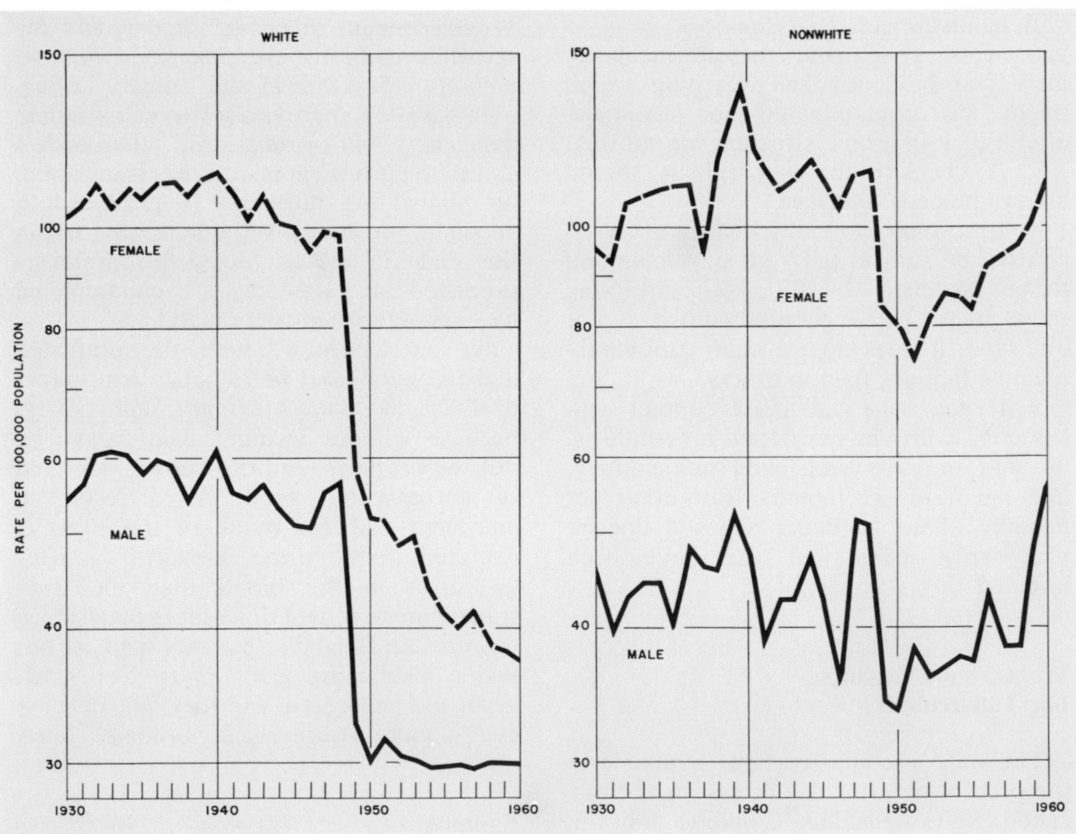

Figure 19–4. Death rates for diabetes, in the 54 to 64 year age group by color and sex. (From *Vital and Health Statistics,* Series 3, No. 1, 1964.)

Table 19–2. Incidence of diabetes in the United States

Classification	*Number*
Known diabetics	1,000,000
Undiagnosed diabetics	1,000,000
Potential diabetics	4,750,000
Genetic carriers of diabetes	40,000,000

sometimes shown a 1:1 ratio of known to unknown cases.

M. Margolin and his associates of Omaha, Nebraska, found that 38 per cent of the hidden diabetics they diagnosed were overweight, 45 per cent showed a positive family history of diabetes, and 62 per cent were over 40 years of age.[5]

The longevity of the diabetic has improved tremendously since the advent of insulin, better understanding of the disease, and improved methods of treatment. But the diabetic must still anticipate a shorter life than that of the general population.

Diabetes is a serious risk for women of the childbearing age, and it affects the fertility of males. Alan Rubin of the University of Pennsylvania reported that about 25 per cent of diabetic men in the 30 to 34 year age group are impotent, and that by the age of 50 to 54, this figure increases to approximately 54 per cent. Also, the wives of diabetic men had significantly more spontaneous abortions and miscarriages than the wives of a control group of nondiabetic men.[6] Potency may return when the disease is stabilized.

The hazards of childbearing in diabetic women are very high. Excessively large fetuses occur in more than 50 per cent of diabetic pregnancies, and spontaneous abortion is considerably greater than in nondiabetic mothers. There are also more complications during pregnancy and a higher proportion of congenital defects in the babies. Although it is still considerably greater than in nondiabetic women, maternal mortality in diabetics dropped 25 to 50 per cent to values of 1.5 to 2 per cent with the advent of insulin. The baby has a better chance of being saved, too, if the diabetes is detected and treated before pregnancy.

Vascular Complications

One of the complications of diabetes which even insulin has not controlled is the development of *arteriosclerosis* in diabetics who have had the disease for 10 to 15 years. This explains the extreme importance of controlling infections in the diabetic, especially in the extremities. A decreased blood supply to the feet is very common; the feet are cold and there is slow healing of injuries, sometimes leading to ulceration and gangrene. Diabetes is a significant cause of blindness, because arteriosclerosis of the retina causes a gradual dimming of vision, and in a certain percentage of cases, complete loss of sight. It can also affect the blood vessels of the heart and the kidneys.

Treatment of Diabetes

Until about 40 years ago, the only therapy for diabetics was to try to eliminate sugars and starches from their diet. The small amount of insulin manufactured in all but the most severe cases might then be enough to control sugar metabolism. This treatment is still the best and simplest one for mild, borderline cases in adults, but diet alone cannot cure severe diabetes or diabetes in children. In the past, they were doomed to waste away or die in coma.

Now that insulin is available, even the most severe types can be controlled. Diabetic children can grow to healthy adulthood and lead normal, active lives. The individual who cannot manufacture his own insulin can obtain the identical hormone extracted from animal glands.

Insulin is useless if taken by mouth and must be injected under the skin. Fortunately the preparations available today release insulin very slowly, and only one or two injections a day are needed. If too much insulin is taken, however, or too little food eaten after it has been injected, the blood sugar may fall to a subnormal level and bring on tremors, cold sweats, a feeling of acute hunger, and, in extreme

[5]*Nebraska Medical Journal, 41*:419, 1956.

[6]Studies in Human Reproduction, *American Journal of Obstetrics and Gynecology, 76*:25, 1958.

cases, *insulin shock*. This type of reaction calls for emergency treatment: the simplest one is for the patient to eat a few lumps of sugar or drink sweetened orange juice.

Diabetic acidosis is just the opposite of an insulin reaction and is caused by too much sugar and not enough insulin. It may develop if injections are neglected or too much food eaten, and the symptoms are deep breathing, tremendous thirst, and dryness of the skin and tongue, as well as nausea and vomiting.

Oral Substitutes for Insulin

There has always been a great deal of interest in an oral insulin preparation or a substitute for insulin which could be taken by mouth. In recent years, studies of several derivatives of the antibacterial sulfonamides have shown that they have an insulin-like action. This led to the synthesis and trial of other compounds with similar action. Two which have received a good deal of attention and publicity are called *Orinase* and *DBI* (the latter is not a sulfonamide derivative).

Specialist in diabetes have varied reactions to these drugs, ranging from great enthusiasm to complete rejection. The present feeling is that they are neither cures for diabetes nor substitutes for insulin. They appear to be helpful in treating older diabetics, but not young diabetics, nor individuals who acquired the disease when they were young. However, this research is moving in a very hopeful direction, and perhaps an effective oral insulin substitute for all diabetics will someday be made available.

Indeed, Panayotis G. Katsoyannis headed a research team at the University of Pittsburgh that, in 1964, produced synthetic insulin for the first time. This accomplishment opened the door to a better understanding of some of the unresolved problems of diabetes.

APPENDICITIS

In the lower right abdomen, at the junction of the small and large intestines, is a little wormlike appendage called the *vermiform appendix*. (*Vermiform* literally

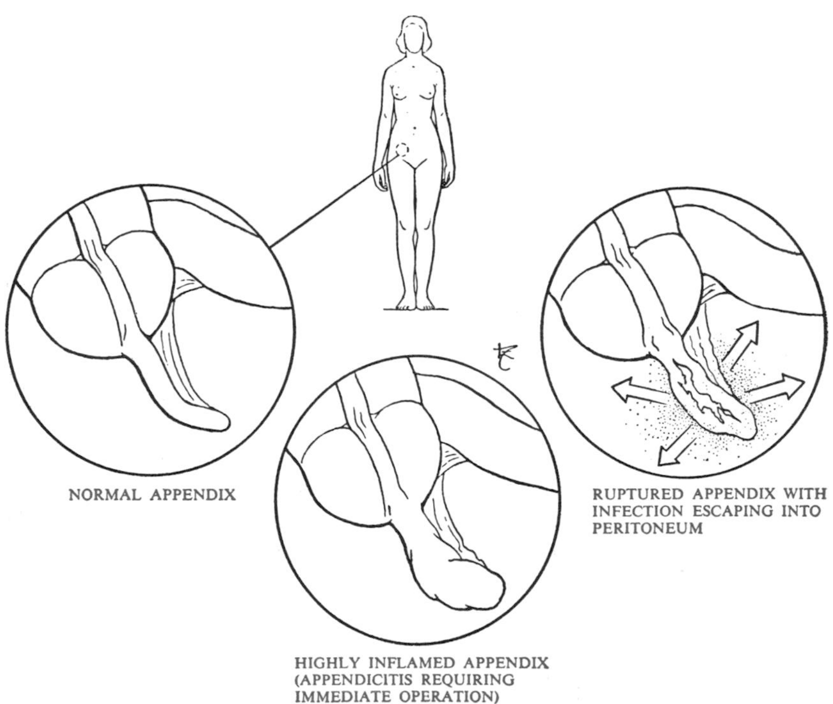

Figure 19–5. Appendicitis and ruptured appendix.

means "shaped like a worm.") This structure is part of the digestive tract in herbivorous animals, and it is often as long as the entire large intestine. But in humans it is a useless and potentially dangerous vestigial organ which we no longer need.

The appendix is a hollow tube, which sometimes becomes plugged by fecal matter or other material. This prevents the normal drainage from taking place, and the appendix then becomes susceptible to infection by bacteria. It is a fertile soil for bacterial activities, and when they multiply they can cause a severe inflammation. You can visualize the situation as a sort of boil which will rupture into the peritoneal cavity unless the body's defenses overcome the infection or the surgeon removes the inflamed appendix before the boil breaks and discharges its pus.

When the appendix becomes inflamed and infected, the process can spread so fast that gangrene and rupture may set in within a matter of hours. The chief danger from this is that rupture of the appendix may lead to peritonitis, one of the most serious of all diseases. In the past 25 years, the death rate from appendicitis has been reduced by 90 per cent. Still, in 1963, 2000 Americans died from this infection and most of them could have been saved if they had obtained early treatment. This death rate could probably be reduced almost to zero by prompt recognition of an inflamed appendix and by avoiding certain hazards in treating it. Unfortunately, the infection cannot be prevented, but early diagnosis makes medical therapy and surgical removal of the organ possible before complications set in.

Appendicitis ranks high in the list of killer diseases for children between the ages of 10 and 14, but it is most prevalent from the ages of 10 to 30. However, no age is completely immune. Fortunately, it is extremely uncommon in the first two years of life. Otherwise pediatricians who see so many intestinal upsets in infants would be even more harassed than they are now.

The three main symptoms of appendicitis are *nausea, abdominal pain* which starts to localize in the lower right part over the appendix area, and mild *fever* in adults. In young children the fever may be very high, and there may also be vomiting, constipation, or diarrhea.

In addition to these symptoms, the doctor looks for positive evidence of an inflamed appendix, such as tenderness over the appendix when pressure is exerted, or pain in the region of the appendix during an examination through the rectum, or through the vagina in the female patient. A laboratory test, the white blood count, is also helpful in making the diagnosis.

Peritonitis and *abscess* formation are the major complications of appendicitis.

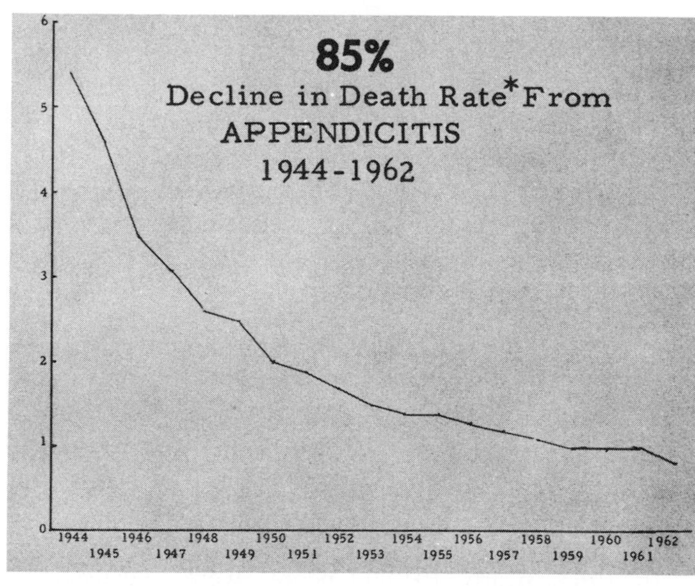

Figure 19–6. Decline in death rate from appendicitis. (From *Facts on the Major Killing and Crippling Diseases in the United States Today.* The National Health Education Committee, Inc., 1964.)

Acute appendicitis is usually treated by removing the diseased appendix surgically. In certain cases, especially mild, chronic inflammations, the physician merely uses bed rest, no food, and plenty of antibiotics. Many cases treated in this way will settle down, and not require surgery.

One of the major dangers in appendicitis is the use of laxatives. Statistics show that when a person with appendicitis takes a laxative, his chance of dying is three times as great as it would be otherwise. With more than one dose of a laxative, the possibility of dying is seven times as great. This is due to the fact that laxatives or cathartics increase intestinal activity and may also increase the pressure within the little sac. The more pressure, the more likelihood that the sac will burst. The same is true for enemas. Delay in operating also lessens the chance of a cure.

Any abdominal pain lasting for more than three or four hours may be appendicitis. There are five common sense rules to follow if appendicitis is suspected.

1. *Call your doctor immediately.* If you have no doctor you can obtain a thorough examination for appendicitis in the emergency room of any reliable hospital. You should be taken there by auto or taxi, if possible.
2. *Lie down and remain as quiet as possible.* Do not massage the abdomen.
3. *Take NOTHING by mouth—no food, water, or medicines. Especially avoid cathartics or laxatives.*
4. *Don't take an enema.*
5. *Don't use a hot water bottle.* If the pain becomes very severe, apply an ice pack.

ACCIDENTS

The tremendous advances in medicine since the turn of the century have added 22 years to our life span. A child born today can expect to live 71 years, as compared to 49 years in 1900. Unfortunately, these advances in medicine have had little or no influence on death or injury by accidents.

From the ages of 1 to 25, accidents represent the leading cause of death. More than 50 per cent are now due to motor vehicles.

In 1963, nearly 101,000 people were killed and 10.1 million injured in all types of accidents, the majority of which were preventable. Motor vehicles are the major cause, followed by falls, drowning, and fire. Males have about twice the chance of being either killed or injured in accidents as have females.

The cost of accidents exceeds 16 billion dollars in wage losses, hospital and medical fees, and damage to property.

Most people, especially younger ones, take a fatalistic attitude about these figures. "I'm not a statistic," they say. "It won't happen to me." Unfortunately, statistics do not selectively examine our dreams and aspirations before including us.

By knowledge and preventive action, we can reduce the chances of becoming an "accident statistic." Therefore, as individuals and as a nation, we must recognize the magnitude of this tragic health problem, and give to accident prevention the serious attention and study it deserves.

AUTOMOBILE ACCIDENTS

The National Safety Council reports a motor vehicle death every 12 minutes and a motor vehicle injury every 20 seconds during the past five years. The death rate today is about the same as that in the Korean War, and has increased from 1700 per year in 1910 to over 43,600 per year in the past few years. For every person killed in an automobile accident, nearly 37 were injured and sometimes permanently disabled. In 1963, this added up to 43,600 deaths and 1,600,000 injuries.

Not until automobile manufacturers and drivers decide to forego increased horsepower and speed *for every possible safety measure* will we reduce our annual gruesome toll. Doesn't it make you shudder to read before every long holiday weekend how many deaths and accidents are predicted, when you know that almost all of these, except those due to unavoidable mechanical failure, could be prevented?

Rural Versus Urban

About three fourths of automobile-caused deaths occur in rural areas, as

Table 19–3. Leading causes of all deaths

Leading causes of all deaths

	No. of Deaths	Death Rate*
All Ages	1,813,549	961
Heart disease	707,830	375
Cancer	285,362	151
Vascular lesions	201,166	107
Accidents	**100,669**	**53**
Motor-vehicle	*43,564*	*23*
Falls	*19,335*	*10*
Fires, burns	*8,172*	*4*
Drowning	*6,347*	*3*
Other	*23,251*	*13*
Under 1 Year	103,390	2,535
Postnatal asphyxia	17,934	440
Immaturity	17,857	438
Congenital malformations	14,581	358
Pneumonia	11,739	288
Birth injuries	8,954	220
Accidents	**3,514**	**86**
Mechanical suffocation	*1,200†*	*29*
Ingestion of food, object	*812*	*20*
Motor-vehicle	*321*	*8*
Fires, burns	*271*	*7*
Falls	*145*	*3*
Other	*765*	*19*
1 to 4 Years	16,571	99
Accidents	**5,174**	**31**
Motor-vehicle	*1,670*	*10*
Fires, burns	*1,069*	*7*
Drowning	*717*	*4*
Poisons (solid, liquid)	*393*	*2*
Falls	*277*	*2*
Other	*1,048*	*6*
Pneumonia	2,236	13
Congenital malformations	1,803	11
5 to 14 Years	16,524	43
Accidents	**6,962**	**18**
Motor-vehicle	*3,063*	*8*
Drowning	*1,410*	*4*
Fires, burns	*758*	*2*
Other	*1,731*	*4*
Cancer	2,616	7
Congenital malformations	1,063	3
15 to 24 Years	29,321	106
Accidents	**15,889**	**57**
Motor-vehicle	*11,123*	*40*
Drowning	*1,517*	*5*
Firearms	*620*	*2*
Railroad	*413*	*2*
Other	*2,216*	*8*
Cancer	2,334	8
Suicide	1,663	6
25 to 44 Years	107,156	230
Heart disease	21,721	47
Accidents	**20,529**	**44**
Motor-vehicle	*11,356*	*24*
Fires, burns	*1,310*	*3*
Drowning	*1,206*	*3*
Falls	*1,084*	*2*
Other	*5,573*	*12*
Cancer	18,747	40
Suicide	6,545	14
45 to 64 Years	443,389	1,170
Heart disease	175,964	465
Cancer	103,440	273
Vascular lesions	32,608	86
Accidents	**21,262**	**56**
Motor-vehicle	*9,506*	*25*
Falls	*3,015*	*8*
Fires, burns	*2,022*	*5*
Drowning	*971*	*3*
Other	*5,748*	*15*
Cirrhosis of liver	12,380	33
Pneumonia	9,599	25
65 to 74 Years	440,362	3,882
Heart disease	199,296	1,757
Cancer	83,922	740
Vascular lesions	51,050	450
Pneumonia	11,746	104
Diabetes mellitus	10,774	95
Accidents	**10,194**	**90**
Motor-vehicle	*3,786*	*33*
Falls	*3,190*	*28*
Fires, burns	*1,036*	*9*
Drowning	*302*	*3*
Other	*1,880*	*17*
General arteriosclerosis	6,152	54
Cirrhosis of liver	4,255	38
75 Years and over	656,836	10,533
Heart disease	308,951	4,954
Vascular lesions	111,779	1,792
Cancer	72,371	1,161
General arteriosclerosis	29,266	469
Pneumonia	27,391	439
Accidents	**17,145**	**275**
Falls	*11,120*	*178*
Motor-vehicle	*2,739*	*44*
Fires, burns	*1,348*	*22*
Ingestion of food, object	*189*	*3*
Drowning	*145*	*2*
Railroad	*135*	*2*
Other	*1,469*	*24*
Diabetes mellitus	10,761	173
Hypertension, not heart	6,385	102

Source: Deaths are for 1963, latest official figures from National Vital Statistics Division.

*Deaths per 100,000 population in each age group. Rates are averages for age groups, not individual ages.

†Estimated.

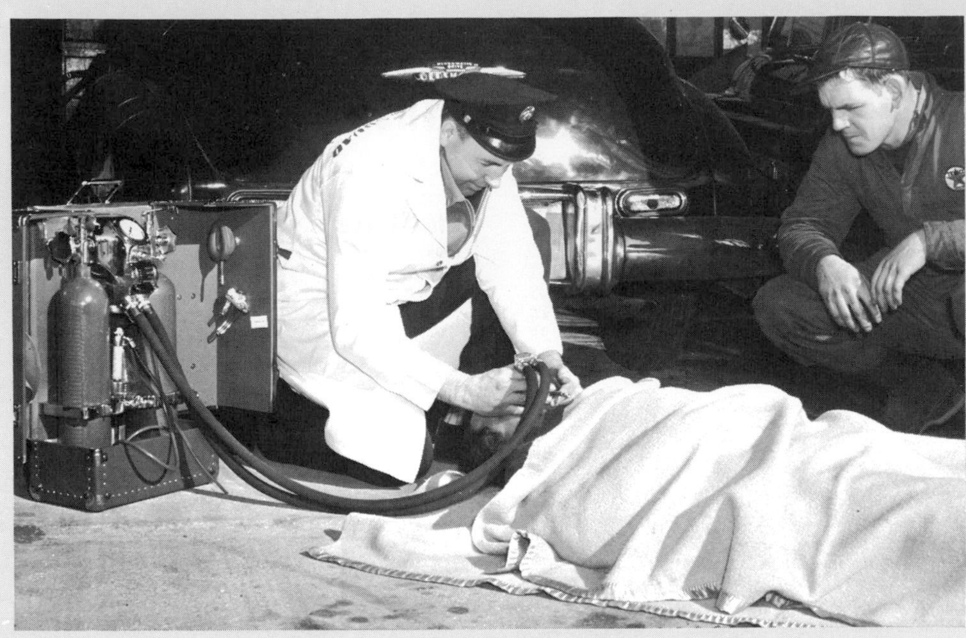

A member of a police rescue squad uses a portable resuscitator to revive a victim of carbon monoxide poisoning. Instructions for three methods of artificial respiration that do not require any equipment are given in the article ARTIFICIAL RESPIRATION.

compared with large cities. (In 1963, these figures were 31,100 and 12,500.) This is not unexpected because our cars attain higher speeds on interurban highways and country roads.

Vehicle Versus Pedestrian Accidents

Nearly four times as many deaths, 35,400 in 1963, result from collision between motor vehicles as compared with pedestrian accidents, 8200.

The Time of the Day and the Time of the Year

In both urban and rural areas, night driving is considerably more hazardous than driving by day. Throughout the United States, for every *four* deaths during the day per 100,000,000 vehicle miles driven, there were *ten* at night. The most hazardous hours for driving are shortly after midnight. At this time the fatal accident rate is ten times as high as the low rate for the day, which occurs during the late morning.

Factors Contributing to Accidents[7]

1. Three of ten drivers involved in fatal accidents were traveling at excessive *speed.*
2. The most comprehensive study to date of postmortem blood alcohol determination revealed that 62 per cent of drivers responsible for accidents had been drinking. Moreover, 53 per cent were under the influence of alcohol.

[7]This information was obtained from *Accident Facts,* 1964 Ed., National Safety Council.

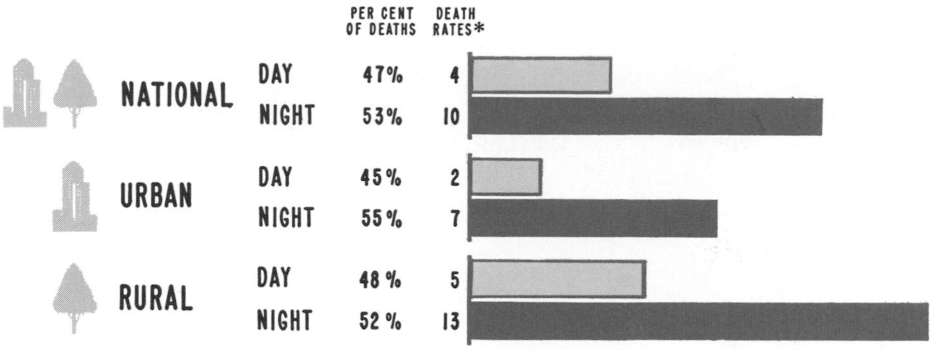

Figure 19–7. Day-night mileage death rates. (From *Accident Facts.* National Safety Council, 1965.)

3. Of the approximately 95½ million licensed drivers in the United States, the highest accident and death rate is in the under 24 age group. This means that students of college age are in the highest fatal accident age group.
4. In 1963, there were 60 million male drivers and 35½ million female drivers. Men drivers were responsible for nearly twice as many fatal accidents as women (79 per 1 billion miles driven as compared to 36 for women). These figures might be different if the sexes were compared under similar driving conditions, but more males drive during the rush hour, on rural roads, during holidays and at night.
5. *Throughout the year, Saturday and Sunday are the worst days to be on the road.* Your chances of being in a fatal smash-up are nearly twice as great on Saturday as they would be, for example, on Monday.
6. Most motor-vehicle-caused accidents are due to collisions with other automobiles. Of the 43,600 deaths from this cause in 1963, 17,600 resulted from collisions between motor vehicles, 13,900 from noncollision in the roadway including overturning and running off the road, 8200 from pedestrian accidents, 1900 from collisions with fixed objects, 1340 from collisions with railroad trains, and 90 from other collisions.
7. A driver's physical condition is related to his safety on the road. Defective vision and hearing are contributory factors, but nearly half of all accidents attributable to health and physiological factors must be blamed on the driver's actually falling asleep at the wheel. About 15 per cent result from fatigue and its concomitant inattentiveness and slowed-down reflex action.
8. The condition of the road surface may determine highway safety, and wet and icy roads present special hazards.

Suggestions That Will Make You a Better Driver

1. *Don't exceed the recommended rate of speed for the type of road you are traveling.* If the road is wet or icy, reduce your speed to the point where you have complete control over your car.

2. *Alcohol is the most dangerous traveling companion. Don't drink before or while driving.* Even a single highball affects the driving skill of some people.

Table 19–4. Motor-vehicle deaths by days and months, 1964

Day	1964 Deaths by Day		Total Deaths by Month and Average Deaths by Day											
	%	Ave.	Jan.	Feb.	Mar.	Apr.	May	Jun.	Jul.	Aug.	Sep.	Oct.	Nov.	Dec.
Total	100%	47,700	3,230	3,260	3,510	3,450	3,830	3,950	4,300	4,840	4,090	4,590	4,160	4,490
Daily Ave.		130	104	112	113	115	124	132	139	156	136	148	139	145
Monday	11%	101	81	87	88	89	96	103	108	121	106	115	108	113
Tuesday	10%	92	74	79	80	81	88	93	98	110	96	105	98	103
Wednesday	11%	101	81	87	88	89	96	103	108	121	106	115	108	113
Thursday	12%	110	88	95	96	97	105	112	118	132	115	125	118	123
Friday	16%	147	118	127	128	130	140	149	157	176	154	167	157	164
Saturday	22%	202	162	174	176	179	193	205	216	242	211	230	216	225
Sunday	18%	165	132	142	143	146	157	168	176	198	173	188	176	184

Source: Based on reports from 23 state traffic authorities.

(From *Accident Facts.* National Safety Council, 1965.)

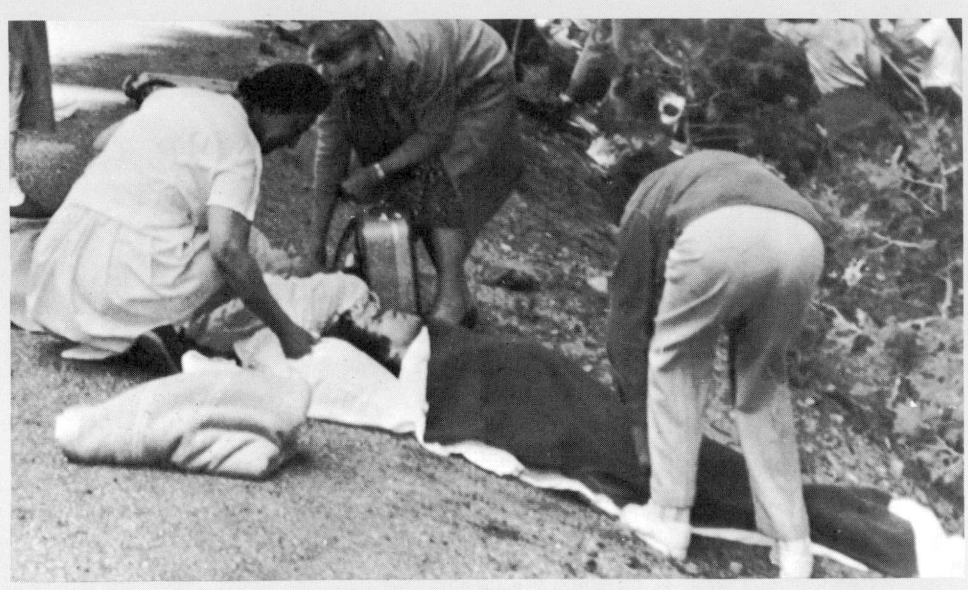

An injured person should never be moved unless absolutely necessary. Above, the patient has been covered and made comfortable, but has not been disturbed, although the feet are lower than the head.

3. *Don't trifle with fatigue.* If you are drowsy, you are a menace to yourself and all other motorists. Pull off the road and sleep.

4. *Stop driving during a heavy storm; wait until it lets up.* You can't find the center of the road if rain or snow reduce visibility to 10 per cent of normal.

5. *Turn on driving lights even during daytime if rain or snow obscures visibility.*

6. *Be on guard on Saturdays and holiday weekends for the highway demons who want to get there before anybody else.*

7. *Keep the mechanical parts of your car in perfect working order, and take advantage of every possible safety device for your car.* Use turn signals. Check brakes and tires regularly. Snow tires and antiskid tires are good investments in most parts of the country.

8. *When you see a car behind you preparing to pass, slow down.* Get ready to stop quickly, if you have to.

9. *Keep a safe distance behind the car in front of you, especially if you are traveling at high speed.*

10. *If your car is in trouble, get off the road.* Keep driving until you find a safe turn-off, even at the risk of ruining a tire which is flat. The loss of a tire is better than a collision and risk to your life.

11. *Don't ride behind a sand truck from which loose sand hits your windshield.* The glass may get so pitted that you won't have clear vision for night driving.

Safety Features for Cars

Research over the past 10 years on safety features for cars has made it perfectly clear that thousands of lives could be saved by making a few inexpensive changes in our cars. These would not prevent all the deaths and accidents that occur, but could reduce the numbers enormously. For example, a comparison of 81 car accidents in which occupants were wearing seat belts to a similar number of almost

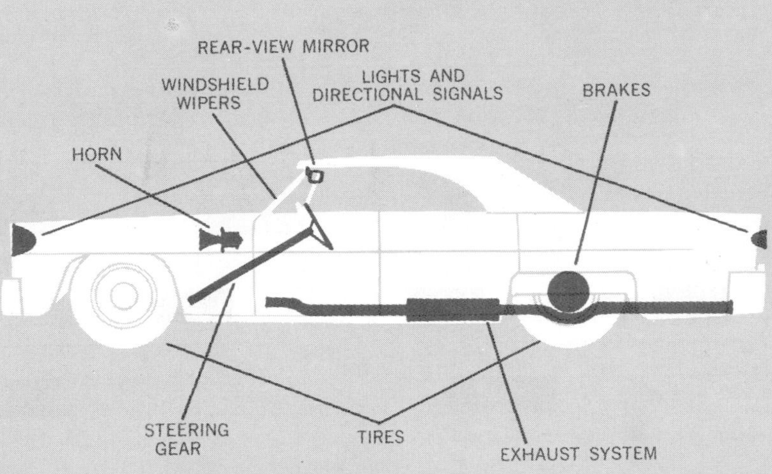

Defects in the automobile parts labeled above are responsible for the greatest number of traffic accidents caused by mechanical failure. Cars should be checked at regular intervals, and even minor defects should be attended to immediately.

Seat belts are having a dramatic effect in reducing driving accidents. They guard against three common situations which cause a driver to lose control of his car—pitching on a sudden stop or minor collision, sliding on too quick a turn, and bouncing over a bump or hole in the road.

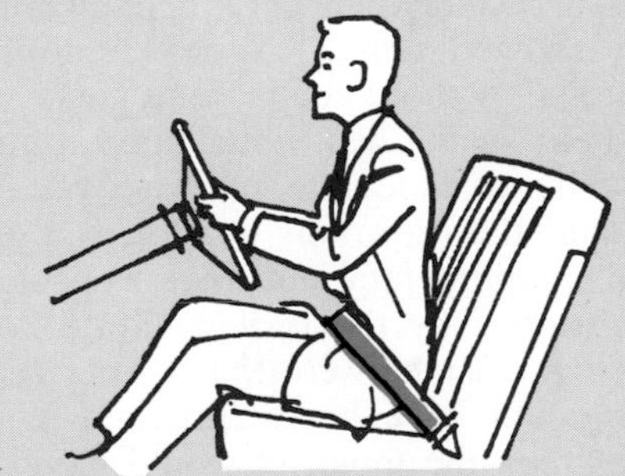

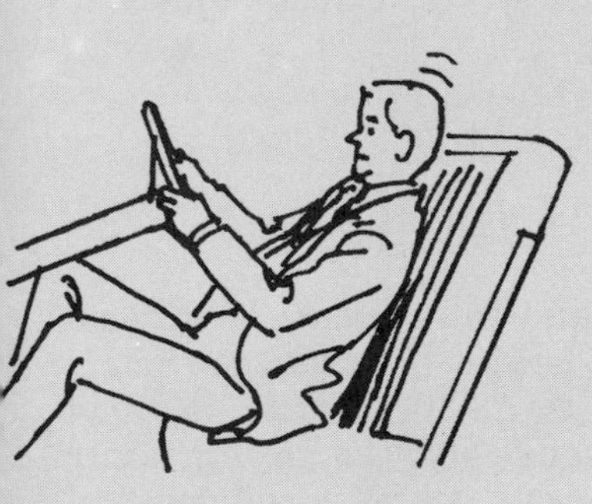

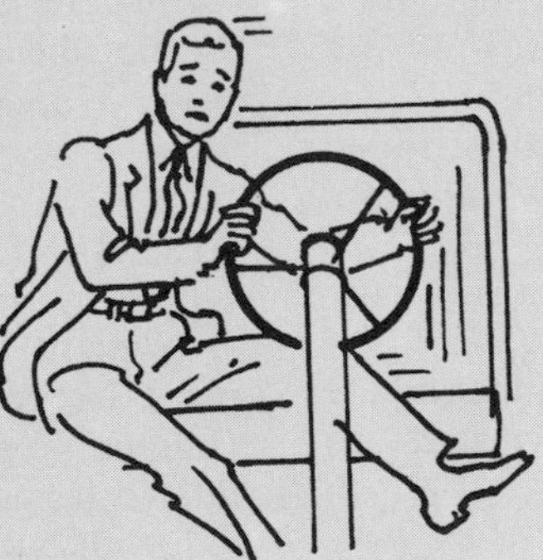

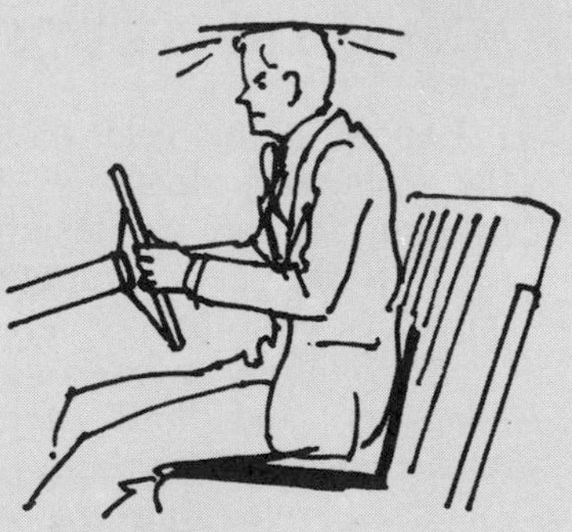

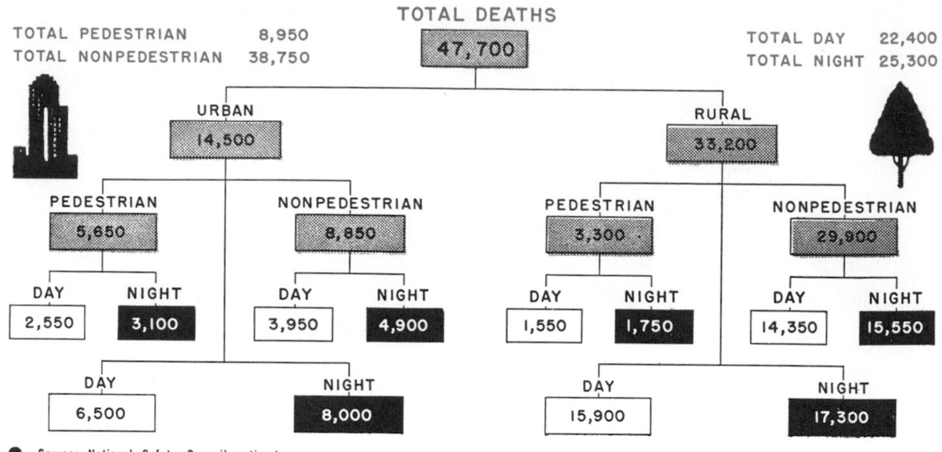

Figure 19–8. Accidental death statistics in the United States. (From *Accident Facts*. National Safety Council, 1965.)

identical accidents where belts were not worn showed that 75.5 per cent of the motorists without belts and only 29.9 per cent with belts sustained injuries. The ratio of moderate injuries was 23 to 9.2 and the ratio of deaths, 3.6 to 1.

Six hundred fatal automobile accidents were studied by the Indiana State Police. Their conclusions were that 16 per cent of these could have been classified as non-survivable—the motorist would have been killed whether his car was safety-equipped or not. *However, proper car design could have saved the lives in 503 cases (84 per cent).*

Experts in this field[8] have recommended the following features as a *minimum* program for safe car design:

1. *Reinforced bumpers* to absorb the impact of collision.
2. *Smooth car exteriors,* eliminating the "daggers" and "fins" of modern cars, so dangerous to pedestrians.
3. *Rearview mirrors mounted at mid-fender for better visibility.*
4. *White tops and dark bodies* for all cars for good visibility at night and in fog.
5. *Fully padded dashboard* to protect the driver in a collision.
6. *All equipment removed from beneath the dashboard.* Heaters could be designed so as not to protrude into the car, thereby removing a hazard to the passenger.
7. *Padded steering wheel column.*
8. *Padded doors and roof.*
9. *Better door safety locks* which wouldn't fly open on impact and let passengers be thrown out.
10. *Air vents removed from the front of car* where they suck in exhaust fumes of the car ahead.
11. *Mandatory seat belts.*

ACCIDENTS IN THE HOME

When it comes to accidents, there's no place like the home. The National Safety Council reports 28,500 *deaths* in 1964 due to home accidents. The great majority (11,900) were due to falls, and most of these occurred in elderly people. Fires destroyed 6300 and were the leading single cause of death resulting from home accidents among persons aged 1 to 64 years. Mechanical suffocation claimed 1300 victims, mostly young children.

[8]Bell, J. N.: One man's fight for safer cars, *Today's Health*, April 1959.

More than four fifths of all fatal *accidental poisonings* occur in the home, accounting for 1000 deaths. Children aged one to four are the most frequent victims. Barbiturate poisoning (sleeping pills) was most often the cause, but even aspirin tablets can be a deadly poison when eaten in large numbers by young children.

The woods take their share of human victims during hunting season, and so do our homes. Half of all fatal firearm accidents occur in the home. There were 1200 fatalities in the home from this cause in 1964.

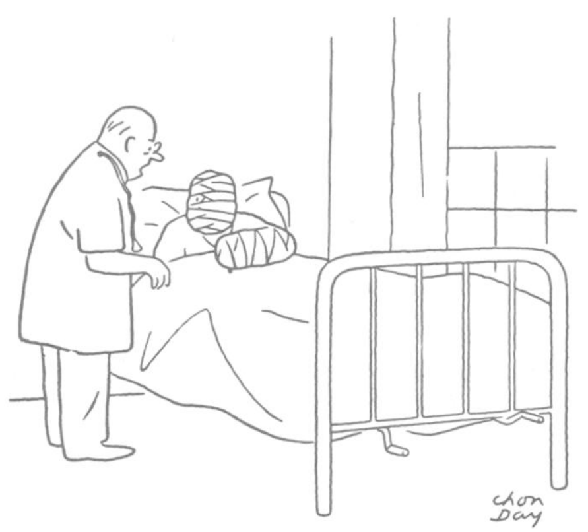

"Hmm—I don't like the looks of that eye."
(Drawing by Chon Day, Copyr. ©1948, The New Yorker Magazine, Inc.)

THE PRINCIPAL CAUSE OF DEATH IN CHILDHOOD

In both the United States and Europe, accidents are the leading cause of death among children. The risks differ from one country to another. For example, poisoning is common in countries like the United States where many chemicals are kept in the home. The fireplace, in England, and open coal heaters in Spain are definite hazards. Drowning is very frequent in Scandinavia, the Netherlands, and in France.

"DO-IT-YOURSELF" ACCIDENTS

The exciting spirit of "do it yourself" has sent the American male shopping for a host of wonderful, but potentially dangerous power tools and other equipment. Among the worst offenders are power lawnmowers, especially the rotary type, and the chief danger is injury from the rapidly moving blade to fingers, hands, toes and feet. Sharp objects thrown by the mower are also responsible for injuries, especially to the eyes.

Power saws and drills can be a menace in the hands of amateurs because these tools can saw or drill through bone almost as easily as through wood. They also carry the usual hazards of any electrical tool, and must be well grounded and never used by anyone standing on a wet surface.

Amateur plumbers do not always realize when they melt a pot of lead that it is extremely heavy and extremely hot, and it may get out of hand. If it spills, it usually lands on the feet, and can cause a very severe burn.

Ladder accidents during painting, roof repair, and television aerial installation are considerably more common among amateurs than professionals because their equipment is not so sound and reliable as

Table 19–5. Deaths from home accidents by type and age, 1964

Type of Accident	ALL AGES	0-4 Years	5-14 Years	15-24 Years	25-44 Years	45-64 Years	65-74 Years	75 Years and Over
Total	**28,500**	**5,900**	**1,500**	**1,300**	**2,400**	**3,600**	**3,200**	**10,600**
Falls	11,900	400	90	60	250	900	1,900	8,300
Fires, burns, and deaths associated with fires	6,300	1,250	750	250	900	1,400	750	1,000
Suffocation—ingested object	1,500	950	50	50	80	180	70	120
Suffocation—mechanical	1,300	1,150	50	20	20	30	10	20
Poisoning by solids, liquids	1,700	350	30	200	500	450	100	70
Firearms	1,200	70	250	300	300	200	60	20
Poisoning by gases, vapors	1,000	50	50	150	250	300	100	100
Other	3,600	1,680	230	270	100	140	210	970

Source: Estimates by National Safety Council, based on data from National Vital Statistics Division and state health departments.

that which the professional can afford to buy.

FARM ACCIDENTS

The farm may appear to be the healthiest place in the world to live, but it is definitely not the safest. Actually, rural Americans have a very high accident toll. The lessened danger from street traffic is counterbalanced by the frequency of accidents from farm machinery and other hazards. Farmers seldom have much hard cash, and understandably try to save money by not buying expensive new equipment or by not repairing materials in use. This may prove to be a dangerous economy because accidents become more frequent when machinery and vehicles become outmoded or worn out.

In 1963, for example, there were 14,200 occupational deaths throughout the United States, and 3300 of these were connected with farms. Farmers represent only about 7 per cent of the total work force. This means that their accidental death rate is almost *four times as great as the national average*. In fact, the on-the-job fatal accident rate ranks farming as the third most dangerous occupation, exceeded only by mining and construction.

HAZARDS IN INDUSTRY

Although accidental work deaths and injuries are still extremely high, they are declining because of vigorous enforcement of safety measures in good industrial establishments. Between 1912 and 1963, the accidental work death rate was reduced 62 per cent. Nevertheless, 14,200 workers lost their lives in 1963 (a death rate of 21 per 100,000 workers) and nearly two million sustained injuries at work—nearly 3 per cent of the working force. It has been pointed out by an eminent physician that there is probably no other field of medicine which offers greater scope for prevention than does the industrial field.

DROWNING

In 1963, the drowning bell tolled for 4200 Americans. The most hazardous years were 15 to 24. Almost all these lives could be saved by following the "Ten Basic Tips on Water Safety" which the American Red Cross recommends:

1. *Don't go beyond your depth,* either in the water or in a boat, until you have learned how to swim.
2. *Limit your stay in the water.* Come out before you start feeling tired or chilly.
3. Before diving in a new place, *test the water for depth* or concealed rocks or logs.
4. *Stay out of the water if you are overheated* or overtired from other exercise.
5. *Don't swim immediately after meals.* Wait an hour.
6. *Learn how to swim properly,* with a qualified instructor.
7. *Don't attempt a long swim on your first dip of the season.* Your swimming muscles have lost their strength through the winter. Train gradually.
8. *Be accompanied by a boat on a long swim.*
9. *Don't swim alone,* especially in an isolated place. Take along a water buddy.
10. *Learn how to apply artificial respiration.* Don't wait for a doctor or a mechanical respirator.

In connection with underwater swimming, you should take only two or three deep breaths before going down. Hyperventilation (excessive breathing) blows off too much carbon dioxide causing constriction of the arteries that supply the brain, and this can result in blackout when swimming increases the need for oxygen.

Also, as a matter of personal safety, every college student should learn the important technique of drownproofing.[9]

ACCIDENT PRONENESS

Surveys of accident rates in industry made it clear a number of years ago that some individuals are more likely to have accidents than others. This has directed attention to the phenomenon of accident proneness, which explains why certain people seem to have repeated accidents—at home, at work, while driving, and even

[9]Lanoue, F. R.: *Drownproofing*, Prentice-Hall, Englewood Cliffs, N.J., 1963.

when they are just relaxing and enjoying themselves.

For example: A follow-up study on subsequent accident rates was made on two groups of taxi drivers. The first group selected had a high accident rate, and appeared to be definitely accident prone; the second group rarely had accidents. In the period under study, additional legal violations due to traffic accidents were reported in 34 per cent of the accident-prone group, and in only 1 per cent of the accident-free group.[10]

This is a problem which makes certain workers a danger to themselves and others around them. Some children also show a marked accident proneness. The explanation isn't completely worked out, but many psychiatrists feel that it does indicate some emotional disturbance. Frequently, accident-prone people show signs of more marked aggressiveness, impulsiveness, immaturity and resentment of restrictions and safeguards than do their accident-free counterparts.

Questions

1. What are two important means of transmission of tuberculosis?
2. What endocrine deficiency is responsible for diabetes? What causes diabetic acidosis? insulin shock?
3. Indicate the chief dangers in appendicitis and how to avoid it.
4. What is the main objection to the BCG vaccine?
5. List six useful rules for the prevention of tuberculosis.
6. Define pneumonia. Why is the treatment of bacterial pneumonia usually more successful than the treatment of viral pneumonia?
7. What are some of the factors that motivate suicide?
8. List some premonitory symptoms of suicide.
9. What is the role of psychiatry in the prevention of suicide?
10. Discuss possible causes of suicide among teen-age individuals.
11. What are the major causes of automobile accidents?
12. Indicate five ways to reduce automobile accidents.
13. Why do you think there are more accidents on Saturdays and Sundays than other days of the week, and on holiday week ends, as compared with other week ends?
14. What safety features for cars do experts recommend to reduce the toll of automobile accidents, and how could they affect this rate?
15. How could you reduce accidents in the home?
16. What precautions should you exert to prevent drowning?
17. Define "accident proneness."
18. If an employer recognizes that one of his employees has a high degree of accident proneness, what should be done to protect the employee and other workers in the plant or industry?

[10]Tillman, W. A., and Hobbs, C.: The accident-prone automobile driver, *American Journal of Psychiatry, 106*:321, 1949.

Topics for Discussion

Accidents in industry—cause and prevention.
Common accidents of babies and small children.
National Safety Council.

Reading Suggestions

Diabetes as a Way of Life, T. S. Danowski. Coward-McCann, New York, 1964. An interesting and informative account of the problems encountered by the diabetic. Common questions and answers are included.

Conquest of Tuberculosis, Selman A. Waksman. University of California Press, Berkeley, 1964. A good summary of what we know about tuberculosis and how that knowledge can be used.

Safety Education, A. E. Floria and G. T. Stafford. McGraw-Hill Book Company, New York, 1962. A basic textbook on safety.

Today's Health Guide, American Medical Association, Chicago, 1965. An authoritative, up-to-date, and readable account of all the conditions discussed in this chapter. Each condition is described by an expert in that field. An important source book for college students.

The Story of Insulin, G. A. Wrenshall. Indiana University Press, Bloomington, 1962. A vivid description of the triumphant discovery of insulin and its historical use. Also discussed are the most up-to-date ideas on diabetes mellitus and its management. An authentic and highly readable book.

Suicide, Louis I. Dublin. The Ronald Press, New York, 1963. This book is a revised edition of the earlier and well known book—*To Be or Not to Be: a Study of Suicide*. It contains an extraordinarily brilliant discussion of the environmental and emotional factors involved in suicide.

Suicide and Scandinavia, Herbert Hendin. Grune & Stratton, New York, 1964. A physician reports on studies of suicide in Denmark, Sweden, and Norway. A remarkable report of the "Scandinavian Suicide Phenomenon." The relationship of culture to character and behavior are vividly discussed.

Accident Research: Methods and Approaches, William Haddon, et al. Harper & Row, New York, 1964. An excellent source book to aid the student in the critical evaluation of accident statistics. Many significant studies are analyzed and evaluated in this comprehensive volume.

People are Accidents: A Treatise On Highway Acci-

dents, Howard Chester. Pageant, New York, 1965. A thought-provoking book on traffic accidents.

Victory over the Sugar Sickness, Charles H. Best and J. D. Ratcliff. Today's Health, March 1964, p. 56. A description of our victory over diabetes by one of the researchers who discovered insulin.

Survival for Diabetics. Today's Health, February 1963, p. 88. A plan for survival in the event of a large-scale disaster.

Doctors' Wives Tackle the Suicide Problem, Marilyn Benson. Today's Health, May 1964, p. 60. Description of a project to aid in the problem of suicide by the Woman's Auxiliary to the American Medical Association.

Suicidal Adolescents and Children, Albert Schrut. Journal of American Medical Association, *188:* 1103, 1964.

Accident Facts, National Safety Council, Chicago. Published yearly. A compilation of accident statistics.

Is Your Car Child-safe?, Harry and Phyl Dark. Today's Health, July 1963, p. 15. A well written article every prospective parent should read.

How the Experts Shop for Seat Belts, Today's Health, April 1963, p. 20. An up-to-date description of how to select seat belts.

You Can Prevent Poison Accidents, Robert M. Hendrickson. Today's Health, October 1961, p. 36. A discussion of the prevention of serious accidents to children.

Appendicitis—the Forgotten Killer, Theodore Berland. Today's Health, May 1964, p. 23. A well written account of a nearly forgotten killer.

Danger! T.B. Is on the Rise, Don Murray. Reader's Digest, June 1964, p. 79. A report on a disturbing increase in new cases of tuberculosis. Also, an excellent description of the current status of our knowledge regarding this disease.

Textbook in First Aid, American Red Cross. Doubleday, Garden City, N.Y., 1957. A standard textbook of first aid.

Hidden Factors in Auto Deaths, Gordon-James Stewart. Reader's Digest, June 1962, p. 124. Research into the cause of auto deaths.

Juvenile Diabetes and Its Management: Family, Social, and Academic Implications, D. D. Etzwiler and L. K. Sines. Journal of the American Medical Association, *181*:304, 1962. An informative article that can be read by the layman.

Diabetic Child, W. H. Grishaw. NEA Journal, *51*:16, 1962. An important article for the future teacher.

SECTION SEVEN

EDUCATING THE CONSUMER FOR HEALTH

20

MEDICINES

Medicine is not only a science; it is also an art. It does not consist of compounding pills and plasters; it deals with the very processes of life, which must be understood before they may be guided.

Die Grosse Wunderartzney (1530)
PARACELSUS

What primitive man could not understand, he ascribed to a force outside himself—a god or a demon. This was just as true with diseases, as it was with thunderstorms, earthquakes, eclipses, the passage of the sun, and the motion of the waves. Sickness was caused by an evil spirit, perhaps from a dead person, from a plant, or from a neighboring hill. Before man hit on any notion of treating illness, he empowered a sorcerer to drive the evil spirit from the sick person's body. When treatment began to be applied, even in a most rudimentary form, its effectiveness was considered the gift of a god. Frequently, in the myths and legends of early cultures, simple treatment of disease was embedded in many rich layers of embellishment, to be dug out patiently and with difficulty centuries later by historians, philosophers, and anthropologists.

About 15,000 years before the Christian era, someone drew on the walls of a cave in the Pyrenees a picture of a witch doctor, clothed in animal skins and wearing deer antlers for a headdress, his legs heavily marked with bright colors. In ancient Egypt—one of the earliest known cultures—many stories grew up around gods and goddesses, ascribing to them a power of healing. One such story has to do with Isis—goddess of fertility and motherhood, whose tears caused the Nile to rise—and with her son, Horus. The boy, playing in the swamps near the river, contracted swamp fever, or malaria. Isis lifted the child between her thighs and bathed his body with her urine. Soon afterward, Horus was cured of his illness. Such mythical embellishment of a simple treatment (for urine therapy was one of the earliest used and reported by ancient man, and one of the most effective) runs through the accounts left by early civilizations.

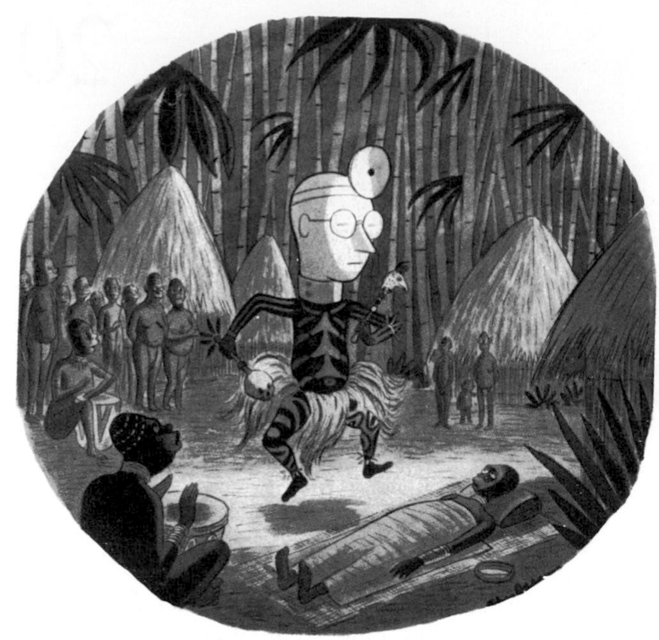

(Drawing by Chas. Addams, Copyr. © 1952, *The New Yorker Magazine,* Inc.)

The early Christians were not above blaming devils for human ills. St. Augustine attributed all disease to demons, who "chiefly torment the fresh-baptized, yea, even the guiltless newborn infant." Comparable superstitions, in an endless variety of forms, are found in the practices and beliefs of every group at an early stage of its development. Belief in an evil spirit that causes an illness and a benevolent spirit that relieves or cures it was inevitable, humans being what they are. The body, unaided, can heal most common afflictions through its own mechanisms. Also, many diseases are psychosomatic; there is no easy dividing line between the influence of the mind and the reactions of the body. Under the circumstances, the chants, prayers, masks, bells, snakes, mud, paint, roots, teeth, skulls, dung, shrieks, groans, and prayers of the medicine man, brought to a suffering person whose body, unknown to him, already was successfully fighting a disease, of course appeared effective. The principles of the medicine man were simple: attract the patient's attention, gain his confidence, possibly even deny the presence of the disease, and inspire him with faith in his recovery. Frequently, the medicine men were successful, and contemporary faith healers succeed as often, for reasons that have not changed for thousands of years.

Early medical treatment and faith healing were barely separable. At one time or another, almost anything had magical healing powers attributed to it. When the potato, for example, was introduced into Europe, it was sold as a medicine rather than as a food, and it was claimed to be effective as an aphrodisiac for curing impotence. From time to time and in various places, pearls, musk, crocodile dung, the head of a raven, children's feces, sarsaparilla, powdered vipers, the gall of a black ox, the skin of an elephant, and human fat, in addition to endless herbs and flowers, were used in treating illness. Human superstition, gullibility, and the desire to be cured certainly account in large measure for the acceptance of such medicines. Another reason is surely that well known love of medication, one of the few traits that distinguishes humans from other animals. Colored pills and liquids, in particular, seem to be prized for their curative powers. D. T. Atkinson, in his book, *Magic, Myth and Medicine,* comments:

> Red was a favorite color with our Stone Age ancestors as a means of restoring vigor to the body, as it still is in many parts of the world. A red light or red hanging in the sickroom of a patient with smallpox is still thought by many to prevent scarring. Inflamed joints are still wrapped in red flannel . . . and there are also some who believe that sore throats should be encased in red flannel. . . . *Perhaps it is because of this age-old superstition that chemists are still prone to color their pills and tablets red.*

Early medicine was irrational and unmethodical, but folk medicine often worked because the herbs and roots that were ground or extracted and used in certain illnesses contained substances that only recently have been refined and compounded into potent drugs. Mercury for syphilis, iodine for goiter, quinine for malaria, ipecac as an emetic, digitalis for heart pain, colchicum for gout, papaya juice for healing wounds, and opium for pain—all are derived from roots and herbs, and many were used centuries before the Christian era. Even penicillin, derived from bread mold, is new only in its refined form—peasants in the Black Forest region of Germany applied poultices from moldy bread to cure infected cuts and other wounds.

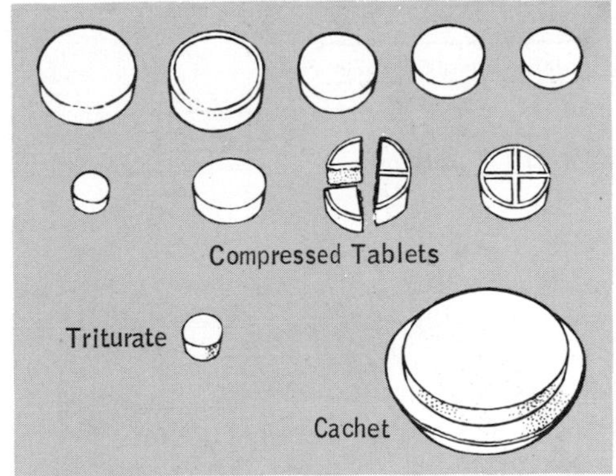

Figure 20–1. Types of tablets. (From Culver and Brownell: *The Practical Nurse*. 6th Ed., Philadelphia, W. B. Saunders Co., 1964.)

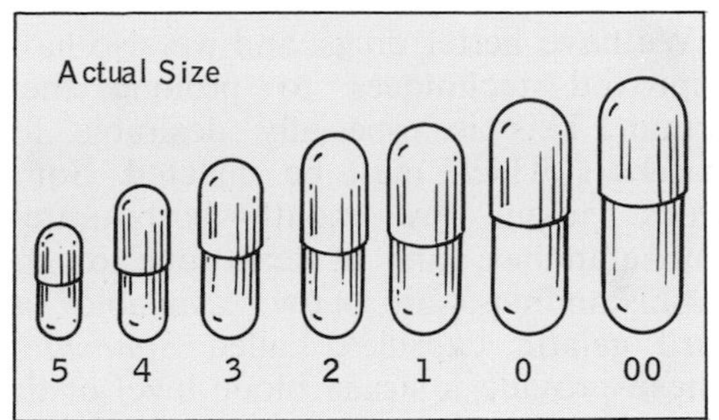

Figure 20–2. Sizes of capsules. (From Culver and Brownell: *The Practical Nurse*. 6th Ed., Philadelphia, W. B. Saunders Co., 1964.)

MODERN MEDICINES

Advances in medicine, the discovery and manufacture of new drugs that have effectively and dramatically reduced infection, and controlled disease and lengthened life have characterized medical science since World War II. It is only since 1943, when penicillin was made available, that antibiotics have been deliberately and methodically prepared in the laboratory, although antibiotic substances are present in man's blood, sweat, and tears, as well as in the natural world around him. Control of many harmful and dangerous bacteria is now medically practical. Many diseases that were dreaded a generation ago are now rare, and many ailments, once major threats to health, have been reduced to mere inconveniences and fairly easily controlled. The life expectancy of the general population in the United States has risen to 70 years (from 47 years in 1900), and the mortality rate has dropped in the same two-thirds of a century by nearly 45 per cent. More than 90 per cent of the prescriptions written today are for drugs that were not on the market 25 years ago. Reduction in certain death rates is shown in Table 20-1. This reduction can be correlated very closely with the introduction of the antibiotics and other highly effective medicines.

Table 20–1. Reduction in death rates from specific conditions between 1944 and 1962.

Polio	100%
Acute rheumatic fever	90 (1944–1961)
Influenza	88
Tuberculosis	87
Appendicitis	85
Maternal deaths	85
Syphilis	82
Acute nephritis	62 (1951–1962)
Infant deaths	36
Pneumonia	25

The economic effects of the drug revolution have been vast. From 1951 to 1963, the annual sales of drugs manufactured in the United States rose from $1.75 billion to $5.5 billion; the drug industry is one of the most rapidly expanding and one of the most profitable in this country.

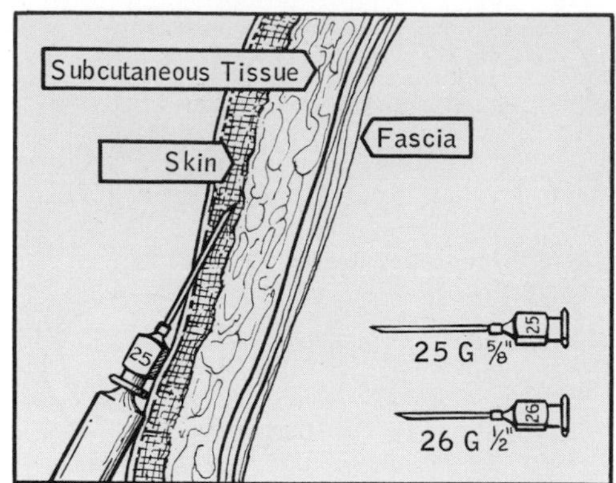

Figure 20–3. Intradermal injection. (From Culver and Brownell: *The Practical Nurse*. 6th Ed., Philadelphia, W. B. Saunders Co., 1964.)

We have better drugs, and we also have improved techniques to prolong their action. This is especially desirable for materials which must be injected. Some drugs taken by mouth–barbiturates, amphetamines, and at least one of the antihistaminics–are now available as hard gelatin capsules, called *Spansules*. These provide a steady blood level of the drug for sometimes as long as 24 hours, because the drug granules are covered with a hard coating, and only a few granules disintegrate at a time. Another method is to combine the drug with what is called an *ion-exchange resin*. This delays release of the drug in the small intestine, and promotes slow absorption, over a long period. The same effect is achieved by using the synthetic, plastic-like polyvinyl acetate.

Other techniques used with drugs taken by mouth are to add compounds which delay the excretion of the drug by the kidney (a compound penicillin tablet is available in this form) or to convert the medicine into a closely related chemical derivative, which is still effective, but not so rapidly destroyed or excreted by the body.

Highly effective, slow-acting insulin preparations containing zinc are now available, some of which are effective for as long as 30 hours. *Lente insulin* is an example. This means greater safety and far fewer injections for the diabetic, a particular boon for young children with diabetes.

Long-acting penicillin and steroid hormones depend on the synthesis of insoluble derivatives of these compounds, which are

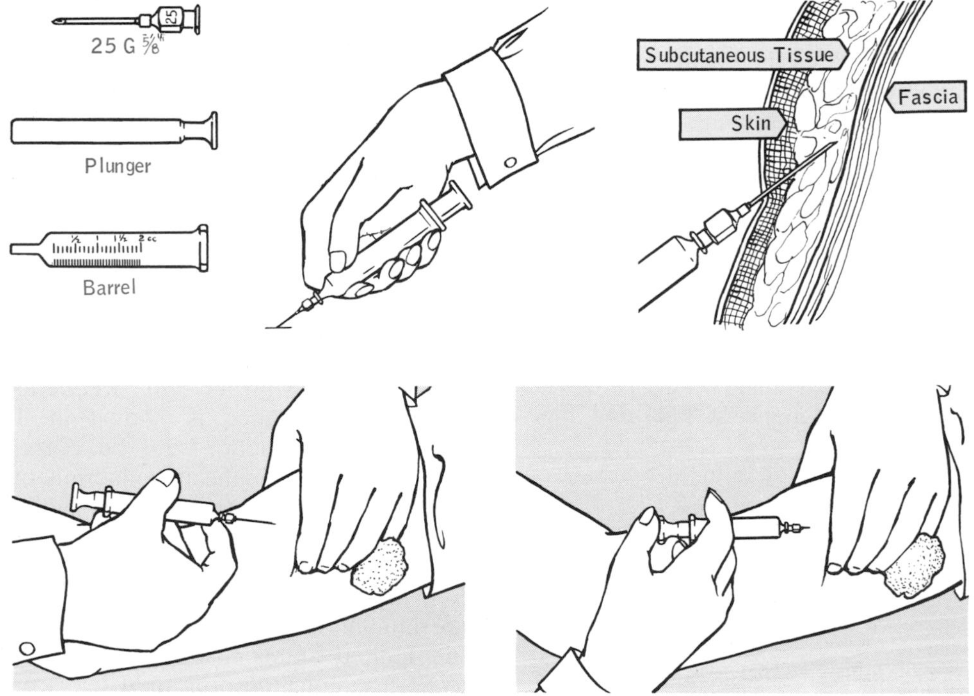

Figure 20–4. Hypodermic injection. (From Culver and Brownell: *The Practical Nurse*. 6th Ed., Philadelphia, W. B. Saunders Co., 1964.)

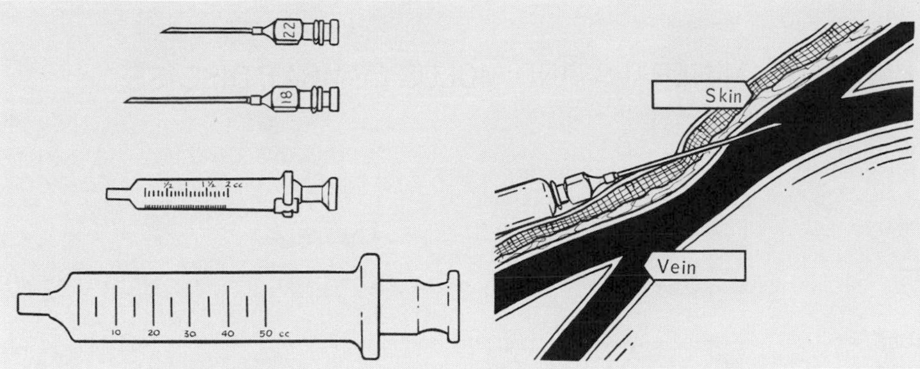

Figure 20–5. Intravenous injection. (From Culver and Brownell: *The Practical Nurse*. 6th Ed., Philadelphia, W. B. Saunders Co., 1964.)

then injected as water suspensions, or in an oil base. One penicillin preparation on the market is said to provide an assayable blood level of penicillin for 14 days after a single injection. Another interesting technique for prolonging the action of certain drugs is to prepare sterile pellets containing the active material. The pellet can then be implanted in subcutaneous or muscle tissue. This method has been used with some of the sex hormones, like estradiol, progesterone, and testosterone. It eliminates the need for frequent intramuscular injections or oral administration.

A dramatic advance in antibiotic medicine, which may lead to even more specific penicillin derivatives, was recently announced by four British scientists. This was the isolation and identification of the parent substance of five natural forms of penicillin. The new compound was named *6-amino penicillanic acid* by its discoverers. Today, all penicillin is produced by a fermentation process, using a specific mold which synthesizes the antibiotic. In the future, penicillin may be synthesized in the chemical laboratory. Perhaps new derivatives will be developed to overcome the sensitivity some patients have to penicillin, and to eliminate the resistance many bacteria have developed to this antibiotic as well. Bacterial resistance to antibiotics is a problem of particular concern at the present time and is probably the chief reason for alarming increases in infection by staphylococcic organisms.

OTHER USES OF THE NEWER MEDICINES

Antibiotics have proved to be very valuable in animal medicine, as well as for humans. They have saved the lives of thousands of pets, and livestock animals. In addition, they have virtually revolutionized animal nutrition. Small quantities of Terramycin, penicillin and other antibiotics have an extraordinary effect on animal growth. The liquids discarded during the production of these drugs are now added to certain livestock feeds, and help bring hogs, chickens, turkeys, and other animals to their desired market weights weeks earlier than ordinary diets would.

Certain crop diseases, such as halo blight of beans and fire blight of apples and peaches, can be controlled by antibiotics.

Germination and early growth of sweet corn and certain other plants can be speeded up as much as 100 per cent by trace amounts of Terramycin.

Cockerels can be castrated with artificial sex hormones, the process called *chemical caponization*. Milk production can be increased in cows after sex hormone treatment, and pregnant sows can be stimulated to deliver their young hours earlier if labor is induced with a hormone called *oxytocin*. This saves the farmer long nights of "sow-sitting" in the pig house.

PLANTS, MINERALS, AND MOLDS COMBAT DISEASE

Highlights in the History of Pharmacy

PLANTS were probably man's first source of medicine. The Chinese were said to have compiled a catalogue of medicinal herbs as early as 3000 B.C. Egyptian apothecaries, in 1500 B.C., knew how to compound herbs, mineral salts, and animal substances into salves, gargles, powders, and purgatives.

DIOSCORIDES, a 1st century Greek physician, compiled a herbal treatise that became a standard text on medicines for more than 1500 years. He described the narcotic effect of the mandrake root, which resembles the human body. Because it was believed that while being dug up the plant emitted screams that could cause madness, dogs were used to uproot it.

THE FIRST DRUGGISTS were Arabs. By the 12th century, pharmacy had become a specialty with its own code of standards. Arab druggists invented "sugar coating" by mixing bitter medicines with rose water and fruit syrups to make them palatable.

PARACELSUS, an early 16th century doctor and alchemist, was the first to propose that chemical medicines could be used to combat specific diseases. About the same time, products from the New World and from the Indies, cinnamon bark, guaiac, and cinchona bark, became popular ingredients in Europe.

POISONS, such as belladonna, have long been used for medicinal purposes. In the 1780's, William Withering developed digitalis from the foxglove plant for the treatment of heart diseases. In the early 19th century, experimental pharmacology was pioneered by French physicians François Magendie and Claude Bernard, when they studied the action of curare and other arrow poisons.

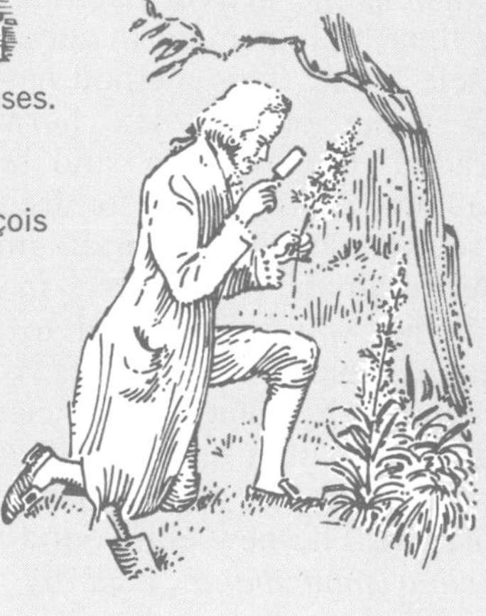

MEDICINE SHORTAGES during the Civil War led to the widespread manufacture of quack patent medicines, and to the overuse of such harmful drugs as calomel. Many of these abuses continued until the early 20th century when the Pure Food and Drug Acts were passed.

MODERN PHARMACOLOGY began in 1909 when Paul Ehrlich, a German bacteriologist, introduced Salvarsan for the treatment of syphilis. With the discovery of the sulfa drugs and the antibiotics (such as penicillin), the pharmacist has been equipped with a wider range of medicines to aid the medical profession in its fight against disease.

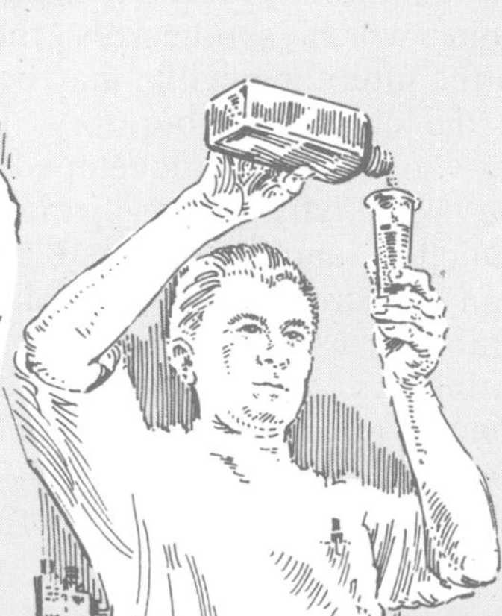

Veterinarians have found that tranquilizers make their lives much easier. Specially designed tranquilizers are now available for pets and these medicines have solved the problem of the dog who barks all night when his owners leave him at the vet's. Bandages and surgical dressings also stay in place on the dog who has been tranquilized after surgery. Cornell University veterinarians prescribe these pills for dogs who suffer from car-sickness or who hide in terror during thunderstorms. Even the ones who roam about all night in search of romance can now be tranquilized and persuaded to sit at home by the fireplace.

Tranquilized cows are easier to milk, and tranquilized beef cattle and turkeys are calmer and lose less weight on their trip to market. Steers treated with tranquilizers face death more calmly and provide more tender steaks.

THE DISEASES OF MEDICAL PROGRESS

The pharmacologic revolution that has taken place in the 1950's and 1960's, like some other revolutions, has had a great impact for the general good, but it has also meant injury and illness for some. Like all other revolutions, it can be modified but it cannot be undone. The antibiotics and other new drugs that appear yearly have side effects, some of them trivial, some serious, a few dangerous and occasionally fatal. A new category of disease has arisen—*iatrogenic disease*—meaning a disease attributable to medicine. It is an irony of contemporary life that perhaps 250 iatrogenic diseases have been recognized and that their identification, prevention, and treatment now are beginning to comprise still another medical specialty.

Some side effects of medicines are extensions of the therapeutic effects themselves—such as oversedation from barbiturates or bleeding from excessive anticoagulants. The side effects that can be predicted and safely handled do not cause complications; but many scientists and physicians fear the unknown complications that many drugs now on the market have a potential for causing.

Medications can cause trouble in many ways—the substance by itself, in combination with other drugs, or in combination with nondrug factors. For example, patients on long-term steroid therapy run considerable risk if they undergo surgery. For some, there are social complications. Persons receiving certain drugs for treatment of cancer are especially sensitive to some infections and may have to be isolated from their friends and families until their bone marrow can regenerate and their resistance can improve. The increasing concern over iatrogenic illnesses has resulted in numerous recommendations for the protection of the patient. Among these are:

Better data on drug toxicity.

More effective publicity about such information.

An upgrading of research.

An increased emphasis on iatrogenic ailments in medical schools.

Avoidance of the temptation to overprescribe.

In the recent past, medicines tended to be innocuous; at least they did no harm. If it comes down to a choice between letting the body fend for itself, or taking a carefully calculated risk of damage from side-effects, the physician really has only the second choice.

There are, however, new methods by which physicians can be forewarned about dangerous drugs. In August 1964, the American Medical Association and the Food and Drug Administration agreed to pool their resources to create a nationwide drug alert system, to detect the potentially adverse side effects of thousands of pharmaceutical products on the market, and to relay this information to physicians quickly. The AMA agreed to expand its efforts to obtain drug reaction reports from its 200,000 members, and the FDA arranged to concentrate on collecting data from 600 military, Veterans Administration, and other government hospitals plus 500 teaching hospitals. The reports are placed on punched cards and stored in data processing equipment of the AMA. An extension of this warning system to the international level was suggested nearly a year later. In May 1965, the United States delegation to the World Health Organ-

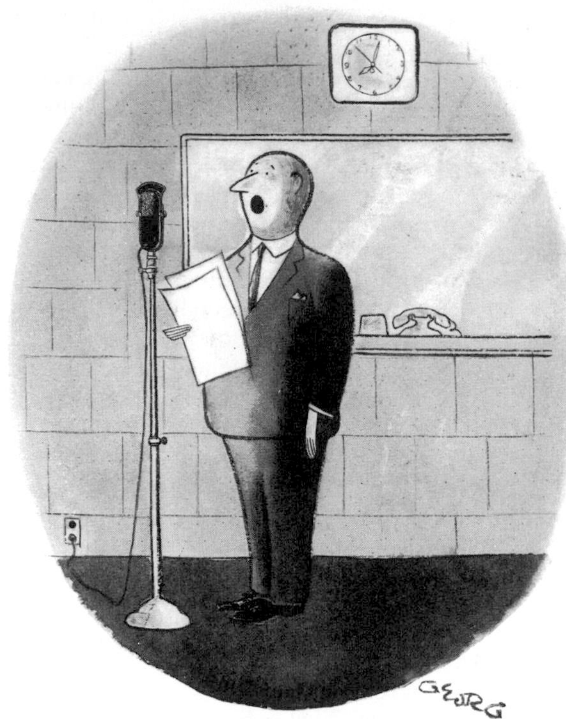

(Drawing by George Olden, Copyr. © 1944, *The New Yorker Magazine,* Inc.)

"Insist on Pasfo! Remember that when you drop the first letter and interchange the next two, simultaneously substituting an 'e' for the final 'o,' it spells 'SAFE.' Yes, Pasfo is the safe way to counteract the annoying discomfort that so often accompanies the common head cold."

ization brought to WHO's Geneva headquarters a proposal by the U. S. Department of Health, Education and Welfare that an international system for monitoring and reporting adverse reactions to drugs be established.

While most discussion of iatrogenic diseases remains on a professional level, occasionally a substance produces side effects of such a shocking nature and on such a scale that every reader of a newspaper and every viewer of television knows about it. Such a drug was thalidomide, which caused thousands of infants to be terribly congenitally deformed in Germany, England, France, Belgium, Australia, and Canada. Thalidomide—a drug that induced a deep and restful sleep—was introduced in Europe in the summer of 1959. In some places, particularly in Germany, it was sold without prescription. Beginning in 1960, its effects began to become apparent—newborn babies had rudimentary, sometimes little more than flipper-like arms and legs. An FDA medical officer, Dr. Frances Kelsey, who was suspicious of the drug and who for 19 months resisted an American drug company's pressure to license it for sale in this country, saved American women from the same shattering experience.

The results of the thalidomide affair were tangible and beneficial in the United States. First, it stirred physicians to exercise even greater care before prescribing new preparations. There was increased pressure for more federal controls to protect the public. The Senate Subcommittee on Antitrust and Monopoly under the chairmanship of Senator Estes Kefauver, which had been mostly investigating the pricing policies of drug houses, increasingly turned its attention to testing and sales policies. In the spring of 1962, the committee's bill to control drug sales more stringently had been seriously watered down, but news of the work of Dr. Kelsey resulted in restoration of the stronger provisions and the addition of some new ones. The Kefauver-Harris

Drug Amendments Act of 1962 requires drug manufacturers to prove their claims of effectiveness before marketing the compound; it empowers the Secretary of Health, Education and Welfare to remove from the market any drug that appears hazardous; it requires extensive animal testing of a drug before it can be tested on humans; it forces advertisers of drugs to list both therapeutic and side effects; and in several other ways the Act adds to the government's authority to protect the public from these adverse side effects, which are an ironic concomitant of the contemporary pharmacologic revolution.

The story of thalidomide was particularly shocking because of the permanent crippling it caused. Less severe, but still serious and much less publicized are the side effects of other drugs, most of which have a proper and necessary place in medical treatment, as long as they are used with caution. Some of these substances and the problems they may present are presented in the following paragraphs.

Tranquilizing preparations have been a tremendous boon to mental hospitals, making even violent patients calm and manageable. They have been used successfully in allaying the severe withdrawal symptoms of narcotic addicts and delirium tremens in alcoholics. Certain psychosomatic illnesses, such as high blood pressure and some skin diseases, are helped considerably by them because they relieve emotional tensions. But perhaps the greatest market for these drugs is the average man and woman, not mentally ill nor suffering from a psychosomatic disease, and not addicted to narcotics or alcohol.

Many people have come to rely upon tranquilizers simply to bring peace of mind to their lives. More than $3.5 million worth of tranquilizers were sold in 1962, many of them to essentially healthy people. Anything to reduce the anxiety and tensions generated in the process of earning a living in a competitive world, of caring for a houseful of children, of assuming the inescapable responsibilities of adult life.

"Yesterday," said M. G. Martin of the Regina General Hospital in Saskatchewan, Canada, "the doctor prescribed a vacation for his emotionally upset patient, and today he prescribes a chemical vacation." According to Aldous Huxley, "Most people lead lives at worst so painful and at best so monotonous, that the urge to escape is one of the principal appetites of the soul."

Tranquilizers *can* provide temporary escapes, especially for people who feel that they are justified in eliminating all struggle, killing all pain, and getting happiness free. But even tension and restlessness, within limits, have their good aspects. They often lead to highly creative, productive undertakings. We might resemble fairly inert vegetables if we didn't have some tensions and drives.

These, however, are not the most important medical hazards of the tranquilizers. In a sizeable number of patients, some of these drugs have had alarming side effects, producing sometimes fatal jaundice, nausea, rashes, severe tremor, and even mental depression and suicidal tendencies.

In addition, people taking tranquilizers, sedatives, barbiturates, and certain soporific antihistaminic pills are serious hazards on the highway. The driver may develop a semi-drowsy, very relaxed, "don't care" attitude, which can slow down his alertness and cause dangerously careless driving.

In a small percentage of patients, the prolonged use of one of the effective *antiepilepsy drugs* (Tridione) is responsible for nephrosis, a kidney disease, as well as undesirable reactions in the central nervous system, and impairment of the blood-forming organs.

Antibiotics have been lifesaving in many diseases—and also death-dealing. Penicillin is responsible for severe allergic reactions in sensitive individuals. Neurological disturbances, including permanent deafness and loss of equilibrium, have resulted from high levels of streptomycin. Chloramphenicol has produced serious diseases of the blood-forming organs. Cycloserine, an antibiotic used against tuberculosis, has an extremely narrow margin of safety: a slight overdose can cause epileptic convulsions and severe emotional damage.

If used for prolonged periods of time, many effective antibiotics will kill off harmless bacteria in the intestine. This permits the resistant ones, some of them really harmful, to run wild and cause extremely serious illnesses. A corollary to this is that antibiotics can be responsible for severe, uncontrolled bleeding if they destroy too many intestinal bacteria. We depend on these to synthesize our supplies of vitamin K, the vitamin needed for blood clotting.

A major hazard in careless dosage or self-medication with antibiotics is that when the dose is too low, blood levels may not be high enough to kill the offending organisms. This encourages development of *resistance* to the antibiotic.

According to Jesse D. Rising of the University of Kansas, many medications used in the treatment of *high blood pressure* have dangerous side effects. Some of these are respiratory difficulties, severe anxiety or depressions, and epilepsy-like convulsions. Symptoms resembling rheumatoid arthritis have been produced in 10 per cent of patients treated for high blood pressure with one of these preparations.

No *steroid* has been discovered which is completely effective against diseases like rheumatoid arthritis and is without potential serious side-effects, according to Drug and Therapeutic Information, Inc. Some of the hazards from cortisone and similar steroids are: peptic ulcers, decreased resistance to infection, activation of quiescent infections such as tuberculosis, weakening of the bones, leading to repeated fractures, excitability ranging to outright psychoses, and aggravation of diabetes.

Nevertheless, Rising concluded in his report, no thoughtful physician would think of abandoning these useful and often lifesaving drugs. At the same time, he should prescribe them with discretion and exert every effort to understand the harmful effects that might result from their use.

Between those drugs that are obviously useless (see the discussion of quackery in Chapter 21 and those that are beneficial but must be used with caution, there is the category of drugs for which great claims are seriously and persistently made, but for which the claims have yet to be proved.

Questions

1. Where can physicians find information about new drugs they are considering prescribing?

2. What attempts are made by professional and government groups and agencies to publicize instances of dangerous side effects produced by new drugs?

3. "Almost any treatment is sometimes successful." Is such a statement meaningful or nonsense? If it is meaningful, why should this be so?

4. Cite some instances of medical superstition in early civilizations you have studied.

5. Name some substances used effectively today for treatment of illness that were well known hundreds or thousands of years ago.

6. What complications or side effects can you describe that result from medicines that were used in ancient times? Do you think that iatrogenic diseases are a new problem or an intensified and more complex form of an old source of concern?

7. Describe several ways that drugs may adversely affect a patient.

8. The dangers of some compounds have been well publicized. Does such publicity in general make people more careful about self-medication with over-the-counter drugs?

9. What are the essential differences between prescription and proprietary drug preparations?

10. What does the word *antibiotic* really mean, and what is the essence of its effect?

11. What do we spend annually for drugs and medicines in the United States?

12. Describe several ways to make medicines more effective by altering the form in which they are administered.

13. What are some of the hazards of *tranquilizers? antibiotics? steroid hormones?*

Topics for Discussion

Effectiveness of faith healing.

The amount of risk justified in treatment with new drugs.

Desirability of public control over testing and application of new medicines.

Dangers of upsetting the "balance of Nature" with antibiotics and other drugs.

Recent decline of major causes of death, such as fatalities from bacterial diseases.

Instances of cooperation between government and professional agencies and organizations.

Extent of governmental protection of the public—whether existing laws are sufficient and what new ones may be needed.

Adequacy of controls over proprietary medicines.

The problem of the cost of many new drugs.

Reading Suggestions

Magic, Myth and Medicine, D. T. Atkinson. Fawcett Publishers, Greenwich, Conn., 1956. An absorbing account of the development of modern medicines.

Devils, Drugs and Doctors, Howard W. Haggard. Pocket Books, Inc., New York (paperback). An extremely interesting, well written and well illustrated popular book.

Science Book of Wonder Drugs, Donald G. Cooley. Pocket Books, Inc., New York (paperback). De-

scribes how the newer medicines were discovered, and how additional ones are being developed.
The Medicine Show, by the editors of Consumer Reports. Simon & Schuster, New York, 1961 (paperback). A blunt account about some popular remedies for everyday ailments.
Wonder Drugs, Helmuth M. Boettcher. Lippincott, Philadelphia, 1963. An account of antibiotic substances from earliest times to today.
The Real Voice, R. Harris. MacMillan, New York, 1964. Detailed information about the American drug industry; in particular, the facts and issues raised by the Kefauver Committee investigation.
Medicines, D. McDonald and H. Ratner. The Fund for the Republic, 1962.
Curiosities of Medicine, Berton Roueche. Little, Brown, & Co., Boston, 1963. An anthology of unusual cases or phenomena, some of them going back several centuries in medical literature.
The Diseases Drugs Cause, Louis Lasagna. In *Perspectives in Biology and Medicine,* Vol. VII, University of Chicago Press, 1964.
Man Against Pain, Bernard Seeman. Chilton, Philadelphia, 1962.
First Facts about Drugs, FDA Publication No. 21, August 1964.
Drugs, Medicines and Man, Harold Burn. Scribner's, New York, 1962. For the lay reader, an account of how drugs act on the human body. Also, a historical survey of drugs and medicines.
Creative Minds in Medicine, William C. Gibson. Charles C Thomas, Springfield, Ill., 1963. Scientific, humanistic, and cultural contributions by physicians.
The March of Medicine, Hermann S. Glasscheib. Putnam, New York, 1963. Historical perspective on the emergence and triumph of modern medicine.
Great Adventures in Medicine, S. B. Rapport. Dial Press, New York, 1961.
Drugs in Our Society, Paul Talalay, ed. Johns Hopkins Press, Baltimore, 1964. A compilation based on a conference sponsored by Johns Hopkins University.

21

MEDICAL AND SURGICAL CARE

> The medical art consists of three elements—the disease, the patient, and the physician; the physician carries out the dictates of the art, and the patient must combat the disease with the physician.
>
> Art is long, life short, opportunity fleeting, experiment hazardous, judgment difficult, nor is it sufficient that the physician should attend to his work, but it is also necessary that the patient and those around him should do theirs, and that surrounding conditions be adjusted in general to the same end.
>
> HIPPOCRATES

To maintain optimum health and improve one's chances for enjoying our tremendous gains in potential longevity, everyone should have a clear idea of the following:

1. How to choose a doctor and when to consult a specialist.
2. Why regular medical checkups are important.
3. What goes on in hospitals and clinics, and the reasons for various tests and procedures.
4. What mysterious things happen during surgical operations.
5. The differences between private and group practice.
6. The costs of medical care and insurance plans.

HOW TO CHOOSE A DOCTOR

No matter how healthy you are, you should have a doctor, or at least know how to find one. Someday you may need him. Preventive medicine is even more important. A doctor can help people *keep* their good health—especially as they grow older—and make it possible for them to benefit from all the modern medical discoveries.

Most colleges and universities have well organized medical care programs for resident students. However, the day student or married student is often faced with the problem of selecting his own physician. Or you may need a doctor sometime when you are visiting in a strange city. And you will certainly need a reliable physician after graduation.

How Do You Go About Selecting a Doctor?

It's risky to make your choice on the casual recommendation of a friend, or because the doctor's office is conveniently located. This gives you no real indication of his ability, and, in medicine, as in other professions and trades, some men have considerably greater skill and better training than others.

1. One of the best ways to find a reliable doctor is to consult a relative or close friend who is in the medical profession. Dentists, medical students, pharmacists, and medical and social workers also have better opportunities of getting accurate information than the average lay person.

2. If there is a medical school in your community you can obtain a catalogue of its faculty by writing to the dean. You will most likely want to choose someone in the Department of Medicine (the others will probably be too specialized).

3. Another way is to write or telephone the superintendent of an approved local hospital for suggestions. A physician's appointment to a hospital indicates approval of his ability, for a good hospital will not staff a man who is incompetent. Furthermore, a hospital keeps the doctor in contact with new medical developments, and with the facilities of the laboratory and modern equipment.

The amount and quality of training that a doctor obtains after graduation from medical school is an important indication of his ability. Almost every physician has had at least one year's hospital training, and most doctors now take at least two or three years of hospital work before entering practice. If a doctor has graduated from a good medical school and has trained at one of the better hospitals in the country, you can feel more confident that he will render the service you want.

Make certain the doctor you choose is on the staff of a good hospital. Many people do not realize that fully one-third of the doctors in most large cities cannot admit their patients to the best hospitals. Ask your prospective doctor what hospital he would send you to, and make sure it is a recognized, accredited institution.

4. You can obtain a list of licensed physicians from your county or state medical society, or from the American Medical Association, 535 North Dearborn Street, Chicago, Illinois 60610. This is a national society which sets standards for the medical profession, and also exposes impostors in the field of medicine.

5. Your board of health or county health officer can also advise you in the selection of a doctor. This might be especially helpful if you live in a rural area, some distance away from a large hospital or medical school.

6. If you move from a community where you have had a physician in whom you feel confidence, you can ask him to recommend a doctor in your new community. Your final judgment should be based on how you, personally, react to the physician. Go and talk to him—professionally, not at a social gathering. This will give you an impression of him in the role you may want him to assume permanently. Do you think you can develop a warm personal relationship with him? This is most important since you must be willing to respect and follow your physician's advice in serious decisions, perhaps even in matters of life and death. Do you think you could like him? Naturally you don't expect him to resemble a Hollywood movie star, but you do want to feel easy and comfortable in his presence, and be able to talk to him about any kind of problem that might arise. Above all, *does he inspire confidence in you?* Remember that you are not looking for the ideal man, but for a doctor you can trust.

Honor a physician with the honor due unto him for the uses which ye may have of him.

ECCLESIASTICUS

What Kind of Doctor Should You Select?

Although specialists are becoming increasingly important in modern medical practice, the family physician is still the key figure. Sixty-seven per cent of the physicians in this country are in general practice, and the remaining 33 per cent have specialized in some field, or hold hospital, teaching, or administrative positions. The family physician in general practice is still the medical advisor and manager for four of five people, and for many he is the only contact with the medical profession.

The reason for this is fairly obvious. You don't want too specialized a doctor for your family physician. You want someone whom you can call if illness strikes you or any member of your family, someone who will *suggest* a specialist if he can't handle a condition adequately. An ophthalmologist, for example, would not treat your bronchitis, nor would he be expected to diagnose heart disease; he has obtained very special training to fit him for diagnosing and treating eye conditions only.

You might choose a *general practitioner* or an *internist* for your family doctor. The general practitioner is trained to take care of most adult illnesses and to do a certain amount of surgery. He also delivers babies, takes care of infants and children, and usually sets broken limbs.

The *internist* is more specialized; his field is medical diagnosis and treatment; he handles most medical conditions but usually does no surgery. A good internist or general practitioner will realize when his knowledge is not sufficient to cover a certain problem, and he will refer you to the proper specialist. It's better for the physician to decide when a specialist is needed than for the patient to do so.

How to Develop a Good Relationship with Your Doctor

When you're consulting a physician, tell him everything, no matter how unimportant it may seem to you. Avoid diagnosing your own illnesses and prescribing your own remedies, and follow his directions exactly. Remember that many physicians don't always know what questions are disturbing you; ask him specific questions such as which pharmacy *he* would use to have a prescription filled, which surgeon *he* would select if he were going to have a major operation, or whether *he* would recommend Dr. — — to deliver his own children.

Medical fees are moderately expensive these days—like everything else—but this doesn't excuse the common habit of getting a free consultation every time a patient meets his physician in a social gathering or walking along the street. The story is told of one physician who developed a sure-fire technique to handle such situations. Whenever anyone stopped him in the street to ask casually what remedy one should take for such and such a disease, he had a very effective response. "Undress," he would say. "I need to see you naked in order to answer your question."

How Many Doctors Are in Practice?

Although there are more than 257,000 physicians in the United States, many more still are needed. Most rural areas suffer from a shortage of doctors. Metropolitan centers, especially those with medical schools, generally enjoy a higher physician-population ratio than smaller communities, and the wealthier areas of the country inevitably attract more doctors than do the poorer sections.

There is one physician for every 780 persons in the United States, but in several other countries, the population load on the individual physician is lower.

Other nations are not so fortunate. The number of persons per physician is much greater in many of these countries (Table 21–1). In these nations, physicians are concentrated in the cities, as they are in the United States, so that for great numbers of the world population most illness must go unattended or be treated with superstition or home remedies by unskilled laymen. Lack of transportation and prohibitive cost of travel and care pose additional barriers to skilled treatment in many areas.

Who Are the Specialists?

In order to become a bona fide specialist, a doctor must be accredited by the specialty licensure board in his field. This indicates that he has had the necessary extra training to become expert in a particular branch of medicine.

If you are to consult them at some time you should know something about the principal specialists in medicine and related fields, and what they do.

Table 21–1. Number of persons per physician in several countries*

Country	*No. of Persons per Physician*
Ethiopia	96,000
Congo	63,000
Indonesia	48,000
Laos	41,000
Afghanistan	36,000
Haiti	11,000
Pakistan	11,000
Burma	10,000
Morocco	9,700
Turkey	6,800
India	5,800
Algeria	5,500
Iraq	5,400
Bolivia	3,900
Brazil	2,500
South Africa	2,000
Chile	1,600
Venezuela	1,400
Portugal	1,200
Sweden	1,000
United States	**780**
Belgium	740
Romania	720
West Germany	680
Argentina	670
Italy	610
Austria	550
USSR	510
Israel	390

*From World Health Organization, *Epidemiological and Vital Statistics Report,* 1961.

The *obstetrician* delivers babies and takes care of the pregnant patient during the months before the baby is born.

The *pediatrician* takes care of infants and children up to the age of between twelve to fifteen.

The *internist* is an expert in diagnosis and treatment of medical conditions of the entire body. (He is often referred to as a diagnostician or medical man, though neither of these terms defines him precisely.)

A *surgeon* specializes in performing operations. He may be a *general surgeon* or may restrict himself to one of the following branches of surgery: The *gynecologist* treats illness of the female reproductive organs. The *urologist* specializes in kidney conditions as well as problems relating to the male genital organs. For example, he would usually be the doctor to operate on a diseased prostate gland. An *orthopedist* specializes in diseases of the bones and joints. The field of orthopedics comprises the setting of fractures, treatment of crippling from infantile paralysis, and many other conditions which interfere with the normal use of bones, joints or muscles. An *otolaryngologist* deals with ailments of the ears, throat, sinuses and nose. An eye specialist who has the degree of M.D. is called an *ophthalmologist,* and his province is surgery and diseases of the eye.

An *optometrist* is *not* a medical doctor. He has been trained to examine the eyes for the purpose of prescribing eyeglasses. The *optician* fills the prescriptions made by the ophthalmologists or optometrists, and he is the counterpart of the pharmacist who fills prescriptions for medicines. Neither the optometrist nor the optician is trained to treat diseases of the eye.

The *dermatologist* specializes in diseases of the skin, hair, and scalp.

An *allergist* treats such conditions as asthma, hay fever, hives, and allergic reactions to food.

A *psychiatrist* is a doctor who is trained to take care of the mentally ill. Usually, however, only a small fraction of his time is spent with the insane. Mostly he treats individuals who have some behavior problem or neurosis. Psychiatrists are sometimes referred to as "psychologists," "nerve specialists," or "psychotherapists" to spare the feelings of individuals who still do not realize that treatment by a psychiatrist does not imply insanity.

Organic diseases of the nerves and brain are treated by a *neurologist,* who is more properly a "nerve specialist" than is the psychiatrist. Some doctors are qualified to practice both neurology and psychiatry.

The *gastroenterologist* treats diseases of the stomach and intestines.

The *radiologist* is a specialist in taking and interpreting x-rays. He is also trained to treat cancer and other diseases with radium, x-rays, and other radioactive substances.

Should Operations Be Performed by the General Practitioner or the Surgical Specialist?

This is one of the most difficult problems facing both the patient and the medical profession. Many general practitioners are competent to handle major surgery; others have not had the necessary training and experience. Certain operations, such as removal of the gallbladder, partial removal of the thyroid gland, or stomach surgery for ulcer require a high degree of skill and experience, and even an appendectomy can be a difficult procedure when it is performed on a very obese person.

The wisest and safest plan would be to ask your doctor to select the surgeon with the greatest experience in the particular operation to be performed.

What About Osteopaths, Chiropractors, and Christian Science Healers?

Osteopathy was founded on the theory that most diseases are caused by a misalignment of the bones, and should be treated by manipulations rather than by other methods such as the use of drugs. Today most osteopathic schools are making a real effort to improve the quality of the training they offer, and many recently trained osteopathic doctors are using modern drugs and techniques. In some states, osteopaths now legally and professionally enjoy the same status as M.D.'s.

Chiropractors believe that diseases are caused by pressure on the nerves because of faulty alignment of the vertebrae, in particular. According to this concept, such diseases can be cured by manipulation, and there appears to be little inclination toward moderation and modernization among most chiropractors.

Christian Science is based on the theory that, "Spirit is immortal Truth; matter is mortal error," and consequently, evil, disease, and death are temporary and unreal.

Most of us feel that there is adequate evidence today that disease and death *do* exist, and that both disease and death result from definite causes, many of which can be prevented or cured. We are all entitled to the best that modern medical science can offer against disease – vaccinations, x-rays, antibiotics, and other specific medications, and skilled surgery for operable conditions. The people who are best qualified to provide accepted modern scientific medical and surgical care are graduates of recognized medical schools, and possess the M.D. degree. You have the freedom of choice in this matter, but it is important to learn to distinguish between religion, fads, and science, when it comes to the healing art.

MEDICAL QUACKERY

The Dangers of Quackery

The medicine man – the peddler of snake oil – is now a popular stereotype of early America. Behind this slightly comical image, though, is the reality, the fact that many people have died because they turned to quacks, that many more have thrown away their savings in the pursuit of false hopes for their health. The blatant claims of the roadside peddlers have been superseded by the more polished – and much more effective – advertising, promotion and sale of worthless "medicines" and devices by clever charlatans. The Food and Drug Administration estimates that today the American public pays more than $1 billion a year to support quackery in all its forms.

Although some protection is provided at the local and state levels, these agencies are often so small and so understaffed that they cannot always act forcefully. Much more effective protection for the public is available through three federal agencies: the Post Office Department may act against anyone who uses the mail to defraud; the Federal Trade Commission may move against false and misleading advertising, and the Food and Drug Administration may take the most direct action of all – from examining a product before it is marketed, through warning physicians and consumers of dangerous drugs and devices, to seizing shipments of products that cross state lines.

The American Medical Association and the Food and Drug Administration, each of which has been active for many years in the battle against quackery, from time to time work together against the common enemy. For example, in 1961 and again in 1963, the AMA and FDA cosponsored a

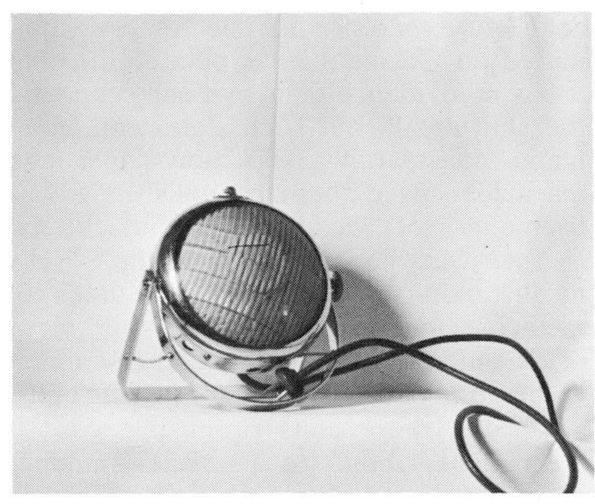

Figure 21–1. Depoloray. (Courtesy of the American Medical Association Bureau of Investigation.)

National Congress on Medical Quackery. At the 1963 meeting, physicians, educators, publishers, and representatives of government agencies whose responsibilities involve various aspects of public health, discussed some of the more recent frauds and some of the steps taken by the sponsoring organizations to combat them. Among the instances of quackery cited by George P. Larrick, Commissioner of Food and Drugs of the U.S. Department of Health, Education and Welfare, at the 1963 meeting were these:

A fake diagnostic instrument, known as the Ellis "Micro-Dynameter," was sold to more than 5000 people, who paid as much as $875. Numerous booklets, leaflets and reprints were distributed to promote this machine, which the manufacturer claimed enabled the operator to diagnose practically every variety of disease. Actually, the only condition it could measure was the amount of perspiration on the patient's skin. The Federal Government won a court fight to stop the distribution of the machine and promotional literature; then the FDA undertook a year-long campaign to seize and destroy as many of the Micro-Dynameter devices as possible.

Food faddism and nutritional quackery also find a large and enthusiastic audience in the United States. The case of Nutri-Bio is illuminating. This substance was promoted as the answer to practically all human ills—anemia, arthritis, cancer, diabetes, frigidity, heart trouble, infections, and nervousness. At one point in the early 1960's, more than 75,000 full and part-time agents were selling Nutri-Bio at $24 per package, a six-months' supply for an individual. Many persons invested their savings for the opportunity to set up a Nutri-Bio sales system. The government acted on the grounds that the substance was misbranded—when it was shipped and while it was held for sale after interstate shipping.

The American obsession with losing weight has enriched many manufacturers and promoters of worthless over-the-counter drugs and of more or less questionable food specialties. It has also made possible the sale of more than 2 million copies of a book, *Calories Don't Count,* which was based on a previously known, but discredited theory that an obese person may lose weight by undertaking a high fat diet without restricting calories. The first 11 printings of *Calories Don't Count* included a sales announcement for safflower oil capsules, marketed by Cove Vitamin and Pharmaceutical, Inc., of Glen Cove, New York. Coincidentally, safflower oil was recommended in the book as an aid in reducing and in lowering blood cholesterol, treating arteriosclerosis and heartburn, increasing resistance to colds and sinus trouble, improving sexual drive and for other desirable purposes. The FDA seized both the book and the safflower oil capsules when they were displayed together, charging that the capsules were misbranded as a result of false claims in the book. The drug company first filed an answer to the charges but then withdrew it, basing their decision on the fact that the publisher, Simon and Schuster, and the author, Herman Taller, M.D., refused to support the claims made in the book.

The facts behind *Calories Don't Count* were surprising in a number of ways. The publishers had had Dr. Taller's original draft revised by a nonmedical editor to make the book more salable, less scientific sounding. A company was formed to market the capsules for which the book, it was hoped, would create a demand, and the limited group that acquired an interest in the company included Dr. Taller. Also, two vice presidents of the publishing house

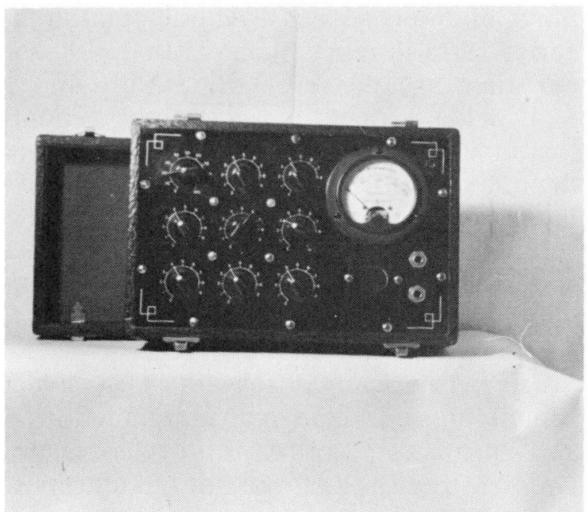

Figure 21–2. Drown Instrument. (Courtesy of the American Medical Association Bureau of Investigation.)

took options to purchase stock, but only one of them exercised his option. All in all, the sordid story of *Calories Don't Count* makes a classic account of medical quackery—the sales approach based on popular appeal, the theory that sounds medically plausible, the physician's name behind the promotion, and the financial maneuvering designed to line the pockets of a few backers.

The anxiety that many people experience concerning their health is pointed up in that equipment, drugs, and foods or food supplements have been sold easily, no matter how far-fetched the claims made for their efficacy. The inventor of the Drown Radio Vision Instruments and the Homo-Vibra Ray instruments claimed that the machines could take blood counts, determine temperatures, and diagnose and treat illnesses. The patient didn't even have to be there; all that was needed was a drop of blood, which would produce the necessary "emanations." In the cosmetic field, health is generally not at stake, although the pocketbook is. For example, several manufacturers have put about 20 cents' worth of "royal jelly" (the substance on which queen bees feed; it is a mixture of ordinary proteins and vitamin B complex) into about 25 cents' worth of cold cream, and they have sold the combination for $10 an ounce as an aid for the appearance of women's skin. The AMA's Committee on Cosmetics has pointed out that it has no evidence that royal jelly can help the skin at all, but such statements command considerably less newspaper and magazine space than the polished advertisements of cosmetic manufacturers.

Americans have been called the world's most credulous people in the areas of medicine and health. Still another piece of evidence supporting this odd distinction is the number and strength of healing cults. Typically, these cults promise a cure if the patient submits to a sufficient number of treatments and maintains faith in the system. Because many bodily ailments tend to subside without any help at all, given enough time, the cultists can often claim success.

Who Buys Quackery?

As effective as government action against quacks may be, a more basic method of halting the cruel practice of medical fraud would be to educate the public both to recognize irregular medical treatment and to stay away from it. Most in need of such indoctrination are the miracle-seekers and the uninformed, two groups that do not necessarily overlap, for many well educated and intelligent men and women have a soft spot in their head for the peddler of medical blue sky.

The danger frequently is delay. A typical miracle-seeker (and many hospitals have dozens of such case histories) discovers a lump in her breast. Immediately diagnosing it as incurable cancer, she consults a religious cultist, who may recommend applying a prayer cloth to the breast daily. When she finally consults a doctor, several months later, she finds that she indeed has cancer, now in an advanced state, and that nothing can be done except possibly to make her comfortable during the terminal stage.

A surprisingly large number of uninformed people do not realize that there is a considerable difference between a doctor with an M.D. degree and a practitioner of dubious arts who may actually call himself "doctor."

Quacks also owe much of their success to

the impatient person, who disagrees with a physician when he recommends surgery, or who cannot afford the time necessary to have a battery of hospital tests. Such a person often prefers a nonmedical practitioner who cheerfully supplies pills and ointments from the first visit.

Of course, the most tragic customers of the quacks are those patients whose diseases are incurable. Told by their own physician that nothing more can be done, they frantically and desperately grasp at any straw of hope, from any source, and at any price. A side effect of this is that charlatans are kept in business and can continue to jeopardize the lives of patients with curable illnesses. In most such cases, the physician can prevent a patient from seeking the aid of quacks, if he is sufficiently considerate, persuasive and able to convince the patient that everything that can be done has been or will be attempted.

The AMA, with more than a half a century of supplying public and professional information about quacks, has a set of ground rules for spotting the frauds. These rules are:

Beware if . . .

he uses a special or "secret" formula or machine that he claims can cure diseases;

he promises a quick or easy cure;

he advertises, using "case histories" or testimonials to impress people;

he clamors constantly for medical investigation and recognition;

he claims medical men are persecuting him or that they are afraid of his competition;

he tells you that his method of treatment is better than surgery, x-rays or drugs.

Action against Frauds

Not until 1906 did Congress pass laws empowering the U. S. Government to protect its citizens against foods and drugs detrimental to health. The original laws were enacted only in the face of powerful opposition, and further legal action since those early days has been successful, again, only after the expression of much hostility and attempted countermeasures by those whose interests were affected. In 1938, after a series of deaths from an inadequately tested drug, Congress strengthened the 1906 laws. The Federal Trade Commission that year was given increased jurisdiction over advertising claims by manufacturers of foods, drugs and cosmetics. In the three decades since then, not only have the drug and pharmaceutical industries done much to clean their own houses, but the FDA, the FTC and the Post Office department have moved more aggressively against fraudulent practices.

In addition, professional societies have been alert and active. The AMA's Department of Investigation, Committee on Cosmetics, and other cognizant groups constantly check reports of false claims and notify both physicians through professional publications and the public through magazine and newspaper releases and a series of leaflets written on a layman's level. The American Dental Association's Council on Dental Therapeutics performs an analogous role with regard to dental preparations.

In 1959, the Senate Subcommittee on Antitrust and Monopoly (Senator Estes Kefauver, chairman) began an investigation of the practices, profits and products of American drug companies. (See Chapter 20, *Medicines,* for an account of another facet of the committee's work.) The hearings continued into 1960 and 1961, and the next year new enforcement laws were passed. The FDA then was able to work more effectively to enforce legislation against quackery. Possibly encouraged by the more aggressive role of the Federal Government, and probably motivated by growing public concern about fraudulent practices, many state law enforcement agencies also began to show their strength.

The problem of quackery is almost certainly unending. Concern about health, the state of one's body, is universal and legitimate. Physicians and scientists will never be able to supply all the answers, and the troubled, the innocent, the gullible, and the desperate will always hope for an answer elsewhere if a qualified source can no longer satisfy them. For long-term control of the problem of quackery, joint efforts through public education and public protection by professional and government agencies are a continuing necessity.

MEDICAL CHECKUPS

Regular medical examinations are desirable for everyone, regardless of age, sex, occupation, or physical condition. Merely for the guarantee against tuberculosis, which is one of the chief causes of disability and death among adolescents and teenagers, it is worth whatever time and money it may cost.

However, it pays other dividends besides the guarantee against the development of serious illness. It gives your doctor an invaluable, continuous record of your health. If a change in blood pressure developed, for example, he would be alerted because he would know the previous readings.

Another important benefit of a periodic examination is the opportunity it gives the patient to talk to an expert about emotionally disturbing situations. There are fears and problems which are not easily discussed with relatives or friends, but a sympathetic doctor can be extremely helpful in this area. It is much easier for the patient if he has been seeing the same doctor year after year, and feels he is an understanding friend as well as a capable physician.

How Often Is a Checkup Necessary?

Most doctors feel that if you are in your twenties or early thirties, every two or three years is sufficient, provided you have a tuberculin test for tuberculosis and your urine tested to detect diabetes every year. People over 50 should have a checkup once a year, and older people, or individuals with a strong family history of cancer, twice a year. Infants and young children need very frequent examinations.

The value of periodic health examinations is dramatically illustrated by the results obtained in the first such examination provided for the University of Michigan faculty. Two hundred and ninety-four persons were examined within a year; 239 were found to have a total of 465 defects or illnesses they didn't know they had, and 245 of these were serious enough to require immediate treatment. These included nine malignancies which were, fortunately, still curable, plus 37 proved and 31 suspected cases of diabetes.[1]

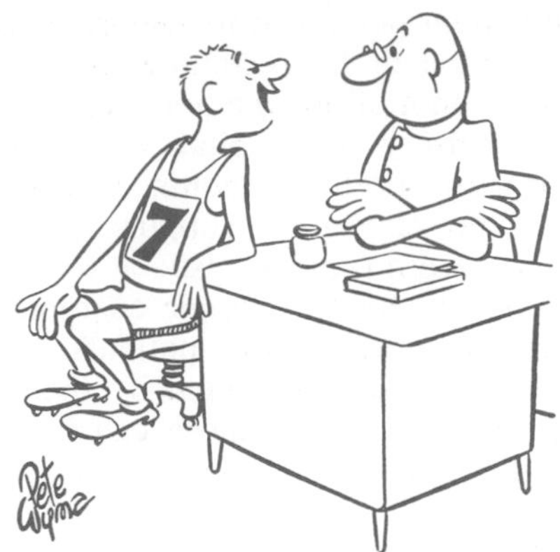

"I just stopped by for my 1,000-mile check-up."

(Courtesy of *Modern Medicine.*)

HEALTH AND X-RAY RECORD

Because of the increasing concern about the maximum tolerable dose of radiation over a lifetime, many physicians believe that it would be wise for everyone to keep a record of all the radiation he has received for diagnostic and therapeutic purposes. This would include dental x-rays, fluoroscopic or x-ray examination for tuberculosis, and the like. Also, it is useful to know what diseases you have had and when, the dates of various immunizations and medical examinations, as well as the kinds of medications you have taken.[2] It's hard to remember when you get older, whether you did or didn't have the mumps or the measles. An actual record kept from birth on will be written proof.

---

[1]Tupper, C.J., and Beckett, M.B.: Faculty health appraisal, University of Michigan, *University of Michigan Medical Bulletin, 24*:35, 1958.

[2]A very useful and inexpensive little booklet for this purpose is the *Personal Health Record* by Carl A. Dragstedt, published by the Military Service Publishing Company in Harrisburg, Pa., which has pages for listing all this information. Your physician can help fill in this booklet.

MODERN HOSPITALS

You probably have a vague idea of the many different kinds of hospitals there are—from small ones resembling private homes and accommodating only a few patients, to tremendous, imposing structures that look as though they could house an entire city. You may know hospitals that specialize in certain conditions and others that accept all kinds of patients.

However, every hospital falls into one of two groups: those that are *accredited* and those that are not. An accredited hospital is one which has been approved by the Joint Commission on Accreditation of Hospitals, which means that the hospital has met the following standards:

1. The physicians and surgeons are organized as a medical staff, and membership on that staff is restricted to doctors who are graduates of medical schools approved by the American Medical Association, are legally licensed to practice in their respective states, and are competent in their respective fields.
2. The medical staff has adopted rules and regulations to govern the professional workers in the hospital, and the staff meets at least once a month.
3. Members of the medical staff review and analyze their clinical experience at regular intervals.
4. A medical records department keeps records on all patients.
5. Diagnostic and therapeutic facilities such as a clinical laboratory and an x-ray department, with skilled men directing them, are available.

Types and Financing of Hospitals

General hospitals are organized to take care of essentially all types of illness,

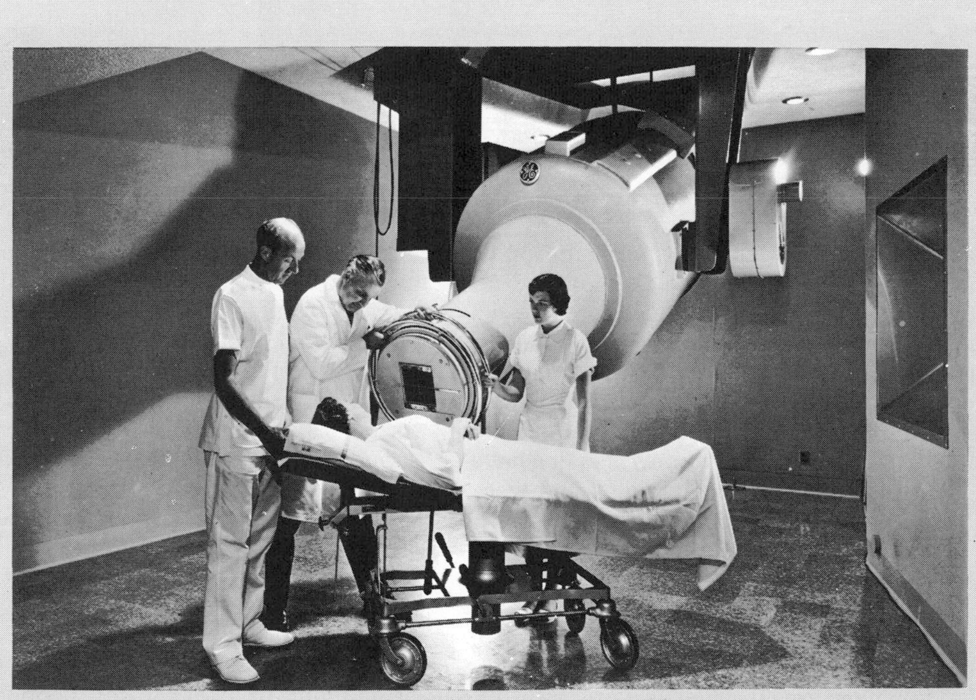

Among the larger pieces of equipment which modern hospitals use in the treatment of deep-seated malignancies is a 2,000,000-volt X-ray unit.

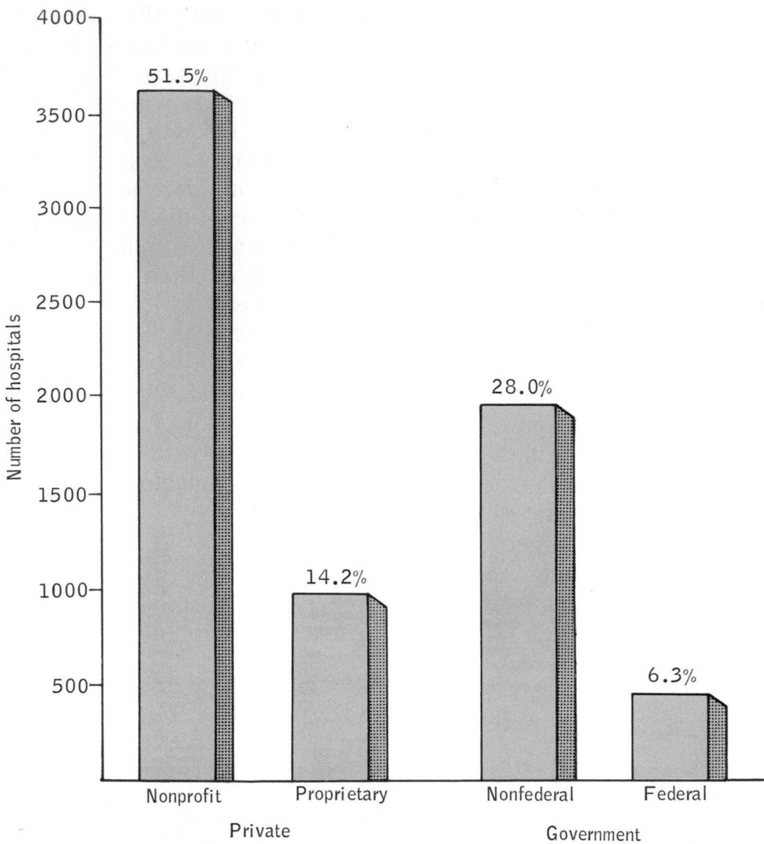

Figure 21–3. Distribution of types of hospitals in the United States.

accidents and surgery; *specialized* hospitals are usually limited to one type of medical problem. For example, there are special institutions for tuberculosis, mental illness, rheumatic fever patients, cancer, chronic diseases of the aged, orthopedics, maternity, children, and the eye, ear, nose and throat. Smaller communities usually have general hospitals, and big cities, with very large patient loads, tend to specialize.

Another modern plan, usually found in large cities, is the *medical center* in which specialized hospitals are grouped within the space of one or two blocks about a main general hospital.

Hospitals are financed in various ways. A small number, the *proprietary* hospitals, are privately owned, with any profits accruing to the owners, and they are rarely as well equipped or staffed as other types of hospitals. *Government* hospitals, such as those operated by the Veterans' Administration, are manned and completely financed by the federal government. Many large *city* and *county* hospitals are supported by the municipal or county government, or both. *Voluntary* hospitals are run by private nonprofit corporations organized for charitable purposes; they are usually supported by endowments and gifts, supplemented by community funds. Church-affiliated hospitals belong to this group.

The Widespread Use of Hospitals

One out of every eight people in the United States will go to a hospital this year, more than 25 million people, and this will include major operations, maternity cases, tonsillectomies and patients admitted merely for observation and special diagnostic tests. Nevertheless, some people

FROM TEMPLE TO MEDICAL CENTER

Highlights in the History of Hospitals

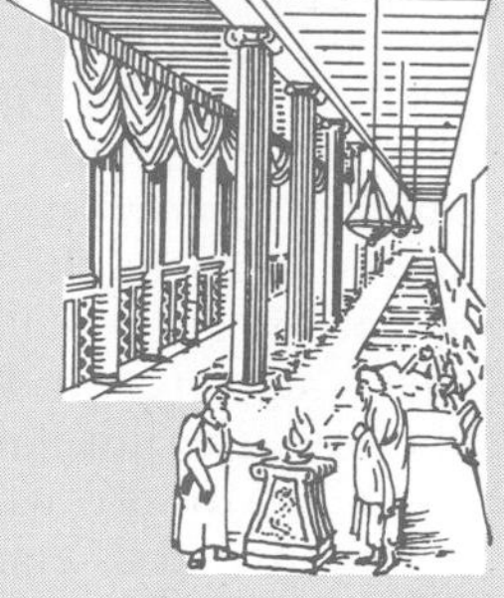

TEMPLES were used by the ancient Greeks to house their sick. Dedicated to Asclepius, the Greek god of medicine, these temples were often built near medicinal springs in which patients were ritually bathed and massaged. Treatment also included rest, special diets, and recreation.

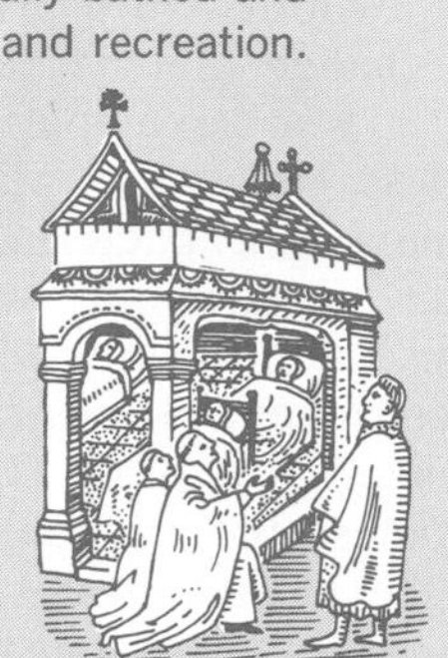

FIRST CHURCH HOSPITAL was built in A.D. 369 at Caesarea (now part of Turkey) by St. Basil, a father of the early Christian church. As Christianity spread, the sick became the concern of the church, and monasteries established hospitals for lepers, cripples, the blind, and the poor.

MEDIEVAL HOSPITALS were elaborate institutions that provided extensive care for the sick and the poor although little treatment for their diseases. In France, the Hôtel-Dieu de Beaune was typical. Architecturally beautiful, it offered privacy, cleanliness, and the opportunity for patients to attend Mass in bed.

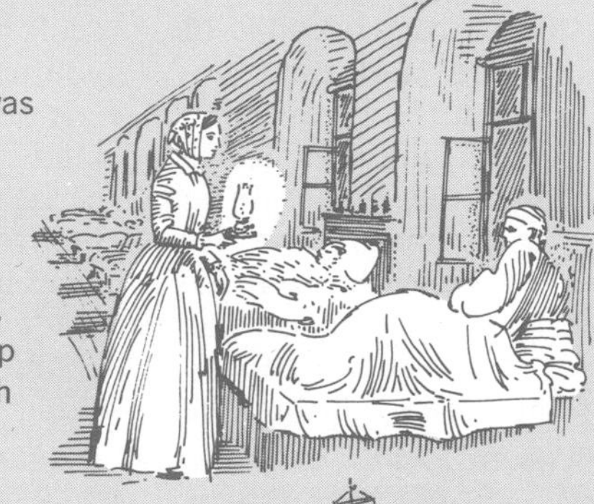

HOSPITAL REFORMS were started in 1853 by Florence Nightingale, who was appalled at the neglect into which hospitals had fallen. With 38 nurses, she scrubbed clean the British military hospitals in the Crimea and washed all the linen the patients wore. She was called The Lady with the Lamp because every evening she walked with a lantern among the hospital buildings, making her inspections.

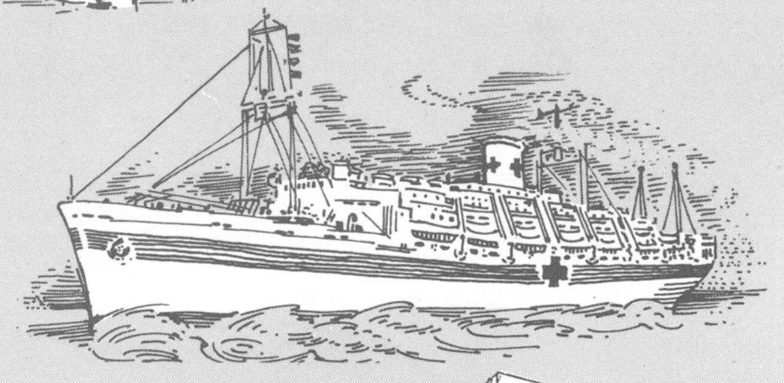

MOBILE HOSPITALS were developed during both World Wars. Doctors, nurses, and supplies followed troop movements and set up field hospitals near the front lines. After emergency treatment, wounded soldiers were evacuated by airplane, ship, or train.

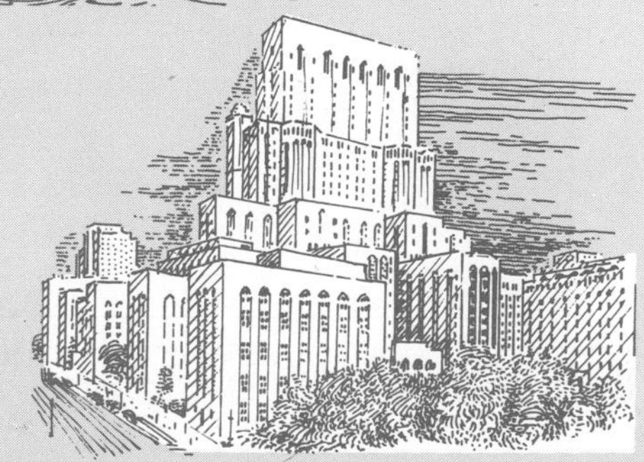

MEDICAL CENTERS that combine hospital, research, and teaching facilities are a modern development. These centers not only provide excellent medical care, but also train many doctors and do important research in the prevention and treatment of disease.

still fear hospitals because ancient prejudices die slowly. There *was* justification for this in the old days, but it is hard to find any resemblance between the modern hospital and the "pesthouse" of the past. The tremendous progress of medical science is nowhere exhibited to a greater degree than in the change that has taken place in hospitals. For example: 80 years ago (even less, in many places) doctors did not know that bacteria had anything to do with diseases or wound infections, and consequently they didn't even wash their hands before performing an operation or delivering a baby. There were no trained nurses; the first nurses' training school in the United States was established in 1872. Once, hospitals were primarily for people who were too poor to be cared for in their homes; but now both wealthy and poor take advantage of hospital facilities.

As Figure 21–4 shows, more than twice as many people used hospitals in 1963 as in 1935. Yet, the average stay has been reduced by almost 40 per cent because of advances in medical care and improvements in hospital procedures. Nevertheless, the increase in cost to the patient has been much sharper than the reduction in the hospital stay. The average cost per patient stay was $85.45 in 1946; in 1955, it was $180.34, and by 1963, it had risen to $299.61. These costs outweigh the declining value of the dollar during the same period.

WHAT HAPPENS WHEN YOU GO TO A HOSPITAL

Let us assume that you are going to the hospital for special diagnostic tests. Your doctor suspects hyperthyroidism, but he cannot be sure of this diagnosis without making use of the equipment and facilities the hospital affords.

Your physician calls the hospital with which he is affiliated and arranges for you to stay there, indicating the time of arrival and the type of accommodations you want.

You arrive at the appointed time with a few personal effects such as pajamas, slippers, robe and toilet articles. The admitting officer, if she thinks you are well enough, takes time to tell you the hospital rules and to ask you a few questions so she can complete her hospital records. She will also discuss your plans for paying the hospital bill. After that she calls a student nurse or orderly to take you to your room, and notifies the information desk and attending hospital physician that you have arrived.

You may have seen nurses in different kinds of uniforms. *Probationers* are in the early months of their training and perform the routine hospital tasks. After passing an examination, a probationer becomes a *student nurse* for the remainder of her course, which usually takes three years. When she graduates, she is a *trained* or *graduate* nurse, and becomes a *registered*

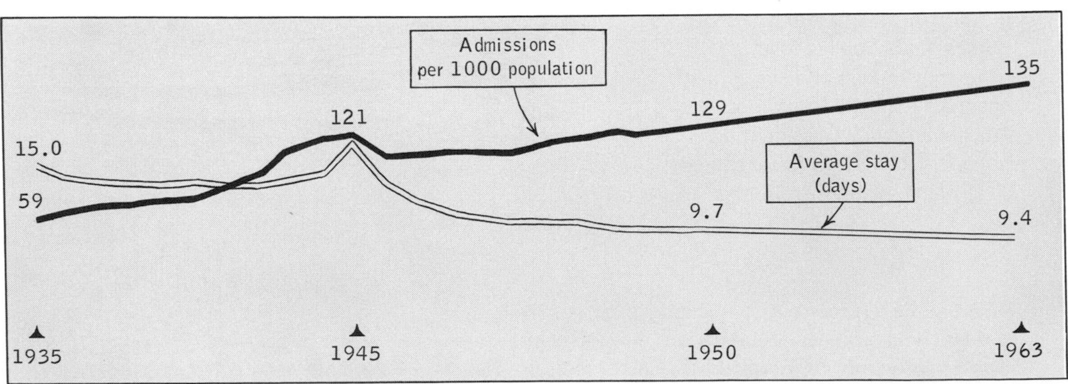

Figure 21–4. Utilization of general and special hospitals, United States, 1935–1963. (Adapted from *Health Information,* May, 1958.)

nurse, or "R.N.," after she passes the state examination. Many nurses take additional courses to fit themselves for specialty nursing.

The supervising nurse on your floor greets you and helps you change into hospital bed clothing.

First on your schedule is *hospital routine*. The attending nurse checks your weight, temperature, pulse and respiration, and records them on your bed chart. She also orders your diet, according to your doctor's instructions.

A nurse will answer your call if there is anything you need, and a circulating library service is usually at your disposal if you feel like reading. In most hospitals, you can also arrange to rent a radio or television set.

The hospital, you soon discover, is a busy place. From the managing board to the janitors, the hospital crew is working around the clock. Here is what goes on behind the scenes.

Staff physicians and young doctors rounding out their medical education assist your doctor in visiting the patients, and administering the prescribed treatments.

Not every young doctor who lives in the hospital is an intern. Today, in the larger hospitals, doctors frequently spend three to five years in training after they are graduated from medical school. For one or perhaps two years they are called interns; then they become assistant resident doctors, and finally in their third, fourth, or fifth years, chief or senior resident physicians. The chief resident has had seven to nine years of training from the time he entered medical school; that is why your own doctor has great confidence in him. If it becomes necessary, the chief resident will call the family doctor to the hospital outside of his regular hours there.

Most doctors visit their hospital patients once or twice each day. They try to keep these visits on a regular timetable so that

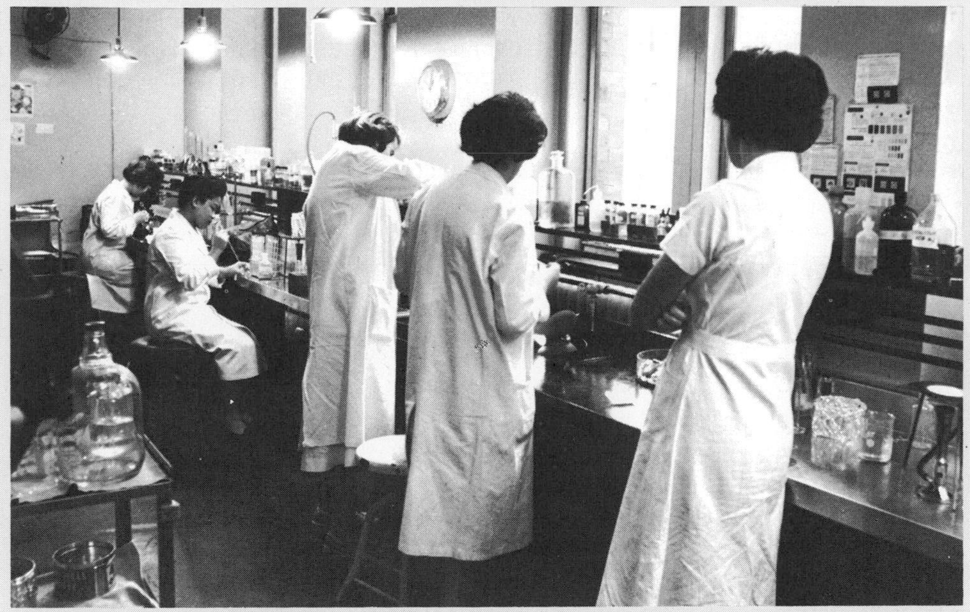

Urinalysis performed in a hospital laboratory. Chemical examination of urine is important in the diagnosis of many diseases, such as diabetes mellitus, liver and kidney diseases, and bladder infections.

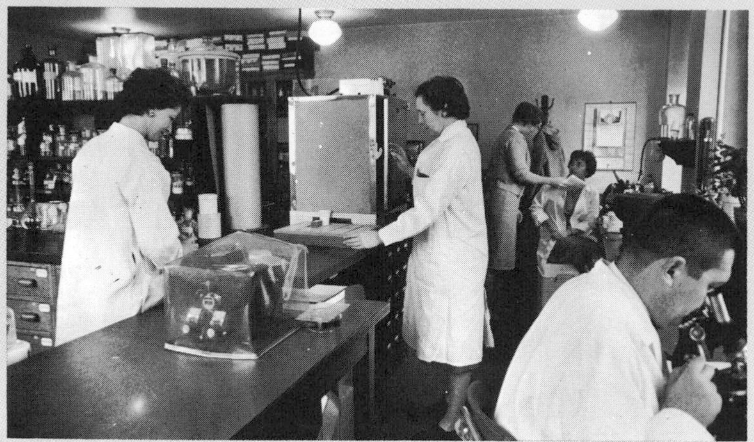

Hospital parasitology laboratory where analyses of feces and other body substances are made to determine if they contain evidence of internal parasites. Other hospital laboratories help diagnose diseases by studying such substances as blood, urine, and samples of tissue taken from patients during surgery.

they can meet their office appointments and schedule of home calls.

Not far from the wards are the *clinical* and *pathology laboratories*. Here a *pathologist* and his staff of technicians use modern scientific instruments and chemicals to help them determine patient progress, diagnose disease, and discover new means of combating disease. In these laboratories, with the aid of radioactive iodine and basal metabolism tests, your doctor will be able to determine whether you are really suffering from hyperthyroidism (our hypothetical diagnosis).

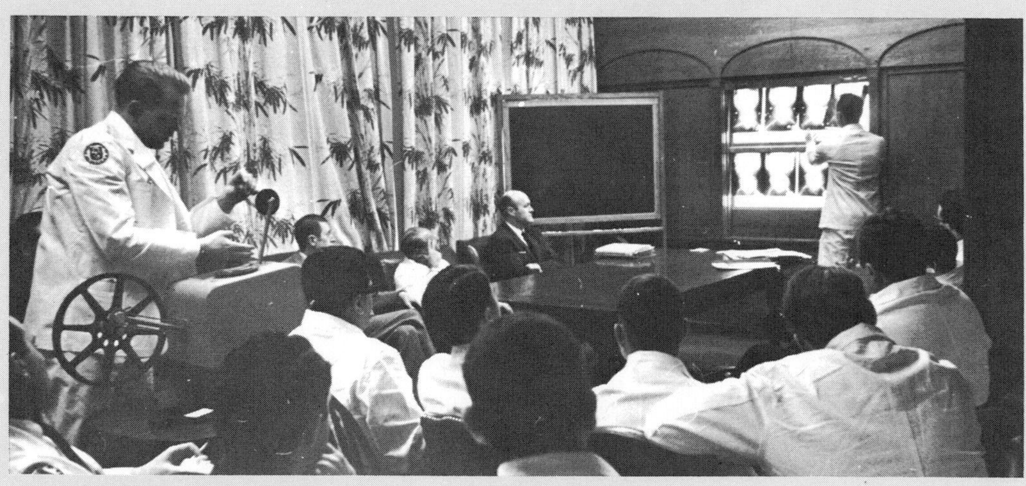

Hospital seminar in which interns learn to interpret X-rays. Many medical schools associate with hospitals because of the experience they provide for their students.

The hospital may also have a department for *physical* and *occupational therapy*. The directors of this department are usually graduates of physical or occupational therapy schools approved by the Council on Medical Education and Hospitals of the American Medical Association. Physical therapists render massage treatment and the like to persons crippled by polio or suffering other physical defects or ailments. Occupational therapists train disabled persons for new skills and jobs that are compatible with their disabilities; occupational therapy also includes crafts and other work that helps the morale of patients.

In another part of the hospital the *dietitians* are at work. They prepare nutritious meals and at the same time consider the special needs of individual patients. Licensed pharmacists in the hospital fill prescriptions for the drugs and medicines staff physicians order for their patients.

The x-ray department is another busy section of the hospital. Here *radiologists* are taking x-rays and reading them for diagnostic purposes; they are also trained and equipped to administer x-ray treatments for many types of disease.

If your hospital is a large, modern one, it probably has a dental clinic with highly trained *dentists* to take care of emergency dental work.

Another vital part of the hospital is its *blood bank*. Many pints of blood, carefully typed and drawn under sterile conditions, are stored here, to be used for accident victims, or patients undergoing operations or suffering from diseases which require blood transfusion. About 5400 hospitals now have such blood banks. In addition, there are 75 banks for mother's milk, 800 for bones, 475 for arteries, 150 for eyes, and 100 for skin tissue, to be drawn on for transplanting these organs or tissues.

Large quantities of medical equipment such as oxygen tents, portable mechanical "lungs," and infant incubators, are also kept in the hospital for special emergencies.

The hospital is a closely integrated unit. Unseen workers, such as housekeepers, carpenters, engineers, electricians, plumbers, bookkeepers, and secretaries, perform the duties that are necessary to keep the hospital running smoothly.

The Outpatient Department

This branch of the hospital provides medical care to ambulatory patients, as well as help and guidance to patients who have been dismissed from the hospital.

Doctors in the outpatient department treat accident and emergency cases which may come in during any hour of the day or night; in addition, they diagnose and treat the various diseases of entering patients. This department is usually arranged according to the specialties of medicine, with divisions for heart disease, cancer and other illnesses, as well as for prenatal, baby and child care. In these clinics, patients can secure the valuable services of specialists they might not be able to afford otherwise.

Clinic patients receive a preliminary examination in which trained men diagnose their ailments and, if necessary, send them to specialists for treatment. However, some patients go directly to the specialists, when they are referred by their own family doctor. Treatment in these clinics is by appointment. Some hospitals maintain free clinics or charge only a nominal amount.

It is important to realize that there is no stigma attached to using a hospital clinic, and it doesn't imply that you are unable to pay for your medical care. The diagnostic techniques required in some illnesses have become so technical, or the treatment so specialized and extensive, that hardly any but a very well-to-do person can be expected to assume the entire cost.

Social Service

Another important section of the hospital is the *medical social service* department. Here patients are helped to solve personal problems, such as home conflicts that interfere with recovery, or difficulty in paying the hospital bill or securing a job after being discharged from the hospital. Medical social service workers are also concerned with restoring the patient to his place in the community after he has left the hospital.

WHAT YOU NEED TO KNOW ABOUT SURGICAL OPERATIONS

Nearly 13.5 million people had some kind of surgical operation last year, and 60 per cent of all hospital patients are scheduled for surgery. Women account for more operations than men, because the figures (70 per cent compared to 30) include delivering babies.

Preparation for a Surgical Operation

Before an operation is undertaken the patient is carefully examined to make certain he is in sufficiently good condition to undergo it. X-rays are taken and other tests made to be sure he doesn't have tuberculosis, diabetes, nephritis, or some other serious illnesses. How good the patient's health should be varies with the type of operation he is facing. Modern surgical methods have made it possible to operate successfully on many patients who are not in good health, but such a procedure is undertaken only when it will subject the patient to less serious risks than those involved in failing to operate. The doctor carefully weighs all the factors.

Blood tests are also made to be sure the patient's blood clots normally, and to determine his blood type in case he should need a tranfusion. Allergies to various medications are noted and called to the attention of anyone who will be attending him.

A nurse or attendant shaves and thoroughly washes the part of the body to be operated on, and after a good night's sleep, the patient is ready for surgery.

Anesthetics

The operation is painless because of anesthetics—drugs that induce sleep or otherwise cause loss of feeling. We have come a long way from the days when the patient was given a stiff drink of whiskey or something to bite on—and withstood the pain as best he could.

Although such crude help was common enough under frontier conditions, for example, this by no means implies that a primitive anesthesia was unknown to ancient peoples. Early Egyptian surgeons exerted pressure on nerves or blood vessels to anesthetize a local area. A Babylonian clay tablet from 2250 B.C. gives the ingredients of a compound to relieve an aching tooth, and the *Iliad* tells of "pounded roots" that acted as an anodyne to soothe a wounded warrior. Nevertheless, only since the 1840's, when ether was first used, has the use of anesthesia become a science. Leading medical schools now have departments of anesthesia, with well trained specialists in charge, and there are many kinds of anesthetics, from *general,* which affect the whole body, to *local,* which anesthetize only the part to be operated on.

General anesthetics put the patient to sleep. *Ether,* which is administered through a cone or mask, is the most common, and it permits the patient to sleep throughout even a long operation. *Nitrous oxide* ("laughing gas") is sometimes given for short procedures or before the patient is given ether, because it induces sleep more pleasantly. *Chloroform,* once used as a general anesthetic, is now considered dangerous because it may damage the liver.

Cyclopropane, another of the inhalation anesthetics, is a gas that is pleasant smelling and quick-acting and results in rapid recovery after surgery. Still another new inhalant is *halothane,* a modern chemical relative of chloroform. In exceptional cases, it may cause liver damage. Nevertheless, it is popular with anesthetists, although they must use it with special caution. Several other commonly used inhalants produce deep or light sleep—*ethylene* is used when profound sleep is not necessary.

Another class of general anesthetics is given rectally. One of these is *paraldehyde,* which is sometimes prescribed for seriously disturbed alcoholics and psychotics. It is administered like an enema, and the patient is quickly anesthetized by absorption of the drug through the colon.

Intravenous anesthetics are general anesthetics which are administered through

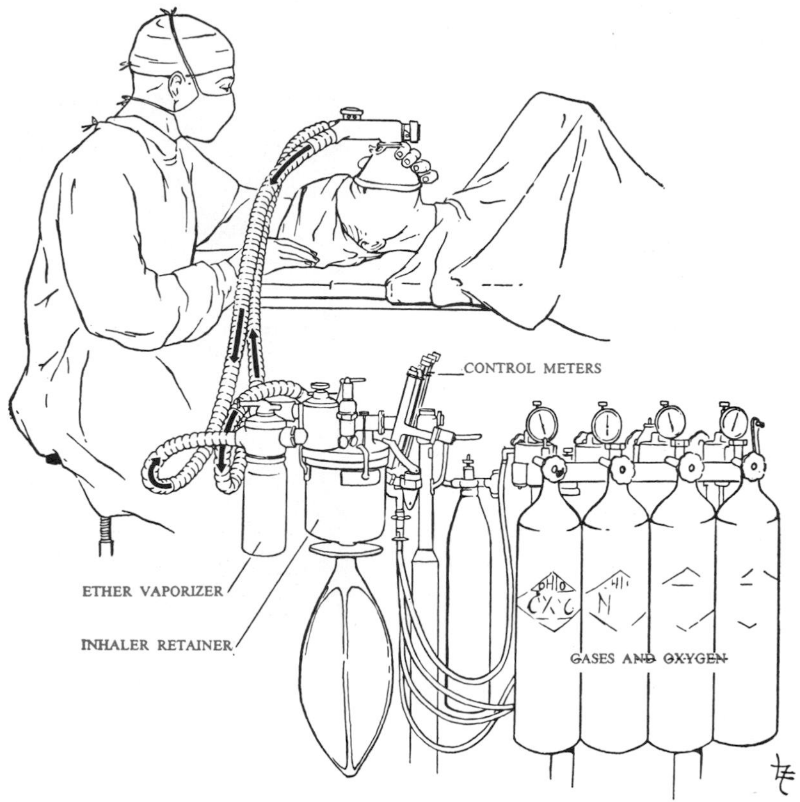

Figure 21–5. General anesthesia, using ether or other anesthetic gases.

a needle inserted into a vein. For very short operations, a barbiturate can be used because it has the effect of a superpowerful sleeping pill. An intravenous anesthetic may also be given to induce sleep quickly before ether or some other general anesthetic is administered.

Dental work and operations on the skin or tissues just under the skin are frequently performed with *local* anesthetics. In this method an anesthetic solution, such as *Novocain* or *procaine,* is injected into the operative area. In about 10 minutes all the pain nerves are deadened, and the surgeon can cut and sew without pain to the patient.

If a main nerve supplies the area to be operated upon, the doctor will inject the anesthetic directly into the nerve. This procedure is called a *nerve block*. In the lower jaw, for example, it is possible to inject directly into the main nerve and block pain from all the lower teeth on that side of the mouth. However, the main nerve trunk to the upper teeth is not so readily accessible, and the dentist has to infiltrate the anesthetic around the tooth by injecting it in several places.

Spinal anesthesia is a type of local anesthesia used in such cases as tuberculosis of the lung for which a general anesthetic might be extremely irritating to the lungs. In this procedure, the doctor first injects the skin and tissues under it with Novocain so that the patient will not feel any pain when he inserts the needle with anesthetic solution into the space around the spinal cord. This deadens all the nerves below the point of injection. This type of anesthesia is frequently used for operations in the lower part of the body, such as appendicitis, hernias and hemorrhoids. However, operations on the stomach and gallbladder are rarely performed under spinal anesthesia.

Caudal anesthesia or *continuous caudal* analgesia is sometimes used during childbirth. A needle is inserted into the *sacral canal* and a "painkiller" such as *procaine* is injected, which will numb the nerves of the uterus. The mother does not feel any pain although she remains completely conscious, and the child is not affected.

Finally, there is the comparatively rarely used anesthetic technique called *hypothermia,* involving the chilling of the body or of the part to be operated on. Chilling may be accomplished by ice packs, electrical units, or ice blankets through which cold alcohol circulates. The special purpose of hypothermia is, through lowering the body temperature, to slow down the heart action for cardiac and vascular operations. A general inhalant anesthetic is usually administered first.

Some physicians let the specialist in anesthesiology choose the anesthetic, because he makes his choice only after considerable study of the individual patient's constitution, condition, medical problem, and often only after consultation with the family physician.

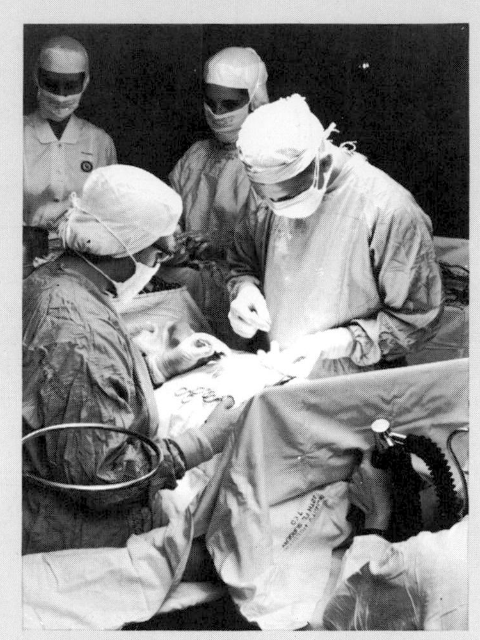

An operation in progress. All instruments and all equipment have been sterilized.

Sterilization and Asepsis

Before starting the operation, the surgeon scrubs his hands for a full 10 minutes to rid them of dirt and bacteria, perhaps also using an antiseptic solution. He is meticulous about this step because his rubber gloves might break or might already have an invisible hole through which bacteria could enter the operative area. All the instruments and everything that touches this area must be sterilized, and every doctor and nurse who assists must go through the routine of scrubbing and putting on sterile clothes. Each person in the operating room wears a cap over the hair and a mask over the nose and mouth to prevent bacteria from entering the air.

Before the surgeon incises the skin, he sponges it carefully with a disinfectant such as iodine or alcohol. Then he takes his position at the operating table along with his assistants and prepares the operative field.

The Operating Team

An operation involves the teamwork of several highly skilled people. The chief surgeon has the big job of planning the incision, opening the operative area, finding the trouble and repairing it. In an extensive operation, he is usually assisted by an experienced doctor (perhaps the head resident physician in surgery), and other doctors to help with various maneuvers during the operation. The anesthetist is responsible for the anesthesia, and there are usually two nurses to hand instruments to the surgeon and perform other incidental jobs.

The Operation

The surgeon or an assistant covers the body with sterile sheets, encircling the area upon which he will work with towels and special cloths. When he is ready to begin, only the operative area is exposed.

He first cuts the skin with a special knife called a *scalpel,* and then pulls back

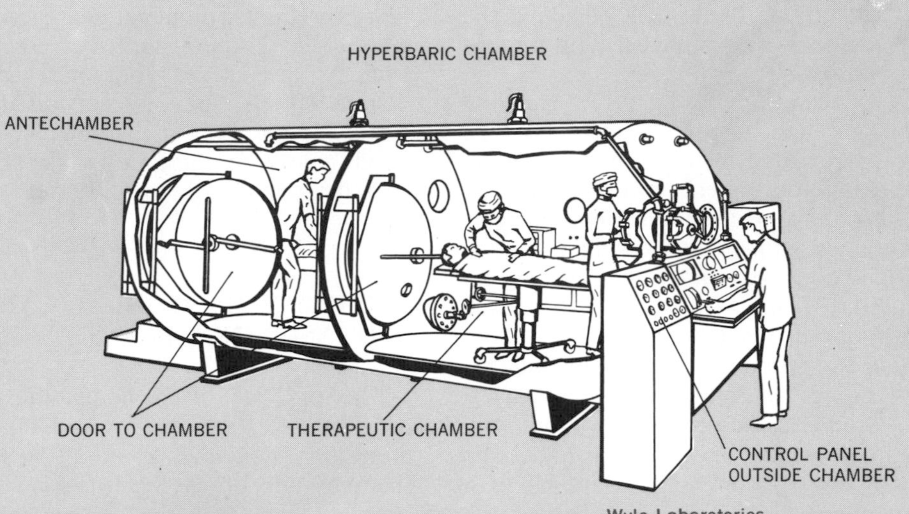

Wyle Laboratories

Diagram, above, shows a hyperbaric chamber and control panel of a hyperbaric system. Surgical procedures in the therapeutic chamber are shown below. To eliminate possible danger from too rapid changes in air pressure, patient, doctors and nurses are "decompressed" in the antechamber before leaving enclosure.

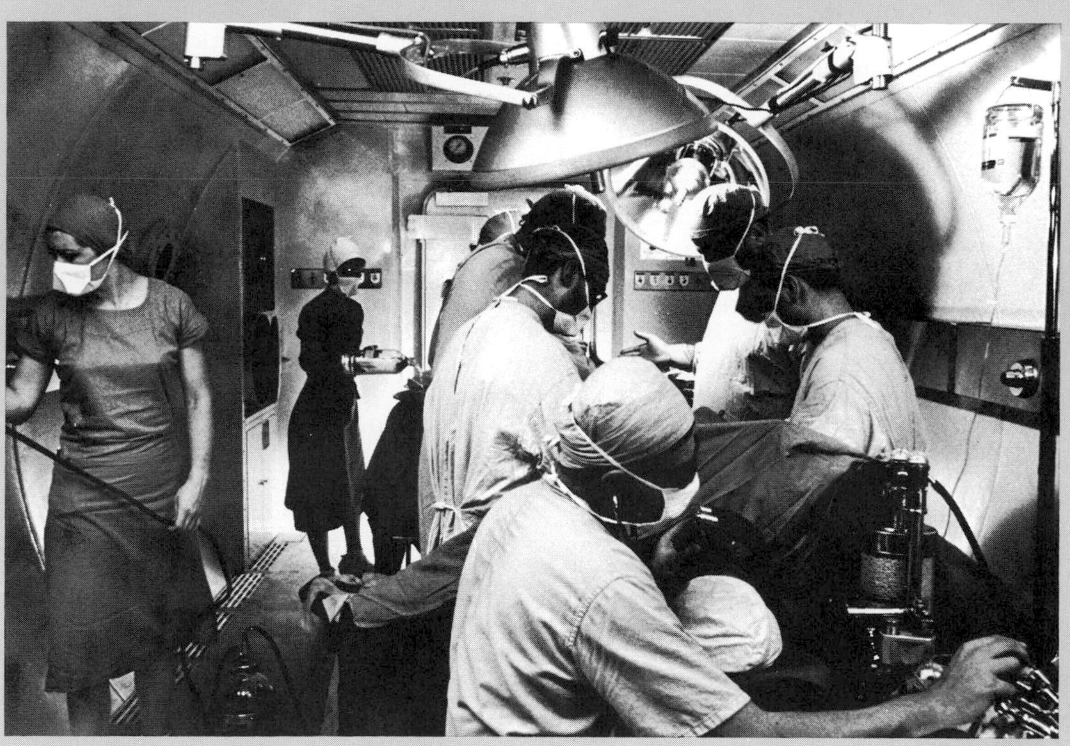

the edges of the skin with *retractors*. Next he methodically cuts into the area he wishes to operate upon. If there is bleeding, the blood vessels are clamped off with forceps called *hemostats*.

The surgeon works deftly, handling the tissues and organs as little and as gently as possible to avoid bruising them or shocking the patient. Even though the operation may be a simple one—a clear-cut case of appendicitis which he has performed countless times—he is always on the alert. There *could* be something different about this patient.

When the surgeon has completed his job, he ties or cauterizes bleeding vessels. This is tremendously important in internal operations which involve cutting large arteries. For example, the removal of a kidney necessitates the severance of the main renal artery. If this vessel were to open and start bleeding after the operation, a serious internal hemorrhage would develop that could threaten the life of the patient. Surgeons anticipate such dangers and prevent them by tying important arteries twice.

After a careful check to make sure that no sponges or instruments have been left in the operative site comes the final step in the operation, closing the incision. This is done with thread sutures or, sometimes, with metal clips, which leave an almost imperceptible scar.

In some operations a drainage tube may be led out from the area of operation through part of the incision. This is to help siphon off pus, or excess fluid, or to drain the bile temporarily in operations on the gallbladder. It is usually removed in a few days.

After the Operation

Modern surgery has made phenomenal advances in recent years, including the prevention of complications after operations. Blood clots in the lungs, once a much feared danger, may arise from blood clots in veins of the lower part of the body, if parts of these clots break off and travel to the lungs, blocking a major blood vessel. *Early ambulation,* which is the practice of getting patients out of bed and having them walk even the first or second day after a major operation, helps prevent complications of this kind. This, plus other improved techniques, such as the use of antibiotics and intravenous fluids, pays good dividends in getting patients out of the hospital, in good condition, and in remarkably brief periods compared to previous decades.

THE COSTS OF MEDICAL CARE AND INSURANCE PLANS

The practice of medicine, the costs of medical care, the quality and quantity of attention available to the public, and the methods of paying for good health—all have changed in kind and in degree since Colonial days. It cost only $7.50 to deliver a baby in New Jersey in 1784, and a pioneer doctor in Bangor, Maine, would make a house call for $1. In 1885, Buffalo Medical College charged $150 for a "medical education ticket." In contrast, annual tuition rates at American medical schools today range from $300 at the University of Texas for state residents to $1750 at Harvard. Total expenses of course are much greater—the Council on Medical Education and Hospitals of the American Medical Association reports that in addition to the $1285 median tuition charge, students pay $900 for room and board and another $150 for books and supplies, not including microscopes.

In the 1950's and 1960's, the question of the quality of medical care was largely resolved. Advances in medical science ensured the highest quality medical care, consonant with the attention given to medical education and training. What was controversial was the precipitous rise in the cost of medical care and by what methods the public should be expected to pay for it.

The Cost of Medical Care

Both the quality and quantity of medical care today are higher than ever before, and the trend is still upward. The generally rising standard of living and the increased cost of good health combine to make good medical attention expensive. The costs, particularly hospital costs, are such that many economists and sociologists—plus, of course, the average head of a household who must meet these bills—have urged a closer look at medical charges. (The Reading Suggestions at the end of this chapter include some critical and controversial studies and recommendations.)

Total expenditures for medical care, public and private, were nearly $33 billion in 1964. This was an increase of $19 billion, or a rise of more than 1½ times, over a 12-year period. On a per capita basis, medical costs rose from $97 in 1958 to $127 in 1963. Today, the average consumer spends 6.3 per cent of his income on medical care. He spent 5.3 per cent five years previously, and 3.7 per cent in 1929. In 1963, according to the American Hospital Association, the American public spent 58 per cent more on hospital care than it did five years previously—this was more than twice as much as the public paid for hospital care in 1953.

The trend of all costs has been upward since World War II, and the costs of medical care over the years have risen faster than the costs of any other item of personal expense. Figure 21–6 shows the percentage of costs in various expense categories.

Of course, the amount spent for medical care rises with income, and conversely, it represents a declining proportion of personal income. In the most recent United States National Health Survey, the average medical expenditure by a person earning less than $2000 annually was $112, or 5.2 per cent.* For the person earning $7000, it was $153, or 2.1 per cent. More than 30 per cent of those families with incomes of less than $2000 reported no medical expenses at all for a year, however, while only 11 per cent of those earning $7000 incurred no such expenses.

The way the medical dollar is divided also has been changing. (See the illustration, Distribution of the Medical Care Dollar, p. 310.) Hospital room rates rose by 38 per cent in the period 1959–63, while physicians' fees increased by 14 per cent. Drugs represent an increasingly significant portion of the medical dollar, while medical insurance plans of all kinds are, by necessity, becoming more popular, thereby consuming a greater share of the overall costs of medical care.

Thirty-three billion dollars for medicine, or for anything else, is a sum too large to be grasped easily. But it makes for interesting comparisons with other expenditures on a national scale. Of the $33 billion for medical care, $23.7 billion represented private expenditures, and the remainder, public outlays at all levels of government. Compare to this the nearly $30 billion spent in 1963 on clothing, accessories and jewelry; the nearly $16 billion spent on recreation, and the $36 billion for transportation. Such statistics do not negate the hardship that mounting medical expenditures present to families caught in crises, but they do suggest that, on a national scale, some value judgments need to be questioned, as well as the costs of health.

Insurance Plans for Medical Care and Hospitalization

Most people resent spending money for medical and dental care, even though they are extremely grateful to their physicians when they are helped through a critical illness or accident. Part of our reluctance to pay doctor bills is that there isn't any pleasure element in seeing a doctor. His job is to correct something that's gone wrong, and to bring our bodies back to working the way they're supposed to. It is curious that we take our irreplaceable bodies for granted, and expect so much more from these fragile skin and bone structures than we do from a reinforced steel automobile.

The sad truth is that the human body, remarkable though it is, *does* need care and attention. The best and most economical way to provide regular, high-quality medical care—as three of four American

*The National Health Survey is a continuing research project of the Public Health Service, U. S. Department of Health, Education and Welfare. The Survey seeks out and reports statistical information like that cited here.

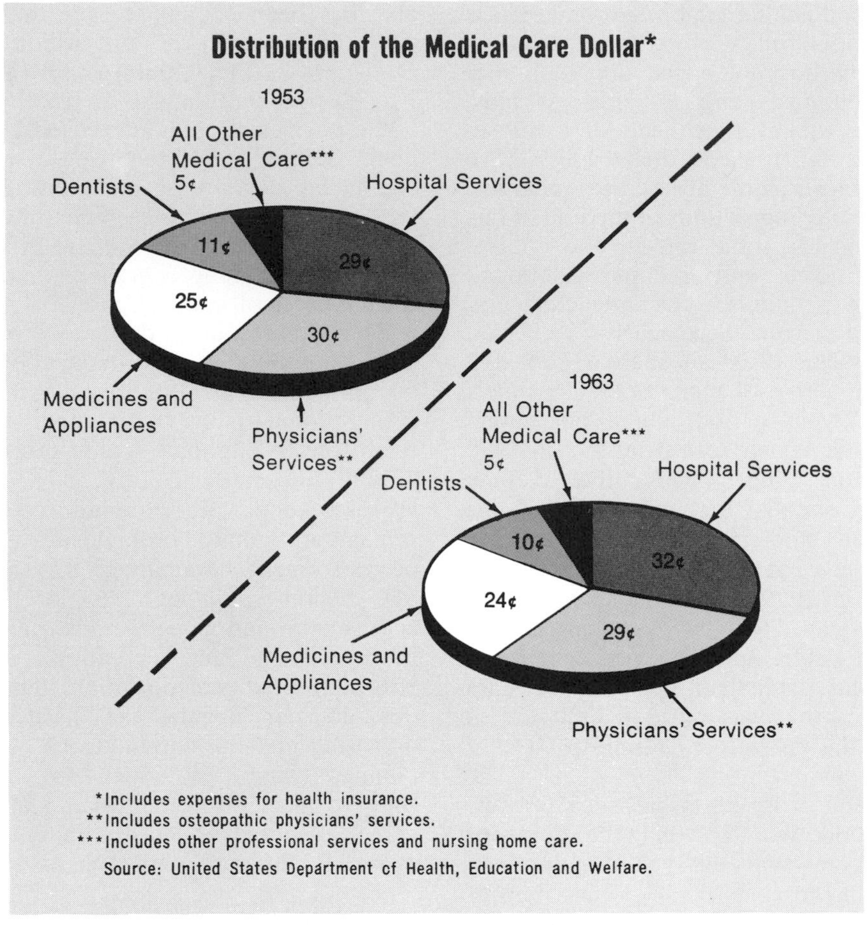

Figure 21–6. Distribution of the medical care dollar including expenses for health insurance.

families have learned—is through some form of insurance.

Suppose every time you needed a package of cigarettes, you stopped at your neighborhood drug store and told him to "put it on the cuff." Eight years—and 2920 days later—the clerk had reached the limit of your credit, and handed you a bill for $876. You would be shocked.

The same economic danger applies to your health. Unless you put something aside for the possibly very rainy day, you may at some time in your life be faced with a ruinously high medical or hospital bill, which could keep you in debt for many years. This has happened to so many people that medical and hospital insurance policies have become very popular purchases.

Of the five major types of health insurance—covering hospital expenses, surgery, regular medical charges, major medical bills, and loss of income—the first is the most popular, although public acceptance of all five continues to grow. In 1963, more than 145 million Americans, 77 per cent of the population, had some form of health insurance. In both absolute and percentage terms, such insurance has become more widely accepted than ever before. By 1960, 121 million Americans had hospital insurance policies, about 70 per cent of the population. Some of these hospital plans (Blue Cross, for example) pay the hospital directly; many compensate the patient in cash.

Surgical expense protection is nearly as popular. In 1963, just under 135 million persons carried such insurance. More than 102 million held regular medical expense insurance, which provides payment for physicians' fees for nonsurgical care in the office, in the hospital, or at the patient's home. Some of the plans also cover diagnostic x-ray and laboratory expenses.

The fastest growing form of insurance is major medical. Forty-two million persons now own these policies, which provide broad protection against almost every kind of health care outlay prescribed by a doctor, both in and out of a hospital. These plans also usually pay the expenses of special nursing care, x-rays, prescriptions, medical appliances, nursing care in the home, and ambulatory psychiatric care. Such policies typically underwrite a large percentage of these costs—perhaps 80 per cent—after the patient pays the first $200 or so. This protection against catastrophic illness, major surgical procedures and serious accidents has saved many families from economic ruin and long-term indebtedness.

Loss-of-income policies, which help replace salaries and wages when a man or woman is unable to work because of illness, are the oldest form of voluntary health insurance. Nearly 47 million wage earners obtained such protection for themselves and their families—or had it provided through their employer—in 1963. In some states, including California, New York, New Jersey, and Rhode Island, this protection is guaranteed by law, and the nation's railroad workers, among others, are sheltered by loss-of-income insurance.

In spite of these advances, insurance payments are much less than private outlays. Insurance benefits cover about one-half of hospital and physician charges, which together account for 53 per cent of all private medical expenditures. The 30 per cent of the population who are uninsured include many poor and elderly persons in serious need of more medical attention because of their position and age who are unable to afford either insurance or attention. The question of individual ability to pay for health insurance, the problem of medical costs, and the complex and troublesome relationships among physicians, patients, hospitals, insurance companies and the government have led to pressures for some variety of national health insurance, a system adopted by most other Western nations, in some cases several generations ago. Such pressures resulted in the introduction of frequent bills in Congress, but until 1965 none were ever passed. Extremely strong and effective opposition historically has been exerted by professional groups, most notably the American Medical Association, and by powerful private insurance companies. In 1965, however, the first steps were taken to provide medical care through a national insurance program, the care to be forthcoming on the basis of medical need rather than financial need, through the mechanism of Social Security. How this legislation will affect private plans is not predictable, but that it will have considerable impact is without question.

In the Summer of 1965, President Johnson signed into law a Medicare bill that included these provisions:

Hospital care—up to 60 days for each period of illness, after payment of the first $40.

Nursing Home Care—20 days in each period of illness, at no cost to the patient.

Home Nursing Care—up to 100 visits by nurses or technicians, at no cost to the patient.

Out-patient Service—80 per cent of hospital diagnostic service costs after the first $20 for each diagnostic study period up to 20 days.

In addition to this basic coverage, the bill provided supplementary coverage, to be paid voluntarily by the patient and federal funds. This coverage augments the basic services.

All services under Medicare are for men and women 65 years of age or older. The financing mechanism is through Social Security, and the money will come from higher Social Security levies.

PRIVATE VERSUS GROUP PRACTICE

The doctor in private practice, especially if he has no assistant, leads a very difficult life. Tremendous demands are made on

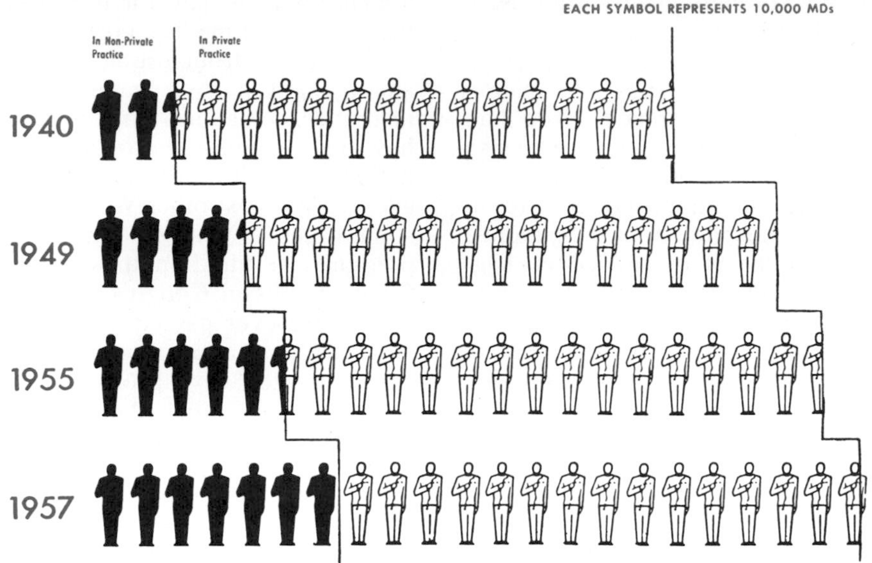

Figure 21–7. Private versus nonprivate practice. (From *New Medical Materia,* January, 1959.)

his time and energy, and, if he is a good doctor and a popular one, he has very little time he can call his own. He is usually awakened by a sick or worried patient—often after making calls in the middle of the night—and goes steadily all day, with house calls, hospital visits, office hours, hospital visits, and house calls again. Often he feels his responsibility to the community he serves so keenly—sometimes he is the *only* doctor serving a relatively large area—that he can't take time off for a much needed vacation. Equally important, he cannot get away for refresher courses, so essential today because of the rapid advances in medical knowledge.

These are the reasons more and more doctors are going into group practice, or full-time salaried positions.

In many communities, particularly in the North Central and Western part of the United States, physicians are teaming up into groups. Such groups will vary in size, in the number of specialists, and, of course, in the kind and quality of services they offer. For example, a small group might consist of a diagnostician, a surgeon, a pediatrician, and a laboratory specialist. A large group might have at least one specialist in almost every important branch of medicine and surgery.

A combination of this type can often offer unusually good medical care because of the close cooperation between its various members. They can provide laboratory tests and the services of specialists at reasonable rates. Some groups provide service on a monthly prepayment basis for the entire family, which includes annual medical checkups without extra charge.

In 1962, 66 per cent of physicians were in private practice. Most of the remaining 34 per cent were in groups of one sort or another. This compares with 86.5 per cent in private practice in 1940.

Questions

1. If you became sick in a strange city, how would you find a competent doctor?
2. Name five types of specialists, and describe what medical or surgical work they engage in.
3. Why is it sensible to keep a record of all x-ray examinations and treatments?
4. What is meant by an "accredited" hospital?
5. How does an intern's medical work differ from that of a practicing doctor?
6. Describe the differences between general and local anesthetics.
7. Why do surgeons go to such extremes of caution to maintain completely sterile conditions during an operation? Describe some aseptic techniques employed in the operating room.

8. How does the annual expenditure for medical care compare with the amounts spent for liquor and entertainment?
9. Describe some of the insurance plans for doctors' and hospital bills.
10. What is the difference between private and group practice?
11. Cite some methods of detecting a medical fraud.
12. Why do so many people turn to charlatans for medical advice and treatment?
13. What obstacles have confronted attempts to legislate medical protection for the American public?
14. Differentiate between health fads, health rackets, and health cults. Do you think one is more or less culpable than another?
15. What legislation, if any, do you think is desirable and necessary for additional protection against quacks?

Topics for Discussion

Types of hospitals in your community.
Osteopathy and chiropractic.
History of sterilization and asepsis.
The trend toward more medical specialization.
The problem of increased costs for medical care.
Effects of medical insurance on hospital occupancy.
How physicians can help wipe out quackery.
The psychology of joining health cults.
How qualified physicians may unwittingly drive patients to seek help from quacks.
Responsibility of government versus professional groups to protect the public against frauds.
Defense of health cults or food fads because they may offer some limited help.
The future of Medicare.
Pros and cons of government health insurance.

Reading Suggestions

You and Your Doctor, Martin S. Gumpert. Bobbs-Merrill Co., Indianapolis, 1952. A guide to show you how to be a good doctor's good patient.

Science and Surgery, Frank G. Slaughter. Perma Books, Pocket Books, Inc., New York, 1956 (paperback). How the surgical wonders are performed that bring added health and longevity to modern man.

Understanding Surgery, ed. by Robert E. Rothenberg. Pocket Books, Inc., New York, 1955 (paperback). Describes the nature of surgical operations and the reasons for them, and answers many questions about surgery.

Devils, Drugs and Doctors, W. H. Haggard. Pocketbooks, Inc., New York, 1959 (paperback). The dramatic story of healing, from medicine man to modern physician.

Economics of Public Health: Measuring the Economic Impact of Diseases, Burton A. Weisbrod. University of Pennsylvania Press, Philadelphia, 1961. An economist's analysis of health costs and of techniques to determine the appropriate level of such expenditures.

A Commonsense Guide to Doctors, Hospitals and Medical Care, Richard H. Blum. Macmillan, New York, 1964. A detailed handbook answering the usual and some unusual questions that arise on this topic.

The Economics of American Medicine, Seymour E. Harris. Macmillan, New York, 1964. The $35 billion cost of all medical care is analyzed critically and often sharply by an influential economist.

The Doctor and His Patient, Samuel W. Bloom. Russell Sage Foundation, 1963. The doctor, the patient and their complex relationship from a sociologist's viewpoint.

Doctors, Patients, and Health Insurance, Herman M. Somers and Anne R. Somers. Anchor, Doubleday & Co., New York, 1961 (paperback). A detailed study of private medical care, in all its ramifications.

Family Spending Patterns and Health Care. Progress in Health Services, Vol. 9, Health Information Foundation, 1960.

The Management of the Doctor-Patient Relationship, Richard H. Blum. McGraw-Hill, New York, 1960.

Patients' Views of Medical Practice, E. Freidson. Russell Sage Foundation, 1961.

Medical Care Financing and Utilization. Health Economics Series No. 1, U. S. Department of Health, Education, and Welfare, Public Health Service, 1962.

The Rising Cost of Hospital Services. Progress in Health Services, Vol. 12, No. 3, Health Information Foundation, 1963.

You and Your Doctor, William H. Potter. Duell, Sloan & Pearce, New York, 1961. A popular guide through the forest of medical specialties and varieties of care.

How to Get the Most out of Medical and Hospital Benefit Plans, Ruth Brecher and Edward Brecher, Prentice-Hall, New York, 1961.

Changes in Family Medical Care Expenditures and Voluntary Health. O. W. Anderson and others. Harvard University Press, Cambridge, 1963.

Medical Care and Family Security, Karl Evang, D. Stark Murray, and Walter J. Lear. Prentice-Hall, New York, 1963. A comparative examination of medical care insurance programs in Norway, the United Kingdom, and the United States.

The History of Surgical Anesthesia, Thomas E. Keys. Dover, New York, 1963 (paperback).

The Medicine Show, by the editors of *Consumer Reports,* Simon and Schuster, New York, 1961. A down-to-earth account of some common ailments and problems, and of the remedies sold to treat them. A good summation of current frauds, outrages, and quackery.

The Toadstool Millionaires, James Harvey Young. Princeton University Press, 1961. An historical account of patent medicine promotion in the United States prior to national legislation.

The Doctors' Dilemmas, Louis Lasagna. Harper, New York, 1962. A frank discussion of many of the "follies, fads and frauds" of medicine, as well as of some of its achievements.

The Natural History of Quackery, Eric Jameson. Charles C Thomas, Springfield, Ill., 1963.

"Proceedings," Second National Congress on Medical Quackery, sponsored by the American Medical

Association and the Food and Drug Administration, October 1963.

Medical Care, Health Status and Family Income: United States: National Center for Health Statistics. Vital statistics on personal health expenditures, health insurance coverage, use of medical and dental services, chronic and acute illness, based on data from the National Health Survey of the U. S. Department of Health, Education and Welfare, 1964.

How to Get Good Medical Care, Irvin Block. Public Affairs Pamphlets No. 368 (381 Park Ave. S., New York, N. Y. 10016), 1965. Criteria for judging a doctor's competence and good hospital care.

22

THE TOBACCO HABIT

Despite the publicity given the report of the Surgeon General's advisory committee that "cigarette smoking is causally related to lung cancer," 70 million persons in our country still continue to use tobacco on a daily basis. Obviously, we Americans are highly susceptible to the "tobacco appeal."

If the present trends continue lung cancer will claim the lives of more than 1,000,000 present school children before they reach the age of 70 years.

THE AMERICAN PUBLIC HEALTH ASSOCIATION

DISCOVERY OF TOBACCO

The tobacco plant belongs to the nightshade family, which also includes the tomato, the Irish potato, and belladonna, from which many important medicines are extracted. It belongs to the genus *Nicotiniana,* and is thought to have been named after the French ambassador to Portugal, Jean Nicot, who sent tobacco seeds as a gift to his queen, Catherine de Medici, in the sixteenth century.

The Persians were apparently familiar with tobacco for a long time, and there is even an old Persian proverb which says, "Coffee without tobacco is meat without salt." However, the widespread use of tobacco apparently came to the continent of Europe from the newly discovered America.

In November of 1492, Columbus sent out a party of men to explore the island of Cuba, and they returned with reports of brown people there who puffed or smoked lighted firebrands.

Ramon Pane, a Franciscan who accompanied Columbus on his second voyage, described the habit of snuff-taking. Tobacco-chewing was first seen by Spanish explorers in 1502 on the coast of South America.

It soon became apparent, when the American continent was opened up, that smoking tobacco was a widespread and very important custom, apparently associated with solemn tribal ceremonies.

The name did not derive from the plant itself but from a **Y** shaped instrument, called "tabaco" by the natives of San Domingo. The two points of the **Y** were inserted into the smoker's nose, and the other end of the **Y** was held in the smoke of burning tobacco. This is how the fumes were inhaled.

Ralph Lane, the first governor of Virginia, and Sir Francis Drake brought the plants and the implements for smoking from America, and gave them to Sir Walter Raleigh. He is credited with popularizing smoking in England, where the custom spread despite enormous opposition resulting in severe penalization and even capital punishment.

The virtues and the faults attributed to tobacco have been many and varied. The plant was at first believed to possess such miraculous healing powers that it was commonly called *"herba santa," "herba panacea,"* and by Edmund Spenser, "divine tobacco."

In 1659, a Dr. Everard in London recommended the use of tobacco leaves, extracts, ointments, powders and lotions to cure an almost endless list of human ills, which included headaches, deafness, toothaches, coughs, stomach pains, burns, wounds, worms, and mad-dog bites.

On the other hand, Dr. Tobias Venner in 1620 expressed his extreme distrust of tobacco as follows:

> It drieth the brain, dimmeth the sight, vitiateth the smell, dulleth and dejecteth both the appetite and the stomach, disturbeth the humors and spirits, corrupteth the breath, induceth a trembling of the limbs, exsiccateth the windpipe, lungs and liver, and scorcheth the heart.

In 1624, the Pope held the threat of excommunication over the heads of snuff-users. The Turks imposed the death penalty for smoking, and the Emperor of Russia ordered smokers to have their noses slit, after which they were whipped and deported to Siberia.

Yet the habit persisted, and the newly formed American Colonies raised tobacco as their chief crop. In fact, it was considered so valuable that it often served as a form of currency among the early settlers. Today, despite continuing controversy and warnings about its dangers, it is more popular than ever before. Tobacco now represents one of the nation's chief sources of farm income, and tobacco growers receive well over a billion dollars a year for their crop.

NICOTINE IN TOBACCO

The effective ingredient of tobacco, responsible for some of its appeal and hazards, is *nicotine*. This is a highly poisonous substance, which the chemists call an "alkaloid."

Nicotine is so toxic that the amount in one cigar is enough to kill two men, if it could be directly injected into the blood stream. Fortunately, we don't extract all the nicotine in cigarettes and cigars when we smoke.

Over a single five year period recently, almost 300 cases of nicotine poisoning were reported. It is a common component of some insecticides and plant sprays, and humans who suffered excessive exposure to such sprays have become ill as a result.

The concentration of nicotine varies considerably in different tobaccos. It runs as high as 6 to 8 per cent in Virginia and Kentucky tobacco, and from 1.3 to 4 per cent in Cuban, Maryland, German, and Austrian tobacco.

Low-nicotine cigarettes fall into two categories: those made from specially bred tobacco strains with a low nicotine content; and the so-called "denicotinized" ones from which part of the nicotine has been removed by extraction with solvents or treatment with steam. Some, but not all, denicotinized cigarettes reduce the nicotine to about 50 per cent of that found in regular cigarettes.

Cigarettes made from specially bred tobacco with low nicotine content may have as little as 15 per cent of the nicotine found in standard brands. However, they contain an analogous substance, *nornicotine,* not normally found in tobacco. The physiological effects of this compound are similar to nicotine, but it is only one-half to one-tenth as toxic.

The so-called "strength" of a tobacco does not depend on its nicotine content. It derives from other aromatic substances

FROM CEREMONY TO CONTROVERSY

Highlights in the History of Smoking

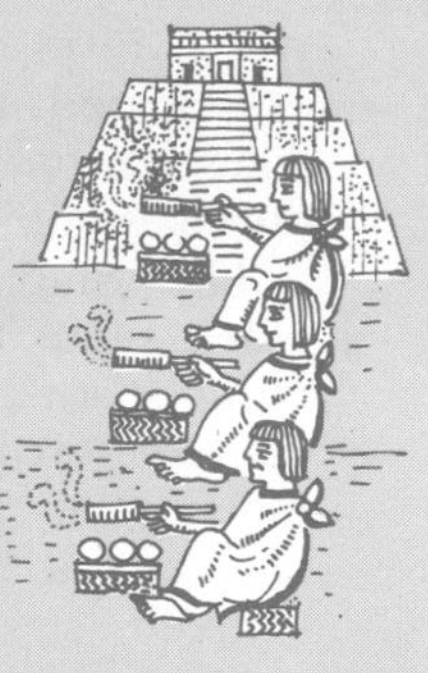

INDIANS OF NORTH AND SOUTH AMERICA were the first people to cultivate tobacco. They used it ceremonially in the ratification of treaties, and believed it to have medicinal value. The Mayans of ancient Mexico made the first cigars. They wrapped cured and fermented tobacco in its own leaves and smoked it during religious ceremonies.

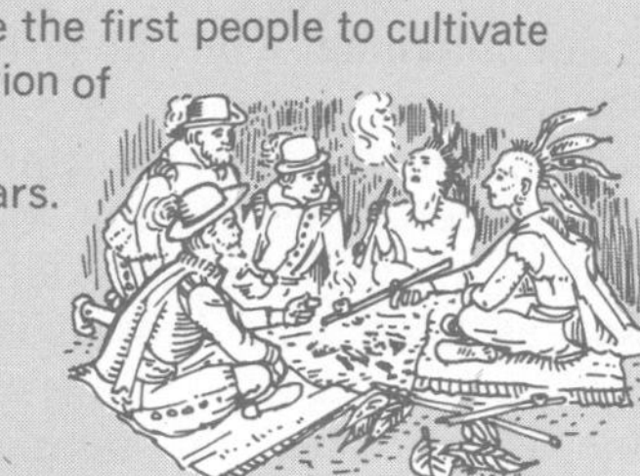

JEAN NICOT, French ambassador to Portugal, is believed to have introduced tobacco to France about 1555, with a gift of seeds he sent to Queen Catherine de Medici. The plant genus, *Nicotiana,* to which tobacco belongs, is named after him.

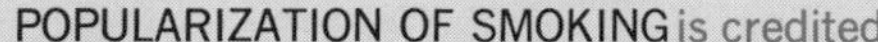

POPULARIZATION OF SMOKING is credited to Sir Walter Raleigh who learned the practice from the Indians. In Europe, men and women of all classes began to use tobacco in its various forms. James I, of England, strongly opposed its use and tried in vain to stop it.

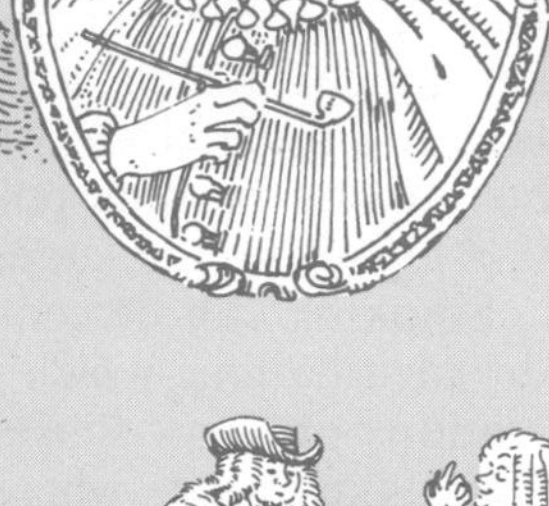

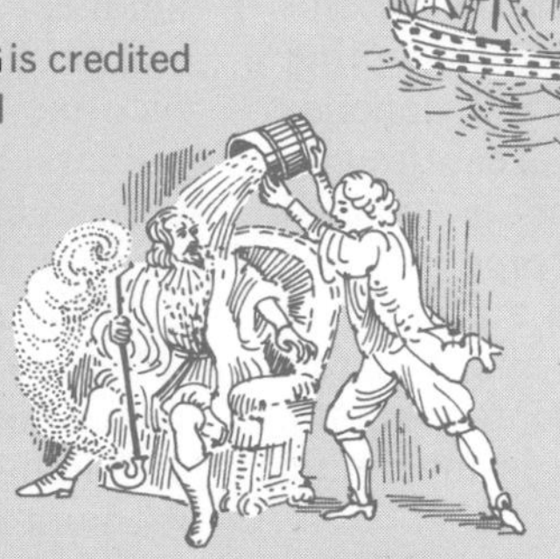

INHALING SNUFF, or finely ground tobacco, became widespread throughout Europe during the 18th century. At first, people carried small tobacco grinders in their pockets. Later, ground tobacco was sold and snuffboxes to hold it were made by jewelers in richly ornamented gold, silver, and ivory.

THE TOBACCO INDUSTRY, in 1963, rated annual world production of tobacco at about eight billion pounds. In the United States, in 1963, about 70 million Americans spent eight billion dollars for more than 523 billion cigarettes and more than 7 billion cigars.

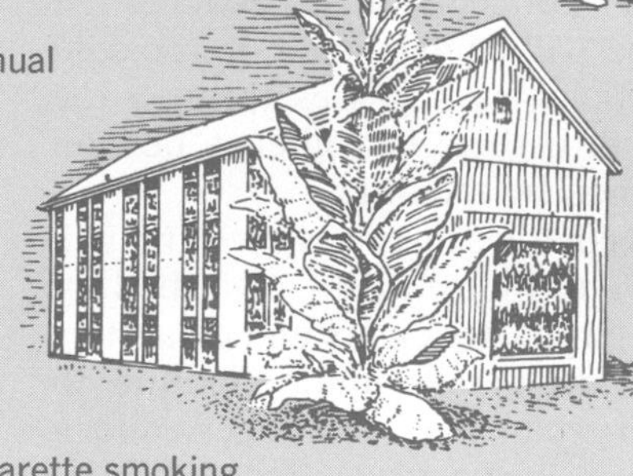

CONTROVERSY over the health hazards of cigarette smoking began in 1895, when an obscure French doctor noted the coincidence of the use of tobacco with cancer of the mouth, tongue, and lips. In January 1964, a committee appointed by the Surgeon General of the United States reported to the Public Health Service, after 14 months of study, that it believed cigarette smoking was associated with cancer of the lungs and the esophagus. It also related chronic diseases of the lungs and of the heart to smoking.

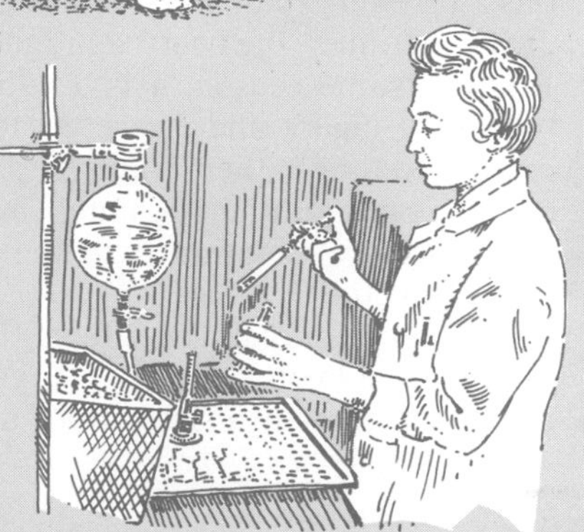

which form during the fermentation process carried out after the leaves are cured. These aromatic materials are volatilized during smoking.

The amount of nicotine you absorb when you use tobacco depends on a number of factors, chiefly the nicotine content of the tobacco, the amount of moisture it contains, whether it is smoked, chewed, or taken as snuff, and how it is smoked.

More nicotine is absorbed in taking snuff than in chewing or smoking, and tobacco chewers swallow more nicotine than smokers do.

Cigarette smoke contains only 14 to 33 per cent of the total nicotine in tobacco, and cigar and pipe smoke contains considerably more. The chief reason for this is that the amount of nicotine and other substances which are volatilized depends largely on the size of the hot area, directly behind the burning point. This is smallest in a cigarette and largest in a pipe.

Smoking can be considered a process of dry distillation, which means the transformation of dry substances into vapors. This takes place where there is maximum heat, at the glowing zone.

Fortunately, about 25 per cent of the nicotine is destroyed at the glowing area, and about 30 per cent is sent out into the atmosphere. The remaining 45 per cent passes through the cigarette or cigar, but only about 15 per cent actually reaches the mouth. Some will be deposited on the cold tobacco particles as it passes through the cigarette, and, if there is a filter, a portion will be retained by the filter.

If the passage is short, less nicotine will be retained and more will be absorbed by the smoker. Short, fat cigars and cigarettes retain less and permit more nicotine to pass through than long thin ones, and a cigar becomes "heavier" as it gets shorter. For the same reason, it is a poor practice to smoke cigars and cigarettes to the very end, or to relight them when they have gone out. A butt contains a much higher concentration of nicotine than the front end of a cigarette.

How you smoke also affects the amount of nicotine you take in. If you smoke rapidly, you will absorb more smoke and pass less out into the so-called "sidestream" than if you smoke slowly. Cigarette smokers who inhale absorb as much as 60 mg. of nicotine from a single package of cigarettes, as compared with as little as seven mg. for noninhalers.

Filter tipped cigarettes have become very popular in recent years because they are supposed to precipitate out and retain some of the harmful ingredients of the smoke as it passes through. Today a high percentage of the cigarettes sold are filter tipped, and new filtering agents are constantly being introduced.

Many filter tips that are used today are no more effective than an equivalent length of plain tobacco in a cigarette. This, too, absorbs some of the noxious materials in smoke.

The stem of the average pipe removes nicotine very poorly. Pipes and cigarette holders with removable and replaceable cartridge filters allow somewhat less smoke to pass through, and take out some of the nicotine and other volatile chemicals from tobacco. However, studies by W. A. Wolman showed that a cigarette holder using an unlighted cigarette as the filtering medium reduced the tar and nicotine concentrations more than any other type of filter tested.[1]

NOXIOUS GASES

In 1604 James I of England expressed his violent distaste for tobacco in the following words: "Herein is not only a great vanity, but a great contempt of God's good gifts, that the sweetness of man's breath, being a good gift of God, should be wilfully corrupted by this stinking smoke."

Besides nicotine, tobacco smoke contains a number of other very toxic substances, fortunately in only small amounts. These include carbon monoxide, ammonia, pyridine, hydrogen sulfide and hydrogen cyanide.

Fritz Kahn has commented in his book

[1]*Journal of the American Medical Association*, *152*:917, 1953; *154*:678, 1954.

Table 22–1. Consumption of tobacco products per person aged 15 years and over in the United States, selected years, 1900 to 1962

Year	All tobacco, pounds	Cigarettes, number	Cigars, number	Pipe tobacco, pounds	Chewing tobacco, pounds	Snuff, pounds
1900	7.42	49	111	1.63	4.10	0.32
1910	8.59	138	113	2.58	3.99	.50
1920	8.66	611	117	1.96	3.06	.50
1930	8.88	1,365	72	1.87	1.90	.46
1940	8.91	1,828	56	2.05	1.00	.38
1950	11.59	3,322	50	.94	.78	.36
1960	10.97	3,888	57	.59	.51	.29
1961	11.15	3,986	56	.59	.51	.27
1962	10.85	3,958	55	.56	.50	.26

Source: Department of Agriculture, Economic Research Service.

Man in Structure and Function that if Miguel de Torre had returned to Columbus from his expedition to Cuba with a chemical analysis of tobacco smoke as part of his report on smoking, no one would have believed him. As Dr. Kahn says, "It is in fact extremely surprising that man can inhale a truly 'hellish' gas mixture such as tobacco smoke for hours daily over a period of years and decades without poisoning himself."

WHO SMOKES AND WHAT DO THEY SMOKE?

A government survey of smoking habits in the population over 18 showed that more than half of all males and about one fourth of all women over that age smoke regularly, and most of them smoke 10 to 20 cigarettes a day.

In the past 15 years, cigarette smoking has increased 50 per cent, cigar smoking has decreased about 13 per cent, and the use of pipe tobacco has declined 66 per cent. The number of women smokers has increased greatly in recent years.

Nearly as much tobacco is chewed a year as is smoked in pipes—about 75 million pounds. Some of this is used by workmen in industries where they are not permitted to smoke. The consumption of tobacco products since 1900 is summarized in Table 22–1.

THE EFFECTS OF TOBACCO

Nicotine has a number of very definite, and sometimes disastrous, effects on the body, depending on the amount absorbed. Tobacco also contains other substances that have been demonstrated to cause cancer in experimental animals.

Digestive System

Nicotine very definitely increases intestinal peristalsis, and many smokers use a cigarette as a laxative. In some individuals, however, smoking may cause indigestion and constipation and even chronic colitis (an inflammation of the intestinal tract). And a significant statistical relationship has been established between cigarette smoking and peptic ulcer.

Smoking can dull the appetite and even spoil it, because it inhibits the production of gastric juice and increases blood sugar levels.

Respiratory System

Excessive use of tobacco is frequently irritating to the respiratory system, and it is the cause of very common cigarette cough. This is due to a chronic irritation of the respiratory mucous membranes, and may lead to an actual thickening of the mucous membrane of the bronchial tubes, demonstrable by x-ray. Too much smoking increases the severity of tuberculosis and other infections of the respiratory tract.

Cancer

"Cigarette smoking is causally related to lung cancer . . . ." reads the 1964 Report of the Advisory Committee to the Surgeon General of the U.S. Public Health Service. This statement results from a careful synthesis of the many studies of the relationship of smoking and lung cancer.

Because the critical student will want to carefully evaluate the facts for himself, the authors have attempted to summarize some of the evidence that prompted the Surgeon General's Report. Study this evidence carefully, note what the experts conclude, and then make your own decision about smoking.

Facts that Suggest Cigarette Smoking Causes Cancer.

1. Cigarette smoking became a common habit in the United States and England about 1900. In 1920 a national epidemic of lung cancer began and has increased each year.

2. In the early years of tobacco usage, women were forbidden the use of this "noxious gas." Accordingly, they had a lower incidence of lung cancer. *Today, more women smoke than men; if this trend continues, it is possible that it may result in a higher incidence rate of cancer among women than men.*

3. Lung cancer was rare in Iceland before 1940. Then cigarette smoking became a popular habit. In the following 20 years, lung cancer increased five-fold.

4. To this day, lung cancer is a rare disease among nonsmokers.

5. When smokers and nonsmokers are compared as statistical classes, there are numerous studies from more than a dozen countries that clearly indicate an increased incidence of lung cancer among smokers.

6. There is a highly significant correlation between the amount of tobacco consumed in the various countries of the world and the incidence rate of lung cancer.

7. Within a given country, there is a highly significant correlation between the amount of tobacco consumed on an individual basis and the incidence of lung cancer.

8. Persons who inhale have a higher incidence of lung cancer than persons who do not inhale.

9. Individuals who stop smoking cigarettes have a lower rate of lung cancer than those who continue to smoke cigarettes.

10. There is a significant correlation between the number of years a person has smoked and the incidence rate of lung cancer.

11. The earlier one starts to smoke the more likely he is to develop cancer of the lungs.

12. Tobacco smoke contains at least eight substances that have been demonstrated to cause cancer in animal experiments.

What Do the Experts Say About This Evidence?

1957—"The sum total of scientific evidence establishes beyond reasonable doubt that cigarette smoking is a causative factor in the rapidly increasing incidence of human epidermoid cancer of the lungs."

Joint Report of a Study Group of The American Cancer Society
The American Heart Association
The National Cancer Institute
The National Heart Institute

1959—". . . the evidence available today was reasonably interpreted as indicating that cigarette smoking is a major causative factor in the increasing incidence of human carcinoma of the lung."

Report of a Study Group of The World Health Organization

1960—". . . The clinical, epidemiological, experimental, chemical, and pathologic evidence . . . indicates beyond a reasonable doubt that cigarette smoking is the major cause of the unprecedented increase in lung cancer."

The American Cancer Society

1960—" . . . cigarette smoking is a major cause of lung cancer."

The National Tuberculosis Association

1962—"The strong statistical association

between smoking, especially cigarettes, and lung cancer is most simply explained on a causal basis."

Royal College of Physicians
London

1964—The following statements are from the 1964 Report of the Advisory Committee to the Surgeon General of the U.S. Public Health Service.

Lung cancer.

"Cigarette smoking is causally related to lung cancer . . . the risk of developing cancer increases with the duration of smoking and the number of cigarettes smoked per day, and is diminished by discontinuing smoking."

Oral cancer.

"The causal relationship of the smoking of pipes to the development of cancer of the lip appears to be established."

Cancer of the larynx.

". . . cigarette smoking is a significant factor in the causation of laryngeal cancer in the male."

Cancer of the esophagus.

". . . the evidence of tobacco-esophageal cancer relationship supports the belief that an association exists. However, the data are not adequate to decide whether the relationship is causal."

Cancer of the urinary bladder.

"Available data suggest an association between cigarette smoking and urinary bladder cancer in the male but are not sufficient to support a judgment on the causal significance of this association."

Heart Disease

There are serious effects of smoking on the heart and circulatory system. Most physicians recommend that patients with angina pectoris or who have suffered heart attacks give up smoking because of the undesirable action of nicotine.

Heart rate and blood pressure, and sometimes heart pain, are increased by smoking. It also causes spasm, or contraction of the arterioles, the very small blood vessels, in the extremities. Aggravation of the condition known as *Buerger's disease* (*thromboangiitis obliterans*) can result from this contraction.

Table 22–2. Summary of physiological changes resulting from the use of nicotine

1. Increased heart rate (15-25 beats per minute).
2. A rise in systolic blood pressure (10-20 mm. Hg).
3. A rise in diastolic pressure (5-15 mm. Hg).
4. Increased cardiac output (0.5 liters/per minute/ per square meter).
5. A decrease in peripheral blood flow.
6. A decrease in finger and toe temperature.
7. An increase in adrenalin.
8. An increase in intestinal peristalsis.
9. An increase of free fatty acids in the blood.
10. An acceleration of the còagulation of blood.
11. An inhibition of the production of gastric juices.
12. A dulling of the appetite.

This disease eventually leads to actual obliteration of the arteries and arterioles of the extremities. Gangrene can then set in, and the loss of fingers or toes, a foot, or even a leg, may result. Buerger's disease occurs only among smokers, and its severity can be arrested by a very simple measure—*stop smoking.* As soon as smoking is resumed, symptoms of the disease reappear.

The relationship of tobacco to Buerger's disease is unequivocally established. It may be related to the fact that during smoking, the rate of blood flow slows down—and may even stop—in the extremities. Skin temperature of a finger may drop more than 5° F. after smoking an ordinary cigarette because blood flow to that area is reduced.

Many denicotinized cigarettes and a variety of filter tipped cigarettes on the market have almost exactly the same effect as ordinary cigarettes on skin temperature and on the severity of Buerger's disease.[2] The ordinary degree of denicotinization and the use of filter tips in cigarettes are not enough to offer significant protection against the effect of nicotine on the heart and circulation.

It is interesting that Buerger's disease has been a very rare disease among women. About 99 per cent of the cases are found in men. However, signs of this disease are fairly high among Puerto Rican women, who smoke short, cigar-like cigarettes with a very high nicotine content.

[2]Wright, I. S.: *Journal of the American Medical Association, 155*:666, 1954.

Another disease of the circulatory system in which tobacco is implicated is *Raynaud's disease*. In this condition, there is a spasm of the small blood vessels in the extremities which causes blanching of the skin after exposure to cold, or from anxiety and certain other factors. This spasm may be brought on by smoking only one or two cigarettes, and most doctors strictly forbid smoking for patients with this disease. The chief danger is that the more serious Buerger's disease may develop later.

There have been many studies on the relationship of smoking to death from heart disease. Although different experimental procedures were employed and the studies were conducted in many different countries, the results are remarkably consistent: cigarette smokers have a much higher incidence of heart disease than nonsmokers. Further, it has been found that the incidence of heart disease increases progressively with the rate of daily cigarette consumption and the amount of inhalation.

The mechanism whereby cigarette smoking leads to an increase in the incidence of heart disease has not been elucidated, but a number of theories are being investigated. For example, it is clearly demonstrated that nicotine by its effect on the nervous system produces a temporary sympathetic preponderance, with the effects shown in Table 22–2. Also of importance may be the finding that smoking increases the concentration of free fatty acids in the blood. This increase in blood lipids could possibly be a contributing factor in arteriosclerosis. Dr. Orville Horwitz and Donald S. Waldorf of the University of Pennsylvania Hospital have found that smoking accelerates the clotting time of blood and increases the toughness of the clot.

Although the mechanism is not clear, the statistical evidence leaves little doubt that cigarette smoking unfavorably affects the cardiovascular system. The most convincing study in this connection was conducted by Dr. Joseph T. Doyle and Dr. Thomas R. Dawber. In their painstaking studies, over 3000 persons between the ages of 30 and 62 years were studied for a 6 to 8 year period. Prior to the study, all the subjects were judged by medical examination to be free of heart disease. Thereafter, the onset of heart and circulatory disorders were observed in both smokers and nonsmokers. The results indicated that among heavy smokers the incidence of heart disease was three times as high as that among nonsmokers. There are many other studies to support this finding.

High Blood Pressure

Nicotine and smoking both increase blood pressure. For this reason, physicians often recommend that individuals suffering from hypertension (high blood pressure) give up smoking.

Fatigue

Certain people seem to be inordinately sensitive to tobacco as far as general health and energy are concerned. Doctors have frequently commented that some patients who seem well, physically and emotionally, nevertheless are easily exhausted and seem to drag around at ordinary tasks. They complain of many fairly mild but unpleasant symptoms like chronic fatigue, headaches, rapid pulse, indigestion, nervousness, and restlessness. Most of these patients are smokers, and frequently feel much better and often completely well when they give up smoking.

Smoking and Longevity

Most specialists in this field agree that smoking influences longevity. Extensive studies by the noted statistician, Raymond Pearl, indicate that a moderate consumption of tobacco has a slight but definite effect on the life span, but that heavy smoking has a very marked effect.[3] For example, among heavy smokers about 25 per cent fewer survive to the age of 50 than among a corresponding group of nonsmokers. Hammond and Horn found

[3]Pearl, Raymond, *Scientific Monthly*, *87*:216, 1938.

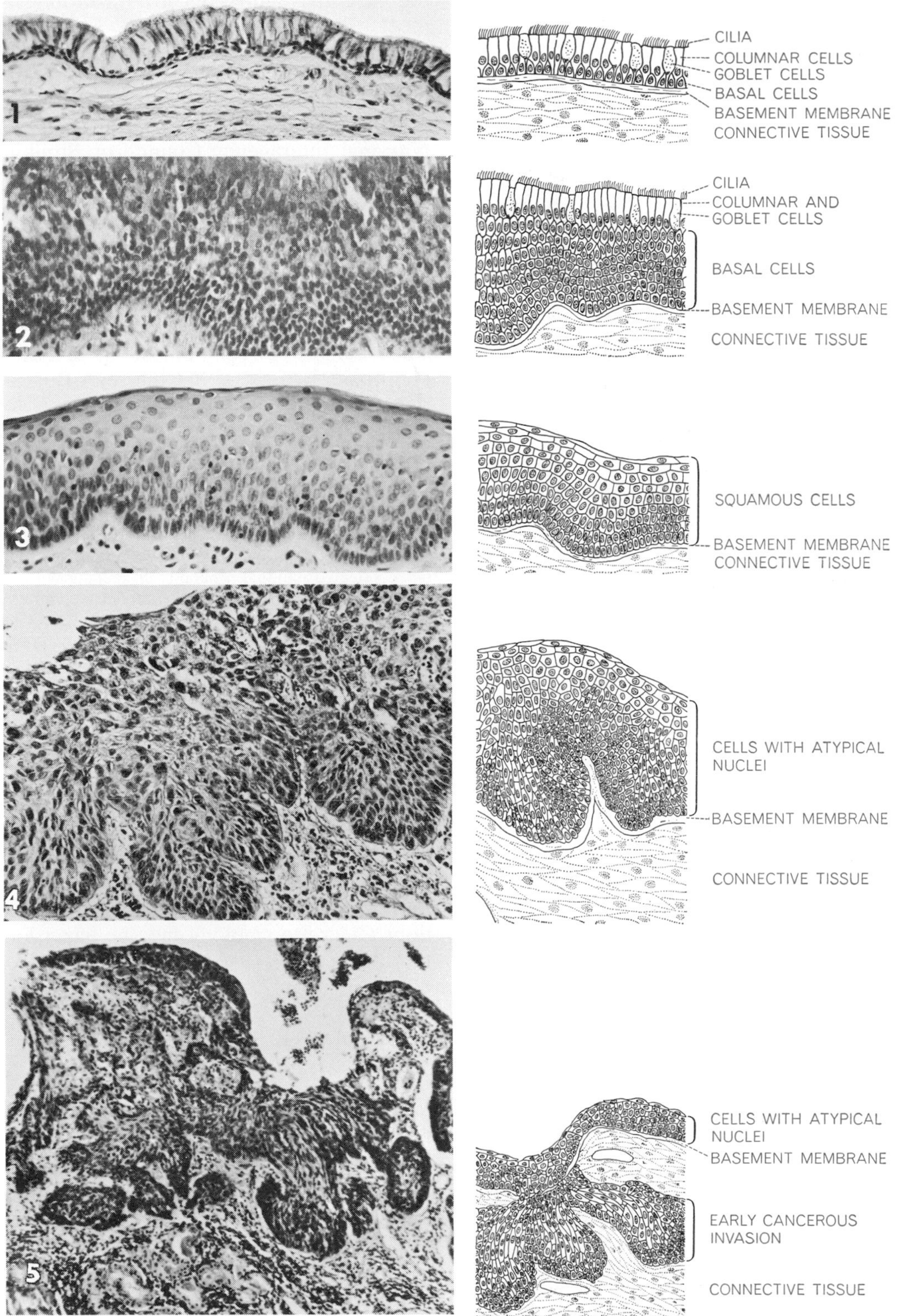

Figure 22–1. Examples of normal and abnormal bronchial epithelium. (From Hammond, E. C.: *Scientific American, 207*:39, 1962. Photomicrographs by Dr. Oscar Auerbach.)

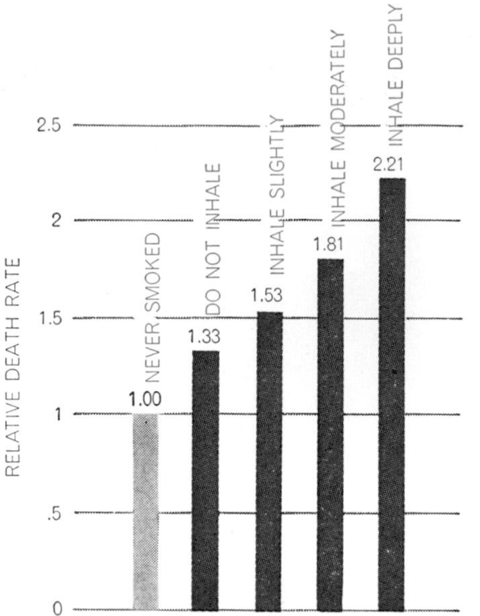

Figure 22–2. Degree of inhalation among cigarette smokers is charted against relative death rates from all causes. Rates are based on Dr. Hammond's new study of 1,079,000 men and women, which was begun in 1959. (From Hammond, E. C.: *Scientific American, 207*:39, 1962.)

75 per cent more deaths among a large group of heavy smokers than would have been expected among nonsmokers (Fig. 16–3).

Public Reaction to Report on Tobacco-Cancer Relationship

Public reaction to the 1964 Report of the Advisory Committee to the Surgeon General of the U.S. Public Health Service followed a classic pattern. Cigarette sales decreased sharply and then within six months returned to their previous level. In the interim, tobacco companies placated the public by bringing out six new brands with "activated charcoal" filters. The implication that the new filters make smoking less hazardous has widespread public appeal, but it is without scientific evidence.

Although the evidence included in the 1964 report may have scared the investigators, it apparently has had little lasting effect on the average smoker. Nevertheless, the scientists and educators continue to meet President Lyndon B. Johnson's plea to find "new techniques for making man's knowledge serve man's welfare." One of the most encouraging developments in this regard has been the formation of a National Interagency Council on Smoking and Health. This council, developed to combat the hazards of smoking, represents the following agencies: the American Cancer Society, the American Heart Association, the American Public Health Association, the Association of State and Territorial Health Officers, the National Tuberculosis Association, the U.S. Public Health Service, the U.S. Children's Bureau, the American Dental Association, the American Association of School Administrators, the National Congress of Parents and Teachers, and the U.S. Office of Education. The council states that it will act to:

1. Identify, approve, stimulate, promote and publicize selected national programs in keeping with the finding of the Surgeon General's advisory committee that "cigarette smoking is a health hazard of sufficient importance in the United States to warrant appropriate remedial action."
2. Give careful attention to the harmful effects of the use of tobacco in other forms.
3. Assist in evaluating national independent or interagency programs designed to combat smoking.
4. Identify, collect, evaluate, and disseminate information on existing and emerging programs aimed at combating smoking.

Also as a result of the recent emphasis on the cancer-tobacco relationship, the Federal Trade Commission has ordered that all cigarette labels should state "Caution: Cigarette smoking may be hazardous to your health."

WHY DO WE SMOKE?

Why then do we continue to smoke, even in the face of mounting evidence about its hazards?

There is no real beneficial physiologic action from smoking, therefore we must smoke for other reasons, and the most obvious of these is that it gives us some kind of emotional satisfaction.

If we're nervous, it gives us something to do with our hands or mouth. In small amounts, tobacco seems to quiet the nerves

Table 22–3.* Age-adjusted death rates per 1000 men for variables that may be related to mortality

Type of smoking	Long-lived parents and grandparents	Short-lived parents and grandparents	No previous serious disease	Previous serious disease
None	14.8	21.1	11.5	42.5
Cigarettes [1]	27.1	44.8	22.3	65.0

Type of smoking	Single	Married	Use tranquilizers	Do not use tranquilizers
None	26.0	18.9	29.1	18.2
Cigarettes [1]	50.1	33.0	52.4	31.8

Type of smoking	Educational level				
	No high school	Some high school	High school graduate	Some college	College graduate
None	22.7	20.0	16.9	18.3	15.8
Cigarettes [1]	35.2	34.5	35.5	34.2	29.4

Type of smoking	Degree of exercise [2]			
	None	Slight	Moderate	Heavy
None	23.8	14.7	11.0	9.5
Cigarettes [1]	34.1	25.5	20.8	19.7

[1] Smokers of more than a pack per day who inhaled moderately or deeply.
[2] Confined to men with no history of heart disease, stroke, high blood pressure or cancer (except skin) who were not sick at the time of entry.

*From *Smoking and Health.* U. S. Department of Health, Education and Welfare, Public Health Service.

and help to sedate us. A cigarette in the mouth possibly provides oral satisfactions of a type most of us have been seeking since infancy. Young people find it makes them feel more grown-up. So, for whatever reason, smoking gives us a lift.

When the mounting body of evidence with its case against cancer began accumulating, cigarette consumption did fall quite drastically. However, by now we are smoking more than ever before.

Part of the rise in cigarette consumption is due to greater prosperity and increasing population. A greater part is because we have somehow recovered from the cancer scare. "It won't hit me; it will affect only the other fellow." Or we try to convince ourselves that the evidence is statistical and therefore not absolutely conclusive. Or we rely on filtered cigarettes to protect us. Or we simply don't care and love smoking too much to give it up.

WHAT CAN WE DO ABOUT IT?

If you insist on smoking, give yourself the benefits of the absolute knowledge we do have:

Don't inhale.

Don't smoke your cigarettes to the very end.

Don't relight cigarette butts. They're loaded with nicotine.

Filters or cigarette holders may help.

It's very difficult to state unequivocally whether it's safer to smoke cigarettes, cigars or pipes. Cigars and pipes have a greater fire area, are hotter, and release more nicotine than cigarettes. Also the tobacco content of the average cigar is equal to five cigarettes or three pipefuls. However, most cigar and pipe smokers don't inhale, and many devotees of the pipe smoke more matches than cigarettes.

The Railway Conductor warned the passenger that he was not sitting in a smoking car. "I'm not smoking," the man said. "You have your pipe in your mouth." "Sure," the man said. "I have my shoes on my feet, too, but I'm not walking."

If you really accept the dangers of smoking and want to stop, or if your doctor tells you that you must stop, there are several ways of going about it:

The Trial Run

The first thing to do is to discover how confirmed a smoker you are. You may find out that you can cut down from a pack of cigarettes a day or the continual puffing on a pipe, to one smoke after each meal. Smoking that little is almost always harmless. If this doesn't work—and it usually doesn't—cut out smoking entirely. Some people find to their surprise that they can stop without much difficulty simply by making up their minds to do so. If you can't and find yourself getting tense, go back to smoking again for a few days. Then set the day, preferably a Monday, when you will come to grips with habit, and try to break it by the following technique.

Day 1. No smoking in the morning, except for one cigarette after breakfast. Don't smoke your favorite brand, but substitute a cigarette you don't care for, preferably one that is denicotinized, or has a filter; or use a cigarette holder with a filter.

Day 2. No smoking in the morning. No smoking in the afternoon except for one cigarette after the noon meal, again substituting for your favorite brand.

Day 3. No cigarettes, except one at night if you really need it badly. Plan a busy day and evening and avoid social gatherings which encourage smoking. Go to a movie or some other place where smoking is impossible or difficult.

General Suggestions

Eating, chewing gum and sucking on candy are usually helpful. Don't worry about gaining weight during the first week or so when you are breaking the smoking habit. It also helps to find something to do with your hands, such as knitting, twirling a key ring or simply handling the coins in your pocket. If you find yourself nervous and jittery, especially on **days 4, 5** and **6** when you have no cigarettes at all, take some aspirin or phenobarbital, which your doctor can prescribe for you.

Day 7. If you are not proudly boasting that you have broken the smoking habit, but are going around biting your nails and feeling a "nervous wreck," then you will either have to make it by sheer will power or, preferably, with your doctor's assistance. He can help you better than anyone else over the difficult withdrawal period with heavier sedation and the encouragement he can give.

Years ago, Mark Twain said that giving up smoking is easy. He had done it hundreds of times. If none of the techniques described work any better than that for you, perhaps you will be one of the lucky ones who benefit from *lobeline* pills. G. W. Rapp of Loyola University Medical School in Chicago found that 23 out of 25 smokers could be eased off the smoking habit entirely with pills containing a chemical called lobeline sulfate. They experienced none of the usual withdrawal symptoms, and were able to give up smoking entirely after a week or two. Lobeline is related to nicotine, and is actually obtained from a plant similar to the tobacco plant.

Smoking is a powerful mistress. When Mark Twain was courting his beloved Livy Langdon, he encountered serious opposition from her family. One reason was that he was a chain cigar smoker, and the Langdons found this a particularly objectionable habit.

Mark Twain responded to the intense Langdon pressure by limiting his cigar smoking to one a day, and in the course of this proved how injurious reform can sometimes be.

> "I kept the cigar waiting until bedtime," he wrote, "then I had a luxurious time with it. But desire persecuted me every day and all day long; so, within the week I found myself hunting for larger cigars than I used to smoke, then larger ones still, and still larger ones. Within the fortnight I was getting cigars *made* for me—on a yet larger pattern. They still grew and grew in size. Within the month my cigar had grown to such proportions that I could have used it as a crutch. It now seemed to me that a one-cigar limit was no real protection to a person, so I knocked my pledge on the head and resumed my liberty."[4]

[4]Allen, J.: *The Adventures of Mark Twain,* Little, Brown & Co., Boston, 1954.

Questions

1. What is the origin of the word, tobacco?
2. What are the effects of nicotine on the digestive system? the respiratory system? heart disease? high blood pressure? longevity?
3. How are "low-nicotine" cigarettes made?
4. How convincing to you is the evidence that smoking is related to cancer, especially lung cancer?
5. If you smoke cigarettes, how can you reduce the amount of nicotine and other toxic components of cigarette smoke you absorb? Why do experts urge, "Don't smoke butts!"?
6. Why should lip and tongue cancer be more common among pipe smokers than among the general population?
7. What determines whether you absorb more nicotine and other volatile components of smoke from cigarettes, cigars or pipes?
8. Why *do* people smoke if it has so many unpleasant and even dangerous effects?
9. Why do you have to indulge yourself in so many other ways, e.g., eating candy and other food, chewing gum, etc., in order to break the cigarette habit?
10. Name a disease that is definitely benefited when the patient stops smoking.

Topics for Discussion

Should smoking be prohibited by law?
Buerger's disease.
Raynaud's disease.
Oral leukoplakia.

Reading Suggestions

Smoking and Health, Report of the Advisory Committee to the Surgeon General of the Public Health Service. U.S. Department of Health, Education and Welfare. For sale by Superintendent of Documents, U.S. Government Printing Office, Washington, D.C. 20402, 1964. This publication consists of a compilation and syntheses of the currently available evidence related to the hazards of tobacco.

Smoking and the Public Interest, A Consumers Union Report. Mount Vernon, New York, 1963. One of the best written and most informative books yet published on the topic of smoking.

Science Looks at Tobacco, John E. Gibson. Today's Health, February 1964, p. 33. A number of important and interesting questions are covered in this article. It consists of nine questions and answers.

The Effects of Smoking, E. Cuyler Hammond. Scientific American, July 1962, Volume 207, No. 1. An excellent scientific report on the effects of smoking on the human body.

Psychosocial Aspects of Cigarette Smoking, M. Powell Lawton. Journal of Health and Human Behavior, fall 1963, p. 163. An informative article on smoking behavior.

Stress, Tobacco and Coronary Disease in North America, Henry I. Russek. Journal of the American Medical Association, April 1965, p. 89. A research report on a survey of 12,000 men in 14 occupational groups. This article can be easily understood by the college student even though it appears in a medical journal.

The Biologic Effects of Tobacco, Ernest L. Wynder, ed. Little, Brown & Co., Boston, 1955. A definitive, readable exposition.

How to Stop Smoking, Herbert Brean. Pocket Books, Inc., New York, 1954 (paperback). Useful as an aid in breaking the smoking habit.

Science Looks at Smoking, E. Northrup. Coward-McCann, New York, 1957. The effect of smoking on cancer, heart disease and other medical conditions presented intelligently and in a good, readable style.

23

ALCOHOL AND ALCOHOLICS

O thou invisible spirit of wine! if thou hast no name to be known by, let us call thee devil! . . . O God! that men should put an enemy in their mouths to steal away their brains; that we should with joy, pleasance, revel, and applause, transform ourselves into beasts.

SHAKESPEARE, *Othello,* Act II

Alcohol is usually considered a stimulant, but it is actually a depressant substance. It *appears* to lessen fatigue and make us feel lively or gay because, in effect, it takes the brake off emotional restraints. Even a small amount of alcohol lessens our habitual inhibitions.

This property of alcohol has been known to man since ancient times, and highly valued. Practically all peoples, even very uncivilized ones, have observed that sweet juices ferment when allowed to stand. It is unimportant that they attributed the process to magic, instead of to the yeasts which fell from the air, transforming the sugars or starches into alcohol.

According to the *Old Testament,* practically the first act of Noah after the waters of the flood receded was that he "began to be a husbandman, and he planted a vineyard. And he drank of the wine, and was drunken."

Certain primitive tribes were so impressed by what wine did to them that they regarded it with awe, and believed one of their gods had gotten into it.

Both the early Christians and the early and present-day Hebrews use wine in their religious ceremonies. However, in later periods, excesses in drinking were frowned upon by the Calvinists and the Lutherans, and, essentially, this attitude has persisted to the present day.

This reflects realistic thinking. In moderation, the average person can tolerate alcohol with no ill effects. However, when drinking becomes immoderate, it can have disastrous and far-reaching medical, economic, emotional, and social effects.

The "pleasures" of alcohol constitute one of its greatest dangers. Its ability to create an easy atmosphere by reducing tensions and releasing inhibitions is too often and too easily followed by its being used to excess, so that reason is impaired, will and self-control are eroded, and physical ability and endurance are undermined. The persistence and popularity of alcohol, in many forms, from as far back in the shadowy beginnings of organized human activity as anyone has been able to trace, strongly suggest that neither warnings, lectures, nor laws are going to turn men and women away from it. Education for moderation in its use and improved methods for relief from the sequels of its misuse are much more likely to prove effective.

ALCOHOL AND CALORIES IN VARIOUS BEVERAGES

Beer contains less alcohol than wine because the fermentation process is checked before all the sugar has been changed to alcohol. The various types of beer and ale are made by using different kinds and amounts of cereals, and processing them in a different way. Gin, whiskey and brandy, however, are distilled drinks and contain up to 50 per cent alcohol. After the grain mash has fermented, it is heated to boiling, permitting the alcohol and certain bouquet-conferring chemicals to be distilled off, just as steam distills off water when it boils. Alcohol has a lower boiling point than water, and the alcohol vapor will distill off first, leaving a good deal of the water behind. In this way, a beverage of high alcohol content can be obtained.

A fluid ounce of alcohol is equivalent to about 150 calories, and the various common alcoholic beverages have the following caloric value:

Beverage	*Amount*	*Calories*
Beer	8 oz. glass	120
Wine	1 wine glass	75
Gin	1 jigger	115
Rum	1 jigger	125
Whiskey	1 jigger	120
Brandy	1 brandy glass	80
Cocktail		150

We are able to metabolize this alcohol in our bodies just as we do sugars and fats, and use it for energy. If you are on a 1500 calorie diet to lose weight, remember that six bottles of beer a day represent more than 700 calories.

Confirmed alcoholics often find that alcohol satisfies their hunger and sustains their energy demands. Unfortunately, it doesn't provide the essential proteins, minerals and vitamins. This is why chronic alcoholics frequently suffer from malnutrition and even severe vitamin deficiencies, such as polyneuritis from thiamine, vitamin B_1, deficiency.

PHYSIOLOGIC EFFECTS OF ALCOHOL

No matter how much or how strong an alcoholic beverage you might drink, 1 per cent or 50 per cent, the alcohol in the blood stream never exceeds 0.5 per cent in concentration. This is because the digestive juices dilute it five- to tenfold, and it is further diluted by blood and other body fluids when it is absorbed. From a concentration of near zero to 0.5 per cent, however, a drinker can experience quite a variety of symptoms and effects—from mild exhilaration and tipsiness, to death.

The alcohol level in the blood depends on a number of factors, such as the amount of food in the stomach, the kind of beverage and the individual's tolerance to alcohol. Food slows down alcohol absorption, and one drink on an empty stomach usually has more effect than several drinks taken after a hearty meal.

The most important effect of alcohol is on the highest nervous portions of the brain, because it is here that motor coordination and control, judgment and speech are regulated. As already stated, and very contrary to popular opinion, alcohol is not a stimulant, but is a *depressant* of brain function at every concentration.

At blood levels as low as 0.05 per cent, the areas of the brain which control inhibition and restraint function less effectively. This is the reason a single drink can give an individual a pleasant feeling of exhilaration and gaiety. He may become very talkative and foolishly long-winded, because his critical faculties and judgment are dulled, and he doesn't know when to stop.

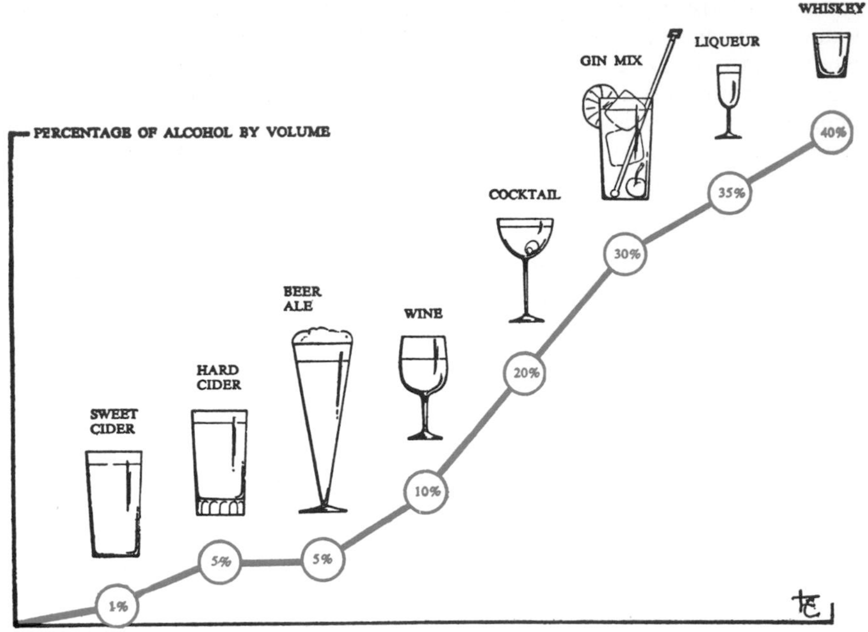

Figure 23–1. Alcoholic content of beverages.

When blood concentration of alcohol reaches 0.1 per cent, motor control is affected. The drinker often boasts he can still "walk the straight line," but what was previously a completely automatic performance is now accomplished only with careful attention. Under New York State law, 0.1 per cent alcohol in the blood is *relevant* evidence, and 0.15 per cent is considered *legal* evidence of intoxication.

As the concentration of alcohol in the blood increases, more definite evidence of

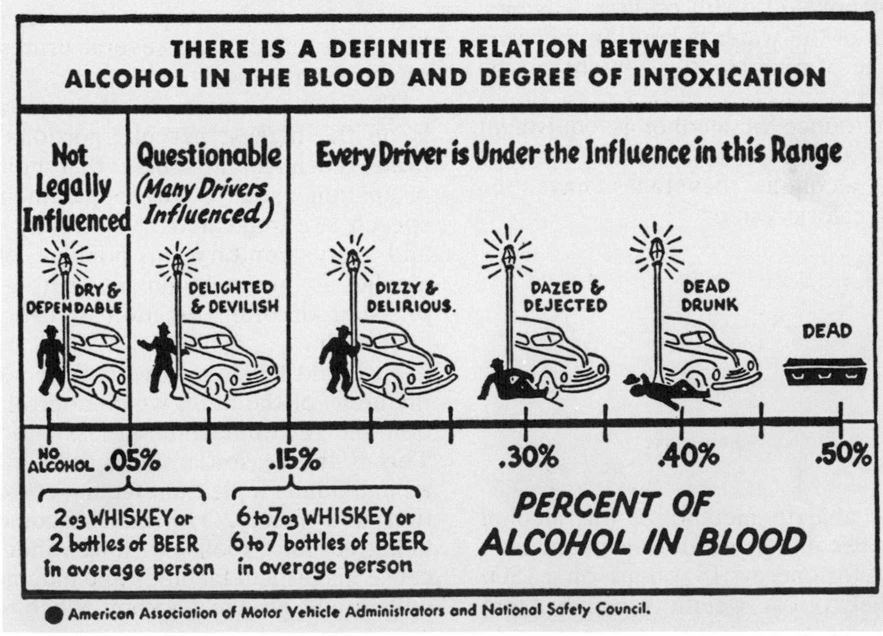

Figure 23–2. Diagram of the probable effect of certain percentages of alcohol in the blood.

impairment of function appears. Alcohol is an anesthetic substance, essentially little different in this respect from anesthetics like ether and chloroform. At 0.20 per cent, the horizontal position is preferable. It is too difficult to stand up. Even coordinating enough to undress and take off one's shoes becomes a major effort.

The presence of 0.3 per cent alcohol in the blood, usually reached after a pint of whiskey, induces a condition of stupor. The senses are so dulled that the drunken individual doesn't know what is happening around him. At 0.4 per cent he is in coma; and at concentrations above this, the areas of the brain which control breathing and heartbeat can no longer function, and death follows.

ILLNESSES CAUSED BY EXCESSIVE DRINKING

Intoxication is not the only physiologic result of excessive drinking. Alcohol is very definitely related to certain diseases. For example, about 5 per cent of all complete mental breakdowns are due to alcoholic psychoses, sometimes of an extremely serious and irreversible nature. Nearly 15,000 people in this country are afflicted with insanity due to alcoholism.

Delirium tremens, the so-called DT's, sometimes follows an extensive drinking bout. This is actually a prolonged delirium, and a kind of temporary insanity. The individual talks incoherently and in a typically delirious fashion, and usually has hallucinations of hearing and of vision. He is frequently terrified by imaginary strange animals, horrible sights and sounds. Thousands of patients are hospitalized each year or cared for in sanitoria or at home because of alcoholic psychoses.

Some physicians have had very good results with certain tranquilizers and adrenal cortical extract or adrenocorticotrophic hormone (ACTH) in treating delirium tremens.

Other fairly common manifestations of alcohol as a nerve poison are neuritis, tremor of the hands and visual disturbances.

Liver disease is frequently observed in heavy drinkers, because continued exposure to alcohol produces definite changes in the liver and its normal functioning. Hardening or *cirrhosis* of the liver may be the final result, with such extensive damage in the final stages that death from liver failure results. Other organs, such as the kidneys, heart and arteries, may also show serious degenerative changes.

The desperate need for alcohol often drives confirmed alcoholics to extremely dangerous substitutes, of which the commonest is methanol, or wood alcohol, a highly poisonous substance which can cause blindness. Doctors are constantly amazed by what skid row inhabitants of major cities will drink: hair tonics, radiator antifreeze, and Sterno.

Alcohol is actually useful in certain diseases, although harmful in others. Many doctors recommend an occasional cocktail for patients with diseases of the circulatory system, because alcohol has the effect of dilating or expanding peripheral blood vessels, which is helpful in the treatment. The use of alcohol is definitely harmful, however, in heat stroke and snake bite. (The well meaning first-aider who automatically administers a sip of whiskey for all types of injured persons may do great harm.)

IS MODERATE DRINKING HARMFUL?

There is no evidence that *moderate* drinking causes any disease, injures the general health or shortens the life of the average adult. The moderate drinker may consume a few highballs or a quart of beer a day. However, he chooses the best time for drinking, and he drinks for relaxation, not from necessity.

Drinking before or after dinner, in a social gathering, during a party, or during convalescence from an illness should certainly have no ill effects if it is done in moderation. However, drinking should be strictly prohibited in any jobs or activities which require judgment, discrimination, clarity of thought and vision and complete mental alertness. It stands to reason that the mountain climber, the locomotive engineer, the driver of a bus or automobile, the pilot of a plane, and people in the many other occupations that require constant alertness, should not drink at all.

CONSUMPTION OF ALCOHOLIC BEVERAGES

According to the 1964 report of the Food and Nutrition Board of the National Academy of Science, the average American consumes 76 calories a day in the form of alcohol. The total annual consumption of alcoholic beverages in the United States is 3.4 billion gallons, and approximately 17.3 gallons are consumed each year for every man, woman, and child in the nation. We spend over $11.6 billion a year for alcoholic drinks, more than $124 per person.

THE MAGNITUDE OF THE ALCOHOLISM PROBLEM

Of the approximately 75 million Americans who drink, 5 million are chronic alcoholics, and 1.25 million of these suffer the medical complications of alcoholism in their most severe form. The rate of alcoholism in the general population has been rising steadily for a generation—from 1956 to 1963 alone, the number of alcoholics per 100,000 adults rose from 4520 to 4760, in an estimate made from data supplied by the National Office of Vital Statistics. Men outnumber women in this unfortunate grouping nearly 6:1.

Some commonly accepted suppositions about alcoholism and alcoholics are upset by these carefully compiled statistics. The notion that alcoholics mostly are found on the skid rows of America is entirely wrong; only 7 per cent of alcoholics are derelicts; most of the remainder (except those in hospitals) are found in homes, offices, or factories. Seven out of ten alcoholics have held jobs involving considerable skill or requiring special responsibilities, and nearly 60 per cent had steady employment on a job for at least three years.

As one might expect, however, the highest incidence of alcoholism is in the large cities. The American cities with the highest rates of alcoholism are, in order: San Francisco, Boston, Los Angeles, Cleveland, Washington, Philadelphia, St. Louis, New York, Detroit, and Baltimore. In these cities, the problem of alcoholism is concentrated in the lowest and the highest economic and social strata.

In one survey, reported in the scholarly *Quarterly Journal of Studies on Alcohol*, the following observations were among those made on 2000 male patients in nine outpatient clinics:

1. Over 80 per cent of the patients were under 50 years of age. The average age was 41.2 years, and most of the patients were between 30 and 49 years old.
2. More than half were married and living with their wives.
3. Three out of four were living in an established household.
4. Nine out of ten had lived in their present community for at least 2 years.
5. Twenty-five per cent had held steady employment on a job for at least 10 years.

DEFINITION OF CHRONIC ALCOHOLISM

Chronic alcoholism is a disease of addiction, and not really profoundly different from the craving for narcotic drugs. The habitual drinkers usually evolve gradually from certain social drinkers. Eventually they reach the stage at which they are dependent upon alcohol, drinking regularly and excessively, ultimately disrupting their work, social and family life, and normal relationships with other people. The extent of the craving and the effect of gratifying it are brilliantly described in Charles Jackson's *Lost Weekend*.

Most people drink because under the influence of alcohol they lose some of their inhibitions, and feel happier and more socially accepted. This is why Shakespeare said, "Drink down all unkindness." The habitual drinker is usually a badly adjusted person emotionally, a basically unhappy individual who seeks happiness or escape from unhappiness by drinking. "Let him drink and forget his poverty, and remember his misery no more," is the explanation we find in *Proverbs*.

Table 23-1. Drinking among fatal motor-vehicle accident victims from nineteen California counties, 1964*

Victims	Number Tested	Number of Alcohol Positive Victims					
		Total		Blood-Alcohol Content			
		Number	Per Cent	.01-.04	.05-.09	.10 & Over	% Over .05
Total Drivers	**1,134**	**621**	**55%**	**41**	**55**	**525**	**51%**
Responsible	879	567	65%	31	43	493	61%
(One-car accidents)	(522)	(362)	69%	(20)	(23)	(319)	66%
Not responsible	173	31	18%	9	9	13	13%
Resp. undetermined	82	23	28%	1	3	19	27%
Total Pedestrians	**353**	**159**	**45%**	**11**	**13**	**135**	**42%**
15-64 years old	215	126	59%	5	10	111	56%
65 years and over	138	33	24%	6	3	24	20%

*From *Accident Facts*. National Safety Council, 1964.

Many people use alcohol because of deep philosophic or psychological needs.

Drink! For you know not whence you came, nor why.
Drink, for you know not why you go, nor where.
(*The Rubaiyat* of Omar Khayyam,
Edward Fitzgerald)

Unfortunately, as Bertrand Russell has pointed out, "Drunkenness is . . . temporary suicide; the happiness that it brings is merely negative, a momentary cessation of unhappiness."

ALCOHOL AND ACCIDENTS

According to an investigation carried out recently by the Police Department of New York City, 55 per cent of motor vehicle operators who were killed at the wheel or who died of injuries within 24 hours after an accident had taken considerable amounts of alcohol before the accident. This is considerably higher than the generally accepted figure, that a third or fourth of all fatal road accidents are connected with drinking.

Likewise, a California survey conducted in 1963 revealed that of the adult pedestrians killed in accidents, 40 per cent had been drinking and 32 per cent were under the influence of alcohol at the time of the accident.

Unfortunately, no figures are available for the relationship of drinking to other types of accidents. It is a reasonable assumption that *all* types of accidents are greater among drinkers than nondrinkers.

ALCOHOLISM AND THE JOB

Drinking during working hours is not only unwise, but definitely unsafe. There is a significant reduction in efficiency and output, and a definite increase in accident hazards. Wage and salary losses resulting from absenteeism caused by alcoholism are estimated at about $450 million a year. Of course, much additional loss results from personal and professional deterioration, but this loss cannot be calculated.

Many industrial corporations have found that most of their disciplinary problems center around people who have been drinking excessively. Alcohol is notorious for the way it loosens the tongue and makes people pugnacious. Several large industrial firms, including Consolidated Edison, Bell Telephone Company, and Allis-Chalmers, have instituted rehabilitation programs for problem drinkers in their employ. When industries have made a large investment in training employees to do highly skilled jobs, it is often cheaper for them to attempt rehabilitation than to train a new person. The program is essentially one of sympathetic counselling and positive aid, coupled, when necessary, with psychiatric guidance and introduction to Alcoholics Anonymous. The significant feature of these programs is that they indicate a marked change in attitude toward alcoholism. It is not regarded as a moral disgrace, but *as a disease, or the symptom of a disease.*

LIFE EXPECTANCY AND DRINKING

Heavy drinking definitely shortens life expectancy, according to extensive studies by Raymond Pearl, the biostatistician, and others. Moderate drinking seems to have little or no effect.

VENEREAL DISEASE AND DRINKING

Army physicians and student health physicians in colleges have repeatedly emphasized the relationship between drinking and venereal disease. Most men who contract venereal disease acquire it from prostitutes after they have been drinking. Unfortunately, alcohol in small amounts stimulates sexual desire, releases inhibitions and diminishes precautionary measures.

SOCIOLOGICAL ASPECTS OF CHRONIC ALCOHOLISM

For every alcoholic, at least two other groups of individuals, wives and children, are adversely affected. Severe social, financial and emotional insecurity is created in the families of chronic alcoholics who are unable to function as providing parents. Confusion and family crises, poverty, broken homes, serious emotional disturbances and retardation of the children in school are the common pattern in such families.

In some instances, the very existence of a family and responsibility creates too great an emotional pressure for the already tempted individual, and drives him to escape in chronic alcoholism. In others, the family represents a rehabilitating influence and support in his efforts to conquer his illness.

It costs our country more than $13 million a year to care for alcoholics in mental hospitals. Society spends over $25 million annually to care for drunkards in jail. Crimes involving habitual drunkards involve sums as high as $175 million a year.

WHY DO WE DRINK?

Alcohol, like tea and coffee, has very pleasant social and psychological effects in small doses. Unfortunately, it can be extremely harmful when used excessively. We seek outlets of this kind and sometimes depend on them because they permit us to escape from the tensions and problems of the extremely complex world in which we live. For example, a young man or woman entering maturity may have to assume considerable responsibility and make many decisions. If he is unable to solve all his problems realistically or if he finds himself too frustrated in the fulfillment of his desires, he may turn to some powerful escape from reality, such as alcohol or even narcotics. Unfortunately, these escapes will only make him so nervous and physically exhausted that he will have to indulge further. Finally a desperate, almost inescapable cycle is created, and the chronic alcoholic or drug addict emerges.

It is chiefly the emotionally immature individual who seeks release and solution to his problems in alcohol. It has been aptly said that, "Alcohol has the quality of rosily blurring the hard, forbidding outline of reality, and if enough alcohol is taken, it has the power of effacing reality altogether. It is the quickest solvent known to man. It is fantasy in a bottle. It produces this magic quickly, and for a long time the drinker escapes social reprisal and stigma. And it is readily obtainable anywhere in this country."

Many teen-agers and adolescents drink for "kicks," or because they think it's a mark of manhood. Often, they hope it will overcome some of the natural shyness of this age period and "lubricate" social situations. However, *the potential dangers in drinking are the same for young people as they are for any other age group. These hazards should be the primary considerations in deciding when, where and how much to drink.*

THE PREVENTION AND TREATMENT OF CHRONIC ALCOHOLISM

As Smiley and Gould have pointed out: "It would . . . seem that every effort should be bent toward building a society where the worries, tensions and discomforts are not so numerous or so great as to necessitate drowning them in strong drink, and where the members of society have learned through early training how to get release and recreation without having recourse to a drug."[1]

Unfortunately, this perfect society is still in the future, and we need other, immediate measures.

Legislation was tried when the Volstead Act was enacted in 1920, prohibiting the sale of alcoholic beverages. However, this was apparently too restrictive a measure, and after strong opposition, it was repealed in 1933. It appears that the sale and acceptance of liquor in present-day society may be swinging too far in the other direction. The number of alcoholics (per 100,000 adults) has increased nearly 50 per cent since 1940, and there is a greater proportion of confirmed alcoholics and youthful drinkers today than ever before.

Prohibition failed to solve the problem of alcoholism because it never got close to the heart of the problem. The constitutional ban on alcohol simply made drinking more attractive than ever. A more effective approach to preventing alcoholism lies in creating a home environment that excludes, so far as possible, severe stresses and strains on young children. One of the most significant statistics concerning alcohol and alcoholism is that 22 per cent of the alcoholics in this country come from homes broken by death or separation of parents before the child has reached the age of ten. If parents can help their children grow up as stable and mature adults, able to meet life's problems and demands with some resilience, the number of persons likely to become alcoholics will be considerably reduced. Alcoholism develops more frequently in those whose lives from infancy to adulthood are subjected to many emotional jolts. Serenity is not a characteristic of contemporary American life, but parents can do much to help their children become the kind of adults who can cope with troubles without seeking the bottle for a crutch.

Another consideration for prevention of alcoholism may be the development of an atmosphere in which drinking is accepted as a social function, to be practiced in moderation, rather than banned as an evil. It is interesting that the lowest incidence of alcoholism in the United States occurs among members of three groups whose customs make alcohol fully acceptable. These three are the Italians, the Jews, and the Chinese. Among these peoples, as different as they are in most other respects, attitudes toward alcohol are quite similar. Drinking has a fixed place in meals, in religious rituals, and in family or holiday occasions. By contrast, consumption of alcoholic beverages in many other groups is either prohibited or viewed with a mixture of alarm and hypocrisy. The analogy here with the American experience during Prohibition is clear.

Any disease brought about by habitual drinking must be treated by a doctor. The disease exists just as truly as though it were caused by bacteria, a virus or some constitutional defect. *Simply giving up alcohol is not enough, and may even be inadvisable.*

Some of the minor effects of drinking can be cured or improved by medical care and proper diet. Injections of vitamins may be required.

The treatment of *alcoholism* itself is a complicated matter. Doctors prefer the term "rehabilitation" to "cure." The three most widely used methods are: drug therapy, organizational methods, and psychotherapy.

[1]Smiley, D. F., and Gould, A. G.: *Your Health,* The Macmillan Co., New York, 1951.

Drug Therapy

The use of drugs has meant that physicians, although still unable to cure alcoholism, can frequently control its symptoms, quiet the patient, or help repair some of the damage the confirmed alcoholic has inflicted on his body. Not all medical treatment involves drugs, of course. Alcoholics tend to become dehydrated, which is corrected by introducing a saline solution and dextrose or fructose into his system. Steady consumption of alcohol, with an accompanying lack of attention to a balanced diet, usually causes nutritional deficiencies that must be corrected, possibly by vitamin therapy. But drugs themselves can be classified in several ways:

Drugs That Stimulate the Central Nervous System and Counteract Depression. Caffeine, dexedrine, benzedrine, and other compounds are often used to help the drowsy or depressed alcoholic.

Drugs That Depress the Central Nervous System. If the drinker is overexcited, restless, or irritable, he may be helped by some of the growing number of tranquilizers, such as reserpine, chlorpromazine, or meprobamate. These drugs generally quiet him, control his nausea, and let him get some rest.

Drugs That Relax the Muscle System. Preparations in this category tend to be powerful and therefore potentially dangerous. They have been useful, though, in helping the alcoholic who is severely agitated, and perhaps afflicted with severe trembling.

Glandular and Hormonal Products. Those suffering from severe alcoholism may have delirium tremens or severe glandular malfunctioning. Such conditions may be treated with ACTH or with thyroid extract.

Aversion Drugs. Much publicity has been given to the use of medications that induce vomiting, either just before or with an alcoholic drink. The hoped-for result is that the patient will come to associate the vomiting with the drink and accordingly develop a dislike or aversion for the liquor. This drastic method presents a number of hazards, however, ranging from severe discomfort (in addition to the nausea), to temporary mental illness, to death in a few cases, when the patient already had a heart or liver ailment.

The criticism most frequently made about drug therapy, especially the aversion drugs, is that of all the methods of treating alcoholism, they come least close to the heart of the problem. In their defense, however, it must be realized that many of these medications at least help the alcoholic physically, for this disease may damage the body in many serious ways, in addition to what it does to the drinker's soul.

The Organizational Method

Alcoholics Anonymous (or AA) is the best known organizational method, a banding together of individuals who have overcome or are trying to overcome their own habitual drinking and want to help others. AA was founded in 1935 by a doctor and a stockbroker, whose mystical experience in attaining sobriety was, in their opinion, something to be shared with other sufferers. AA membership is based on acceptance of Twelve Steps and Twelve Traditions, the first Step being an admission that "we were powerless over alcohol—that our lives had become unmanageable." From this point of departure—actually, a recognition that the alcoholic can never again take a drink—the AA member moves ahead in his quest for sobriety, through his own efforts, sustained by his fellow-sufferers. AA has been recognized by many authorities as an effective approach, and as the authors of *Alcoholism and Society* point out,

> "The very size of AA is socially significant. It is a reflection of the ostracism that always has plagued alcoholics. Morally shunned, punitively treated, the alcoholic's only hope for help lay in one person helping another. It is a sad commentary that even to this day the sick must lead the sick because of ignorance and bias. What we are suggesting is that because we failed the alcoholic, AA came into being."

A more recent organization is the Al-Anon Family Group Headquarters, Inc. Al-Anon evolved to meet the needs of the entire family of the alcoholic, and its membership is primarily made up of the husbands and wives of alcoholics. Although Al-Anon has no formal ties with AA, it does have a spiritual relationship and an approach that also stresses the importance of recognizing the problem and working as a group for the welfare of each member. Its focus, like that of AA, is on helping oneself by helping others.

Psychotherapy

Psychotherapy may be used alone or in conjunction with medical treatment, organizational help, or both. The general goal of psychotherapy here, as in other areas, is to help the patient gain insight and to strengthen himself so that he will no longer need to drink. Such a goal is basic, most worthwhile, and difficult to achieve in proportion to its ambition. Because many alcoholics drink owing to their lack of personal security and owing to tensions and conflicts with themselves and their surroundings, alcoholism is also a problem of mental health.

Effective psychotherapy depends first on the establishment of a good relationship between the drinker and the doctor. It also entails learning about the patient in detail, a process particularly difficult sometimes because of the alcoholic's resistance to disclosing much about himself and his reluctance to face the fundamental facts about his personality and his troubles. Finally, the extensive time required for thorough psychotherapy, the expense, and the shortage of qualified psychiatrists all make this form of treatment on a mass scale an unlikely prospect. In fact, the work of AA and Al-Anon represent an effective group therapy situation, although such "treatment" has been criticized as being crude and unscientific. Nevertheless, this particular form of group therapy has worked for many men and women and has displayed large-scale successes that individual psychotherapy cannot claim.

Questions

1. Discuss the physiologic effects of alcohol at various blood concentrations. Why does it appear to be a *stimulant,* although it actually is a *depressant?*
2. Explain the malnutrition and vitamin deficiency effects which are so common in chronic alcoholics.
3. Approximately how many calories could you obtain from four glasses of beer?
4. What are the major illnesses caused by excessive drinking?
5. What factors impel people to drink excessively even when they recognize the consequences of addiction to alcohol?
6. How does alcoholism affect the accident rate, and what proportion of automobile accidents are caused by excessive drinking?
7. Most people have heard or read that it is dangerous to drink while driving. Why do you think we still persist in urging "one for the road" when a party begins to break up?
8. What is the effect of alcohol on *life expectancy?* on contraction of *venereal disease?*
9. What treatments are used in an attempt to cure chronic alcoholism? What is the special significance of Alcoholics Anonymous?
10. What are the warning signals of incipient alcoholism?
11. What are some methods of relieving the tensions of college life other than drinking?
12. Why is drug therapy for alcoholism so frequently successful in the short run but so often a failure on a long-term basis?
13. Why is "moderate" drinking a relative term? If even a small amount of alcohol has some effect on the body and personality, how can anyone decide for himself what is a "moderate" amount?
14. Compare the amount of money spent in the United States for "getting drunk," with the amount allotted on a national scale for *all* medical research.
15. Why do some large industrial firms spend significant amounts of money to try to rehabilitate their alcoholic employees?
16. Compare your observations about drinking on the campus with what your older relatives can recall about drinking at college during Prohibition.
17. Do you think group therapy, led by a psychiatrist rather than an AA member, could help alcoholics? Would you expect alcoholics to respond more readily to psychotherapy in a group situation or with an individual therapist?

Topics for Discussion

Alcoholics Anonymous.

Psychiatric treatment of alcoholism.

Delirium tremens.

An alcoholic's responsibility for his misdeeds or crimes.

Government's responsibility to treat alcoholics.

Effectiveness of legal restrictions on manufacture and consumption of alcoholic beverages.

Relationship between alcohol and personality problems.

Widely varying rates of alcoholism in different countries.

A host's responsibility for his guests' safety, if they are driving.

Increase or decrease in drinking on your campus.

Whether alcoholism is an addiction or an habituation.

The possibility of a society without alcohol.

Alcoholism as a sign of a "weak" personality.

Whether a heavy drinker must necessarily become an alcoholic.

Reading Suggestions

Science Looks at Liquor, John E. Gibson. Today's Health, February 1963, p. 84. Many of the myths about alcohol are exploded in this well written article.

Young People and Drinking: The Use and Abuse of Beverage Alcohol. John Day Company, New York, 1962. The facts about drinking are reviewed in an interesting and scientific fashion.

Alcohol, Berton Rouche. Grove Press, New York, 1962 (paperback). A well written, authoritative account of the history, folklore, and physiologic effects of alcohol.

Alcoholism and Society, Morris E. Chafetz and Harold W. Demone, Jr. Oxford University Press, New York, 1962. The authors examine the causes of alcoholism and discuss how varying cultures have reacted to alcoholism and how they have treated it.

The Cured Alcoholic: New Concepts in Alcoholism Treatment and Research, A. H. Cain. John Day & Co., New York, 1964.

The Disease Concept of Alcoholism, E. M. Jellinek. Hillhouse Press, 1960.

Alcoholic Addiction, a Psycho-Social Approach to Abnormal Drinking, Howard Jones. Tavistock Publications, London, 1963.

Society, Culture, and Drinking Patterns, David J. Pittman. Wiley, New York, 1962.

Alcohol and Civilization, S. P. Lucia. McGraw-Hill, New York, 1963.

Aspects of Alcoholism, preface by Ebbe Curtis Hoff, Lippincott, Philadelphia, 1963.

Drinking and Intoxication, Selected Readings in Social Attitudes and Controls, Yale Center of Alcohol Studies, 1959.

Alcoholism, U. S. National Institute of Mental Health, publication No. 730, 1960.

Recovery from Alcoholism, Karl E. Voldenz. Regnery, Chicago, 1962.

Psychiatric Theories of Alcoholism, J. D. Armstrong. Canadian Psychiatric Association Journal, *6:* 140, 1961.

Some Current Theories of Alcoholism, W. McCord, J. McCord, and J. Gudeman. Quart. J. Studies Alcohol, *20*:727, 1959.

Effects of Alcoholic Drinks, Tobacco, Sedatives, and Narcotics, T. B. Rice and R. N. Harger. Harper & Row, New York, 1961.

Teaching about Alcohol, F. Todd. McGraw-Hill, New York, 1964.

Helping the Alcoholic and His Family, T. J. Shipp. Prentice Hall, New York, 1963.

Social Drinking: How to Enjoy Drinking Without Being Hurt by It, Giorgio Lolli. World Publishing Co., New York, 1960.

Marty Mann's New Primer on Alcoholism, National Council on Alcoholism, New York, 1963.

The Lost Weekend, Charles Jackson. New American Library of World Literature, New York (paperback), 1964. A vivid and illuminating fictional—but realistic—account of chronic alcoholism and of delirium tremens.

Facts About Alcohol, Raymond G. McCarthy. Science Research Associates, Inc., Chicago, 1951. An excellent, informative pamphlet.

Alcoholism. Its Scope, Cause and Treatment. Ruth Fox and Peter Lyon. Random House, New York, 1955. An interesting and well written book by experts in this field.

How to Live Without Liquor, Ralph A. Habas. Farrar, Straus & Cudahy, New York, 1955. Why people drink to excess and how they can be helped, told by an expert psychologist and sociologist.

NARCOTICS AND OTHER HABIT-FORMING DRUGS

I hanker too much after a state of happiness, both for myself and others. I cannot face misery, whether my own or not, with an eye of sufficient firmness, and am little capable of surmounting present pain.

—DeQuincey
(Confessions of an English Opium Eater)

It is the nature of man to be curious, to explore new ideas and territories in the world around him. How and why he behaves as he does is left to sociological and psychological studies. However, actions that may result in damage to the body through careless or uninformed behavior are of concern to all.

In his investigations into his own surroundings, man has made remarkable use of the products of nature in providing for his own basic needs and comforts. Food, clothing, and hundreds of other products have been produced from these natural sources for better living. Not all of nature's gifts, however, are safe. Some plant and animal species contain deadly poisons and other irritants that can cause our eyes to water, our skins to itch and blister, and our noses to run. Some species appear to only lend a wild beauty to our surroundings with their bright colors and unique shapes.

In his early search for useful materials in nature, man discovered certain products that eased pain and infection when consumed internally or applied to his wounds, but they sometimes killed or sickened the user. Refinement and continued study of these products have made available to medical science much of the wonderful supply of drugs and medicines we have today. Unfortunately, many of these products have dangerous and damaging effects on the body if used indiscriminately. The drugs known as narcotics (from the Greek, *narkotikos*—to benumb or deaden) are some of those that man must learn to use wisely.

WHAT IS A NARCOTIC?

Any drug which relieves pain and produces sleep or stupor is usually considered a narcotic. Opium was once called "the divine drug of sleep." Depending on the dosage, narcotics may produce a feeling of well-being and euphoria, or numbness and insensibility. The best-known drugs of this class are opium and its derivatives, such as morphine and heroin.

Narcotics in History

The use of *opium, hashish,* and *cocaine* extends so far back in time that they may have been known to Stone Age man.

Opium was familiar to the Sumerians as early as 7000 B.C., and was employed medicinally by the Egyptians, Persians, and Greeks. Its extensive modern use in China developed during the nineteenth century.

The American Indians extracted desert plants which contained the drugs *mescaline* and *peyote* to enable them to communicate with their dead ancestors. Warriors sometimes smoked hashish to endow them with superhuman strength before battle, and the Indians of the Andes chewed coca leaves, extracting the cocaine, for energy and virility. Drugs were also used by many primitive peoples in tribal rituals, such as puberty rites, and to combat and neutralize various taboos.

WHAT IS ADDICTION?

The narcotic drugs have many desirable features. They relieve pain, produce pleasurable feelings, and dissipate anxiety. Unfortunately, continued use for any of these reasons may lead to addiction.

The Committee of Experts on Drugs Liable to Produce Addiction, World Health Organization, defines addiction as follows:

> "A state of periodic or chronic intoxication detrimental to the individual and to society, produced by the repeated consumption of a drug. Its characteristics include: (1) an overwhelming desire or need (compulsion) to continue taking the drug and to obtain it by any means; (2) a tendency to increase the dose; (3) a psychic (psychological) and sometimes a physical dependence on the drug."

The extent of this physical dependence is perhaps most dramatically illustrated by the fact that a child born to a woman who is a drug addict is also addicted to narcotics. Without them, the child may develop serious, and sometimes fatal, symptoms, and must be given the drug in diminishing amounts until it can safely be withdrawn from it.

THE SPREAD OF DRUG ADDICTION

In the early days of its use as a medicine, opium was taken by mouth in a fairly dilute solution and was not especially harmful. Widespread addiction stemmed from two factors—the development of the hypodermic syringe, and the extraction of morphine from opium and its purification.

The modern hypodermic needle was invented in 1839, although as early as the seventeenth century drugs were sometimes injected intravenously with a quill attached to a small bladder. The first needle addict was the wife of a Dr. Wood, who perfected the hypodermic needle in 1853, and the widespread use of Wood's needle for morphine injection produced many addicts among wounded Civil War soldiers.

It has been estimated that by early 1900, there were from 100,000 to 1 million addicts in the United States. At that time, opiates could be purchased over any drug counter and in many grocery stores, as well as in patent medicines of all kinds, and even in soft drinks. Many infants became partially dependent on opium or its derivatives because the patent medicines sold to soothe a colicky baby contained opiates.

Morphine was isolated from opium in the early years of the nineteenth century, and its dangers were quickly recognized. Searching for a safe substitute, German scientists produced heroin, a derivative of morphine, in 1898. This was widely hailed by the medical profession because it was thought to possess the virtues of morphine without its hazards. On the contrary, heroin proved to be one of the most powerful of the addicting drugs, and its widespread and sanctioned use produced thousands of addicts.

Today, the Federal Narcotics Bureau estimates that the United States has

60,000 heroin addicts. There could, however, be as many as 100,000 because, for obvious reasons, an accurate determination is impossible. More than half the country's addicts live in New York; most of the others reside in the slums of Detroit, Chicago, and Los Angeles. Approximately half the addicts are Negroes; 20 per cent are women.

WHY PEOPLE USE DRUGS

Professional personnel, especially when they are under extreme stress, as in wartime and periods of intense and exhausting hospital training, sometimes turn to narcotics for relief and come to depend on them, because the supply is so readily available. A study by Dr. J. Dewitt Fox has revealed that drug addiction is approximately 100 times more common among physicians than in the general population.

Many persons are introduced to the use of drugs (by their physician) as relief for pain in long periods of severe illness. Constant effort by doctors and hospitals to avoid addicting patients to drugs is maintained; however, experience with drugs and their effect in relieving tension and pain leads many people to ignore the warnings of professional advisors on the dangers of uncontrolled and habitual use, and they try to obtain drugs from other sources.

A major portion of known drug addicts and an increasing number of our youth are introduced to this terrible habit in another manner. Through ignorance of the damaging effect on the body and mind produced by narcotics or because "a friend" or "the gang" uses a narcotic, many individuals are persuaded to undergo their first experience in self-administration of drugs in one form or another. The first few doses or shots seem perfectly safe. The clever peddler or firm addict often supplies the novice free of charge, knowing that once he is addicted he will pay almost any price to satisfy the craving for it. Thus, a vicious cycle is formed. The addict, tormented by a body poisoned from use of narcotics, finds relief only through numerous and more concentrated doses of drugs that are only available if he can pay the price on the illegal market. To obtain the money necessary to support his own needs he is persuaded to introduce others to the use of narcotics.

Having undergone an initial experience in taking a narcotic, the individual's decision to continue its use is moderated by the physiological effect experienced by the user and by his psychological stability.

It is perhaps misleading to state that narcotics produce "some special feeling." According to reports of addicts, it is more accurate to state that narcotics produce an absence of feeling. In fact, one addict has described "the greatest possible high" as death. Whatever the sensation experienced by the individual, narcotics do provide an escape from reality for those who are unable to adjust to the problems of society or environment. Although the world with its problems and frustrations is still there to be faced, the individual is unaware of its existence. The person who continues using drugs as an escape is the most difficult to treat, as his emotional involvement is often very deep-seated. This is the type of person who makes up the hard core of addicts in our society. The remaining individuals, who become addicted through curiosity or group association and who are capable of rehabilitation, are offered hope through continuing research and professional clinics. Whatever the reason leading to uncontrolled use of narcotics and the problems it poses to society, the student should familiarize himself with current preventive measures being employed to overcome this health menace. They are:

1. Education regarding the dangers and effects of uncontrolled use of narcotics on the body and the mind.
2. Improved environment for large masses of our population in depressed economic areas of the nation.
3. A continued effort by local and national authorities to restrict illegal traffic in narcotics and drugs.

WHO ARE THE ADDICTS?

Drug addicts can be found among young and old, rich and poor and every social class, but wherever they are found, predisposing emotional factors will exist. As the psychiatrist S. Bernard Wortis has pointed out:

"Addicts have immaturity of character development—people who like their pleasures without looking ahead to the future, who are very unwilling to postpone pleasure, who even seem to have self-destructive tendencies. The lack of a sense of meaning in life and a desire to escape from reality characterize many of the seriously addicted group. They also have low capacities for dealing with frustration, anxiety and stress. Among the other early factors is emotional deprivation occurring in early childhood because of broken homes or the lack of interest on the part of the parents. Sometimes, overindulgence and lack of disciplinary training during childhood are involved. Sometimes, a child has not been able to identify himself with a respectable parental figure and can't form a proper ideal of what to do in life."[1]

An enormous increase in *juvenile addicts* started in 1949, and children as young as fourteen were admitted to treatment centers. This is still a tremendous problem, especially in the large metropolitan centers, and recent reports indicate that teen-age drug addiction has now spread to the middle class suburbs. A significant trend in this regard indicates that drug use in these communities was not initiated by clever dope peddlers but by a desire for excitement by the young people. Because of this motivation, the teen-age boys and girls visited metropolitan centers, obtained drugs, and returned home to use them. The implications of this type of behavior are quite important to society and to you as future parents.

NATURE'S DANGEROUS GIFTS

Marihuana

The cheapest, easiest and also one of the most frequent ways of developing drug habituation is to smoke *marihuana*. This is the same as hashish, and is obtained from Indian hemp, the plant that provides twine and rope. It is generally smoked as "reefers," but it may also be chewed, or drunk after it has been extracted.

Marihuana can be, and often is, grown in the empty lot in perfectly respectable neighborhoods, and, to the untrained eye, looks like any ordinary weed. Almost all portions of the plant can be used—leaves, flowers, seeds, and woody portion—with no elaborate extraction or purification procedures. It is simply ground into a powder and made into cigarettes.

Because marihuana is so readily available and so cheap, it is frequently sold in places where young people meet—dance halls, pool rooms, and theaters. The dealers can offer this special thrill for just a few cents, whereas heroin costs at least 100 times as much.

The central nervous system reacts to marihuana in a variety of ways, depending on the individual and the amount smoked. At first the drug produces a feeling of exhilaration and well-being: the marihuana smoker usually becomes very gay and talkative, or excitable. As time goes on, however, there is gradual loss of muscular coordination and the development of visual defects, hallucinations, and sometimes, extreme depression or panic.

The marihuana user often shows characteristic jerky movements of his head, shoulders and arms, and finally loses control of muscular coordination completely and becomes stuporous. When he is deprived of the drug, he is apt to be extremely tense and irritable, and may suffer painful headaches and abdominal cramps. However, marihuana differs from heroin because it does not cause withdrawal symptoms, and therefore, in the strict physiological sense, it is not an addicting drug.

Opium

Opium and its derivatives are obtained from the seed pods of the Oriental poppy. These drugs are used in several ways: they may be smoked, injected or taken by mouth.

The crude, dried juice of the seed pod forms a brown, gummy mass which is used in smoking. This produces a deep sleep with apparently extremely pleasant dreams and hallucinations, so desirable that the smoker can hardly wait to repeat the experience. Continued smoking builds up a tolerance to opium, until larger and larger amounts are needed to produce the effect. In essentially every part of the world, opium smoking is illegal and has inevitably led to a considerable traffic in smuggled opium.

[1]Wortis, S. B.: *Modern Medicine,* October 1, 1957.

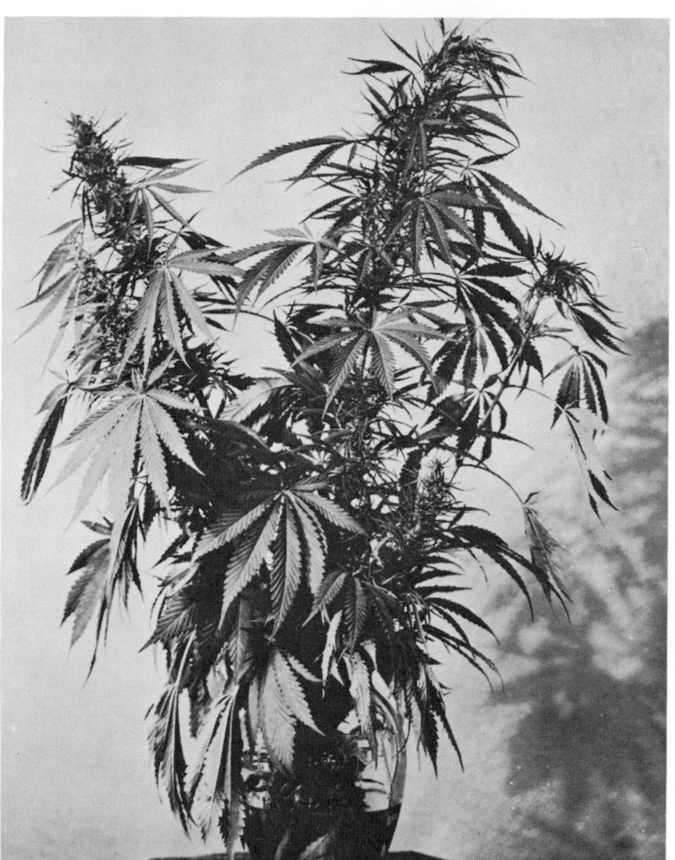

Figure 24–1. Marihuana. (Courtesy of Bureau of Narcotics, Treasury Dept.)

Opium has definite physiological effects, and this is what the addict seeks: it deadens pain, produces a remarkable sense of well-being, and removes all inhibitions. Under the influence of opium, an individual can live in a very pleasant fantasy world, because it is difficult to differentiate dreams from reality.

Morphine and Its Derivatives

The most important compounds found in opium are morphine and codeine, both of which have valuable medicinal uses: they are *analgesics,* or pain-relievers.

Morphine can be taken by mouth or by injection, but, unfortunately, tolerance to this drug is built up very rapidly, and larger and larger amounts are needed for full effect. The addict develops a profound need for morphine, and experiences almost intolerably painful and distressing symptoms when he attempts to stop the habit. The result is that he will resort to *anything* to obtain money for it. *It is not the drug itself which causes crime, but the unbearable craving for morphine.*

For an estimated 60,000 addicts, the cost of drugs per person amounts to well over $10 a day, at least $300 million annually for all addicts. This is far beyond the income of the average individual. Addiction and crime are essential partners; a Senate Committee which investigated drug traffic in the United States concluded that narcotics addiction is responsible for at least 25 per cent of all crimes committed.

In testimony taken by this committee in Philadelphia, they learned from an attractive 25 year old woman that "a friend" had persuaded her to take heroin seven years before. The cost of the habit gradually rose to $10 a day, then to $30. She turned first to shoplifting, then to prostitution, and finally became a peddler of narcotics herself, until she was arrested. This is a quite typical story, and many

Table 24–1. The language of the addict

Works	The equipment needed to inject heroin.
Spike	A small needle.
Cooker	A bottle top used to dissolve heroin.
Dynamite	Good quality heroin.
Garbage	Poor quality heroin.
Copped *Scored*	Having successfully obtained a drug.
Shooting up *Taking off* *Getting off*	Injection of drugs.
Going on the nod	After injection of heroin, the eyelids become heavy and the mind wanders pleasantly.
10 dollar trick	Prostitution to obtain money for drugs.
Speedball	A mixture of a stimulant and a depressant in one shot (e.g., heroin and cocaine).
Snow	A cocaine powder that is inhaled.
Reefer	A marihuana smoke.
Booting	Withdrawing blood into syringe and mixing it with heroin before injecting. This is thought to prolong the initial effects.
Shooting the gravy	If the blood coagulates in "booting," it is heated until it dissolves and the "gravy" is injected.
Pinned	Constricted pupils when heroin addict is high.
Narco	Narcotics detective.
5 dollar deck	Pack of heroin.
Pill heads	Users of barbiturates and amphetamines.
Goof balls	Barbiturates.
Bennies *Pep pills*	Amphetamines.
Pill popping	Taking pills.
Zip-five	A short jail sentence.
Gopher	A middle-man between the pusher and the addict.
Pusher	Dope peddler.
Wild West *New Frontier*	The addict's escape from the real world.
Hooked	Addicted to narcotics.
Tracks	Needle marks.
Wake-up	Morning shot of heroin.
Square	Those who do not use drugs.
Busted	Arrested.
Dealer's band	A rubber band worn by a pusher, which when hooked to a bag of heroin flings it away if the police are spotted.

prostitutes and call-girls are confirmed narcotics addicts. *And every addict is a potential drug peddler.*

In these same hearings, a Texas police official described the history of a nineteen year old boy from a respectable family. This youngster became snared by a pusher who gave him his first heroin free. He became habituated within a few weeks, and the increasing cost of the drugs he needed led to burglaries, muggings and holdups. By the time he was finally arrested, this teenager had become a hardened criminal, and had already involved a number of other young people in the narcotic habit.

Heroin is a synthetic derivative of morphine and is probably the most dangerously addictive drug. About 75 per cent of confirmed addicts use heroin.

Habituation frequently begins by sniffing heroin powder. Later it is generally taken by injection, like morphine. Some of its effects are also similar to morphine, but its chief attraction seems to be the sensation of excitation and euphoria it gives. Heroin is considered so dangerous that its manufacture and sale are forbidden in this country. All traffic in this drug is illegal.

Cocaine is another synthetic compound, familiar to us as a local anesthetic. This property depends on its ability to block the conduction of nervous impulses. However, because of dangers of addiction, cocaine has largely been replaced by Novocaine and related substances.

Cocaine may be injected, but it is usually sniffed in the form of a powder, called "snow" by habitués. Individuals who crave cocaine are not interested in its local anesthetic action, but in its other effects. Unlike the drugs derived from opium, cocaine stimulates, rather than slows down, the nervous system. The result is that cocaine users tend to be restless and highly excitable. There are also other, much less pleasant, symptoms: hallucinations, feelings of persecution, sensations of "something alive crawling under the skin." Nausea, digestive disturbances, loss of appetite, tremors, and even convulsions are common in cocaine addicts.

NONNARCOTIC DRUGS WHICH CAUSE ADDICTION

Many nonnarcotic drugs in common use are known to cause habituation or a quasi-addiction, and should therefore be used with great caution. Among these are *benzedrine* and related derivatives, such as *Dexedrine,* the barbiturates and some of the *tranquilizing drugs.*

Amphetamines

Benzedrine and Dexedrine are derived from a chemical called amphetamine, which is valuable in treating hay fever and colds because it shrinks the nasal membrane. "Pep pills" containing these compounds are sometimes prescribed by doctors because they combat depression, and seem to cheer patients. They also stimulate physical activity, apparently by blunting the sense of fatigue, and have been reported widely used among athletes.

Benzedrine inhalers and stimulants such as Dexedrine have come into fairly common use among college students, especially during examination periods, when the need for stimulants more powerful than coffee is felt.

These preparations are *definitely dangerous,* especially if taken repeatedly and in excessive amount. They produce restlessness and wakefulness, a jittery feeling, and, when taken in very large doses, have actually caused delirium, panic and suicidal or homicidal situations. The Federal Food and Drug Administration has stipulated that sales of amphetamine inhalers be switched from over the counter to prescription only. This action followed a report from Kansas City that young people were soaking the "wicks" of inhalers in warm water, then injecting the resulting solution for "kicks."

Barbiturates

The consumption of barbiturates has also increased at an alarming rate in this and other countries. These preparations are sold under various names, such as Seconal, Luminal, Nembutal, Amytal, and many others. They are very useful remedies to quiet disturbed or tense persons, and also to treat insomnia. *But they should be used only when prescribed by a physician, and should not be taken indiscriminately, because of an occasional restless night.*

Barbiturates are definitely habit-forming drugs, and are not a safe substitute for normal, drug-free sleep. Havelock F. Fraser and his associates at the U.S. Public Health Service Addiction Research Center in Lexington, Kentucky, found that the amount of barbiturates taken determined the degree of physical dependence. In 18 healthy volunteers who took 0.9 to 2.2 grams daily for 1 to 12 months, 14 had convulsions, 12 had delirium, and all had minor symptoms when the drugs were abruptly withdrawn. Of 23 subjects given 0.6 to 0.8 gram daily, three had convulsions, two had hallucinations, and 14 had minor withdrawal symptoms.

Barbiturates often leave a considerable hangover the next day, with blurred vision, poor judgment and indecisiveness, and sometimes they produce rather dangerous intoxication before they induce sleep. In large enough doses, they are fatal. A federal law prohibits dispensing barbiturates without a prescription.

Tranquilizers

Tranquilizing tablets, such as Equanil, Miltown, Serpasil, Thorazine, and many others, are the newest additions to the doctor's medicine kit and have proved to be very powerful therapeutic weapons. They have been used with great success in treating mental disturbances, delirium tremens, withdrawal symptoms from narcotics, and other conditions. However, they are not general panaceas, and even the mildest tranquilizer may be somewhat habituating.

Billions of tranquilizers are sold annually, a great many without a doctor's prescription, merely to quiet tension and anxieties. Unfortunately, although these compounds may reduce anxieties, they also carry with them many dangers. They can be habit-forming, and may induce undesirable side reactions, including intestinal upsets, skin eruptions, jaundice, and sometimes very unusual emotional reactions.

Tranquilizers should be taken only on a doctor's prescription, and should be stopped when the acute need for them has passed.

THE CONTROL AND TREATMENT OF DRUG ADDICTION

Drug addiction is a world health problem, and will probably not be eliminated until there is stringent international control of opium production, and drastic, effective punishment for venal dope peddlers. Law enforcement and education are our most effective weapons. It has been estimated that about 500 tons of opium are needed each year for legitimate medical purposes; yet official sources estimate that as much as 12,000 tons are produced. The difference goes into illegal traffic.[2]

In 1915 the Harrison Narcotic Act was passed; it was originally essentially a revenue measure, defining taxes, special forms and licenses. According to this law narcotics could be prescribed only for medical purposes and not for the continuance of addiction. Violations were penalized.

As a result of this law, ethical physicians and pharmacists refused to write or fill prescriptions for narcotics. Unfortunately, the law was not accompanied by any educational campaign to emphasize the dangers of drug addiction.

A separate bureau of narcotics was established in this country in 1922, and it has become extremely effective. In addition, numerous international conferences on the addiction problem have been held, resulting in the establishment of a Permanent Central Opium Control Board. The purpose of this was to restrict the production of opium to the estimated needs of the participating nations.

[2] *The Illicit Narcotics Traffic*, U. S. Govt. Printing Office, Washington, 1956. Report No. 1440.

Treatment Centers

The first specific treatment center for drug addiction was the United States Public Health Service Hospital, opened in Lexington, Kentucky, in 1935. In a 20 year period, 23,625 patients were admitted a total of 45,058 times.

A similar treatment center was later established in Fort Worth, Texas. However, existing institutions are still inadequate to handle the problem, and in a partial attempt to solve it, a hospital was established in New York City in 1951, specifically for the treatment of juvenile addicts. A number of other cities have also established special treatment clinics.

Once the habit of addiction to narcotic drugs is well established, treatment is exceedingly difficult, and many patients, apparently cured, return time and time again for help.

The withdrawal of opiates from a confirmed drug addict is an agonizing process, but it is essential for the cure.

This is how Eugene Carey, surgeon of the Chicago Police Department, describes a typical narcotic addict picked up by the police:

> He is detained in a concrete-floored, steel-barred cage or cell after he has been catalogued and screened. Then he is left to his own resources to think and meditate. There may be other addicts in the same cell. None knows what is next on the agenda, what is to happen to him, or where he is to go.
>
> In time, the drug within each addict's system begins to wear off. One yawns, then they all yawn. Next follows lacrimation, retching, vomiting, running bowels, twitching, jerking. The vertebral canal seems to fill with ice-water, they say, and soon this chilly ache becomes an agonizing, unbearable, freezing pain, not alone in the back, but all over the body. The pain causes them to cry piteously, scream and convulse.
>
> This condition is withdrawal sickness.[3]

The present method of treatment is to give the patient a medicine, called *methadone,* as a substitute. This is administered in amounts just sufficient to permit the patient to tolerate the symptoms of abstinence from narcotic drugs. After that, it is given in steadily decreasing amounts. Tranquilizers have also been used with considerable success to lessen the agony of withdrawal symptoms.

Complete recovery from addiction takes about four months, and during this period every effort is made to rehabilitate the patient and restore him to good physical shape. In addition, he is given as much support and encouragement as possible, as well as psychiatric help.

Synthetic Morphine Substitutes

An intensive search has been going on for many years to synthesize a morphine substitute, which would be nonaddicting and yet a powerful pain-reliever. Currently, there is a great deal of interest and hope for a compound synthesized at the National Institutes of Health in Bethesda, Maryland. This drug, called NIH 7519, is the result of 25 years of continuous research by a group under Nathan B. Eddy, a physician and pharmacologist. It has been described as "a synthetic pain-killer ten times as powerful as morphine, but far less addicting," and is now being studied extensively in clinical trials with human beings.

Legalization of Narcotic Sales

In certain countries, addicts are registered with physicians or clinics, and can obtain drugs very inexpensively, by legal means. This is the situation in England, for example, and means that incurable drug addicts are not forced to resort to crime to obtain money for their supplies.

There is a strong movement in the United States, supported by distinguished physicians (and opposed just as vigorously by equally distinguished physicians) for the inauguration of similar clinics here.

Narcotics that are no more costly to manufacture than aspirin are currently sold through underworld channels for amounts ranging from $30 to $100 per day. Legalization of their sale would eliminate an enormous amount of crime and help eradicate a whole segment of the underworld which has been enriching itself for decades on illicit narcotic traffic.

[3]*Annals of the New York Academy of Science, 61*:222, 1955.

Herbert Berger, consultant to the United States Public Health Service and former president of the Medical Society of the City of New York, has this to say on the subject:[4]

> Our present punitive legislation has excluded narcotic addicts from any legitimate source of drugs and has driven these sick people away from the medical profession into the hands of criminal traffickers in narcotics. It has done little to prevent the inception of narcotic addiction and nothing to cure it.
>
> The horrible truth that many experts won't face is that dope addicts are not curable. Perhaps 3 per cent of those who have had extensive treatment at Lexington Federal Hospital and other reputable places are able to stay 'cured'—the other 97 per cent return to the habit. That's how the narcotics problem differs from robbery of the mails or any other crime. A dealer or pusher craving for his shots cannot be scared off by the vague threat of a long prison term or even the death chamber. To put a narcotics victim in jail for life is unnecessarily cruel, for many of these men can lead useful lives if they are provided with the drugs they need.

The anticlinic group points out that we already tried such clinics as far back as the 1920's, establishing them in 44 cities, and they failed. According to a Senate Investigating Committee: "They had become little more than 'filling stations' for drug addicts who resorted to fraud and trickery to secure larger doses. When addicts could not satisfy their cravings with the clinic shots, they turned to illicit sources again." The chief opposition to the clinic plan is the fear that drug addiction will spread if it is too readily obtainable.

The opposition group includes such notable figures as Harry Anslinger, the Federal Narcotics Commissioner, Harris Isbell, Director of the Addiction Research Center in Lexington, Kentucky, and its former Medical Director, James V. Lowry.

Lowry expresses his objections to such a clinic as follows:

> I think my function as a physician is to treat people, not to maintain them in a state of disease, and I think in administering narcotics, we cannot forget what happens to that person. The addicted male becomes sexually impotent. The addicted female becomes sterile. If a person receives narcotic drugs he has every need satisfied in terms of blotting out reality. His worries are gone; his responsibilities are gone. Now, what you are asking me as a physician is whether I want to perpetuate a condition of this kind; and I say, no.[5]

Nevertheless, the Subcommittee on Drug Addiction of the New York Academy of Medicine has unanimously recommended the establishment of clinics to dispense narcotics under medical supervision.

Increased Penalties for Narcotics "Pushers"

Effective control of narcotic traffic requires vigorous law enforcement as well as the certainty of stiff punishment. Heavier penalties have proved to be one of the strongest deterrents to narcotic addiction and narcotic traffic. Harry Anslinger has pointed out that the penalty for breaking into a post office is a great deal higher than that for violations of the narcotics law.

In 1951, the so-called Boggs Law, Public Law 255, was enacted, and this appears to be responsible for turning the rising tide of narcotic traffic and addiction. This law, for the first time, imposed minimum mandatory sentences of not less than two years nor more than five years for a first offense; not less than five years nor more than ten years for a second offense; and for a third or subsequent offense, not less than 10 years nor more than 20 years. The average narcotic sentence now is approximately 43 months, nearly three times what it was before the enactment of this law. However, many experts believe that our laws are still too lenient, and a number of states have passed more severe measures for controlling the unlawful use of drugs.

The results in the state of Ohio dramatically illustrate the success of these measures. In the summer of 1955, the State Legislature enacted a severe narcotic control law providing imprisonment for two to ten years for illegal possession of narcotics; 10 to 40 years for illegal possession with intent to sell; and 20 to 40 years for illegal sale.

Major narcotic violations in Ohio have

[4]*Modern Medicine*, March 1, 1959; *This Week Magazine*, Sept. 15, 1958.

[5]*This Week Magazine*, Sept. 15, 1958.

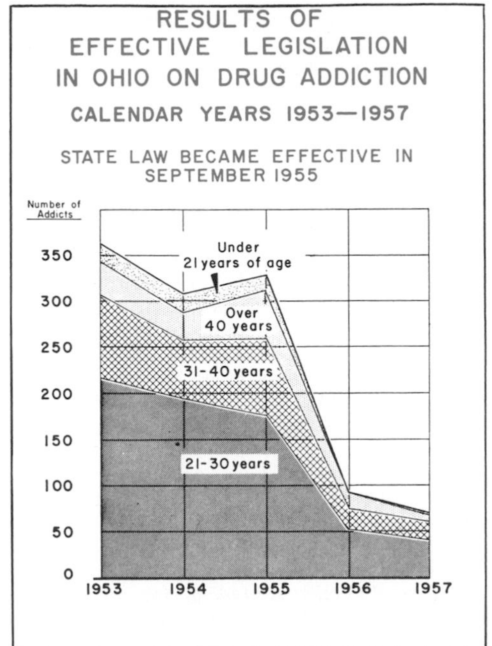

Figure 24–2. (From *Traffic in Opium and Other Dangerous Drugs*. U.S. Treasury Department, 1958.)

been reduced by about 80 per cent since this law became effective, and the Bureau of Narcotics has been able to transfer about half its agents in Ohio to other parts of the country where large-scale criminal narcotic activities still flourish. (Fig. 24–2).

A General Control Program

The program recommended by the New York Academy of Medicine for control of narcotics and addiction was worked out by a committee of experts after careful study and thought. In essence, it is the following:

1. Recognition that the addict is a sick person and not a criminal.
2. Prevention of the formation of new addicts by taking the profit out of drug traffic. Addicts could obtain drugs for withdrawal at low cost under government control.
3. Medical supervision of existing addicts, with emphasis on rehabilitation. Service clinics would be established in conjunction with hospitals to dispense drugs legally and inexpensively to addicts while attempts are made to institute a course of treatment. Adequate controls and safeguards would be established to prevent abuse of the clinic system.
4. Constant efforts toward complete and permanent elimination of illegal narcotic drug supplies and traffic, with provision of drugs for addicts under medical supervision and treatment.
5. Adequate program of education for adults, teachers and adolescents on the danger of narcotic drugs and the need for treatment.
6. Accumulation of more information on drug addiction to learn the magnitude and causes of the disease.

This appears to be a comprehensive program that might succeed in solving the narcotics problem.

Questions

1. What is the proof that addiction is not only a psychological, but also a physiological dependence?
2. Discuss the major causes of drug addiction? Do you think it is correct to say that only "weak" people become drug addicts?
3. Why do you think minority groups in the United States have a disproportionately high percentage of drug addicts?
4. What is the source of marihuana? its effects? Why is marihuana smoking so dangerous?
5. What are the medical uses of morphine, the opium derivative?
6. Why is it said that "every addict is a potential drug peddler"?
7. Why is the sale of heroin forbidden in this country?
8. How are heroin and cocaine taken by drug addicts?
9. Describe the dangers of barbiturate habituation.
10. How is addiction to morphine or heroin treated?
11. Do you feel that robbing a bank or a post office is as serious a crime as selling narcotics? Would very severe punishment of narcotic "pushers" ever solve the narcotics problem?
12. Discuss the pros and cons of the legalized sale of narcotics to known addicts.

Topics for Discussion

Drug withdrawal process.
Current therapy for drug addiction.
Tranquilizers and energizers—uses and abuses.

Reading Suggestions

The Murderers, Harry J. Anslinger and Will Oursler. Farrar, Straus & Co., New York, 1961. A U.S. Commissioner of Narcotics writes the story of narcotic gangs. In the author's words the book "is the record of a world-wide apparatus of criminal conspiracy, civic corruption and murder by appointment. It is the story of the crime syndicate's national and international dealings in commercialized drug addiction."

Narcotic Addiction in Britain and America, Edwin M. Schur. Indiana University Press, Bloomington, 1962. An important book that discusses the consequences of society's reactions to the addict. Addiction policies and addict behavior in the U.S. and Britain are compared. A thought-provoking book.

Drug Addiction: Crime or Disease, Joint Committee of American Bar Association and American Medical Association on Narcotic Drugs. Indiana University Press, Bloomington, 1961. An important discussion of clinics for legal distribution of narcotics, relapse and rehabilitation, foreign practices, legal aspects, and educational needs.

Drug Addiction, Lawrence Kolb. Charles C Thomas, Springfield, Ill., 1962. An informative discussion of the problems associated with drug addiction. Interesting and very well written.

Narcotics and the Law, William B. Eldridge. New York University Press, New York, 1962. A thoughtful book regarding the legal aspects of the narcotics problem.

Narcotics and Narcotic Addiction, David W. Maurer et al. 2nd Ed., Charles C Thomas, Springfield, Ill., 1962. A realistic analysis of narcotic addiction. A useful and authoritative book.

Drug Addiction in Youth, Ernest Harms. Macmillan, New York, 1965. Special problems of young addicts are discussed, including institutional treatment, withdrawal, and use of "Narcotics Anonymous."

Narcotics, Norman Taylor, Dell, New York, 1963 (paperback). A comprehensive and extremely well written account of the various narcotics and their use.

Drugs in Our Society, Paul Talalay and J. H. Minagham. Johns Hopkins Press, Baltimore, 1964. The results of a conference held on this important topic.

Who Live in Shadow, John M. Murtagh and Sara Harris. McGraw-Hill Book Co., Inc., New York, 1959. A vivid, realistic description of addicts, and a discussion of the general problem of addiction.

The Traffic in Narcotics, H. J. Anslinger and W. F. Tompkins. Funk & Wagnalls, New York, 1953. A thorough discussion of the narcotics problem by two experts.

The Addict and the Law, Alfred R. Lindsmith. Indiana University Press, Bloomington, 1964. A sociologist's documented analysis of present practices and recommendations for a more effective public treatment of the narcotics problem.

Film: *Drug Addiction, A Medical Hazard*, 25 minutes. Winthrop Stearns Co., New York.

FOODS AND BEVERAGES

Getting enough to eat is less of a problem in America than in most of the world, and than it has been at any other period in history. Throughout the ages the vast majority of people seldom, if ever, knew what it was like not to be hungry; and in many parts of the world they are hardly any better off today.

Yet there is more to food than the simple matter of satisfying one's hunger pangs. Some people enjoy food so much that they practically "live to eat." Others care little about it, and simply "eat to live." Diets can be inadequate in *both* these groups, sometimes even incompatible with good health.

No one should have to force himself, or be forced, to eat at any meal. But it is not forcing to encourage your appetite by giving time and thought to meals. This means that meals should not only be well prepared, but they should also be served in a pleasant atmosphere and made to look attractive.

WHEN TO EAT

Honest bread is very well—it's the butter that makes the temptation.

DOUGLAS JERROLD
The Catspaw

As a matter of custom and convenience, we eat three meals each day, usually at a regular time, whether we are hungry or not. This practice is consistent with good health only because the stomach is able to act as a storage bin, discharging food slowly into the small intestine. When the stomach is removed, it becomes necessary to eat smaller quantities of food at more frequent intervals.

For many years now, we have been taught to eat regular meals and to avoid snacking between meals. This practice has a logical basis: what one eats between meals is likely to consist of some form of carbohydrate or sweet foodstuff (empty calories), which may spoil the appetite for scheduled nutritious meals. Also, snacking may provide the extra calories that contribute to obesity.

With this exception, however, there is no reason to avoid eating between regular meals. In fact, if the snack consists of nutritious foods, it seems advisable, on the basis of recent evidence, to eat more often than three times daily.

In a study of animals, it was demonstrated that those that ate many times daily were less likely to develop arteriosclerosis than those on regular meals. Also, animals that nibbled all day failed to gain weight, whereas those that ate one meal each day became obese.

Dr. Edgar S. Gordon of the University of Wisconsin Medical School has hypothesized that the consumption of large meals may result in an overly active enzyme system with exceptional efficiency in the conversion of foodstuff into fat. After placing his obese patients on a 48 hour fast to break this faulty enzyme pattern, Dr. Gordon has successfully treated obesity by prescribing a six-meal-a-day diet of 1300 calories. This diet is discussed in more detail in Chapter 26.

How About Breakfast?

Breakfast is a far more important meal than most people realize. All the experts agree that energy and work performance are far better on a well balanced, high-protein breakfast. Unfortunately, some people awaken slowly and painfully. Nothing more than orange juice, black coffee, and a few bites of toast appeals to them. However, many people *think* they don't like breakfast simply because they've never given themselves a chance to enjoy it.

If you awaken slowly, set the alarm ahead by 10 or 15 minutes. Spend *at least* 15 minutes every morning eating breakfast, or just sitting at the breakfast table. Try adding various things that appeal to you, such as a bit of crisp bacon, a small dish of cereal, an extra piece of buttered toast, a small portion of egg, some milk.

Usually by the end of a week or two of this experiment, people find they are enjoying a larger breakfast.

If you have succeeded in eating a larger breakfast, try to convert to a high-protein breakfast. Medical scientists have shown that a high-protein diet provides energy at a more uniform level throughout the morning than do other types of breakfast. The sugar in the blood doesn't fluctuate nearly so much as it does after a high-starch breakfast. These changes in sugar level affect your appetite and energy capacity. Also, because the appetite is satisfied for a longer period after a high-protein breakfast, the actual calorie intake later in the day is reduced, which helps to keep total body weight down.

For the high-protein breakfast, concentrate on *eggs, cereal and milk, meats,* such as ham, crisp bacon, sausages, and *milk* (use skimmed, fat-free milk if you have a tendency to be overweight). Reduce to a minimum the sugary and starchy foods, e.g., toast, jelly, marmalade, pancakes, waffles.

If you can't eat a good-sized breakfast, or if you don't eat sufficient protein, then by midmorning you may possibly feel the effect of a low blood sugar—hunger and even sensations of dizziness and fainting. Before this time arrives, try to take some solid food and a glass of orange juice, or at least a cup of coffee and a doughnut.

WHAT TO EAT

The diet shown in Table 25–1 was prepared by the country's leading experts for the National Research Council. Everything

Table 25–1. Recommended daily diet

Milk	1 pint (1 quart for children)
Egg	1 daily (on days not used, substitute more milk, meat, cheese, peanuts or other protein food)
Meat, Fish, Fowl	1 or more servings
Potato	1 or more
Vegetables	2 or more servings; one green and one yellow
Fruits	2 or more; one citrus fruit or tomato or other food source of Vitamin C
Cereals and Bread	whole-grain or enriched

Sweets, fats, starchy and other foods should be added to complete the meals and to maintain normal weight.

necessary to good health is in this daily diet. If the food you eat in the course of a day includes everything listed here, you can be sure of an adequate intake of vitamins, proteins, calories and minerals.

Tastes vary according to national and regional customs. Some people of Italian descent eat spaghetti almost every day, whereas in parts of the United States dinner consists of meat and potatoes, bread and butter, and pie. Every group has some justification for thinking its dishes are the best in the world. Many of them are, indeed, excellent, and all customs need not be changed.

However, it is important to realize that

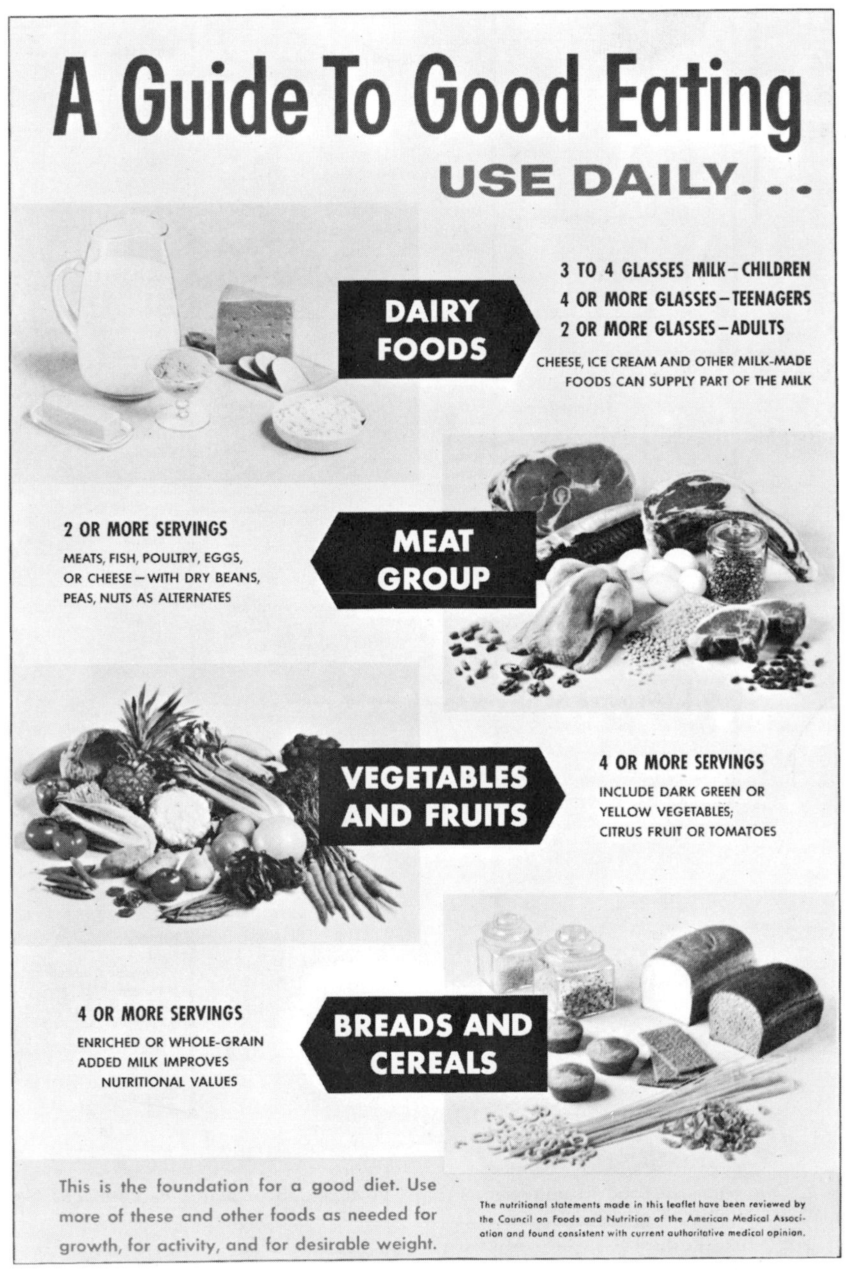

Figure 25–1. Guide to good eating. (Courtesy of the National Dairy Council, Chicago.)

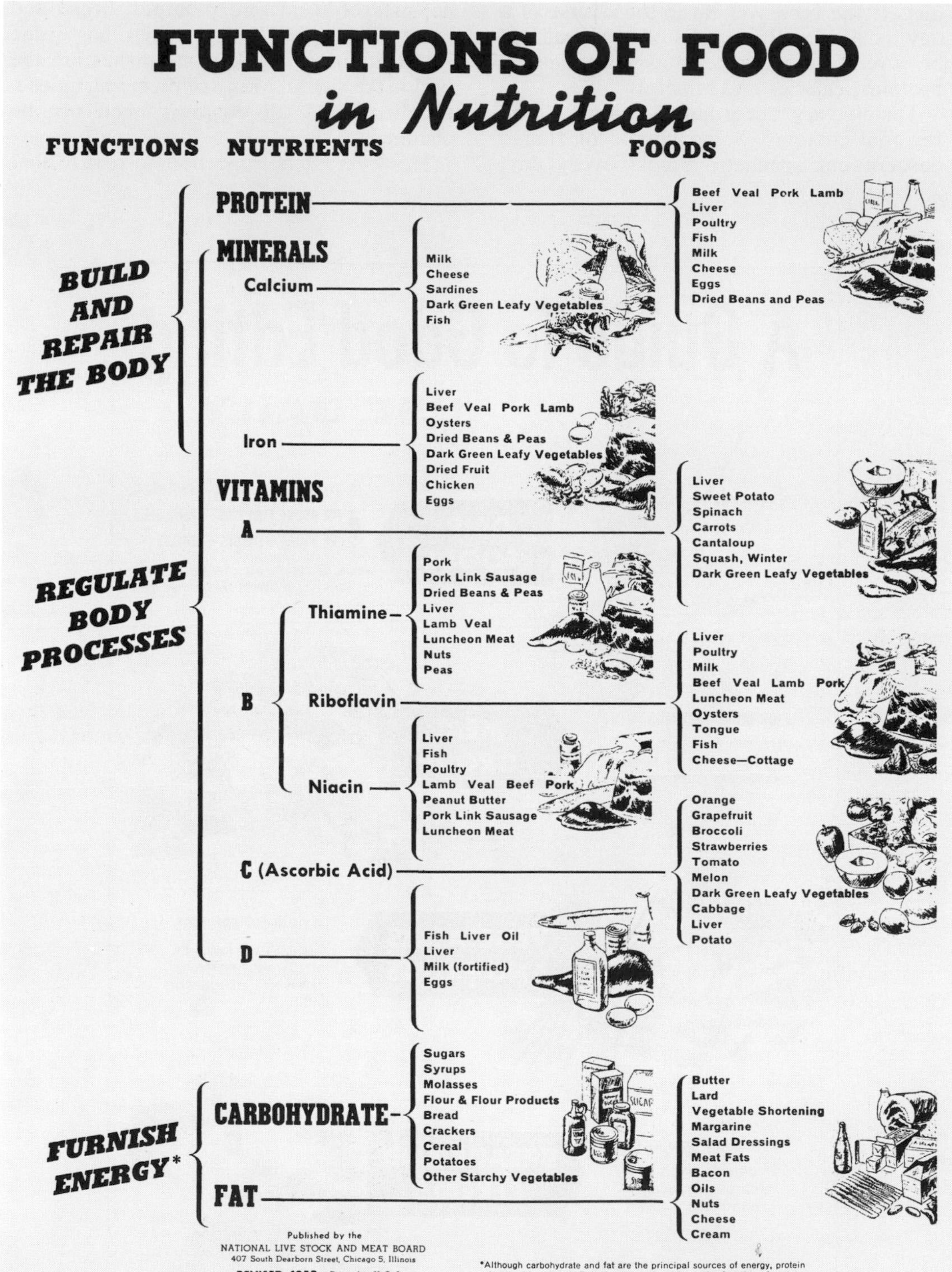

 Figure 25–2. Functions of food in nutrition. (From Culver and Brownell: *The Practical Nurse.* 6th Ed., Philadelphia, W. B. Saunders Co., 1964.)

many groups eat certain food almost exclusively (rice, for example) because they cannot get anything else. Here in the United States we need not limit ourselves. A tremendous number of foods are easy to obtain here, and equally inexpensive, because of transportation, refrigeration, and canned and frozen foods. The many national groups that have contributed to the melting pot of American cookery have made it possible to enjoy the best and most varied dishes in the world. A restaurant in the United States may serve French onion soup or Russian borscht, lamb cooked with vegetables in the Greek, Armenian, or Turkish manner, American corn on the cob, Chinese chop suey, East Indian curried rice or Hungarian goulash.

Why You Need a Balanced Diet

Food provides the body with four essentials: energy, repair materials, growth materials (from infancy through the period of active growth), and vitamins and other special substances.

The framework of the body is largely muscle and bone, and it must be built out of the food you eat. It is to build up the muscles and other vital organs, such as the heart, liver, and kidney, that the child and growing adolescent need plenty of proteins. A high-protein diet is especially important during pregnancy for the rapid growth of the baby. Meat, fish, milk, and eggs are among the best sources in the ordinary diet.

Even after the period of rapid growth, cells of the body must be constantly replaced, because they are being worn out continuously. That is why adults, as well as children, must have ample protein in their diets. Lacking protein, the body may become weakened and offer lowered resistance to infections.

In addition to the organs and muscles, the body must build its solid framework of bones. They are composed chiefly of the mineral substances, calcium and phosphorus. The best source of these two minerals is milk, either fresh or canned, dried, skimmed, or whole. Milk is a splendid, all-around food because it is rich in both minerals and proteins. Other good sources of calcium are: American and Swiss cheese, molasses, turnip tops, and dandelion greens. Good sources of phosphorus include cereals, meat, and fish.

Minerals and proteins build the bones and flesh. But what supplies the energy? An automobile can't go without gasoline, no matter how good an engine it has, nor can a stove or furnace operate without fuel. The fuel of life is sugar (carbohydrates). Starches are converted into sugar in the body, and the sugar is burned (metabolized) to supply energy.

Sugary and starchy foods provide ready energy. Anyone doing hard physical exercise or labor requires plenty of energy-giving foods, such as bread, pancakes, syrup, jelly, honey, and sugar.

Fat and protein can also be used to provide energy, and these the body can store up and keep in reserve. However, starches and sugars act more promptly in providing energy than do proteins and fats.

Usually your appetite tells you just how much food your body needs. This indicator is so sensitive that some people go for years at almost precisely the same weight. If more food is taken in than is needed for fuel, building and repair, the body stores it as fat. If too little food is consumed, the body burns its reserves of fat and protein.

Calories

The calories, or energy from food, needed per day by persons engaged in different types of activity are shown in Table 25–2. They indicate the number of calories required to maintain weight.

It is evident that the farmer, for example, needs more food than the secretary. He will have to eat a number of extra slices of bread, pancakes, or other sweet or starchy foods to make up the difference in

Table 25–2. Energy cost of different occupations.

Occupation	*Calories Required*
Secretary or office worker	2000
Housewife	2500–3000
Factory worker	3000–4000
Farmer, laborer or lumberjack	4500–5000

Table 25–3. Cost of various activities in calories per minute

Activity	Calories per minute
Recreational Activities and Hobbies	
Painting, sitting	2.0
Playing piano	2.5
Driving car	2.8
Canoeing (2.5 mph)	3.0
Horseback riding (slow)	3.0
Volleyball	3.5
Bowling	4.4
Golfing	5.0
Swimming (20 yd./min.)	5.0
Dancing	5.5
Gardening	5.6
Trotting horse	8.0
Spading	8.6
Skiing	9.9
Squash	10.2
Cycling (13 mph)	11.0
Industrial Activities	
Watch repairing	1.6
Typing	1.8
Armature winding	2.2
Radio assembly	2.7
Bricklaying	4.0
Plastering	4.1
Wheeling barrow (115 lb., 2.5 mph)	5.0
Carpentry	6.8
Mowing lawn by hand	7.3
Felling tree	8.0
Shoveling	8.5
Ascending stairs (17 lb. load, 27 ft./min.)	9.0
Tending furnace	10.2
Household Tasks	
Hand sewing	1.4
Sweeping floor	1.7
Machine sewing	1.8
Polishing	2.4
Peeling potatoes	2.9
Scrubbing, standing	2.9
Washing small clothes	3.0
Kneading dough	3.3
Scrubbing floors	3.6
Cleaning windows	3.7
Making beds	3.9
Ironing, standing	4.2
Mopping	4.2
Wringing by hand	4.4
Hanging wash	4.5
Beating carpets	4.9

the "gasoline" he burns each day. Yet both the farmer and the secretary require the same *basic, essential foods—proteins, minerals and vitamins.*

Vitamins

What is a vitamin? Do we know more about them than that their absence results in some vulnerability of the body to disease or malformation? To understand how vitamins work in the human body, we must first understand something of how the individual cells work.

The human body consists of more than a trillion cells working together to accomplish a variety of chemical functions. Assisting each cell with its respective task are numerous enzymes (biochemical catalysts), each performing its assigned task about 10,000 times a minute. Dr. Philip Handler, a renowned biochemist, has estimated that each cell contains 1000 different enzymes. Some enzymes cannot function alone; they require a co-worker. These co-workers are known to biochemists as coenzymes. It is in this connection that vitamins are important; for many coenzymes are vitamins or require vitamins for their production. Thus, a primary function of vitamins is to aid enzymes in directing and controlling the many chemical reactions necessary for life.

Can one tiny coenzyme be of any real consequence to our well-being? There are 13 vitamins known to be very necessary to good health. An example of their importance is that 1/28,000,000 ounce of vitamin B_{12} taken daily can prevent pernicious anemia. In equally infinitesimal amounts, other vitamins help prevent a variety of diseases and abnormal functioning in the body.

Some of these diseases have been recognized for centuries. *Scurvy* was familiar to seafaring people for hundreds of years before they suspected it had anything to do with the limited diet of sailors on long voyages. Scurvy made them weak, caused their gums to bleed and their teeth to fall out, made their muscles ache, and eventually ended in death. About 200 years ago, Joseph Lind, a British naval surgeon, found that the juice of citrus fruits would cure or prevent scurvy. Lime juice was subsequently carried on British ships so that sailors could have some every day, with the result that scurvy was eliminated, and British sailors came to be known as "limeys." Now we know that the value of the juice was in the *vitamin C* which citrus fruits contain.

Lack of *vitamin A* causes poor vision in dim light (called night blindness).

Without *vitamin D* the bones fail to harden properly, causing *rickets*, one result of which is seen in bowlegs, from which so many children used to suffer.

Lack of *vitamin B* causes susceptibility to several diseases, such as *beriberi* and *pellagra*. Victims of this latter deficiency disease are weakened to the point of helplessness, and their minds are frequently affected. Pellagra is widespread in certain poverty-stricken areas where the population consumes a very limited diet.

In addition to these striking deficiency associated diseases, lack of vitamins can cause milder disturbances that are more difficult to detect. Both the mild and the severe cases can be prevented by a balanced diet which contains all the vitamins.

We have to get our vitamins from foods because our bodies do not synthesize (manufacture) them, with the exception of *vitamin D*. Our bodies can make this vitamin when sunlight falls on the skin. However, we seldom synthesize throughout the year enough *vitamin D* for our needs, especially if, because of climate or our work, the sunshine we receive is inadequate. Thus, we must obtain additional *vitamin D* in our food.

The following listing shows some good sources of each of the principal vitamins:

"But why should I bother with this list?" you may ask. "Why can't I just buy my vitamins at the drugstore?"

In the first place, buying vitamins is more expensive. No one should spend money for vitamins when they can be obtained in standard foods which contain other essential nutrients as well. In the second place, there is still no guarantee that all the purified vitamins are as good as those which nature provides, or that all the vitamins have been isolated and purified. So don't buy vitamin pills, capsules, or other products unless your doctor says you need some concentrated supplements.

Other Dietary Requirements

In addition to vitamins, the body needs small amounts of other valuable materials. Only a fraction of an ounce of *iron* is required, but without this the body develops a form of anemia, a blood disease. The blood's rich redness is produced by hemoglobin, which contains iron and protein. Foods rich in iron include: kidney and navy beans, liver and other meats, turnip tops, beet greens, spinach, whole-wheat bread, and molasses. A trace of *iodine* is necessary to prevent goiter; this can easily be obtained from iodized table salt. Small quantities of *magnesium, manganese, copper,* and other substances are necessary. Fortunately, nature provides these when we have balanced diets.

Salt. Adequate amounts of salt (sodium chloride) are obtained from the average diet, except when a person sweats profusely. Salt is lost in the perspiration, and during hot summer days all of us, especially athletes and workers, should take in more than our usual quota of salt. We can salt food liberally, eat salted nuts or crackers, or add salt to tomato juice. One-fourth teaspoonful of salt in each glass of water is usually enough to compensate for salt loss in excessive perspiration. If salt tablets are taken, they should be specially coated ones which do not irritate the stomach.

How Much Water Should We Drink?

The amount of water needed is usually correctly adjusted by the sense of thirst. Every day the body loses about a quart of water in the invisible perspiration from the skin and the water vapor expired in the air from the lungs. This loss, plus the quart

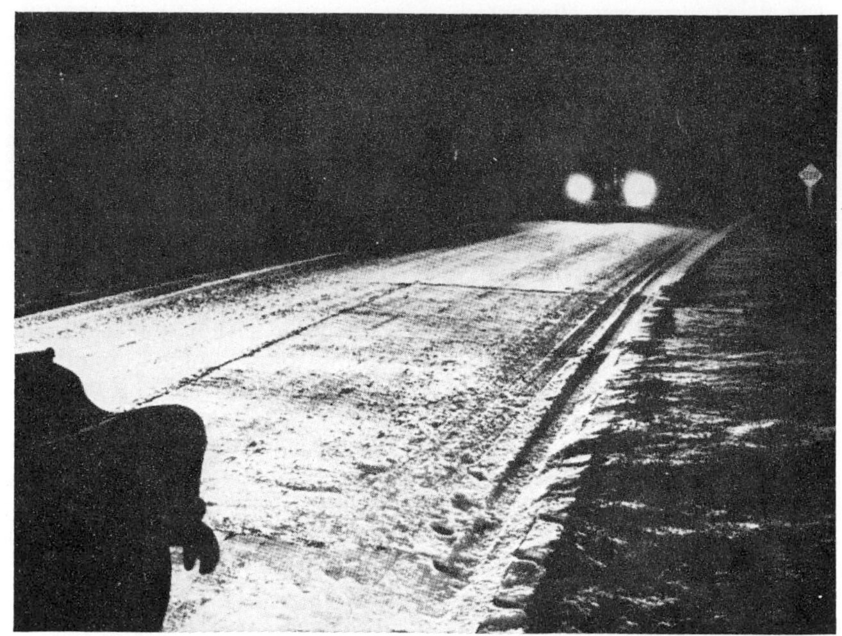

A

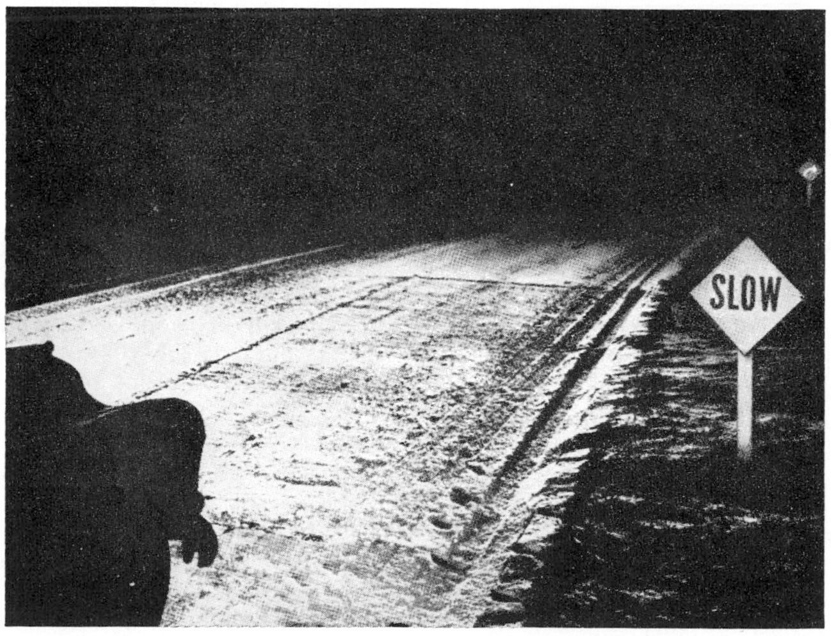

B

(See legend on opposite page.)

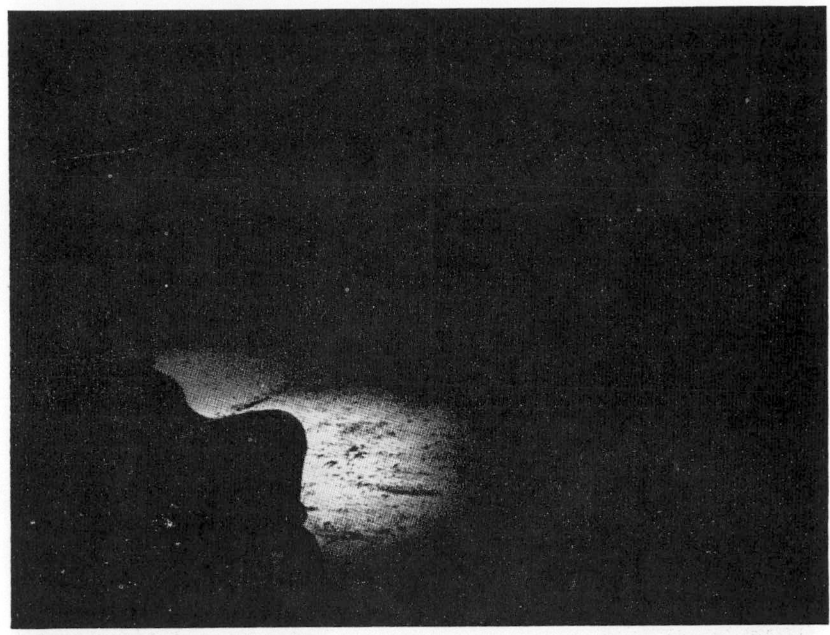

C

Figure 25–3. Vitamin A deficiency—night blindness. **A,** Both the normal individual and the vitamin A-deficient subject see the headlights of an approaching car. **B,** After the car has passed the normal individual sees a wide stretch of road. **C,** The vitamin A-deficient subject, whose view of the road is shown here, can barely see a few feet ahead and cannot see the road sign at all (From *Vitamin Manual.* The Upjohn Company, 1953.)

or more in urine, must be supplied chiefly by:

1. Water in solid foods. Vegetables and fruits, for example, have a high water content.
2. Water in fluids such as milk, soups and beverages.
3. Water itself. This should balance any difference between your intake and output.

In summer, or when you work in a hot area, your body requires more water to compensate for the loss of sweat. The *visible* perspiration may amount to many quarts a day.

In hot weather people have a tendency to drink huge quantities of extremely cold, iced water. This may overload the stomach with too much cold fluid. It is best to take iced water and other iced drinks in small quantities.

Some people have an almost mystical belief that it must be very healthy to drink large quantities of water and other fluids in order to wash "toxins" out of the body, especially through the kidneys. Medical research has shown that this is not true. The food you eat and the amount of water dictated by your thirst provide enough fluid, under normal conditions, to remove all waste products.

In certain diseases, larger amounts of fluid are recommended. For example, if an individual has a tendency to form *kidney stones,* his doctor may prescribe extra fluids. This tends to keep the urine more dilute and prevent the stones from precipitating.

In kidney infections, such as *pyelitis* and *pyelonephritis,* and infections of the urinary bladder, such as *cystitis*, extra water may be useful to help wash out the infection.

In *gout,* there is a tendency for crystals of *uric acid* to precipitate and accumulate at certain joints. Extra water may help keep this compound in solution.

Fluid intake is sometimes *restricted* in diseases where there is *edema,* or water-logging. This is true, for example, in certain

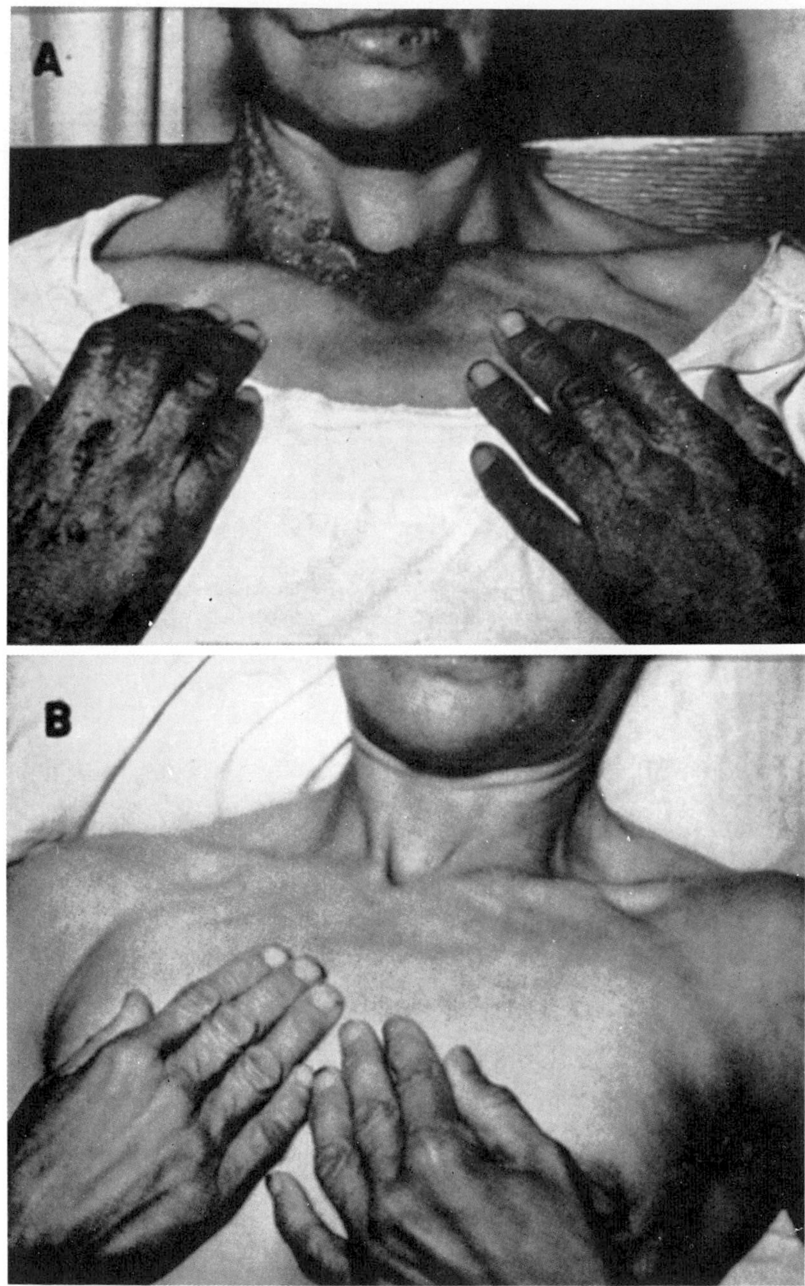

Figure 25–4. Pellagra. **A,** Dermatitis outlining the exposed area of the neck is found, as are the characteristic lesions on the backs of the hands. **B,** Same patient after nicotinamide therapy. (From *Vitamin Manual.* The Upjohn Co., 1959.)

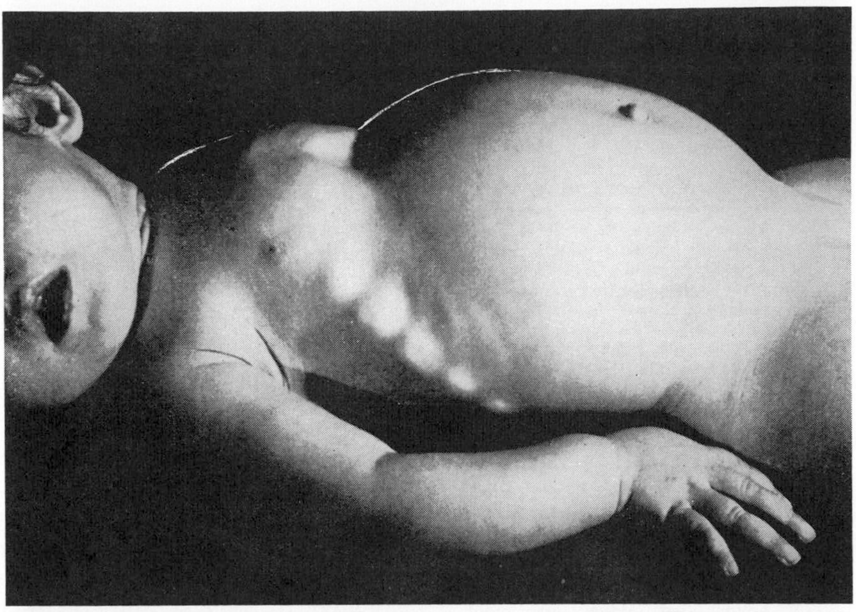

Figure 25–5. Rickets. The rachitic rosary is one of the earliest signs of rickets. Enlargement of the costochondral junctions results in beads or knobs that can sometimes be seen and can always be felt or demonstrated by x-ray. (From *Vitamin Manual*. The Upjohn Co., 1959.)

stages of heart failure, cirrhosis of the liver, and Bright's disease, which is a kidney disease.

Food Fads

Vegetarian Diets. There are three types of vegetarian diets: (1) the strictest is limited to fruit, vegetables, nuts, and the like, and excludes all animal products in addition to the flesh and organs of all animate creatures; (2) the intermediate includes certain animal products, such as milk, cheese, and eggs; (3) the most liberal permits fish and shellfish as well as dairy products.

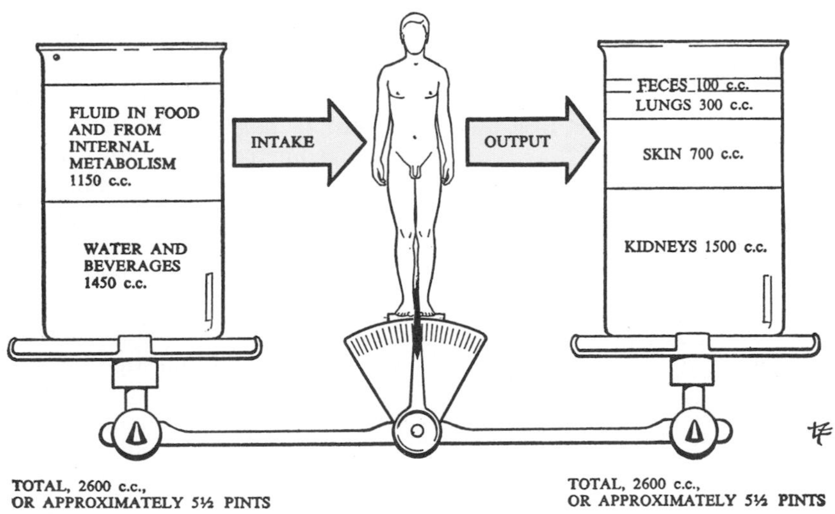

Figure 25–6. Fluid balance of the body. This diagram shows the sources and the quantity of fluids required by the average, moderately active man, and how these fluids are eliminated.

Table 25–4. Important food sources of vitamins*

IMPORTANT FOOD SOURCES OF VITAMINS

VITAMIN	IMPORTANT SOURCES
A	**Animal:** fish-liver oils, liver, whole milk and cheese products, butter, cream, egg yolk. **Plant:** dark green leafy vegetables, yellow vegetables, yellow fruits, fortified margarines.
B_1 (Thiamine)	**Animal:** pork products, liver, milk products. **Plant:** legumes, soybeans, nuts, whole grain and enriched cereals and breads.
B_2 (Riboflavin)	**Animal:** milk, cheese, eggs; liver, kidney, heart, meats. **Plant:** green leafy vegetables; whole grain and enriched cereals and breads.
NIACIN	**Animal:** liver, kidney, lean meat, fish, poultry. **Plant:** whole grain or enriched cereals and breads, peanuts.
B_6 (Pyridoxine)	**Animal:** meat, liver, kidney; small amounts in milk. **Plant:** wheat germ, whole grain cereals, soybeans, peanuts, corn; small amounts in green vegetables.
Biotin	Widespread in many foods. **Animal:** kidney, liver, eggs, milk. **Plant:** most fresh vegetables.
Pantothenic Acid	Widespread in many foods. **Animal:** liver, kidney, egg yolk. **Plant:** most fresh vegetables, whole grain cereals, peanuts.
Folic Acid	Widespread in many foods. **Animal:** chicken livers. **Plant:** vegetables — asparagus, broccoli, endive, leaf lettuce and spinach.
B_{12}	**Animal:** liver, kidneys, oysters, clams, lean beef, veal, lamb, poultry, milk, eggs, cheese.
C (Ascorbic Acid)	**Plant:** citrus fruits (oranges, grapefruit, lemon and limes), berries, melons, tropical fruits (pineapple, guava and others). Green leafy vegetables, broccoli, green pepper, cabbage, tomatoes, potatoes.
D	**Animal:** fish-liver oils, fortified milk; small amounts in butter, fortified margarine, liver, egg yolk.
E	**Plant:** oils of wheat germ, rice germ, cottonseed; green leafy vegetables; nuts; legumes.
K	**Animal:** liver. **Plant:** green leaves of plants (cabbage, spinach, kale), cauliflower, soybean.

*From *Today's Health,* January, 1963.

There is no conclusive medical evidence that vegetarian diets possess any unique virtues, except for the fact that people who adhere to them are apt to be lean, which is usually a good thing. However, for every vegetarian who attributes his healthy old age to his diet, you can probably find an even older person who gives credit to something else, perhaps the fact that he eats beef every day. Also, it is important to recognize that unless enough nuts and high protein vegetables are eaten, vegetarian diets can be dangerously low in protein.

Diets as Cures. We constantly hear about diets to "prevent acid or alkaline stomach," cure constipation, skin disease, cancer, high blood pressure and tooth decay, or to "increase virility and guarantee long life." Some of these systems are advocated by quacks; others by reputable physicians who become unduly optimistic and fail to test their theories sufficiently. For example, Eli Metchnikoff, one of the great pioneers in bacteriology, was convinced that drinking sour goat's milk would extend the span of human life tremendously. Thousands of people followed his advice, unfortunately to no avail.

Some diets are sound. For example, a special diet is essential in a disease like diabetes. Other diets may be helpful in constipation, anemias, acne and other conditions.

Food Fancies

Don't worry about "mixing" foods. There is no truth to the old superstition that something terrible happens when "acid" and "alkaline" foods get together in your stomach, or that you are bound to get sick if you have lobster and milk at the same meal, or ice cream and cherries.

There is no scientific basis for the superstition that eating oysters increases virility, or that fish is "brain food."

You don't need to cut down on the quantity of food you eat in the summer, unless, of course, you cut down on your activity and don't want to gain weight. But foods won't thicken or heat the blood.

Seasonings don't injure foods. The danger from highly seasoned foods in the past came from the fact that seasonings were often added to hide the fact that the food had spoiled.

There appears to be no scientific basis for the Orthodox Jewish interdiction of the simultaneous use of meat and dairy foods. On the other hand the Mosaic Law was very sound in the attitude toward pork, the washing of hands before eating, and the inspection of animals intended for human consumption.

There is no danger in drinking with your meals, as long as this doesn't encourage you to bolt food down without chewing it. Actually, the digestive enzymes work very effectively, even in dilute solution.

The consumption of large amounts of protein or meat in the diet is not at all harmful to the ordinary person. We usually limit the amount of meat we eat because it is one of the most expensive foods. Also, certain religious groups have strong taboos against meat, or against specific meats, such as pork or beef. However, Eskimos and certain African tribes live almost exclusively on meat and fish, and enjoy excellent health. After all, meat is the sole diet of many healthy carnivorous animals, who derive all the protein, fat, minerals, and vitamins they need from it.

Food Allergies

Certain foods cause allergies in sensitive individuals, and the symptoms may range from very mild to extremely severe. Eggs, wheat and milk are most commonly responsible for allergies, either respiratory, gastrointestinal, or skin (hives). However, many other foods, such as fish, nuts, chocolate, peas, potatoes, beans, garlic, and certain other fruits or vegetables, may have the same effect. Often an allergic individual can safely eat a particular food only when it is cooked.

Foods which are responsible for allergic symptoms vary from person to person, from age to age, and from symptom to symptom. One individual may be very sensitive to shellfish, and another only to wheat. Food allergies are often very pronounced in infants or young children, and then outgrown. Strawberries may cause hives, and chocolate may cause headaches in the same individual.

Food Poisoning

Perishable Foods. Meat, fish, cheese, and similar foods must be kept cool. Fruits and vegetables lose some of their vitamin content as well as their palatability if allowed to become stale. Even food in cans will eventually deteriorate if exposed to high temperatures, for example, near hot pipes or radiators.

Moist or liquid foods spoil most rapidly because of contamination by bacteria, yeasts and molds from the air. This process goes like wildfire if the liquid or moist food is slightly warm, the temperature which most microbes like best. Since bacteria do not thrive in cooler temperatures, such foods should be refrigerated.

Milk must be guarded more carefully than almost any other food. It should be cooled when it is delivered to the home or taken from the store, and it should not be allowed to sit around on porches or in halls for several hours getting warmed up before it is put into the refrigerator. It spoils if left in the sun, and may even be dangerous to use because of the increased number of bacteria in it. Exposure to light also destroys some of its precious B vitamins.

Contrary to popular opinion, modern cans are perfectly safe, and food may be left in a refrigerator in opened cans. Some foods, especially tomatoes and pineapple, take on a slightly metallic taste after a few days in open cans, but they do not become harmful.

Ptomaine Poisoning. In past years much was heard and written about "ptomaine poisoning," a diagnosis made on the incorrect theory that mysterious poisons were created during the digestion of some foods.

However, serious *food poisoning* can occur. This may result from contamination of food at its source, for example, milk from a diseased cow, oysters from a polluted bed, or vegetables which have been fertilized with human manure; by food that has spoiled—lobsters, for example—or by contamination of food during its preparation.

Certain foods provide very attractive culture media for various bacteria. Many outbreaks of food poisoning and gastrointestinal upsets have been traced to picnics in which some of these foods were permitted to stand out in the open air too long without refrigeration. This enables the bacteria, chiefly the staphylococcus, to proliferate rapidly until extremely large numbers are present. According to a study made by the U.S. Public Health Service, about 80 per cent of the stomach upsets due to gastroenteritis from spoiled food were caused by the staphylococcus organism.

The foods most commonly implicated in this type of poisoning are pastries, milk, eggs and products of milk and eggs, such as custards and cream fillings.

Meats, particularly cured hams, are also frequent offenders. Cured hams may be safe when they leave the packing house. However, when they are sliced, they are very easily contaminated with staphylococci. At room temperature these organisms may grow very rapidly without producing any change in odor or taste.

Botulism is a special type of food poisoning, caused by a toxin produced by the organism called *Clostridium botulinum.* It differs from the ordinary food poisoning caused by staphylococci, because it doesn't usually produce gastrointestinal distress. Instead, it acts on the central nervous system. Fatigue, headaches and dizziness, muscular weakness, disturbances of vision, and many other symptoms are characteristic of botulism.

The commonest source of this toxin is home canned food, inadequately sterilized. Canned meats and fish, as well as fruits and vegetables, may harbor the toxin, but the organism will grow only in foods which contain protein.

The poisonous botulinus toxin is made by bacteria which are commonly found on fresh foods, in their spore form. The only way to prevent its growth in canned food is by very thorough heating during the canning process, if necessary, heating twice to kill both the organisms and their spores.

Many types of food and milk poisoning result from human contamination. Bacteria can be transmitted to food by men and women who are handling or preparing the foods—cooks and their assistants, canners and meat packers. This is why it is so important to exclude anyone harboring pathogenic bacteria from handling or preparing food.

Contaminated Milk. Milk is one of our best foods, and every consumer is entitled to get clean milk. Unfortunately, in the raw state practically all milk contains more or less dirt and more bacteria than does any other food. Even when the most sanitary precautions are observed in the care of cows, during the milking process, and in the refrigeration of the milk, enormous numbers of bacteria can be introduced. Fortunately, most of these are not dangerous (pathogenic), but some are responsible for serious illnesses.

Milk can convey a greater variety of diseases than can any other food. It may transmit the microorganisms responsible for gastrointestinal upsets, undulant fever, typhoid fever, or bovine tuberculosis. All of these come from the cow itself. An infected milker may also contaminate the milk. For example, two separate outbreaks of scarlet fever in England were traced to raw milk from a single cow which had become infected from a handler with a sore throat.

The only really safe precaution against contaminated milk and milk products, such as cheese, is *pasteurization.* In this process, milk is heated for 30 minutes at 142° F., or at 160° F. for one minute.

Certified milk, meaning milk from inspected cows, is considerably safer than routine raw milk. However, it is still not nearly so safe as pasteurized milk, because the certification of the cow's health is never 100 per cent certain. Also, the milk has to be handled before it is bottled, and the handler may contaminate it. *Pasteurized milk goes directly into sterilized bottles after the heat treatment, and is not touched by human hands.*

Coffee, Tea and Cola Drinks

Stimulants are chemical substances which act on the nervous system and increase its activity. They may also affect other tissues and organs, directly or indirectly. For this reason, a little may be good, but too much, dangerous.

The caffeine which is found in coffee, tea, cocoa, and some cola drinks is such a stimulant, and belongs to a family of compounds called the *xanthines*. Tea and cocoa contain other xanthine derivatives—theophylline and theobromine—in addition to caffeine. All of these have essentially the same effect on the nervous system, but the action of caffeine is the strongest, and coffee is the most stimulating drink of all.

Caffeine in Drinks. Although tea leaves actually contain considerably more caffeine than the coffee bean, a cup of tea or coffee contains about the same amount of caffeine, approximately 120 milligrams. However, coffee is a much more stimulating drink than tea. It may be that the other chemicals in tea weaken the effect of the caffeine. A good deal of tea is consumed throughout the world, but largely because it is a warm pleasant drink, and not for its stimulating qualities.

Cocoa also contains caffeine, as do certain cola drinks on the market. Analyses made in the American Medical Association's laboratories on several popular cola drinks showed that they contain about 40 milligrams of caffeine in 6 ounces.

Caffeine is actually a poisonous substance, and it has been studied carefully in experimental animals. In all probability, 300 to 600 milligrams of caffeine injected directly into the blood of a human would be a fatal dose. Fortunately, not all the caffeine in the coffee we drink reaches our blood stream. Besides, habitual users of coffee build up a considerable tolerance for caffeine, and can safely ingest large amounts.

The use of coffee as a beverage apparently originated in Arabia, and was introduced into Europe during the seventeenth century. This led to violent arguments in the beginning. Was it poisonous or nonpoisonous?

The millions of coffee drinkers have proved that it is possible to drink this beverage without disastrous consequences for the human race. A good part of the world drinks coffee regularly. Americans drink about one-third of all the coffee produced throughout the world. The *average* annual consumption of Americans is 500 cups.

Effects of Coffee on the Human Body. Like many other stimulants people have come to depend upon, coffee is not particularly pleasing to the taste of many persons at first. It is certainly very bitter. Yet its *effects* are so pleasant and desirable that many of us learn to like it very much, and even to rely upon it.

In moderate amounts, coffee and tea are not harmful. However, it should be remembered that what is moderate for one person may be distinctly immoderate for another. If you are not accustomed to drinking more than one or two cups of coffee a day, or if you are unusually sensitive to the action of caffeine, you may react very unpleasantly.

We know that coffee has the following definite effects:

1. Its taste and aroma are very pleasant to confirmed coffee drinkers, and therefore it has definite appetite appeal and usefulness.
2. It is a useful drink, because it stimulates the brain and helps promote better work in many persons.
3. It reduces feelings of fatigue, and can actually give a physical lift when you are tired. It helps promote good conversation and pleasant moods.

Coffee can achieve all these desirable results because of its specific physiological effects on various organs of the body. The most important of these are:

1. It dilates or expands, the blood vessels of the brain. In this way, it increases the circulation of blood in the brain. This may be the explanation for increased mental alertness after drinking coffee, especially if the person is fatigued.
2. It stimulates the action of the heart and improves blood circulation generally.
3. It increases respiration and heat production by the body.
4. It improves muscle tone and strengthens the desire for muscular activity.

Certain other effects of caffeine are not always so desirable. For example, in some individuals it makes intestinal movements more active, and may actually cause indigestion, constipation, or even diarrhea. Also, it stimulates the kidneys to secrete more urine and is therefore called a *diuretic* agent. Several cups of coffee can increase urine flow two or three times. This may be particularly marked at certain hours of the day, especially in the morning.

Unfortunately, the good effects of coffee may be overdone. Excessive amounts sometimes produce restlessness, overexcitability, dizziness, and nervousness. If you develop symptoms like these after moderate amounts of coffee, you are probably inordinately sensitive, and should not drink it.

Exceptionally nervous individuals may find that coffee makes them even more jittery. Even people who are accustomed to coffee often react badly to it late at night. It can produce wakefulness and irritability, and sometimes interferes seriously with sleep and rest.

Should Children Drink Coffee? A surprisingly high percentage of children, especially if they have foreign-born parents, drink coffee regularly. This is undesirable for several reasons. Few children need the stimulus of coffee drinks, because they are usually already stimulated. Even more important, coffee should not be substituted for the milk and fruit juices which are needed to provide vital proteins, minerals, and vitamins. *There are no important nutritional substances in coffee.*

Watch Your Coffee If You Are Overweight! Six cups of coffee a day with plentiful cream and sugar represent about 600 calories. If you like your coffee sweetened and with cream, and have a tendency to gain weight, you'll have to employ restraint or learn to drink it black.

The same is true for some of the cola drinks. Because they also contain caffeine, they have the same advantages and hazards of coffee. Also, they are heavily sweetened. A 6 ounce bottle of a cola drink may contain 4½ teaspoonsful of sugar, which is equivalent to 75 calories. This amount of sweetening is often a very unnecessary caloric supplement and may also accelerate tooth decay.

Questions

1. Why is a high-protein breakfast specially important?
2. What are the essentials of a good, well-balanced diet?
3. What determines the number of calories you must consume each day? What are the high-calorie foods?
4. Discuss the importance to the body's health of proteins, minerals and vitamins.
5. Indicate the chief function of and a good source for the following: vitamin A, vitamin B, vitamin C and vitamin D.
6. Why are natural sources of vitamins better than vitamin pills?
7. What is the chief danger in vegetarian diets?
8. Is there any likelihood, as the food faddists maintain, that all diseases can be traced to our diets?
9. What are the major causes of food poisoning?
10. What is the difference between *pasteurized* and *certified* milk?
11. What are some of the undesirable effects of coffee and other caffeine-containing drinks?
12. Discuss the hazards of cola drinks to the nervous system, weight and teeth.

Topics for Discussion

Intestinal bacteria and digestion.
Specificity of enzymes.
Water loss in diabetes insipidus.

Reading Suggestions

Eat Well and Stay Well, Ancel Keys and Margaret Keys. Doubleday & Co., New York, 1963. A reference guide for food selection and nutrition.

Eating for Good Health, Fredrick J. Stare. Doubleday & Co., New York, 1964. A physician discusses the nutrients that we do and do not need. Highly readable.

Alcohol and Caffeine: A Study of Their Psychological Effects, Harvey Nash. Charles C Thomas, Springfield, Ill., 1962. An up-to-date review of 70 years of research on the topic. Comprehensive.

Nutrition and Physical Fitness, Jean L. Bogert, George M. Briggs, and Doris H. Calloway. 8th Ed., W. B. Saunders, Philadelphia, 1966. A highly sensible guide to nutrition. Good discussion of fads and fancies.

Foods Without Fads, E. W. McHenry. J. B. Lippincott, Philadelphia, 1960. An informative book for the layman. The myths of nutrition are discussed.

Recent Advances in Human Nutrition, J. F. Brock. Little, Brown & Co., Boston, 1961. A survey of current knowledge in nutrition.

Food Becomes You, Ruth M. Leverton. Iowa State University Press, Ames, 1960. A scientific but nontechnical discussion of nutrition written for laymen.

Human Nutrition, V. H. Morttram. Williams & Wilkins, Baltimore, 1963. An up-to-date discussion of what the human body does and does not require in nutrition.

Your Food and Your Health, R. Carter. Harper & Row, New York, 1964. Diets that are compatible and incompatible with good health are discussed. Informative and well written.

Introductory Foods, Osee G. Hughes. 4th Ed.,

Macmillan, New York, 1962. A highly sensible discussion of foods and nutrition.

What Is a Vitamin? Donald G. Cooley. Today's Health, January 1963, p. 20. A well illustrated and accurate description of vitamins and how they work.

How Much Health Is There In "Health Foods"? Ronald M. Deutsch. Reader's Digest, May 1963, p. 57. An informative discussion of unscrupulous health food promoters.

The Food Fanatic's Four Myths of Nutrition, Philip L. White. Today's Health, June 1963, p. 72. The author explodes several myths about nutrition.

Why Not Nibble Like a Rat, Robert Herman. Science Digest, March 1965, p. 53. A popular discussion of recent trends in dieting. Six meals a day are recommended in preference to the usual three.

The Energy Factory: How Food Finally Produces Power. Life, March 29, 1963, p. 48. A well written and understandable discussion of the chemistry of digestion. Beautifully illustrated.

SECTION EIGHT

HEALTH AND APPEARANCE IN DAILY LIFE

26

OVERWEIGHT AND UNDERWEIGHT

Sooner or later almost everyone is faced with the problem of losing or gaining weight—or, at least, wonders whether he or she ought to diet. Medical statistics show that 2½ million individuals in the United States actually consulted doctors during one year recently to ask for help in reducing. Scientific estimates indicate that one-fifth the people over 30 years of age in this country, and undoubtedly a large number of younger people, are overweight.

WEIGHT AND HEALTH

Anyone who is markedly under- or overweight is suffering from a kind of illness. The obese person may be subject to one or more of the following: overworked heart and circulation; shortness of breath, tendency to high blood pressure; tendency to diabetes; poor adjustment to hot weather and changes of temperature; increased strain on joints and ligaments, often leading to chronic back and joint pains; reduced capacity for physical exertion and sometimes for mental work; increased susceptibility to infectious disease; and personality problems due to poor appearance.

Such a person cannot be enjoying good health. And the final proof comes from incontestable medical evidence which shows that *overweight shortens the span of life itself.* For example, the mortality from circulatory conditions is 44 per cent higher in males who are 5 to 15 per cent overweight than it is in men whose weight is what it ought to be. Death rates from *all* causes in men 45 to 50 years old increase 18 per cent in men 20 pounds overweight, 45 per cent in men 40 pounds overweight, and 67 per cent in men 60 pounds overweight. "The longer the waistline, the shorter the life line."

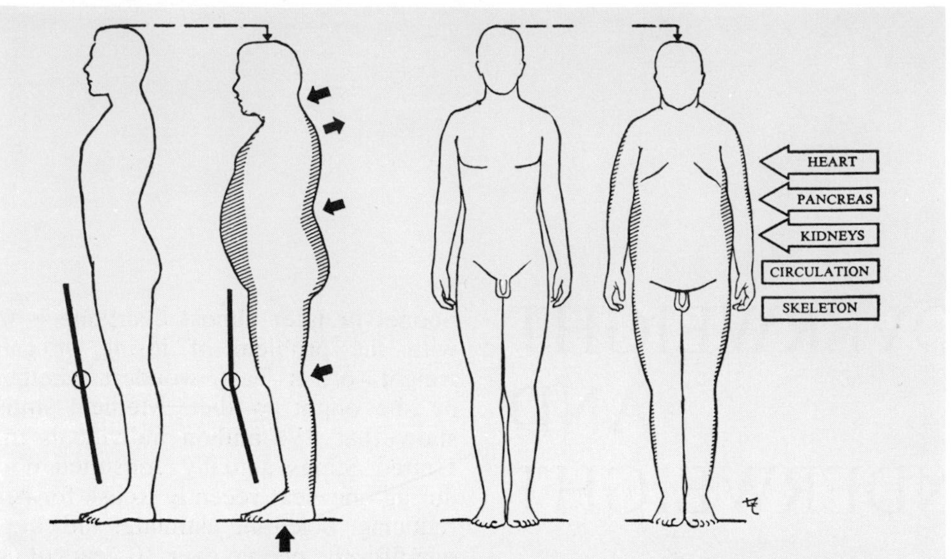

Figure 26–1. Obesity. Note the decrease in height due to increased weight. **Left,** The black arrows indicate the location of the most severe skeletal strain. **Right,** The organs most severely affected.

Obesity should be regarded as a potentially serious type of illness, instead of a subject for jokes and ridicule.

Individuals who are markedly underweight are in less danger, provided, of course, that their condition is not due to illness. However, they often lack energy, endurance, and resistance to infection, being more susceptible to illnesses such as tuberculosis, especially when they are young. To be "skinny" is not funny, either.

Obviously, people in these two groups don't look as well as they would if their weight were normal, and appearances, as well as health, contribute to happiness and success.

Does This Mean You?

Your doctor can answer this question better than anyone else. Usually your mirror has provided you with a pretty good clue. Figure 26–1 and Table 26–1 may help you decide whether or not your eyes have been deceiving you.

This table indicates not the *average,* but the *desirable* weight for various heights and frames. There is a range of approximately 10 pounds in each ideal weight group. Differences of only a few pounds above or below these limits should not be a matter of much concern. However, a variation of 15 or more pounds from the given limits is probably excessive and should be corrected.

The older you are, the more important it is not to be overweight. The younger you are, the more dangerous it is to be underweight.

More Accurate Methods of Assessing Obesity

Although Table 26–1 serves as a useful reference, it is not entirely accurate for determining your proper weight. By this method, an individual with good muscular development could in some instances be classified as obese. Of the available methods of estimating the proportion of fat in the living body, the determination of body density by underwater weighing is probably the most reliable, but this requires heavy and expensive apparatus. Other methods include the measurement of skin-fold thickness, estimation of total body water, and estimation of lean body mass from basal oxygen consumption and study of the urine. Of these, the simplest and the one showing best correlation with body density is the measurement of skin-folds.

Table 26–1. Height and weight charts

Desirable weights for men and women, aged 25 and over, according to height and frame.

WEIGHT IN POUNDS ACCORDING TO FRAME (IN INDOOR CLOTHING)

HEIGHT (with shoes on) 1-inch heels Feet	Inches	SMALL FRAME	MEDIUM FRAME	LARGE FRAME
5	2	112-120	118-129	126-141
5	3	115-123	121-133	129-144
5	4	118-126	124-136	132-148
5	5	121-129	127-139	135-152
5	6	124-133	130-143	138-156
5	7	128-137	134-147	142-161
5	8	132-141	138-152	147-166
5	9	136-145	142-156	151-170
5	10	140-150	146-160	155-174
5	11	144-154	150-165	159-179
6	0	148-158	154-170	164-184
6	1	152-162	158-175	168-189
6	2	156-167	162-180	173-194
6	3	160-171	167-185	178-199
6	4	164-175	172-190	182-204

WEIGHT IN POUNDS ACCORDING TO FRAME (IN INDOOR CLOTHING)

HEIGHT (with shoes on) 2-inch heels Feet	Inches	SMALL FRAME	MEDIUM FRAME	LARGE FRAME
4	10	92- 98	96-107	104-119
4	11	94-101	98-110	106-122
5	0	96-104	101-113	109-125
5	1	99-107	104-116	112-128
5	2	102-110	107-119	115-131
5	3	105-113	110-122	118-134
5	4	108-116	113-126	121-138
5	5	111-119	116-130	125-142
5	6	114-123	120-135	129-146
5	7	118-127	124-139	133-150
5	8	122-131	128-143	137-154
5	9	126-135	132-147	141-158
5	10	130-140	136-151	145-163
5	11	134-144	140-155	149-168
6	0	138-148	144-159	153-173

Courtesy Metropolitan Life Insurance Company

Ideal weights for boys and girls, according to height and age.

HEIGHT Feet	Inches	AGE 14	15	16	17	18	19
4	6	72					
4	7	74					
4	8	78	80				
4	9	83	83				
4	10	86	87				
4	11	90	90	90			
5	0	94	95	96			
5	1	99	100	103	106		
5	2	103	104	107	111	116	
5	3	108	110	113	118	123	127
5	4	113	115	117	121	126	130
5	5	118	120	122	127	131	134
5	6	122	125	128	132	136	139
5	7	128	130	134	136	139	142
5	8	134	134	137	141	143	147
5	9	137	139	143	146	149	152
5	10	143	144	145	148	151	155
5	11	148	150	151	152	154	159
6	0		153	155	156	158	163
6	1		157	160	162	164	167
6	2		160	164	168	170	171

HEIGHT Feet	Inches	AGE 14	15	16	17	18
4	7	78				
4	8	83				
4	9	88	92			
4	10	93	96	101		
4	11	96	100	103	104	
5	0	101	105	108	109	111
5	1	105	108	112	113	116
5	2	109	113	115	117	118
5	3	112	116	117	119	120
5	4	117	119	120	122	123
5	5	121	122	123	125	126
5	6	124	124	125	128	130
5	7	130	131	133	133	135
5	8	133	135	136	138	138
5	9	135	137	138	140	142
5	10	136	138	140	142	144
5	11	138	140	142	144	145

From American Child Health Association.

cut out and post

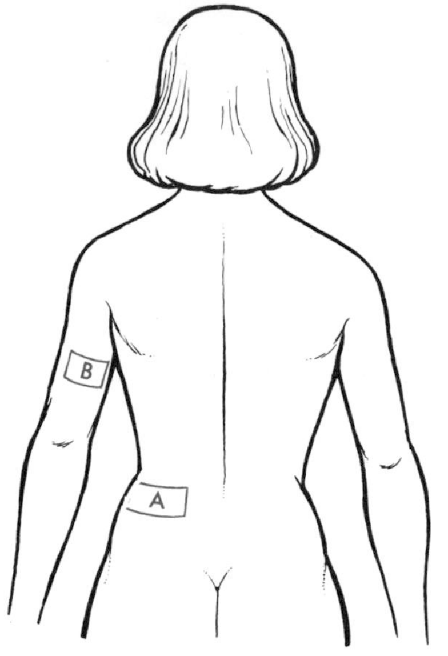

Figure 26–2. Determination of density of body fat in adult women by skin-fold measurement. To determine body density, measure in millimeters the skin-fold thickness at points *A*, and *B*. Then insert the values into the formula: Density = 1.0764 – 0.00081A – 0.00088B. Density is converted into per cent of fat by the formula: Per cent fat = 100 × [(4.950/density) – 4.500]. An average value for college age women is around 21 per cent of the total body weight. (The formula to convert skin-fold thickness to body density is from research by A. W. Sloan and associates, *Journal of Applied Physiology, 17*: 967, 1962. The formula to convert density into per cent fat is from research by W. E. Seri, Donner Laboratory of Biophysics and Medical Physics, University of California.)

Formulas for the determination of body fat from skin-fold measurements of adult men and women are presented in Figures 26–2 and 26–3. The only equipment required is an inexpensive skin-fold caliper.[1]

[1]Your teacher can recommend the nearest supplier.

Food and Weight

For a long time now it has been emphasized that there is a direct relationship between food intake and obesity. But it now appears that this may have been a somewhat oversimplification of a very complex problem. Just as some breeds of

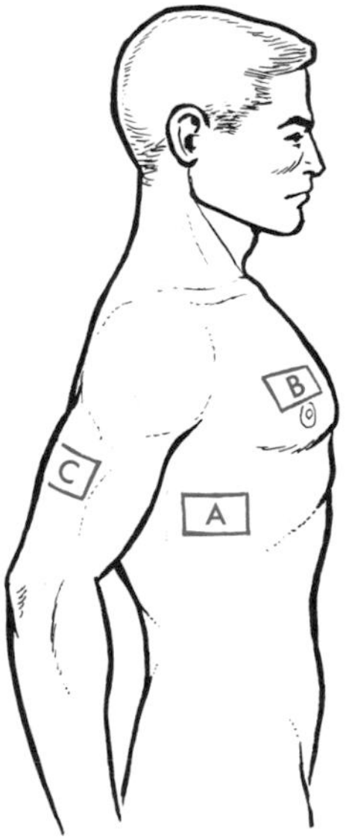

Figure 26–3. Determination of density of body fat in adult men. To determine body density, measure in millimeters the skin-fold thickness at points *A, B* and *C* and insert these values in the formula: Density = 1.088468 – 0.0007123A – 0.0004834B – 0.0005513C. To convert density to body fat, use the formula described for women in Figure 26–2. An average value for college age men is 13 per cent. (The formula to convert skin-fold thickness to density is from research by L. R. Pascale and associates; Med. Nutr. Lab., *162*, 1955.

livestock gain more weight than others from the same amount of calories, so it now appears to be with humans. This comes as no real surprise, because humans differ in so many ways. In fact, Dr. Edgar Gordon and his associates at the University of Wisconsin School of Medicine have listed more than 25 physiological and biochemical differences between obese and normal persons.

One such difference is that, following a period of fasting, the free fatty acids in the blood of normal subjects increase, whereas in the obese patient there is no change. Next to glucose, free fatty acids are the most readily available form of energy for cellular oxidation. On the basis of this finding, Dr. Gordon stated:

> . . . it is evident that there is a peculiar metabolic anomaly about obese individuals that may eventually tend to justify some of their protestations that they 'gain weight even while eating a reducing diet.' This statement is not to be construed as indicating that the behavior of these obese subjects is incompatible with the laws of thermodynamics, but rather that the efficiency of their engine is greater than that of thin individuals, with a difference that is definable in biochemical terms.

An encouraging method of treating obesity has emerged from Dr. Gordon's research. This method consists of an initial period of fasting (water, coffee, and tea only) followed by a diet of 1320 calories a day consumed in a minimum of six daily feedings. The purpose of the initial fast is to break a metabolic pattern in which an overactive enzyme system is thought to be too efficient in the transformation of food (especially carbohydrate) into fat.

Dr. Gordon's dietary method recognizes a qualitative as well as a quantitative difference in food. The emphasis is on a high-protein, low-carbohydrate diet, with fat acting as the main source of energy.

Anyone who "eats nothing and gains weight" may be eating the wrong types of foods at the wrong time of day. The following program described by Dr. Gordon may be of help to those who want to lose weight:

Daily Diet

Protein	100 gm.	400 cal.
Fat	80 gm.	720 cal.
Carbohydrate	50 gm.	200 cal.

Schedule of Feedings

Breakfast
Midmorning
Lunch
Midafternoon
Supper
Bedtime

Dr. Gordon reports that six feedings a day have been acceptable to all his patients, and none have complained of hunger. This regimen, with slight modifications, has been successfully employed in many different medical centers.

Why Do People Eat Too Much or Too Little?

Norman Jolliffe, in his excellent book, *Reduce and Stay Reduced,* has coined a term, *appestat,* for the mechanism that regulates the appetite. According to this concept, the appestat resembles the thermostat on a furnace, supplying heat when the temperature falls below the ideal setting, and shutting off when the proper temperature is reached.

In many people, the appestat is easily influenced or conditioned by habit. Children coming from families that love food and make a happy event out of each meal often grow up to be adults whose appestats are set too high, while those from homes where mealtimes are unpleasant, and the food skimpy and poorly prepared, may have low appestats.

Emotional factors can play a very important part in overeating or undereating. People who feel lonely and unwanted often eat excessively. Women with small children sometimes overeat when they become bored by having to stay home too much. Or overeating may make them calmer and better able to meet problems with the children and other stresses. On the other hand, worry and tension can also *keep people from eating.* Sometimes psychological quirks, like the desire for attention and sympathy, also express themselves in the rejection of food.

Table 26–2. Nutritive values of foods in average servings or common measures*

Food	Weight gm.	Approximate Measure	Calories	Protein gm.	Minerals		Vitamins				
					Calcium mg.	Iron mg.	Vitamin A I.U.	Thiamine mg.	Riboflavin mg.	Niacin mg.	Ascorbic acid mg.
Breads:											
Bread, white, enriched	23	1 Slice, average	63	2.0	18	0.4	0	0.06	0.04	0.5	0
Bread, whole wheat, 60%	23	1 Slice, average	55	2.1	22	0.5	0	0.07	0.03	0.7	0
Doughnut, yeast	30	1 average	121	1.9	15	0.4	67	0.06	0.05	0.5	trace
Griddle cakes, white	45	1 medium, 4 in. diam.	62	2.3	96	0.3	44	0.03	0.05	0.2	0
Roll, white, hard	35	1 av., no milk or butter	95	2.8	8	0.6	0	0.08	0.05	0.8	0
Cereals:											
Corn flakes, Kellogg's	30	1⅓ cups	109	2.2	1	0.5	0	0.12	0.03	0.6	0
Oatmeal, or rolled oats	30	¾ cup, cooked	111	4.0	15	1.3	0	0.17	0.04	0.3	0
Rice, white	28.35	¾ cup, cooked	103	2.1	7	0.2	0	0.02	0.01	0.5	0
Spaghetti, tomato sauce	220	1 serving	271	6.4	23	1.0	1336	0.125	0.076	1.57	19
Wheaties	30	1 cup	105					(mcg.)			
Crackers and similar products				2.9	7	1.3	0	0.15	0.04	1.5	0
Crackers, saltines	4	1 cracker, 2 in. square	17								
Pretzel	20	1 medium	72	0.3	1	0.05	0	trace	trace	0.05	0
Ry-Krisp	6.5	1 double wafer	21	1.8	7	0.3					
Dairy products				0.8	3	0.3	0	0.02	0.01	0.1	0
Butter	10	1 pat, average	72								
Cheese, Cheddar, American	30	1 ounce	113	0.1	2	0	330	trace	trace	trace	0
Cheese, cottage	30	1 rounded tbsp., or ⅛ cup	27	7.1	206	0.3	400	0.01	0.12	trace	0
Ice cream, plain, vanilla	100	⅙ of quart	207	5.5	27	0.1	10	0.01	0.09	trace	0
Milk, whole, fresh	244	8 oz., 1 cup or full glass	166	4.0	123	0.1	520	0.04	0.19	0.1	1
Egg, boiled	54	1 medium	77	8.5	288	0.2	390	0.09	0.42	0.3	3
Fish:				6.1	26	1.3	550	0.05	0.14	trace	0
Halibut steak	90	1 serving, 4 from a pound	205	21.0	15	0.8	497	0.05	0.06	8.8	0
Oysters, raw, meat only	100	5–8 medium	84	9.8	94	5.6	320	0.15	0.20	1.2	
Salmon, canned, red	100	⅔ cup (no bones)	173	20.2		1.2	230	0.04	0.16	7.3	0
Fruits and fruit juices:											
Apple, fresh	125	1 medium, 2¾ in. diam.	72	0.4	7	0.4	112	0.05	0.04	0.25	6
Banana, fresh	125	1 medium	110	1.5	10	0.75	538	0.05	0.06	0.9	12
Orange juice, fresh	185	6 oz., ¾ cup, small glass	81	1.5	35	0.4	352	0.15	0.06	0.4	91
Prunes, stewed	75	4 medium, 2 tbsp. juice	86	0.7	17	1.3	545	0.02	0.04	0.4	trace
Tomato juice, canned	180	6 oz., ¾ cup, small glass	38	1.8	13	0.75	1905	0.09	0.05	1.35	28
Watermelon	600	1 sl. 6 in. diam. × 1½ in.	168	3.0	72	1.2	3540	0.30	0.30	1.2	36
Meats:											
Bacon, cooked	25	3 strips, 6 in. long, crisp	152	8.2	8	0.8	0	0.12	0.08	1.2	0
Beefsteak, sirloin, cooked	100	1 pc. 4 × 2½ × 1 in.	297	23.0	10	2.9	0	0.06	0.19	4.8	0
Lamb chop, cooked	70	2 chops, ¾ in. thick	256	15.8	18	2.2	0	0.09	0.16	3.8	0
Liver, beef, fried	74	2 sl., 3 × 2¼ × ⅜ in.	172	17.5	7	5.8	37,315	0.18	2.56	10.1	20
Pork chop, fried	80	1 medium large chop	310	17.4	12	2.6	0	0.59	0.17	3.6	0
Veal cutlet, breaded	92	1 average serving, baked	217	23.8	22	3.0	0	0.10	0.25	6.5	0

Table 26–2. Nutritive values of foods in average servings or common measures* *(Continued)*

Food	Weight gm.	Approximate Measure	Calories	Protein gm.	Minerals: Calcium mg.	Minerals: Iron mg.	Vitamins: Vitamin A I.U.	Vitamins: Thiamine mg.	Vitamins: Riboflavin mg.	Vitamins: Niacin mg.	Vitamins: Ascorbic acid mg.
Poultry:											
Chicken, fried	85	1/4 bird, fortified margarine									
		used in frying	232	22.4	18	1.8	230	0.07	0.17	9.7	0
Turkey, roasted	100	3 sl., 3 1/2 × 2 1/2 × 1/4 in.	200	30.9	30	5.1	0-20	0.08	0.17	9.8	0
Nuts:											
Almonds, salted	15	12–15 nuts	90	2.8	38	0.7	0	0.04	0.10	0.7	trace
Peanut butter	16	1 tbsp.	92	4.2	12	0.3	0	0.02	0.02	2.6	0
Walnuts, English	15	8–15 halves, 2 tbsp. chopped	98	2.3	12	0.3	5	0.07	0.02	0.2	trace
Sweets:											
Chocolate creams	13	1 avg. pc. (35 to a lb.)	51	0.5							
Hershey's milk chocolate	43	1 bar, 1 1/2 oz.	238	3.2	86	1.1	64	.044	.02	0.14	
Assorted jams, commercial	20	1 tbsp. level	55	0.1	2	0.1	trace	trace	trace	trace	1
Vegetables:				1.4	36	0.7	660	0.07	0.10	0.5	14
Beans, string, fresh	100	3/4 cup, cooked	22								
Beets, fresh, cooked	100	1/2 cup diced, or 2 beets		1.0	21	0.7	20	0.02	0.04	0.3	7
		2 in. diam.	41								
Carrots, raw	50	1 carrot, 5 1/2 × 1 in. or		0.6	20	0.4	6,000	0.03	0.03	0.3	3
		1/2 cup grated	21	2.7	4	0.5	200	0.03	0.05	0.9	5
Corn, sweet, canned	100	2/3 cup, drained solids	85				yellow,				
Potatoes, white, baked	100	1 medium, without skin	98				trace white				
Spinach, cooked	100	1/2 cup	23	2.4	13	0.8	20	0.11	0.05	1.4	17
Tomatoes, fresh	150	1 medium, 2 × 2 1/2 in.	30	2.8	*	1.8	10,600	0.07	0.18	0.55	27
Beverages:				1.5	16	0.9	1640	0.08	0.06	0.8	35
Chocolate milk shake	342	1 regular	435								
Cola drink	170	1 bottle, 6 oz.	78	11.1	362	0.4	708	0.12	0.05	0.37	2
Coffee, roasted	100	3 1/2 oz.						0.09	0.07	8.69	
Beer, lager, American	240	1 large glass	103	1.2				10	72	1.92	
Desserts:											
Cake, chocolate, 2 layers	100	1 pc. iced 1/12 of avg. cake	378	4.4	88	0.5	690	0.02	0.07	0.2	0
Pudding, bread, with raisins		1 serving	205	6.1	99	1.1	349	0.01	0.02	0.98	16
Pie, apple	160	1/6 of medium pie	377	3.8	11	0.5	156	0.05	0.03	0.4	1
Miscellaneous:											
Salad, gelatin with fruit	155	1 serving with lettuce	172	1.9	16	0.3	331	0.02	0.03	0.18	2
Sandwich, bacon, lettuce,											
tomato		1, white toast	306	7.0	38	1.5	776	0.02	0.01	1.78	12
Soup, vegetable, canned											
ready to serve	250	1 cup	82	4.2	32	0.8		0.05	0.08	1.0	8
Stew, oyster	325	1 1/2 cups	287	14.3	353	7.3	714	0.03	0.06	1.30	12

*From Bogert, J. L.: *Nutrition and Physical Fitness,* W. B. Saunders Co., Philadelphia, 1960.

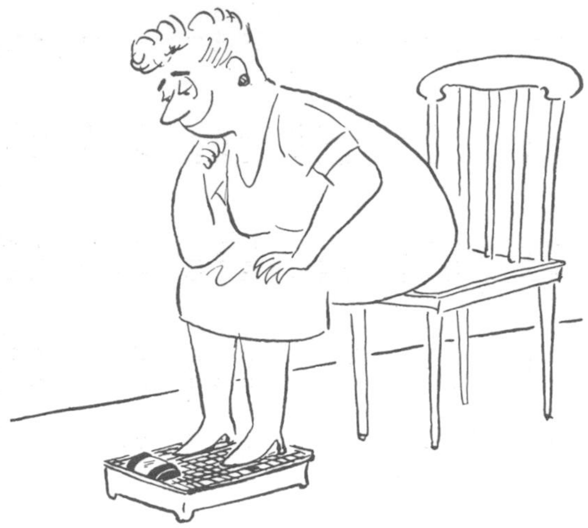

(Drawing by Con Suozzi. Reprinted with permission of *Today's Health,* published by the American Medical Association, March, 1958.)

Should One Take Drugs or Medicines to Reduce?

Only in exceptional cases is it necessary to use medicines in the treatment of obesity. Furthermore, reducing aids should never be taken without a doctor's prescription. A consultant writing in the Journal of the American Medical Association says:

> No known drug or compound may safely be taken without medical advice to cause loss of weight. The word 'safely' deserves emphasis, since some drugs, which have succeeded in taking off pounds, have had the disadvantage of making some people blind and killing others.

Many reducing preparations contain amphetamine, the same stimulant used in "pep pills," and unless properly controlled, this compound can produce a nervous, jittery feeling. Some reducing aids are harmless to most people, but this is no guarantee that they will be safe for all. Besides, such medicines are merely short cuts, with little usefulness in the long run. They can depress the appetite or speed up the metabolism, but are helpful only as long as you are taking them. As soon as you stop, the problems begin again. *The most sensible way to regulate the appetite is to diet properly.*

Can Exercise Reduce Weight?

The role of exercise in weight control was discussed in a preceding chapter. One additional example may serve to emphasize the importance of activity in the control of creeping overweight. The example was cited by Dr. Gordon:

> A stenographer, 63 inches tall and weighing 120 lbs., operating a mechanical typewriter, uses 87.7 calories per hour. She changes to an electrical type-

ENERGY EXPENDITURES PER HOUR —20 YR. OLD MAN

Activity	Calories
Sleeping	65
Lying still	75
Sitting	100
Typing	140
Walking	200
Severe exercise	475
Running	600
Walking upstairs	1100

Extracted from data compiled by M. S. Rose

Energy expenditures of the body vary widely according to activity. As this chart shows, walking upstairs requires approximately 17 times as much energy as lying in bed asleep.

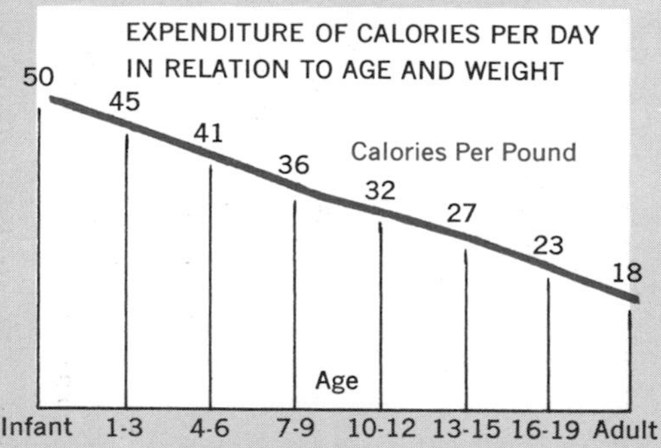

Calorie expenditures per pound fall steadily as a child grows up. During each three years between infancy and adulthood, daily needs per pound decline by about five calories.

writer and her energy requirement falls to 72.9 calories per hour. Thus, there is a saving of 14.8 calories, which for a 6 hour day amounts to 90 calories and in a 5 day week, to 450 calories. If her food intake and physical activity otherwise remain unchanged, she will gain 1 pound of body weight in about 10 weeks, because she has changed to an electrical typewriter.

We might add that this simple change in working habits could result in 25 pounds of excess fat within 5 years.

Can Massage Reduce Weight?

You can't massage away pounds of flesh, but massage may tone up the skin and muscles, and help the body adjust to its new, slimmer contours.

Similarly, sweating and hot baths merely remove water, which is immediately regained. These methods have no permanent effect, and *may* impose a dangerous strain on the heart and circulation in certain individuals.

Fad Diets

New diets are constantly appearing and disappearing with, sometimes, nothing to recommend them except a popular movie star's endorsement. Some of them are based on sensible calorie control, with a harmless "gimmick" added, perhaps a catchy title to make them popular. The main danger in many fad diets is that they tend to encourage people to reduce too rapidly. Some are too expensive or difficult to be practical, while others are based on theories which have not been scientifically proved.

Many fad diets are actually so dangerously low in protein, vitamins and minerals that it is hazardous to stay on them for more than a week or two.

Perhaps the most important consideration, however, is that fad diets fail to teach how to eat properly to *maintain* the optimum weight. *Losing* weight is actually not so very difficult. The problem is *to stay reduced.* As Norman Jolliffe, the eminent nutritionist, pointed out, about 90 per cent of the people who reduce successfully sooner or later regain their hard-lost pounds. The reason is that they never reformed their food habits, and failed to learn appetite control and elementary dietetics. *They never will on fad diets.*

Is It Safe to Reduce Without a Doctor's Supervision?

Anyone who is not more than 10 pounds or so overweight, and is prepared to reduce at the rate of 1/2 pound to 1 pound or so a week can do so perfectly safely on his own. Self-control for a few months is all that's necessary. It took a while to put extra weight on, however, and it should be eliminated at a moderate rate, too. Furthermore, fat lost slowly stays off better than fat that is lost rapidly, and getting rid of only 1/2 pound a week would add up to 26 pounds a year. If weight is lost slowly, the skin adjusts better, and that deflated balloon look doesn't develop.

Weight reduction for the really obese individual, however, is best carried out under the supervision of a physician. This is to guard against too rapid a loss of weight, which can impose a severe strain on the heart and circulation, and to guarantee that the diet used contains adequate amounts of protein, minerals and vitamins to prevent weakening of bones and organs, and lowering resistance to disease.

Suggestions for the Dieter

Tables 26–3 and 26–4 indicate representative diets for 1000 calories a day. For extra calories, snacks may be taken between meals, or sugar and cream may be added to coffee.

Fats. Use skim or powdered milk. These are fat-free. Avoid fried foods, especially French fried. Boil or poach eggs, and eat them on unbuttered toast. Select lean meats and fish, or trim the fat from your meat.

Use vinegar or lemon juice instead of mayonnaise or other fattening salad dressings. If you make "no-calorie" salad dressings from mineral oil, take vitamin pills, because mineral oil slows the absorption of vitamins.

Sweets. Saccharin or other artificial sweeteners, such as Sucaryl, can be used

Table 26–3. 1000 calorie menu A

Breakfast	
Orange juice (1/2 cup)	85
Soft boiled egg	75
Toast, 1 slice	75
Butter (1 tsp.)	30
Coffee	0
with cream (1 tsp.)	30
	295
Luncheon	
Consommé (1 cup)	25
1 Lamb chop	130
Broccoli (1 large stalk)	40
Carrots (1/2 cup)	25
Pineapple slice	50
Coffee or tea	0
with cream	30
	300
Supper	
Crabmeat (3 oz.)	90
Green peas (1/2 cup)	55
Cole slaw	15
with vinegar	0
Apple	75
1 Cookie	75
Skim milk	90
	400
TOTAL	995

Table 26–4. 1000 calorie menu B

Breakfast	
Grapefruit, 1/2	70
Poached egg	75
Hard roll	95
Butter (1 tsp. or half a pat)	30
Skim milk	90
	360
Luncheon	
Bouillon	25
Beef tongue (3 thin slices)	160
Asparagus (6-7 stalks)	20
Summer squash (1/2 cup)	15
Canned peaches (2 halves)	100
Coffee	0
with skim milk	10
	330
Supper	
Clear tomato soup (3/4 cup)	75
Slice of chicken	100
Green beans (1 cup)	30
Eggplant (4 slices)	50
Cantaloupe, 1/2	50
Tea with lemon	0
	305
TOTAL	995

in coffee or tea instead of sugar, as well as in cooking. These are not drugs or medicines, and have no danger in the small amounts you are likely to use.

Take small portions of desserts, or skip desserts entirely. Avoid cookies, candies, and soft drinks, except the ones that contain no-calorie sweeteners.

Starches. Don't fill up on bread and butter. In fact, as far as possible, avoid breads, rolls, cakes, and cookies. Substitute leafy green vegetables and fruits for the bulk you were accustomed to getting from starchy foods.

Snacks. Limit snacks to very low-calorie foods. Take the edge off your appetite with unsweetened tea or coffee, or with clear consommés.

Breakfast. A *high-protein* meal in the morning usually keeps people from being hungry in the midmorning and from eating too much at noon.

Alcoholic Beverages. These are high in calories, and don't satisfy your hunger except when taken in excess. Usually they make you forget you are on a diet.

Nibbling. Nibbling between meals helps some people diet by decreasing their appetite at mealtime. If you try this, keep careful count of calories so you'll know whether or not it is really helping you.

Eating Binges. Just as some people can take a drink without becoming alcoholics, so some dieters are able to go off their diets occasionally without ill effect. Their morale may even benefit from knowing they can do this every month, which is better than constant cheating. But remember, your appestat is probably easily conditioned, or you wouldn't be dieting in the first place, so be very careful.

Table 26–5. Caloric content of various alcoholic beverages.

Alcoholic Beverages		*Calories*
Beer	8 oz. glass	120
Wine	1 wine glass	75
Gin	1 jigger	115
Rum	1 jigger	125
Whiskey	1 jigger	120
Brandy	1 brandy glass	80
Cocktail		150

Talking About Your Diet. This may make people shun you as a bore. Some people will try to get you to break your diet, while others will help you keep it. You have to know which kind you are with before you start discussing your diet. Sometimes it will save embarrassment for you to say that the doctor has told you not to eat certain foods. As a general rule, the best social technique is to avoid attracting attention to yourself and your problem. Simply eat very little of fattening foods that are placed before you.

Importance of Preventing Overweight. It is much easier to prevent overweight than to correct it, easier to lose a few pounds than to readjust the appestat after years of indulgence!

The Bonus You Get from a Proper Diet. Every pound of fat you store ties up about 0.17 pounds of water. When you lose 10 pounds of fat, you will actually lose 11.7 pounds of weight, counting the water that is associated with the fat. If you work off 50 pounds of weight, your bonus will amount to nearly 10 pounds.

UNDERWEIGHT IS NOT DESIRABLE EITHER

Chronic underweight or a sudden loss of weight is not compatible with good health, and may increase susceptibility to illness. It may also indicate the onset or presence of a disease, such as diabetes, an overactive thyroid gland, intestinal worms (especially in children), and many other diseases. Even tuberculosis may be the cause, although contrary to popular opinion, it does not always produce loss of weight.

How to Tell if You Are Underweight

If you are 10 to 15 pounds below the figures in the weight tables, if the bones stick out all over your body, and the muscles don't cover the back, thighs, and buttocks with resilient protection, if your face is thin and drawn, you are very likely underweight. But the figures in this table can't always answer your

Table 26–6. 3500 calorie menu C

Breakfast	
1 Banana sliced	100
with cream (1/2 cup)	120
2 Griddle cakes	200
with sirup and	50
butter (1 tbsp.)	100
2 Sausages	350
Black coffee	0
	920
Luncheon	
Cup of cream of potato soup	250
Macaroni and cheese (1 cup)	300
Apple and nut salad	150
Pie a la mode	400
Cocoa	210
	1310
Dinner	
Fruit cocktail	90
Duck (4 oz.)	350
with gravy	20
Baked potato	90
with butter	100
Green peas	55
Avocado pear salad	250
with mayonnaise	100
Chocolate pudding	200
Tea or coffee	0
	1255
DAILY TOTAL 3485	

Table 26–7. 3500 calorie menu D

Breakfast	
Dry cereal	100
with cream and sugar and	140
1/2 banana, sliced	50
Toast	75
with butter (1 tbsp.) and	100
jelly	100
Coffee or tea	0
with 1 tsp. sugar and	20
2 tbsp. cream	60
	645
Luncheon	
Cup of cream of tomato soup	250
3 Saltines	45
Ham and cheese sandwich	350
2 Celery stalks	15
filled with mayonnaise	100
Milk (half cream) or cocoa	210
Chocolate layer cake	400
	1370
Dinner	
Pineapple juice (4 oz. glass)	55
1 Pork chop or veal chop	235
with gravy	20
Mashed potatoes (1 potato)	100
Creamed broccoli	140
Bread and butter	100
Sweetened applesauce (1/2 cup)	100
Ice cream sundae or lemon meringue pie	335
Milk (8 oz. glass)	170
	1255
Bedtime	
Eggnog	230
DAILY TOTAL 3500	

question, and consultation with a doctor may be necessary. Perfectly healthy individuals with small skeletal framework may appear to be underweight.

If extreme thinness is not due to ill health, it is due to a failure to eat enough of the right food, because of carelessness, ignorance, the desire to be stylishly thin, or a psychological resistance to eating. Most of these factors are readily corrected. But a deep-seated resistance to food, based on some emotional problem, requires medical advice.

How to Gain Weight

Substitution of High-Calorie for Low-Calorie Foods. Concentrate on fattening foods, such as cream soups, chowders, mayonnaise, cereals with heavy cream, sauces made with butter or margarine or thickened with flour, and desserts to which hard sauce or whipped cream has been added. Substitute high-calorie vegetables like peas, potatoes, and lima beans for bulky low-calorie ones.

Use more butter and margarine on your bread, and add extra butter to vegetables and soups. Add cream to your milk. Tables 26–6 and 26–7 show representative high-calorie diets.

Eat More. Try to eat extra bread and butter with your meals, and take second helpings.

Treat Yourself to Snacks. These can include rich cocoa and eggnogs.

Sweets. These are concentrated sources of energy. Unfortunately, candy and other carbohydrate foods, such as jellies, pastry, cake, and ice cream, present a rather ticklish problem. They are essentially "empty calories," because they provide energy and potential fat, but lack valuable proteins, minerals, and vitamins. Also, they may accelerate tooth decay.

Smoking. This may dull the appetite. If you want to gain weight, avoid cigarettes just before meals and at mealtime, and if possible, cut down on the number of cigarettes you smoke or stop smoking entirely.

Alcoholic Beverages. These beverages, such as sherry, are often very relaxing and good appetite stimulants. However, alcohol should not be substituted for food.

Questions

1. Discuss the dangers of obesity.
2. What are some low calorie vegetables? low calorie fruits?
3. How can emotional factors influence one's appetite?
4. Are reducing drugs necessary in weight reduction?
5. How can exercise cause loss of weight? Define the "appestat."
6. Indicate two major objections to fad diets.
7. Show how you must alter your consumption of the following three types of foods to lose weight: fats, sweets and starches.
8. During dieting to lose weight, why is a high-protein breakfast especially important?
9. How many calories do you have to skip to lose 1 pound of weight? What "bonus" do you get when you lose a pound of fat?
10. How would you alter a diet to *gain* weight?
11. Why is smoking undesirable for someone who is underweight?
12. What kind of between-meal snacks should you eat or drink to gain weight?

Reading Suggestions

Reduce and Stay Reduced, Norman Jolliffe. Simon & Schuster, New York, 1952. An excellent, very complete book by an authority in nutrition.

Body Fat, Vincent P. Dole. Scientific American, December 1959, pp. 71–76.

A New Concept in the Treatment of Obesity, Edgar S. Gordon, Marshall Goldberg, and Grace Chasy. Journal of the American Medical Association, October 1963, p. 50. A report of recent research related to the treatment of obesity.

Calories Can Kill, Thomas C. Desmond. Today's Health, January 1961, p. 50. The health hazards of obesity are discussed.

The Great Balancing Act: Eating Versus Activity, Martha F. Trulson and Fredrick J. Stare. Today's Health, June 1963, p. 35. A well written account of "food habits" versus "activity patterns."

Mayo Clinic Diet Manual, Committee on Dietetics of the Mayo Clinic. W. B. Saunders Co., Philadelphia, 1961. A good source reference for planning the diet.

Nutrition and Physical Fitness, L. J. Bogert. 8th Ed., W. B. Saunders Co., Philadelphia, 1966. A good, basic textbook of nutrition. Excellent chapters on overweight and malnutrition.

Your Weight and How to Control It, Morris Fishbein. Doubleday & Co., Garden City, N. Y., 1963. An authoritative and comprehensive discussion of the problems of weight control.

The Strange Case of Calories Don't Count, R. W. Apple, Jr. Saturday Review, Nov. 24, 1963, p. 15. Critical comments on the book and its promotion.

The Overweight Society, Peter Wyden. William Morrow & Co., New York, 1965. An entertaining discussion about the facts and fallacies of weight control. Provides insights into an important problem.

Diets are for People, Caroline W. Shearman. Appleton-Century-Crofts, New York, 1963. A well written text on diet therapy by a dietitian.

Diet is Not Enough, Irving B. Perstein and William Cole. Macmillan, New York, 1963. A highly readable account of weight control by a physician. Discussed are such factors as motivation, habits, diet, appetite, exercise, drugs, and many others.

Overweight: A Problem for Millions, Michael H. K. Irwin. Public Affairs Pamphlets, New York, 1964 (paperback). About causes, effects, and treatment of overeating.

The Overweight Society: An Authoritative, Entertaining Investigation into Facts and Follies of Girth Control, Peter Wyden. Morrow, New York, 1965. An objective analysis of various programs of dieting and exercise, including fads and rackets.

27

CARE AND BEAUTY OF THE SKIN AND HAIR

You never see a man bald-headed on his chin. But his hair! It is a graceful ornament, it is a comfort, it is the best of all protections against certain perilous ailments, man prizes it above emeralds and rubies. And because of these things Nature puts it on, half of the time, so that it won't stay.

MARK TWAIN
Letters from the Earth

It takes time for people to get to know the "real you," and their first impressions usually come from your external appearance—your skin, hair and general grooming. Also, it helps your own morale to have clear, clean skin and attractive hair.

THE SKIN

Normal skin can be kept clean with nothing more than good soap and water, but the soap should be thoroughly rinsed off, and the skin well dried. Germicidal soaps and antiseptics are rarely necessary and they can be irritating. Besides, healthy skin has its own natural protection against bacteria that land on it. Cuts and abrasions, however, may require special care against infection.

Excessive perspiration may be due to poor health. Night sweats, for example, are characteristic of certain diseases. However, if you are in good health, but perspire excessively, especially under the arms, you can probably control it by a commercial antiperspirant deodorant. Most of these preparations contain aluminum chloride, which is usually perfectly safe, unless you happen to be allergic or sensitive to this chemical. However, the newer stick deodorants frequently contain a compound called sodium zirconium lactate, which has produced benign skin growths in some individuals.

It is always wise to try any new preparation cautiously, using very little at first, and stopping if repeated applications cause irritation.

Chlorophyll preparations are deodorants, but they do not check perspiration. They are no more effective than plain bicarbonate of soda (baking soda) used as a powder.

It does no harm to check perspiration in the armpits, the hands, or the feet, but don't take the scare propaganda about "B.O." too seriously.

The medical name for offensive body odor is *bromidrosis*. Truly offensive body odor is rare, and can usually be prevented by bathing with ordinary soap and using a deodorant under the arms.

Dry skin is the result of insufficient fat production by the sebaceous glands of the skin. It often occurs in middle and old age, and encourages wrinkling. If your skin is dry, don't wash it too often with soap and water. Instead, use a cleansing cream or soap substitute, and apply a lubricating cream before going to bed.

Dry skin is apt to *chap* during cold weather or when the air is very dry. A commercial lotion or hand cream will help prevent this by providing extra oils.

Chafing is caused by friction, usually from clothing or body surfaces that are damp with perspiration. Keeping the skin dry and using a plain talcum powder will clear up the irritation.

Prickly heat occurs when the skin is damp and overheated. The best treatment is to keep the skin cool, and use a light powder.

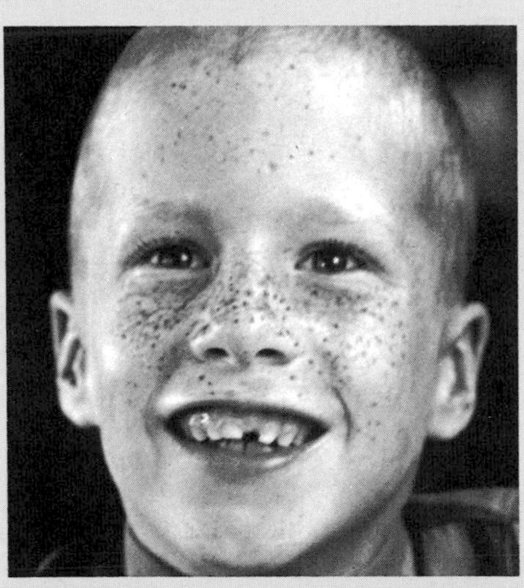

Children with freckles should never be made to feel self-conscious of them. Many people have freckles and those without them seldom consider them unusual, if they even notice them at all.

Frostbite is due to extreme cold and usually attacks the nose, ears, fingers, or toes. The cold part should be warmed very gradually. Rubbing on snow, or massaging the frostbitten area can damage the skin. If the frostbite is severe, a physician should be called, because gangrene can result unless treatment is started in time.

Oily skin can be more distressing than dry skin. To correct it, use plenty of soap and water, and avoid creams and greasy lotions. Go easy on heavy powder or pancake make-up, always washing it off thoroughly at night.

The less *pigment* the skin contains, the lighter its color will be. Those rare people who have no pigment at all are called *albinos*. If your skin produces little pigment, you should guard against sunburn.

White areas that appear on the skin *(vitiligo)* are usually due to a loss of pigment in those spots. If they are conspicuous, the best thing to do is to cover them or avoid getting tanned (which makes them more conspicuous).

Freckles are simply highly pigmented spots. If you are a freckler and have to spend a good deal of time in the sun, expose your skin as little as possible. A heavy suntan lotion or face powder will also help. Avoid "freckle removers." Anything that is strong enough to be effective may cause a severe inflammation. Usually, the best thing to do about freckles is to cover them with face powder or, if necessary, a preparation like *Covermark*. Individuals who are sensitive about disfiguring freckles should consult a dermatologist. Freckles do tend to become less conspicuous after adolescence, but they seldom disappear entirely.

Sunburn

Sunshine is healthful for most people, and usually makes them look and feel better. However, you can easily get too much of a good thing!

No matter how anxious you are to get a

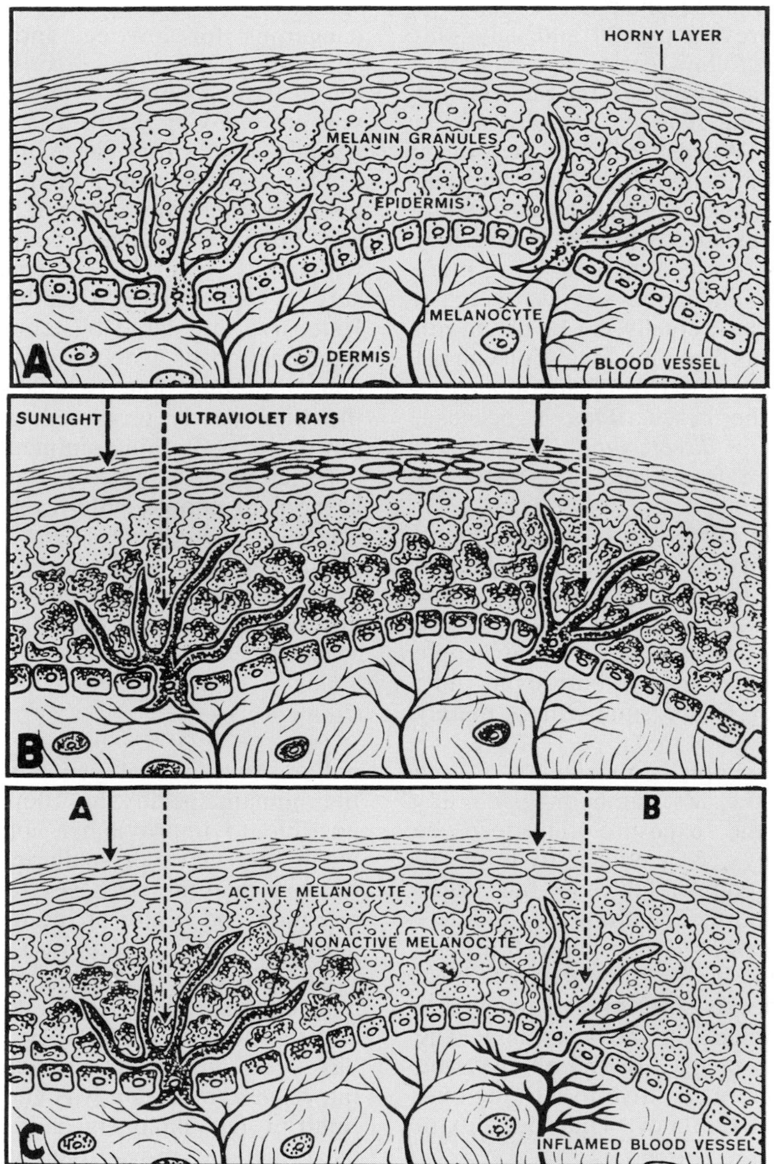

Figure 27–1. **A,** Ordinary skin, not exposed to sun, contains special cells (melanocytes) in the lower epidermis, which continually produce small amounts of melanin pigment. This gives a white skin a pale brown cast while blood vessels add a pinkish cast, creating the color of the skin. Negroes produce much melanin, albinos none. **B,** Suntanned skin under strong sunlight shields itself from burn by producing dark pigment evenly throughout the epidermis. The sun's ultraviolet rays stimulate the melanocytes to convert a chemical that they contain into large amounts of melanin pigment, which is then spread through the skin. **C,** Freckled skin is result of nonactive melanocytes. The melanocyte at the left in the diagram reacts normally to ultraviolet rays and produces melanin granules to form a freckle. Another melanocyte *(right)* does not react to the rays. The skin around it is burned by ultraviolet rays, which dilate blood vessels and redden the skin. (From: Freckles: why do they come? Life, Aug. 25, 1958, pp. 49–50.)

good tan, don't try to get it all the first day. Give your skin time to produce enough of its melanin pigment to absorb the ultraviolet rays of the sun, and protect you.

You can prevent painful and ugly sunburn if you follow certain precautions:

Learn When and Where the Sun Has the Greatest Burning Power. Beware of the noonday sun. When the sun is high overhead its rays are short, direct and burning. Late afternoon is a safer time to start sunbathing, because when the sun goes down, its rays are long and burn more slowly. Even when the sky is overcast, the sun can burn cruelly, so be as careful on hazy days as on bright ones. You can get sunburned on snowcovered mountains as well as at the beach. This is because, *in addition to direct sunlight,* there is *reflected glare* from sand and water, or snow and ice.

Know Your Own Skin. Skins differ in their sensitivity to sunlight. Babies and children burn more quickly than do adults. People with fair skins are more sensitive to sun than brunettes are. Some people never develop a tan, and burn every time they stay out in the sun. Others merely freckle.

For most people, *15 minutes is long enough* for the first sunbath. Each day after that, the exposure time can be lengthened by 15 minutes. Five or 10 minutes are enough for very fair skins. Start with short sunbaths and gradually make them longer to give yourself a good protective tan. If you know that you burn quickly, start exposing yourself to the sun after four o'clock in the afternoon. The face, the skin in front of the elbows, and the legs are more sensitive to burning than other parts of the body. They need extra protection.

Use a Suntan Preparation. Suntan preparations help guard your skin against burning, but even the best ones give only partial protection; so don't fail to watch the clock just because you're using one of them.

Drink Plenty of Water When You Are Suntanning. You will need it to make up for the fluid you lose, even though you may not realize that you are perspiring on a dry, sunny day. *Take extra salt* such as salty crackers or tomato juice with salt in it to compensate for the salt you lose in perspiration.

Getting overheated in the hot sun is dangerous for anyone, and may put a strain on the internal organs, particularly the heart and blood vessels. The fact that you are enjoying yourself is no protection against *heat stroke* or *heat prostration.*

You may be called upon sometime to help a person who has been burned by the sun. Sunburn can make people very sick, with chills, fever, and even delirium. Be sure to call a doctor if the burn is severe. Extensive and large blisters always need the attention of a doctor because there is danger of infection. In mild cases where the skin merely turns red, use a dusting powder or a soothing ointment.

Excessive sunshine is almost certainly harmful to people suffering from diseases such as *tuberculosis of the lungs* (which often becomes worse after injudicious exposure to the sun), *nephritis* and skin diseases like *lupus erythematosus.*

Cosmetics

For thousands of years, the female of the human species has done everything possible to improve her appearance and make herself more alluring—with one primary natural purpose—to attract the attention and desire of the male. The first authentic records, found on papyri in the tombs of ancient Egypt, refer to such cosmetic materials as the fat of the cat and the hoof of the donkey. An alabaster vase containing an ointment of animal fat, resin and balsam was unearthed in the tomb of Tutankhamen, and the Egyptians used metallic ores—green copper oxide, red iron oxide, carbon black, cinnabar and lead ore—to adorn their eyes, cheeks and lips. Some of the famed beauty of Cleopatra must be attributed to these metallic compounds, and to the henna with which she dyed her hair and colored her palms and soles.

The Bible details the recipe for the anointing oil which the infamous Jezebel used along with paints for her face and eyes, and the Babylonians and Greeks enlarged on the number of cosmetics available to alluring females. Hair dyeing, spices and perfumes were very popular with the Romans, who also developed creams to heal blemishes, remove wrinkles and soften the skin.

During the Renaissance, Italy was the center of cosmetic use, but later such preparations were widespread throughout Europe. Some revolt against excesses finally set in. A bill was introduced into the English Parliament in the eighteenth century to restrain women "from beguiling men into matrimony by the use of scents, paints, cosmetics, washes, false hair, false teeth, Spanish wool, iron stays, hoops, high-heeled shoes, and bolstered hips; and making such marriages null and void; and the penalty the same as for witch-craft."

Because our Federal Food and Drug Administration is extremely vigilant, most cosmetics on the market today are safe to use. Lipstick, powder, and rouge are usually harmless unless you happen to be allergic or sensitive to them (often to the perfume they contain).

There is usually no important difference, aside from the appearance, odor and packaging, between expensive and inexpensive cosmetics.

The Food and Drug Administration can protect you from harmful ingredients in cosmetics, but even the Federal Trade Commission cannot always control the false and exaggerated advertising claims of many cosmetic manufacturers. Expensive hormone creams hold out the promise of eternal youth to the dissatisfied middle-aged female, yet they are generally useless. Hormones are medicines. If the commercial hormone creams contained enough hormone to have any effect, they should be dispensed by a physician, not a cosmetician.

Currently, an expensive skin ointment containing a special royal jelly obtained from bees is being sold, with luxurious packaging and glamorous advertising. An expert from the American Medical Association, on being asked about the skin-feeding benefits of this royal jelly answered, "The so-called royal jelly contains protein and sugar principally, and a small amount of sulfur. *This may be of unusual value to a bee, but people can get all of it they need in an adequate daily diet.*" And at a much smaller price.

The American public spends millions of dollars annually in its search for a much publicized beauty ideal. Yet health and cleanliness can usually do more for your appearance than can any cosmetic.

The Skin and the Emotions

The skin is one of the many organs closely linked to the emotions, and just as it may mirror general health, it can also mirror your emotional state. We blush, and we "break out in a cold sweat." Under the stress of unusual emotion, some individuals develop cold white fingers, others, giant hives, and still others manifest so-called "neurodermatoses"–dermatitis of nervous or emotional origin.

It is sometimes very difficult to discover whether emotional factors are responsible for a skin condition, although some cases are fairly obvious. Perhaps you have known someone who gets a rash on the neck when he is embarrassed or angry.

Eczema is a common and troublesome but *not* contagious skin disease of an allergic nature. There are indications that emotional factors may also play a part in both eczema and psoriasis, another chronic skin disease. Unfortunately, neither of these stubborn conditions can be cured as miraculously as claimed by patented or advertised remedies.

Allergies and Sensitivity

In past years, many unfortunate individuals suffered from rashes and other troublesome skin complaints that refused to yield to treatment. Today we know that some of these are due to an allergy (see p. 189).

Itching caused by allergic reactions can be relieved by applications of calamine lotion or by putting one cupful of bicarbonate of soda (baking soda) in the bath water. Of course the best thing to do is to avoid the substance that causes the reaction. Sometimes this is easy. Many of us have been able to discover, by ourselves, that we get hives or "break out" after eating strawberries, taking a certain medicine, putting away winter clothes in moth balls, using a perfumed soap, wearing certain materials, or touching poison ivy. However, in a great many cases physicians with special training in these fields (*dermatologists* and *allergists*) have to do considerable detective work to discover whether the condition is due to an allergy, and if so, what is responsible.

Common Skin Troubles

You have noticed that all skins are definitely not alike. For example, the number of lubricating and sweat glands and the amount of pigment may vary considerably from one individual to another.

Acne is probably the cause of more heartaches and embarrassment than any other skin condition. It affects almost 90 per cent of young people of both sexes at an insecure period of life when they are working hard to establish themselves socially, scholastically and economically. Fortunately, *acne vulgaris,* the proper medical name for what you probably call pimples, whiteheads, or blackheads, is a self-limiting disease. In most cases, the shower of lesions begins and ends in the decade of life between 13 and 23.

By various techniques, modern medicine can usually prevent serious disfigurement, as well as scarring of the body and the soul.

Acne is so characteristic of youth that you often wonder who coined the slogan "Keep that schoolgirl complexion."

As boys and girls approach maturity, their glandular activity, including that of the sebaceous glands of the skin, increases. In girls this may become pronounced at the time of their menstrual periods. It is interesting that two physicians reported they could produce acne at will simply by injecting young women patients with the hormone *progesterone.* This correlates with the aggravation of acne many women suffer during the premenstrual phase when progesterone levels are high.

Certain foods also increase the activity of the sebaceous glands, the worst offenders being chocolate, nuts, sharp cheeses,

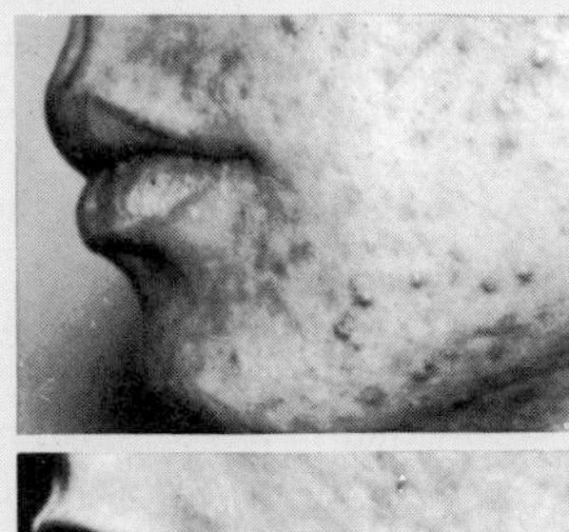

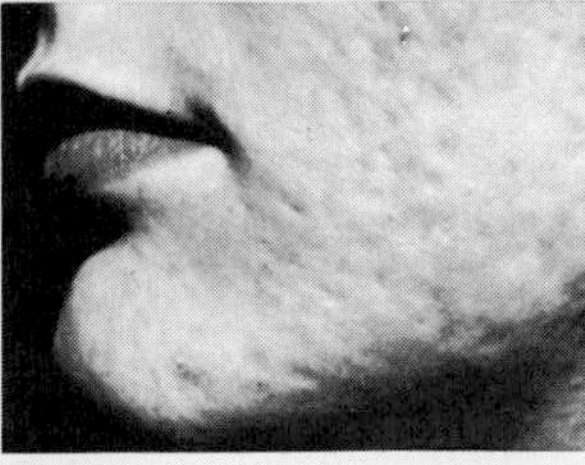

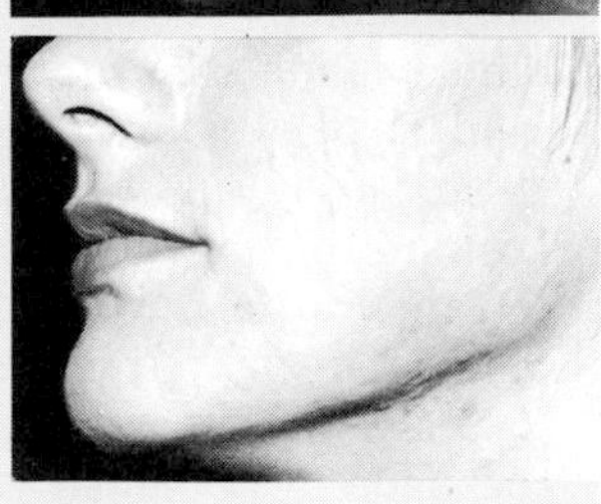

Acne: The first sign of acne is the eruption of pustules and blackheads (top). If acne is neglected, scars may remain after the condition ends; usually, they are in the form of pits (middle). Sometimes this may be remedied by surgical means. The bottom photograph shows the result of proper surgical treatment.

and greasy, fried foods. If the pore opening is small or clogged by dirt or heavy cosmetics, the fatty material released by the sebaceous gland accumulates, and a "bump" appears under the skin—a *whitehead* or a *blackhead* (a *comedo*).

Blackheads are not due to dirt, but to the discoloring effect of air on the fatty material in the clogged pore. If this substance becomes infected, as it often does, a pimple results. The temptation to squeeze the unsightly pimple should be resisted. A hard push, and the membrane around the pimple is broken, permitting the infection to spread to the surrounding tissue. It also spreads on the surface unless it is carefully washed off. The result—more pimples and scar tissue or pits.

If you suffer from acne, try to discover and eliminate any food you feel encourages it. *Don't* arbitrarily cut out all desserts and fats. Just go easy on rich, greasy foods and chocolate—and search for others you should avoid entirely because they irritate *your* skin.

Keep the skin very clean, particularly

the areas where acne is most apt to appear—the face, chest, and back. Plain soap and fairly hot water are best. Scrub with a *clean* washcloth, but not so hard you hurt the skin, and follow by a cold rinse. Change towels at least daily.

Avoid all creams and greasy lotions. Don't plug the pores with heavy make-up or "pore-closing" beauty aids.

If you have pimples, don't squeeze them. Apply a compress soaked with hot water. This will encourage drainage and healing.

The offending spots can be hidden with certain medicated preparations, such as *Acnomel cake,* which also help heal the pimples.

To get rid of blackheads, soak in warm, soapy water to loosen them, and press gently with a *comedo extractor* (which can be purchased at most drug stores). *Don't use your fingers.* If the blackhead comes out easily, touch the spot with rubbing alcohol. If it doesn't come out, leave it alone for awhile.

Severe cases of acne require more complicated treatment, which only a doctor can provide. Unsightly acne has been reported improved or overcome by washing the face with a dry, abrasive paste containing particles of granites, porcelains, or silicates. This dries and scales the skin, opening up oil follicles so that blackheads and pimples disappear. The action is something like the beneficial effects from long exposure to sunlight.

The antibiotic *tetracycline* has been used with considerable success in the treatment of acne, but this should be taken only under a physician's care.

Even if acne has scarred your face, medical science can help you. *Planing* with a high-speed rotary brush is the answer. This removes the outer layer of pitted skin, leaving the portion which contains the glands and hair follicles. New skin, rosy at first and then fading to a normal color, grows in from the bottom up. This technique has also been used successfully in removing some types of birthmarks and disfigurations due to accidents. The so-called *"sandpaper surgery"* for acne scars is not recommended by most dermatologists.

Because of its exposed position, the skin can be infected by microorganisms, including bacteria, such as those causing *boils* or *impetigo*; viruses which cause *fever blisters*; parasites which are responsible for *scabies*; fungi which cause such diseases as *athlete's foot*; and the spirochete germ of syphilis, which causes *syphilitic lesions.*

Athlete's foot (dermatophytosis) is caused by a fungus, a tiny form of plant life. This organism grows on the dead cells that make up the calluses and "old

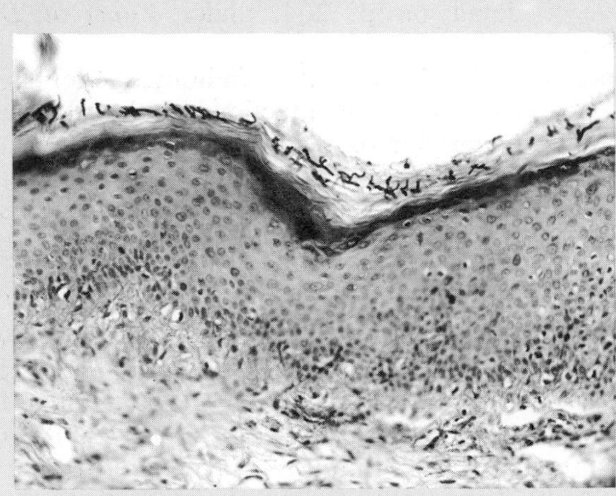

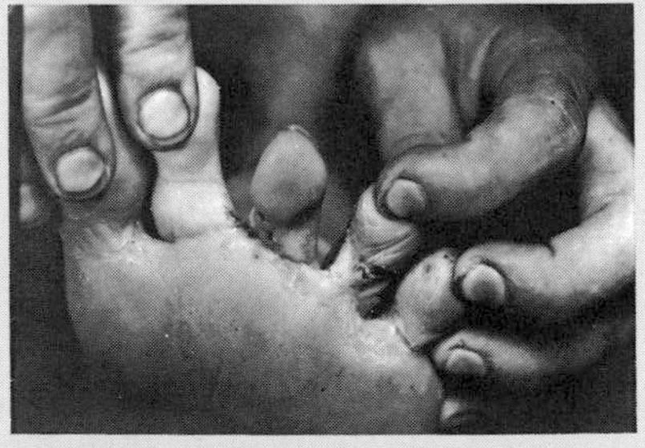

Athlete's foot usually attacks first between the toes (above). It is caused by a fungus which grows beneath the skin. On the left, a microphotograph of a cross section of the skin shows the fungus growing.

skin" of the feet, and thrives on warmth and dampness. It causes itching or burning spots, and often blisters, usually between the toes.

There are safe ointments available today which can cure athlete's foot, but it may recur again and again, on re-exposure to the fungus. Keeping your feet clean and thoroughly dried, and dusting carefully between the toes with talcum powders will discourage this infection.

Boils and *carbuncles* are caused by pus-forming bacteria. These germs are usually present on the skin, but do no damage unless the skin's resistance has been lowered by cuts, irritating friction, poor health, bad nutrition, or diabetes. A carbuncle is more serious than a boil because it is larger, goes deeper, and is accompanied by a general feeling of illness.

Boils and carbuncles respond readily to treatment. A physician can incise and open them, if necessary, or use the proper antibiotic. Boils on the upper lip or nose should be treated by a doctor. But if you have a small boil which is *not* on the nose or upper lip, it is usually safe to try the following:

Wash the boil and the surrounding area with soap and warm water, several times a day, lightly dabbing on 70 per cent alcohol afterward. Cover, not too tightly, with an antiseptic gauze pad to prevent irritation.

Apply hot compresses—as warm as you can stand—every hour, for 10 minutes at a time. Make these compresses by soaking an antiseptic gauze pad in hot water containing as much salt as will dissolve. This helps relieve pain and encourages the boil to drain. Cover with a fresh, dry pad.

If the boil doesn't get better within a few days, see a doctor. *Do not* open a boil yourself or let an amateur surgeon friend do it.

Impetigo is also caused by bacteria, and is quite *contagious,* especially in infants. Typical yellow crusts form, often on the face, that look as though they had been applied to the skin. Impetigo should be properly treated before other infections set in.

Folliculitis is similar to impetigo, except that the infection occurs in the hair follicles or the pore openings of the skin. *Barber's itch* is a special case of folliculitis which affects the beard and makes shaving unpleasant. The medical name for barber's itch is *sycosis vulgaris.*

Fever blisters (herpes simplex) are caused by a virus. They usually occur with a fever or cold, and appear around the mouth and nose; or they can follow exposure to sun and wind. Usually they clear up within a week or so. Spirit of camphor and cold cream may bring relief. Troublesome, recurrent fever blisters should be seen by a doctor who can prescribe more specific medication.

Shingles (herpes zoster) is a very painful infection, also caused by a virus which infects part of a nerve, causing an eruption on the skin.

The itch (scabies) is extremely contagious, but fortunately it yields quickly to treatment. Hands, genitals, and folds in the skin are favorite areas for the tiny itch mite to burrow. However, almost any part of the body may be affected.

Other parasites include *lice* and *"crabs"* (pubic lice), both of which can be eliminated by powders or sprays containing certain very effective chemicals.

Syphilis may be the cause of any sore which appears on the genital regions between three days to three months after sexual intercourse with an infected person. It commonly manifests itself again about six weeks later in the form of a rash resembling measles, accompanied by symptoms somewhat like those of a cold. Syphilis does *not* cause pimples and itching. (Syphilis is described in greater detail on p. 204, under *Venereal Diseases.*)

Erysipelas (St. Anthony's fire) is a streptococcus infection of the skin and underlying tissues.

Glanders, anthrax, and tularemia are serious ailments contracted from animals suffering from these diseases. Skin lesions can be important symptoms.

Rashes can be caused by a number of contagious diseases such as *smallpox, meningitis, measles,* and many of the common diseases of childhood. *Any rash or abnormal skin condition accompanied by a fever or a general feeling of illness is a danger signal.* If there is no fever, the rash may be due to an *allergy* or to a toxic reaction to some chemical.

Never Neglect a Skin Disease

There are literally hundreds of skin ailments. It is important to remember that a skin condition can indicate the presence of a deep-seated disease of the lungs, liver, heart, and many other organs of the body, including the *endocrine glands.* It can also reflect a *vitamin deficiency.*

Always consult a doctor if anything unusual happens to your skin.

Corns, Birthmarks and Warts

Corns and *calluses* are caused by pressure, and may occasionally appear in places other than the feet. They can cause a great deal of suffering, and the best way to avoid them is by wearing shoes that fit. Corns are of two varieties: *hard corns,* usually found on the outside of the little toe; and *soft corns,* between the toes. They are hardened or thickened skin which, unlike a callus, have a central point or core.

Soft corns and calluses can often be removed by paring them off carefully. Hard corns may require expert attention.

Birthmarks include pigmented moles and the vascular birthmarks, such as "strawberry marks." If they are disfiguring, they can be concealed with a cosmetic cream, like *Covermark,* or removed by a surgical operation or electric needle treatment. Most moles are harmless, but any mole that starts to grow or bleed should be seen by a physician.

Warts are caused by a virus. *Plantar* warts on the bottom of the toes or the soles of the feet are very common after adolescence. If they are in a prominent place, or are unusually painful, consult your physician, who can clear them up.

THE NAILS

The nails, like the hair, are really extensions of the skin, and are very closely related chemically. All three tissues contain the same tough, resistant protein—*keratin.*

In general, your nails need little care. In fact, most infections such as *abscesses, whitlows, paronychias,* or *"runarounds"* are usually caused by too much manicuring of the cuticle. Push it back gently. Don't use a sharp instrument for this or for cleaning nails. Dryness encourages hangnails, and oil or a handcream will help correct this tendency. A hangnail will heal over in a few days if protected by a Band-Aid.

Any nail polish is safe provided it does not cause irritation. Always try out a new one on a single nail at bedtime and make certain it is safe to use on your other fingers in the morning. A plastic cosmetic, recently placed on the market, a "press-on" type of nail polish, has been found dangerous and is no longer being sold. In the first six months of its sale, more than 700 women reported to the Food and Drug Administration and the manufacturer that their nails had been damaged in varying degrees.

Nails which are brittle and break off very easily seem to improve considerably if gelatin is added to the diet.

HAIR AND SCALP

Like the skin and nails, the hair too can reflect the condition of our health. For example, an underactive thyroid gland makes the hair dry and coarse. Hair is actually an outgrowth of the epidermis, but differs somewhat chemically. It is more highly *keratinized* than either skin or nails, and more deeply *pigmented,* except in the Negro.

Care of the Hair

Keep your hair clean. Wash it at least every 10 days, more often if it tends to be oily. Washing removes the natural oil in your hair, along with the dirt, and *no* shampoo actually lives up to its claim that it restores these oils. For oily hair, a tincture of green soap is satisfactory. For dry hair, a castile shampoo is good. Don't forget to wash your comb and brush at least as often as you do your hair.

Rinse your hair carefully after washing. If you use hard water, the soap is apt to leave a deposit on your hair. Soapless

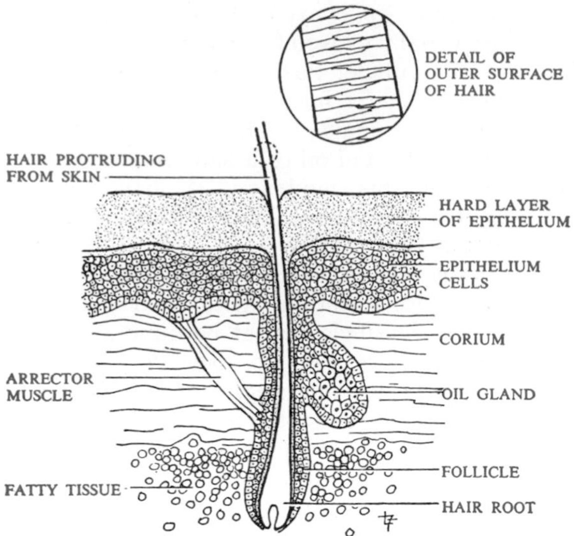

Figure 27–2. Hair and follicle.

detergent shampoos do not leave a film, but they may make hair excessively dry.

Don't rub your hair too hard while drying it. Sunlight or a hairdryer that blows air on the hair is good. So are massage and brushing the hair gently as it dries. The 100 daily strokes with a hair brush which our grandparents used to swear by is excellent for the hair, making it sleek and glossy, and stimulating the sebaceous glands that supply the natural oil.

If your hair is dry, rub in a little pure olive oil or other oil after shampooing. (Lanolin has been very much overrated and won't work magic for your hair.) If your hair is oily, a little alcohol after shampooing, *quickly rubbed off,* will correct this condition. Brilliantines and similar pomades are usually made of mineral oil and keep the hair in place, but that is all they do. Sometimes these pomades are so heavy they clog the gland openings. Don't wet your hair repeatedly to keep it in place. Your hairbrush will do this better without drying your hair.

Singeing does *not* "seal up the ends of your hair nor keep in the oil, coloring and other vital fluids." Sunlight, although good for hair in moderation, will *not* make it grow. Nor do cutting and shaving increase its rate of growth. Keeping it clean and brushed is the best thing you can do for hair.

Dandruff

Dandruff is a very common and troublesome condition, in which the outer layer of the scalp peels off in little white scales. If the dandruff persists, these flakes eventually become larger, greasy, and yellowish. If they block the openings of the sebaceous glands, the hair becomes dry. More often, dandruff is associated with increased activity of these glands, the condition called *oily seborrhea,* and may produce greasy patches of the skin on the face, neck, and body.

A combination of factors is responsible for dandruff, including lowered resistance due to a generally poor physical condition or nervous tension, sometimes an infecting germ, and inadequate care of the hair. You can clear it up by improving the general care of your body and the food you eat. Keep your hair and scalp scrupulously clean by shampooing every few days, and keep your comb and brush even cleaner. A moderate amount of exposure to sunlight may be helpful.

Great care is needed to prevent reinfecting yourself with your comb or brush. Also, be sure than any beauty parlor or barber shop you patronize uses only sterilized combs and brushes, and observes good, sanitary methods.

Almost every type of dandruff, including

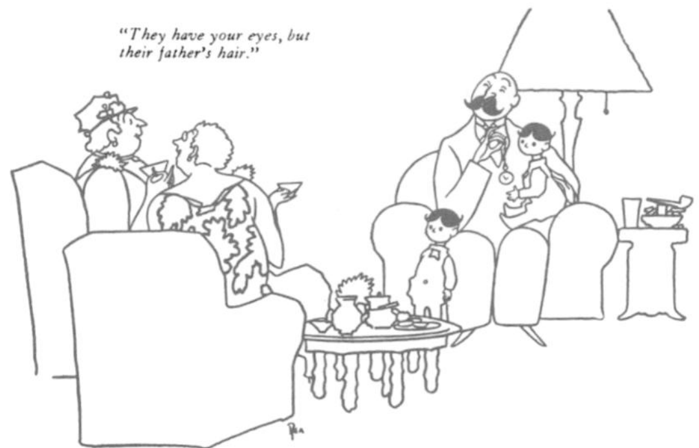

(Drawing by Rea. Copr. © 1931, The New Yorker Magazine, Inc.)

the most severe cases, *improve* when treated with Selsun, a preparation containing *selenium sulfide*. This has been approved by the Council on Pharmacy and Chemistry of the American Medical Association. Fostex is another useful preparation.

Ringworm

This is a fungus infection of the scalp which can be cured without too much difficulty after the fungus responsible for it is identified.

Shaving and Removal of Excess Hair

Until the current interest in beards, our civilization set great store on a smooth-shaven face. As a result, most men shave once, and many, twice daily. This represents a considerable abrasion of a fairly sensitive surface. Fortunately, the skin is well supplied with blood vessels and has enormous recuperative powers, so that cuts and scraped areas heal quickly. The following are good precautions to keep in mind:

Because infections can be carried from the hands to the face, scrub your nails and hands thoroughly before shaving.

Soaking the beard for several minutes with the cream or soap makes shaving quicker and easier.

Aftershave lotions or pure 70 per cent alcohol help keep your skin in good shape.

For infections: Use a new blade each time, and shave the noninfected portions of the face first. If the infection covers a fairly large area, consult a physician.

Hirsutism is the medical term for excessive facial or body hair. Unfortunately, it is unattractive and frequently very embarrassing for women. The time-honored remedies are bleaching with ordinary peroxide, shaving, or chemical depilatories.

Shaving does *not* encourage the growth of hair nor make it coarse. There are electric razors especially designed for women, but ordinary safety razors can also be used. Both are better and far easier to use than rubbing hair off with an abrasive such as pumice, and less painful than pulling hairs out with tweezers. If there aren't too many excess hairs, they can be cut off very short with cuticle scissors.

Most *chemical depilatories* on the market today are relatively safe. However, be careful about the use of a chemical depilatory on the face, and don't get it into your eyes. Always try it on a small spot of skin first to be sure it isn't irritating, and don't use it more often than once every two weeks, discontinuing immediately if the skin becomes inflamed or itches. Wax depilatories are painful, but safer.

No depilatory removes hair permanently. Permanent removal is difficult and tedious and requires an expert. Quacks or people who advertise miraculous methods for removing hair often substitute ugly scars and pits for excess hair.

Most endocrinologists believe that hirsutism is due to an imbalance in certain hormones of the adrenal cortex. A group of physicians from Temple University School of Medicine recently reported that small daily doses of the hormone *prednisone* could correct this imbalance. In most of their patients, excess hair grew at successively slower rates after prednisone therapy and it became sparser and finer with monthly depilations using wax applications. Within a few months, further hair removal was often unnecessary.

Baldness

The time and money women waste on useless "hormone" creams and other beauty aids can probably be matched by what men spend on "cures" for baldness. Unfortunately, there is *no cure for ordinary baldness*. The miraculous ones you read or hear about have nothing to do with normal baldness. In a condition called *alopecia areata,* the hair suddenly falls out, often in patches. In many cases, the hair will grow back again after the illness has subsided. If the sufferer has been using a "hair restorer," he may mistakenly sign testimonials crediting it with his new growth of hair.

Hair normally grows in "spells," a period of growth alternating with a rest period, and on the head the rate is usually about 3/4 inch a month. If it is not cut, it grows to about 25 inches, on an average. Hairs fall out and new ones grow from the same follicles.

Baldness can be caused by general ill health, infections of the scalp, nervous tension, and *temporarily* by a disease such as typhoid fever. However, in most cases, the ordinary baldness of men is due to the combination of sex, age, and inherited factors that result in what doctors call *male pattern alopecia.*

We do not fully understand all the factors that control this condition. We know that the tendency to become bald runs in certain families, and that some racial groups are more susceptible than others. It is often associated with aging, perhaps because the layer of fat between the scalp and the skull tends to disappear in men with advancing years and the hair follicles die. The male sex hormone also has something to do with it.

It is fairly safe to say that baldness results from internal and not external factors, that it cannot be blamed on cutting or not cutting the hair, on wearing a hat or not wearing a hat, on dandruff or other scalp disease, on washing or not washing the hair, or on any one of the large number of harmless things which are frequently implicated.

The distribution of hair in men is related to sexual maturation, and is apparently controlled by the hormone *testosterone.* Testosterone is responsible for secondary sexual characteristics such as the growth of pubic and chest hair.

Some men have very thick hair on their heads and chests, while others have relatively little. Eunuchs never become bald, because baldness is a *normal* sexual change. It is interesting that baldness has been described as a "tertiary sexual characteristic."

Eight out of 10 Americans over the age of 30 suffer from some degree of baldness and from stale jokes, such as

"Say, Joe, you know your
hair's getting thin?"
"So who likes fat hair?"

Irwin I. Lubove, a dermatologist of New York Medical College, feels that aside from old age, the chief reason for dying hair follicles—and baldness—is heredity. Your hairline will probably recede in pretty much the same pattern, at the same spot, and at about the same age as your father's. According to Dr. Lubove, there is no assurance of help from the various advertised salves and ointments because "no salve applied locally to the scalp can be absorbed by the follicles."

The chief hope of researchers in baldness at the present time is that as long as the follicle is hooked up to a healthy blood supply, there may be a chance of restoring the hair. A new and rather unusual experimental animal for baldness studies has just been found—a bald African starling, which loses its hair feathers, starting at the crown and leaving a meager fringe, in almost exactly the same pattern as baldness occurs in man. The androgens, or male hormones, are involved in some way in this bird's baldness, just as they are in man.

Ton Smits—Ben Roth Agency

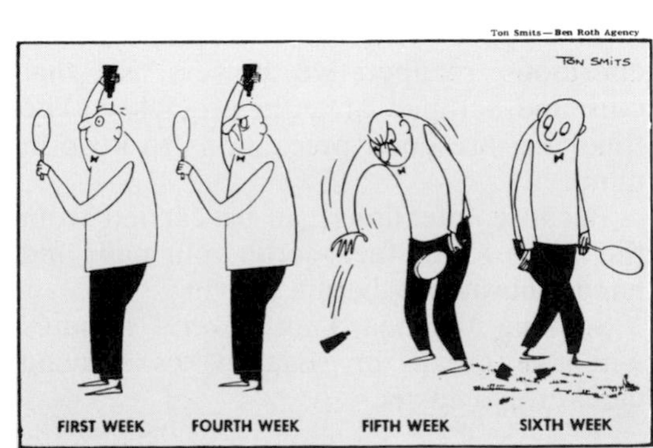

A promising development in the study of baldness was recently reported by Drs. C. M. Papa and A. M. Kligman. These researchers applied a solution of the male hormone testosterone to the scalps of 21 bald men and reported some hair regrowth in 16 of them. However, they emphasized that this is not a long-awaited cure for baldness. It does, nevertheless, open the door to further research.

Gray Hair

The *color* of hair is due to pigment, and *gray hair* develops when, for reasons not completely understood, air spaces form in the hair shaft, and pigmentation diminishes. This usually takes place in middle age, although it can occur prematurely. It does not, however, happen overnight, although illness has been known to cause rapid onset of grayness. Neither vitamins nor anything else so far developed will prevent graying, or permanently darken gray hair.

Bleaching Hair

Hair can be bleached by ordinary hydrogen peroxide to which a drop of ammonia has been added. Sodium perborate bleaches can be harmful, and all bleaching tends to alter the texture of hair, making it coarser and more porous, and usually very brittle. The new hairs and the new portions of hair around the roots will, of course, grow in with their original color.

Hair Dyes

Hair can be dyed or tinted, but no hair dye can confer a permanent, natural color. If you want to have your hair dyed, have a small lock tested first to find out whether you are sensitive to the dye.

The "rinses" and "tints" sold in reliable stores are usually harmless and satisfactory. Although they do not wash off if your hair gets wet, shampooing will remove them.

Never dye *eyelashes* or *eyebrows,* because the skin about them, and the eyes themselves, are extremely sensitive. A temporary darkener like mascara is relatively safe, but even that sometimes produces irritation.

Permanent Waves

Whether your hair is curly or straight depends on its structure. You can't change it *permanently,* because it will grow back in its original form. However, hair is pliable, and it can be stretched and curled, although too much heat will dry it. Kinky hair can be stretched and straightened.

How safe are *permanent waves?* The process depends upon the action of chemicals which make the hair more pliable, permitting it to take the shape of the curler, and a "neutralizing" chemical to make it hold its new shape. These chemicals probably do a *little* harm to the hair, but this isn't important because hair grows fairly rapidly under ordinary circumstances. However, too strong a solution of the chemical *can* injure the hair. Far more important is the fact that some people are allergic or sensitive to these chemicals. *Always* make a "test curl" first to be certain you will not suffer an allergic reaction.

Be careful to keep the waving lotion from the eyes and any cuts or sores, and to remove it promptly if it does touch any sensitive areas. Don't have permanents more often than essential. Bleached and dyed hair is particularly sensitive.

Home permanents contain much the same ingredients as those used in beauty parlors. However, the operators are less experienced! All these lotions are potentially dangerous so *read the directions carefully*. Be sure that your scalp is free of eruptions, and the skin of your hands intact and not chapped. The American Medical Association, although recognizing potential dangers, feels that home-permanent kits are safe for normal use.

Nonneutralizing home-permanent kits depend for their neutralizing action on the oxidation that normally occurs when the waving lotion is exposed to air as it dries. They are probably as safe as the ones with neutralizers, but they may not produce as long-lasting a wave.

Pony Tails

The innocent and attractive pony tails many girls wear are causing temporary female baldness. Many dermatologists have commented on bald patches in ponytail wearers, especially at the hair line near the ears. The damage is due to excessive pull on the hair, which is actually dragged out by the roots.

Questions

1. When would you use soap and water for cleansing the skin? a soapless detergent? a greasy cream?
2. How would you prevent and treat excessive perspiration? chafing? frostbite?
3. What is the difference between freckles and vitiligo?
4. What changes take place in the skin to prevent excessive burning by the sun's rays?
5. Why is it undesirable and uneconomical to get one's hormones from commercial skin creams?
6. Give some examples of skin responses to emotional reactions. Can you understand why some skin diseases are considered "psychosomatic" illnesses?
7. What is acne? When does it appear? How can you reduce its unsightliness?
8. What causes *boils? fever blisters? athlete's foot? scabies?*
9. What are birthmarks? How can they be made less disfiguring?
10. What chemical substance makes up skin, nails and hair?
11. What kind of shampoo would you select for dry hair? for oily hair?
12. How would you treat dandruff?
13. Do you think hirsutism in women means a woman is any less feminine or delicate? How can excess hair in women be safely concealed or removed?
14. What precautions should you take in *bleaching* hair? *dyeing* hair? using *home permanent waves?*

Topics for Discussion

Chemistry of cosmetics.
Albinism.
Neurodermatoses.

Reading Suggestions

What Can You Do About Skin Blemishes? E. T. Wilkes. Parents' Magazine, June 1958, p. 47. Good advice on how to treat or conceal birthmarks, moles and warts.

1001 Questions and Answers to Your Skin Problems, Sidney J. Robbins, et al. Harper & Row, New York, 1964. Medical experts answer common questions regarding acne, allergies, skin cancer, suntan, hair and scalp, syphilis, and miscellaneous other skin conditions. A highly sensible and informative book directed toward the layman.

The Medicine Show, 2nd Ed., Consumers Union, Mount Vernon, N. Y., 1963. An excellent discussion of sunburn, aging skin, deodorants, itches and rashes, and dandruff. Popular products are frankly evaluated.

The Wonderful Human Machine, The American Medical Association, Chicago, 1961. Contains a well written and extremely well illustrated section on the skin.

New Hope for Your Hair: A Scientific Guide to Healthy Hair for Men, Women and Children, Collier Books, New York, 1961. A good discussion of general principles of hygiene for care of the hair.

The Savage Cell, Pat McGrady. Basic Books, New York, 1964. An excellent book about cancer with a section on skin cancer.

Cosmetics and the Skin, F. V. Wells and Irwin I. Lubove. Reinhold, New York, 1964. This authoritative and comprehensive book brings together very timely information regarding face creams, lotions, toothpastes, hair restorers, deodorants, and other products that come in contact with the skin.

Dermatology for Students, Ray O. Noojin. Charles C Thomas, Springfield, Ill., 1961. A helpful discussion of skin and its care.

What Medical Science Can Do About Acne, Bruce H. Frisch. Science Digest, January 1965, p. 61. An up-to-date discussion of a stubborn condition.

Color Her Beautiful, Adolph Rostenberg and Gus Kass. Today's Health, August 1964, p. 14. A professor of dermatology discusses the hair-coloring products.

What to Expect from Your Deodorant, Carol Leth. Today's Health, June 1963, p. 13. This authoritative article, prepared in consultation with the Committee on Cosmetics of the AMA, describes how deodorants work and presents information useful in the personal selection of deodorants.

A Dermatologist Talks About Warts, William R. Vath. Today's Health, March 1963, p. 40. Many important questions are answered in an interview with a dermatologist who has made a special study of warts.

28

THE TEETH, MOUTH AND GUMS

Nature provides two sets of teeth in a lifetime: the 20 deciduous, or baby teeth, and the 32 permanent teeth. And this is all. There is no record that anyone ever developed a third set of natural teeth.

This is not extravagant of nature, because the jaws of an infant just aren't large enough to accommodate the teeth he will need in adult life. Contrary to the usual belief, the first set, just like the second, needs good dental care. If deciduous teeth become badly decayed and too many have to be extracted, the permanent teeth may later align themselves poorly.

Tooth decay, or *dental caries,* is our most common disease, affecting about 100 million Americans. It is the chief cause of toothache, and of the necessity for fillings and inlays; it is the major source of pulp and root abscesses, and a very common reason why teeth have to be extracted and artificial ones substituted.

Among children, defective teeth rank ahead of all other impairments, and almost everyone has experienced a decayed, missing or filled tooth before he reaches early adolescence.

A recent survey made by a government agency led to the estimate that 22 million Americans and 30 per cent of persons over 35 years of age are edentulous, or completely lacking in natural teeth.

In addition to the amount of pain and distress it causes, tooth decay can be a contributory factor in other diseases. Also, poor teeth and the unpleasant odor of an unhygienic mouth are definitely not social or economic assets. Cervantes did not exaggerate in *Don Quixote* when he said that "every tooth in a man's head is more valuable to him than diamonds."

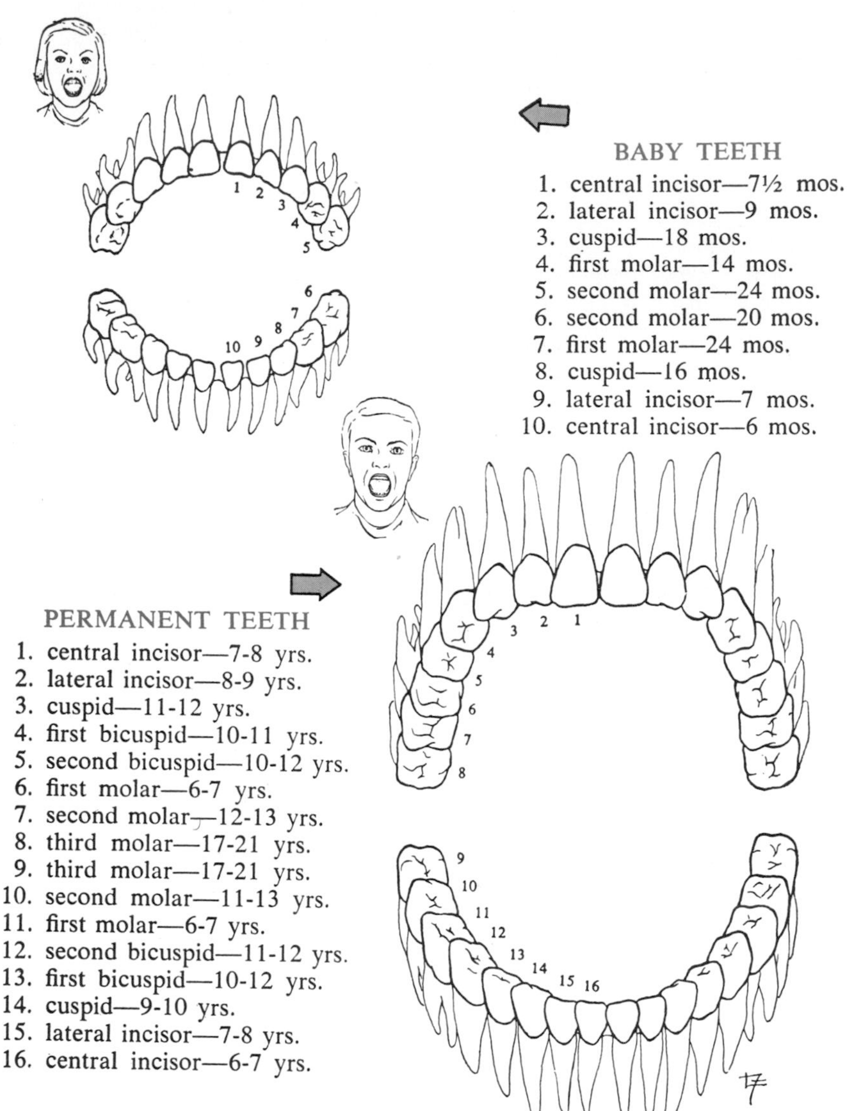

Figure 28–1. Baby teeth and permanent teeth; the approximate time of their appearance.

THE PROBLEM OF DENTAL CARIES

The teeth of men apparently started decaying with the cave man and have continued to do so for thousands of years. The oldest specimens showing decay date from the Stone Age. Furthermore, dental caries is an extremely widespread disease, affecting both civilized and uncivilized nations.

Yet there *are* areas of the world where the inhabitants are practically free from tooth decay: some Alaskan Eskimos, the natives of parts of the Hebrides islands off the coast of Scotland, several tribes of South African Zulus, and a few others. In some areas there is partial immunity, as in certain sections of Texas, Oklahoma, and some other states. Resistance to tooth decay in these areas in the United States appears to be directly related to the fluoride content of the water.

Dental research experts are actively studying the immune areas of the world in an effort to unearth information which will help the caries-susceptible areas.

The Economic Problem

At present, only about 40 per cent of the people who need it are getting dental treatment, yet our dental bills total nearly $2 billion annually. According to the American Dental Association, "to meet the existing dental needs of the population at any given time would require between five and 10 times the annual productive capacity of all the dental personnel in the United States."

Prevention is certainly the best solution to such a widespread disease.

What Is Dental Caries?

Dental caries is best understood if the nature and function of each part of the tooth are first described.

The *crown,* which lies above the surface of the gums, is covered with a coating of *enamel.* Fortunately, this is thickest on the grinding surface where it wears down from use. The *root* lies within the jaw, and is covered with a thin, bonelike layer *(cementum).* Beneath the enamel is the resilient, leathery *dentin,* with a chamber called the *pulp chamber,* and the *root canal.* These contain the blood vessels and nerve fibers which nourish the tooth and maintain its life and sensations.

Dental caries is a disease, not a vague, mysterious "rotting" of the teeth which must be accepted fatalistically. Dental caries *always* start on the outside of the teeth, in the enamel. If we focus a microscope on a section of enamel where the tiniest new cavity is developing, we see a pinhead-sized collection of bacteria and food adhering to the smooth surface of the tooth, much like barnacles gathering on the smooth hull of a ship. Dentists call this collection a *plaque.*

It is generally believed that a good proportion of these bacteria are the kind that thrive best on starchy and sugary foods, which they change into *lactic acid.* Although tooth enamel is the strongest material in the body, able to withstand enormous biting pressures, lactic acid quickly and permanently dissolves it. Eating minute pits and furrows in the

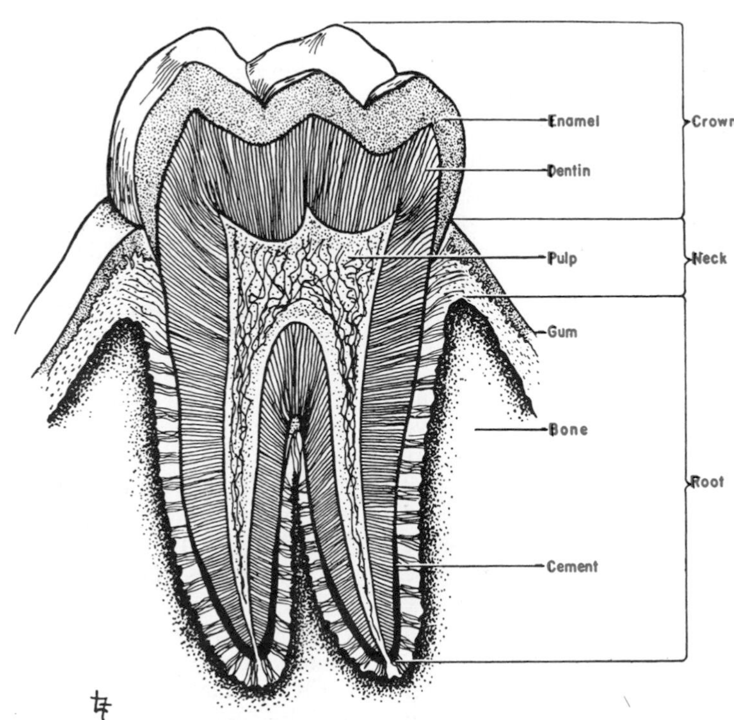

Figure 28–2. Diagram of a section through a human molar tooth. (From Villee: *Biology*. 4th Ed., Philadelphia, W. B. Saunders Co., 1962.)

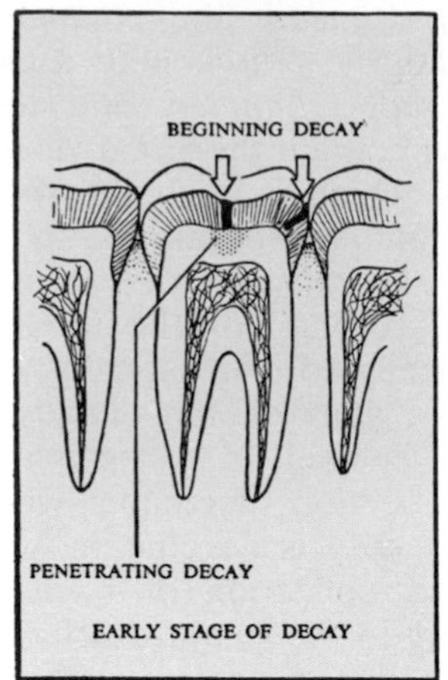

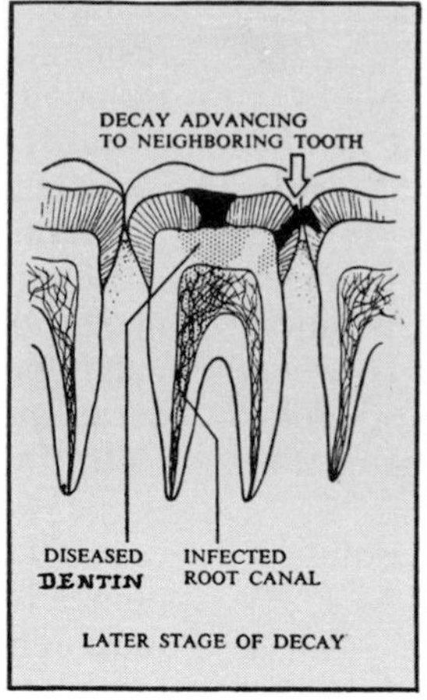

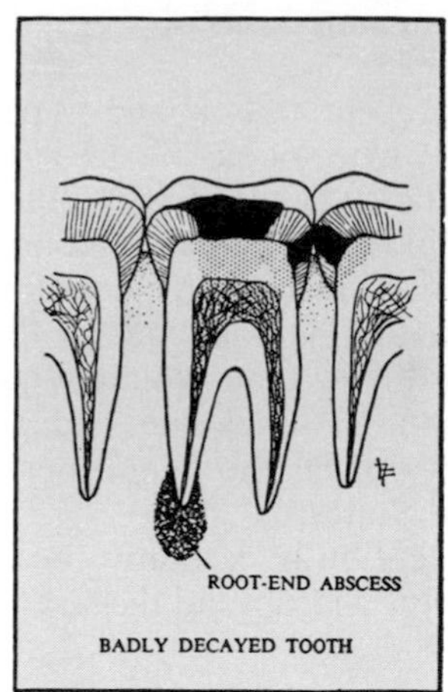

Figure 28–3. Early and late stages of dental caries.

surface of the tooth, the acid opens up new territory for the bacteria. Soon they reach the softer, richer dentin, where they grow faster and spread rapidly. They proceed into the root canal, attacking the nerves and causing great pain.

Unfortunately, enamel that has been destroyed by acid will not grow and come together again. Neither will the dentin of the tooth, eroded by bacterial action. If the decay has not gone too far, the tooth can be saved by removing the diseased portion and filling the cavity. Dentists generally consider a tooth beyond repair, however, when decay has entered the root canal, and affected the pulp. The tooth is usually extracted, although in special cases root canals can be filled.

Immunity to Caries

Some individuals seem to have an immunity to dental caries. Most of us have a partial immunity: the molars may decay while the front teeth almost never get cavities. Also, we may be immune at certain times and not at others. The same patient may have numerous cavities one year and not develop a single cavity the following year. As yet, these types of immunity are not thoroughly understood.

Susceptibility to caries may also differ markedly in a single family. It is not unusual to find one member of a family completely free of dental decay, and another, extremely susceptible. Yet a genetic factor is indicated by the fact that identical twins show very similar patterns of tooth decay.

How Can Caries Be Controlled?

Three major factors which contribute to tooth decay are sweets in the diet, which bacteria of the *Lactobacillus acidophilus* type convert to corrosive lactic acid; mouth bacteria: and acids from other sources, such as soft drinks. Numerous studies have shown that if these can be reduced, the number of cavities which form in the teeth is significantly lowered. A fourth factor is the neglect of dental care.

Reduce Sweets. The mouth always contains large numbers and varieties of bacteria, but the *Lactobacillus* is stimulated to grow only when carbohydrates are available. One of the best ways of conquering an enemy is to starve him. This is an excellent weapon against tooth decay. *All cavities start from the outside.* The bacteria on the tooth surfaces demand carbohydrates for food. *Therefore, if you deprive them of carbohydrates, these bacteria will have nothing to convert to acid, and the enamel will not be penetrated.*

Of course, all balanced diets contain starches and sugars. Nevertheless, reduction or elimination of rich, concentrated, sticky sugars from the diet almost always diminishes the number of new cavities and the spread of existing ones. This includes chewy candies, chewing gums, sweetened, carbonated beverages, pastries, pies, and cookies. *A sweet tooth can ruin all the teeth.*

Another way of starving the acid-forming bacteria is to remove sweets from the teeth promptly so that they won't serve as bacterial nourishment for hours. This may be helped by brushing, rinsing the teeth with water, and use of dental tape or floss to remove large food particles.

Inhibit the Bacteria. A variety of *dentifrices* have appeared on the market in recent years, each claiming remarkable results as antienzyme agents for controlling tooth decay. These contain chemicals ranging from *alkaline agents,* like urea and ammonium sulfate, which might effectively neutralize the lactic acid produced; *detergents* of various kinds which possess some antibacterial activity; *antibiotics* like penicillin, and several types of fluoride compounds.

Insufficient research has been done on these dentifrices in most cases to justify the extensive claims made for them. As one dental expert pointed out, "One must continue to differentiate dentifrices on the *basis of scientific evidence rather than on the basis of magazine, newspaper, radio, and television claims. Unfortunately, most patients see their television sets more frequently than they see their dentists."* Nevertheless, the search for effective antibacterial agents is very worth while.

Fluoridation of Water. The addition of sodium fluoride to dentifrices has not shown remarkable results in reducing dental caries, although a related compound, stannous fluoride, appears more promising. However, *the addition of fluoride in very low concentrations to drinking water* has been thoroughly tested in many communities over a period of years, and holds considerable promise.

Three scientific observations stimulated the extensive and successful use of fluoride: noncarious teeth were found to contain more fluorine than carious teeth, and the highest content was in the enamel, the first tissue destroyed in the carious process; caries is less prevalent in areas where the drinking water contains one part per million of fluoride or more; and the addition of fluorides to the drinking water of experimental animals reduces the number of carious teeth.

Large amounts of fluoride produce a discoloration or mottling of the teeth, but if the fluoride content is low, it does not affect the appearance of the teeth, and it does reduce the incidence of caries.

Many communities are adding fluoride to water supplies as a preventive public health measure. More than 45 million Americans are now getting fluoridated water, and similar programs are operating in 19 foreign countries.

Unfortunately, despite extremely convincing evidence of its effectiveness and safety (see Table 28–1), opposition to the use of fluoridated public water supplies still persists. Sincere opposition will be resolved by public health education. However, much of the more vociferous resistance stems from individuals and groups who take every opportunity to discredit medical science and public health progress, and do not really want to know

Table 28–1. Effects of fluoride on general health as judged from mortality statistics.* †

Cause of Death‡	*32 Cities with Natural Fluoride Drinking Waters (More than 0.7 parts per million)*	*32 Control Cities (Fluoride less than 0.25 parts per million)*
Heart disease	354.8	357.4
Cancer	135.4	139.1
Intracranial lesions	111.5	104.8
Nephritis	21.9	26.9
Cirrhosis of liver	6.6	8.2
All causes	1010.6	1005.0

*From *Fluoride Drinking Waters,* National Institute of Dental Research, U. S. Public Health Service, 1962, p. 359.

†Deaths per 100,000 adjusted for age, race, and sex.

‡No significant differences between cities.

the facts. The most important official and professional groups in this and allied fields have endorsed fluoridation: the National Research Council, the U. S. Public Health Service, the American Dental Association, the American Medical Association, the American Public Health Association, and numerous others.

George F. Lull of the American Medical Association has discussed the principal questions raised by fluoridation opponents, and has answered them very objectively:

> Is there sufficient scientific and experimental evidence that fluoridation is safe? *Answer:* Yes, in the dosages recommended . . . 1 ppm, it is quite safe. There is more than that in many natural waters, and the only bad effect is the harmless mottling of children's teeth. . . . Fluorides in minute quantities are a normal constituent of the human body.
>
> It is claimed that fluoridation of public water supplies is expensive and wasteful because only a small portion of the water fluoridated is consumed by human beings. *Answer:* There is no practical way to fluoridate a public water supply but to fluoridate it all, and the cost amounts to only a few cents per taxpayer per year.
>
> It is claimed by some that the community has no right to force them to take undesirable medication. *Answer:* Fluoridation is not medication; it is adjustment to normal of a deficient fluorine content in water in certain areas where it is needed. No one is forced to use a public water supply; bottled water can be purchased.
>
> It is claimed that fluoridation is dangerous because a breakdown of the mechanical system might cause excessive dosage. *Answer:* Long experience with automatic addition of many chemicals to public water supplies for safety or to remove objectionable tastes, colors and odors has brought machinery for this purpose to a high degree of perfection. If something goes wrong, these machines shut down, resulting in no fluoride rather than too much.[1]

The use of fluoridated water supplies has proved to be of tremendous value as a public health measure in a very important, widespread, expensive, and painful disease. Misguided opponents are doing themselves and the public a serious disservice.

Acids in Soft Drinks. In addition to their high content of sugar which is in all probability a strong offender in dental caries, most carbonated beverages contain acids, especially phosphoric acid. Because these are powerful enough to be quite destructive to tooth enamel, carbonated drinks should be taken in moderation. If possible, the mouth should be thoroughly rinsed afterwards.

IMPORTANCE OF DIET IN THE FORMATION OF TEETH

The formation of sound teeth requires the correct diet, during pregnancy and the child's early life. Because the first teeth start to form in the eighth week of pregnancy, the mother should eat a properly balanced diet to guarantee good tooth development in the child. Foods containing calcium and phosphorus are extremely important because these are the two chief components of teeth. Vitamins A, C, and D are especially important in the development of good tooth structure.

THE IMPORTANCE OF PROMPT AND REGULAR DENTAL CARE

Regular visits to the dentist not only save time, money, and suffering, but they also save your teeth.

A survey made a few years ago showed that people who stayed away from the dentist for three years lost *twice as many teeth* as those who had dental treatment every year; 16.7 per cent of the people in this group had to have *complete dentures* as compared with 1.9 per cent in the group that went every six months to a year.

It is well established that complete oral rehabilitation, which includes restoring and filling all decayed teeth, and extracting all badly diseased ones, causes a sharp drop in the number of undesirable *Lactobacilli* in the mouth. Despite this, the U. S. Public Health Service estimates that only 36 per cent of the population visit a dentist yearly.

How Often Should You See Your Dentist?

Regular periodic dental checkups, including dental x-rays to detect tiny new cavities, are very important. How frequently you need these depends on your susceptibility to caries or other diseases relating to the teeth. If dental decay is on a

[1] *Today's Health, 3*:13, 1955.

rampage, you might need a checkup every few months or even oftener. If you are one of the rare caries-immune, or partially immune, individuals, a yearly visit may be enough. Unfortunately, not more than 36 per cent of Americans follow this advice despite very good public health education by the American Dental Association.

The *choice* of a dentist is also important. Inadequately trained dentists will perform poor dentistry. If a dentist merely covers up an existing cavity, instead of unearthing and digging out the decayed area, you will have spent good money for nothing, and will probably lose the tooth eventually, when the inner decay reaches the root.

Dentistry has made tremendous technical advances in recent years, and dentists are now able to save many teeth they would formerly have extracted. Better instruments and improved techniques make it possible for the dentist to work faster and more gently. For example, air-cooled drills avoid creating the heat which is a major source of pain in drilling, and high-speed air drills shorten the drilling time tremendously.

Years ago, dentists used anesthetics only when extracting teeth. Today most dentists use them for almost all painful procedures, including preparing teeth for fillings. The most popular methods are the injection of procaine, Novocain, and similar compounds into the nerves or gums, or the inhalation of nitrous oxide gas. Although the patient remains conscious and is aware of the drilling, his sensations are dulled so that it does not hurt him.

Future research may bring forth effective remineralizing agents which could be routinely applied to weakened enamel, and prevent caries from developing.

TRANSPLANTING TEETH

Tooth transplants have been in and out of vogue throughout history, but recent research indicates that soon there will be no reason for anyone to have a false or missing tooth. For example, impacted wisdom teeth have been removed and used to replace missing permanent molars. Dr. Ralf Mezrow of Einstein Medical Center in Philadelphia has reported many successful transplants between individuals; some patients were in their 70's.

The tooth transplant operation is performed under local anesthesia and takes about 45 minutes. The new tooth is held in place by a plastic splint until it takes root—generally about 6 weeks. The operation is usually successful, and the new tooth even changes color to match the others.

Dr. Mezrow reports that the body does not reject transplanted teeth as readily as it does other organs. Because transplants have been successful, several tooth banks have been established in this country.

It is of practical importance to remember that knocked-out teeth should be taken to the dentist at once; usually, they can be reimplanted in their original location.

KEEPING YOUR TEETH CLEAN

The need for good oral hygiene is essential and will probably remain so, no matter what miracles future dental research brings. Even the ancient Arabs recognized this 3000 years ago and cleaned their teeth after meals, using twigs for tooth brushes. Yet, according to Herbert K. Cooper, Director of the Lancaster Cleft Palate Clinic: "The human mouth needs more care, and probably receives less . . . than any other part of the anatomy."

Your Toothbrush

A recent editorial in the Journal of the American Dental Association deplores the fact that toothbrushes are used so little and are in such poor condition. "Most toothbrushes in American homes are filling more of an honorary than a serviceable use, judging by the condition of these brushes." A survey of 1000 families possessing 2032 brushes showed 1219 of them to be unusable, almost 100 doubtful, only about 700 that could be considered fit for use.

When you choose a toothbrush, select one that isn't too large, has a flat bristle surface, and a handle long enough to let you manipulate it. Regardless of its size, shape and bristle distribution, no brush can possibly live up to advertising claims that it "conforms exactly to the shape and size of your teeth." The shape and size of everybody's teeth are different.

It is desirable to have two brushes, one for morning and one for evening use, to permit drying in between use. This diminishes rotting and softening of the toothbrush. A toothbrush is not a very expensive commodity and should not be regarded as a permanent possession. It is expendable, and should be replaced as soon as the bristles soften. Stiff bristles have a dual role: they remove food and they stimulate the gums.

The Electric Toothbrush. This device is new and relatively expensive, but dentists who have evaluated it seem to be, for the most part, favorably impressed. Electrical brushing appears to be as effective as proper hand brushing but less irritating to the gums. Also, it is easier, in many cases, to get children to use the electric brush than to get them to use a hand brush.

The efficiency of the electric toothbrush varies with the model, and your dentist should assist you in the selection. An up-to-date discussion of the various types is found in *The Medicine Show,* an excellent book by Consumers Union. According to this report, some are potentially lethal if dropped into a basin of water while plugged in. Safer, battery-operated models are available.

Dentifrices and Mouthwashes

The number of dentifrices marketed and the extensive claims made for them are bewildering and frequently unsubstantiated. Your dentist can suggest a satisfactory and safe powder or paste, which will perform its necessary function of giving your mouth a pleasant, fresh taste, and not be so gritty as to wear down the teeth. Many dentists feel that powders are more effective than pastes, because they are slightly more abrasive, but most dental authorities agree that the effect of any "germicidal" dentifrice is only temporary. Even though it may be able to destroy mouth germs, the first glass of water you drink will wash it away, and so will your saliva.

Mouthwashes, too, have the virtue of imparting a clean, pleasant taste but possess little more value. Their effect is transient. Infections and similar mouth conditions which require the use of some kind of antiseptic will rarely yield to a mouthwash alone. They usually need special dental care.

When to Brush Your Teeth

The most desirable plan would be to brush your teeth every time you eat anything. This would prevent solid food particles from adhering to the teeth or becoming lodged in between them, to serve as nourishment for mouth bacteria until the next time you brushed them. Unfortunately, this is rarely feasible, and the usual substitute is to brush them before retiring, and after breakfast.

If possible, try to brush your teeth, and clean between the teeth with dental floss, after every major meal, or at least swish water back and forth vigorously in your mouth to dislodge food after you have eaten.

Brush Them Properly

Don't brush *across* your teeth in a scrubbing motion. This doesn't get rid of the food particles between the teeth, and may wear down the enamel or injure the gums if you are too vigorous about it. Most dentists suggest that you brush down on the upper teeth, up on the lower ones, holding the toothbrush at an angle that will enable you to avoid sticking the bristles into your gums. Place the bristles against the teeth and pointing toward the gums, at an angle of about 45 degrees. Start high enough, or low enough, to massage the gums as well as brush the teeth. (Massaging the gums may cause them to bleed a little at first, but this shouldn't happen after a few days.) Brush only a few teeth at a time, inside as well as out. Then clean the biting surface by putting the toothbrush square against it and jiggling it around.

Use dental floss, dental tape, Stim-u-dents, or the rubber points on the ends of certain toothbrushes to remove the food from between the teeth.

HALITOSIS

There are many and varied causes for an unpleasant mouth odor: decayed teeth or diseased gums; the residue of certain foods; digestive disturbances; inflamed tonsils or infections in or behind the nose; and diseases such as diabetes and uremia.

Mouthwashes may *temporarily* mask the odor, but they do not influence the basic cause, whose treatment is within the province only of a physician or a dentist.

IMPACTED TEETH

Teeth which are fully formed, but for one reason or another are unable to erupt completely through the overlying gum tissue may cause considerable pain and distress. This happens most commonly with the third molars, the *wisdom teeth,* and may be due to malformation or twisting of the tooth in the gum, or because there is not sufficient space for it to erupt.

Dental x-rays reveal the cause of impaction. Such teeth are usually extracted if they are causing difficulty.

MALOCCLUSION

Teeth which are irregular, overlapping, or protruding at abnormal angles are poorly aligned. Serious malocclusion occurs when the upper and lower teeth do not mesh, and fail to provide a proper biting surface.

There are many causes for poor alignment of the teeth: too narrow a jaw, causing crowding of the teeth; early loss of deciduous teeth because of decay or accident; and failure of the teeth to erupt at the proper time. Prolonged thumb-sucking and lip-biting have also been implicated.

Poorly aligned teeth often cause trouble because the food collects behind them, and the gums become irritated. If only a few of the teeth meet in chewing, they must sustain the entire force of the bite, which may eventually weaken and loosen them.

Perhaps equally important, "buck teeth" or a weak, receding chin caused by malocclusion detract from a person's appearance, and may make him sensitive and self-conscious. Also, these conditions are often responsible for speech defects.

The *orthodontist* is the dental specialist who corrects malocclusion by applying special braces and restraining devices which force the teeth into better alignment. These techniques are most successful with young children, but even older individuals can benefit from skilled orthodonture.

COMMON DISEASES OF THE GUMS AND SUPPORTING STRUCTURES

Gingivitis is an inflammation of the gingival tissue, or gums, which fit snugly around the tooth like a collar. If this tissue is irritated, it may become swollen and tender and bleed easily.

The commonest causes for this disease, sometimes called "bleeding gums," are: *dental calculus* or "tartar"; impaction of food; improper brushing of the teeth and massage of the gums; irregular teeth or badly fitting fillings which irritate the gums; certain allergies; and possibly too soft a diet to keep the gums in healthy condition.

Deposits of tartar, mainly phosphate of lime and food particles, on the margin between the gums and the teeth irritate the gums, causing them to shrink and become a ready prey to infection. Eating fresh fruit may help reduce the amount of tartar which forms, but once it is laid down, only your dentist can scale it off completely.

Vincent's infection, usually called trench mouth because it was so common among soldiers in World War I, is a very infectious disease which affects the gums, but may spread to other parts of the mouth and the throat. It sometimes produces an unpleasant odor and inflammation of the gums, accompanied by tenderness and bleeding.

Trench mouth is still a common infection, and may be brought on by poor mouth hygiene. Vitamin deficiencies and general poor health may also be contributory factors. Local antiseptic treatment by a dentist, and proper diet and care of the mouth usually clear it up. However, Vincent's infection is sometimes a prolonged, chronic condition which needs very careful dental attention.

Pyorrhea, also called periodontal dis-

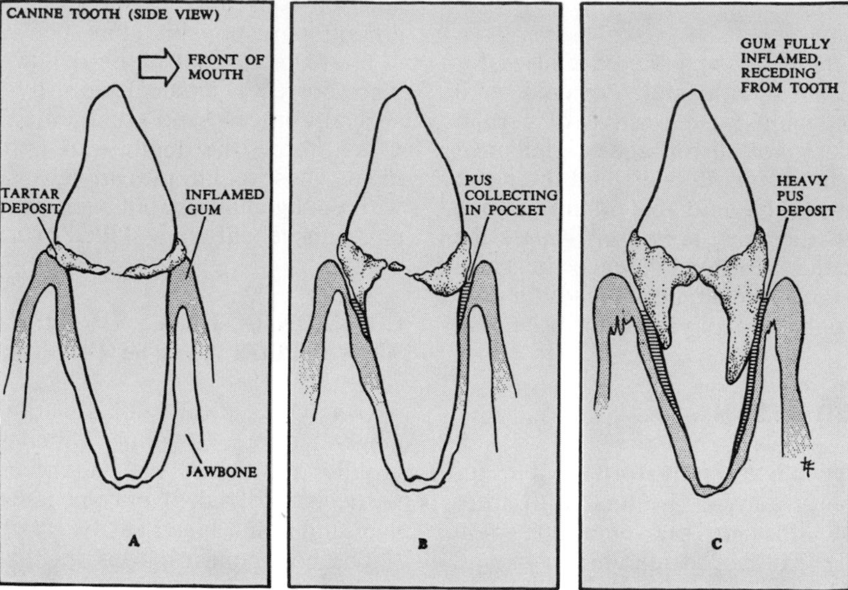

Figure 28–4. Early and advanced pyorrhea.

ease, is a progressive condition which may destroy the attachment of the teeth to the jaw bones, if it is neglected. Even teeth that withstand repeated attacks of decay can be lost in later life by periodontal disease. It causes many more lost teeth in adults than does caries.

The first sign of pyorrhea may be an inflammation of the gums. In the more advanced stage, actual pus is present around the teeth. The bones which hold the teeth in their sockets may be resorbed, and the final result of this disease is loosening of the teeth to the point where they either fall out or must be extracted.

Red, tender, and bleeding gums are a warning signal for an immediate visit to a dentist. Severe gingivitis and pyorrhea can be prevented.

TEETH AS FOCI FOR INFECTIONS

Infected pulps or decaying teeth make excellent breeding places for bacteria. They can cause localized abscesses, and may even enter the blood stream to spread their toxins to various parts of the body. However, doctors are not quite so prone today to blame teeth for generalized illnesses as they once were.

In certain illnesses, such as chronic heart disease and rheumatic fever, no teeth should be extracted without consultation with the physician in charge.

Questions

1. How many deciduous and how many permanent teeth are there? What are they named?
2. What is the fundamental cause of dental caries? Name at least three ways to reduce the incidence of tooth decay.
3. Where does the pain of a toothache originate?
4. Why should studying dental caries among peoples who seem to be immune to it help us reduce our dental caries? Have you any idea how it has already aided us?
5. What is the basis for opposition to public fluoridation of water supplies? Do you think it is justified? Is public fluoridation essentially any more objectionable than *chlorination* of municipal water supplies to remove dangerous bacteria?
6. How does a good diet during pregnancy and the early years of life influence the formation and soundness of teeth?
7. What is the proper way to brush your teeth? How much reliance should you place upon dentifrices? How often should you buy a new toothbrush? What is the value of mouthwashes?
8. Define the terms: *impacted teeth, malocclusion, orthodontist*. How are the first two conditions treated?
9. What is *dental calculus?* How does it lead to gingivitis and sometimes to the more serious pyorrhea? What measures can you take to prevent its formation and end effects?

10. Why do you think extraction of teeth is hazardous in rheumatic heart disease and some other diseases of the heart?

Topics for Discussion

High-speed dental equipment.
Transplanting teeth.
Costs and procedures in orthodontia.
Fluoridation of public water supplies.

Reading Suggestions

Teeth, Their Forms and Functions, Aubrey M. Lauterstein and Thomas K. Barber. Heath, Boston, 1965. An authoritative and comprehensive review of the teeth and mouth in health and disease.

The Medicine Show, Consumers Union, Mount Vernon, New York, 1961. An excellent discussion of dentifrices, mouthwashes, electric toothbrushes, and dental care in general.

Today's Health Guide, The American Medical Association, Chicago, 1965. An authoritative book describing all phases of health including a well written and very well illustrated section on the teeth, mouth, and gums.

Structure and Function in Man, Stanley W. Jacob and Clarice A. Francone. W. B. Saunders, Philadelphia, 1965. An excellent textbook in integrated anatomy and physiology; it contains a good review of the teeth, mouth, and gums.

Teeth, Health and Appearance, 5th Ed., American Dental Association, Chicago, 1961. The proper care and use of the teeth are described in an authoritative, comprehensive and well written book.

Principles of Dental Public Health, James M. Dunning. Harvard University Press, Cambridge, Mass., 1962. Education, prevention, and early treatment are emphasized in this important book.

Fluoride Drinking Waters, F. J. McClure, ed., National Institute of Dental Research, Bethesda, Md., 1962. A selection of public health service papers related to the topic.

Report on the Electric Toothbrush, Bruce H. Frisch. Science Digest, March 1964, p. 35. An informative evaluation of a new device.

Far Worse Than an Aching Tooth, Francis A. Arnold. Today's Health, February 1964, p. 56. An authoritative discussion of periodontal diseases by the director of the National Institute of Dental Research.

Mouthwashes: The Dental Viewpoint, J. Roy Doty. Today's Health, December 1962, p. 6. The American Dental Association's views on mouthwashes are presented.

Fluoridation Fight in New York, Howard A. Rusk. Science Digest, April 1964, p. 30. The study of how America's largest city decided to fluoridate its water.

Tooth Decay, P. J. Sandell and C. M. French. Journal of School Health, December 1962. An important article for those concerned with proper dental care.

Anatomy of a Tooth Ache, Howard Earle. Today's Health, October 1961, p. 32. A well illustrated and authoritative discussion of tooth decay.

29

THE SENSES: THEIR IMPORTANCE IN DAILY LIVING

Man's sight, smell, hearing, sense of locality—how inferior they are. The condor sees a corpse at five miles; man has no telescope that can do it. The bloodhound follows a scent that is two days old. The robin hears the earthworm burrowing his course under the ground. The cat, deported in a closed basket, finds its way home again through twenty miles of country which he has never seen.

MARK TWAIN
Letters from the Earth

Through the long years of evolution, animals have managed to survive because of information received through their senses. Man, the highest of all the animals, is also extensively dependent on his sensory organs.

We literally exist through our senses, because by seeing, hearing, and feeling we avoid danger and death.

We learn through our senses (and imparting learning to a child who is both deaf and mute is enormously difficult).

We are even bound to reality through our senses. Recent experiments have shown that when sensory input, such as sight, sound, and kinesthetic sensation, is reduced to the lowest possible minimum, profound neurotic and even psychotic behavior patterns may result.

At McGill University in Montreal, volunteers were subjected to just such conditions. They were placed in isolated, soundproof, completely dark rooms. All sensations of touch were eliminated by covering the arms and legs. In other words, they were out of communication with the world and its inhabitants, and forced within themselves.

Within a very short time, in some cases less than 24 hours, many of these volunteers signaled that they wished to stop the experiment and be released from their intolerable prisons. They reported experiencing visions and hallucinations, which were sometimes unbearably frightening and disturbing. The subjects couldn't tolerate the experiments even though they were being paid $22 a day.

Since the time of Aristotle, five special senses have been emphasized: vision, hearing, smell, taste, and touch. Today, physiologists subdivide touch, or feeling, into such sensations as pressure, contact, sharp-point pain, deep pain, warmth, heat, cold, muscular pressures, and others. Finally, there is the sense of balance and rotation, which keeps us erect and at equilibrium.

THE EYES AND VISION

Certain patterns of behavior in man and the lower animals are *instinctual,* and the skills needed for their execution are essentially automatic, part of our inheritance. But most of our accomplishments stem from what we *learn and absorb through our senses.* Of these, seeing is probably the most important because it has been estimated that 75 per cent of our learning—and also an inestimable fraction of our enjoyment of life—comes through our eyes.

How the Eye Functions

Whenever you marvel at the performance of a camera, the artistry and detail, remember that its construction was inspired by the human eye.

The eye is a hollow, globular organ, fitting smoothly into a depression of the skull. The white part, the *sclera,* is transparent where it crosses the front of the eye to form the *cornea,* permitting light rays to penetrate. Behind the cornea is the colored *iris,* with the *pupil* in the center. This acts as a shutter, growing larger or smaller, by dilating or contracting, to control the amount of light which enters. The clear, crystalline *lens* located just behind the iris focuses an image on the *retina,* which is the inside coat of the eye, and the *optic nerve* carries this image to the brain. Because of the crisscrossing of light waves as they pass through the lens, the retina receives an inverted image, and it is the responsibility of the experienced brain to set it upright again.

Nature has also devised excellent protective devices for the eye: the *eyelids* are simply two flaps of skin, opened and closed by muscles, to guard the eye against injury or too much light; the *conjunctiva* lines the inside of the eyelid; the *eyelashes* are coarse hairs which can also protect the eye against foreign particles. Finally, tears from the *tear ducts* in the upper, outer corner of the eye continuously lubricate and wash away foreign matter from the surface of the eye.

Day and Night Vision. Our eyes possess several mechanisms for controlling the amount of light which enters: the muscular fibers of the iris contract and constrict the pupils; the lids also blink and shut out light. However, eyeshades or sunglasses should be used to control excessive glare, in summer from the sun and in winter from snow.

We can see surprisingly well at night in dim light because our pupils become dilated—that is, fully expanded to permit all available light to enter. You have probably noticed that a cat's eyes seem to be all pupil in the dark because they are fully dilated.

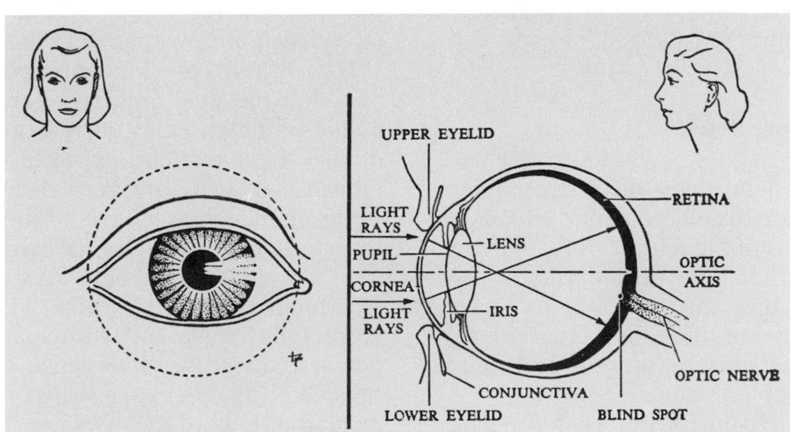

Figure 29–1. The eye. **Left,** Front view. The approximate orbit of the eye is indicated by dotted lines. **Right,** Side view, showing the light rays passing through the lens.

Another factor responsible for night vision is that certain chemical changes occur in one of the eye pigments, *rhodopsin,* or *visual purple.* The reason it takes a few minutes to adapt from bright light to dim light (as in a darkened theater) is that the time is required for rhodopsin to undergo this chemical change.

When a physician puts drops in your eyes to conduct an eye examination, he dilates the pupils. Perhaps you have been struck afterwards by the harsh glare of the sun because your eyes could not adapt to the intense light.

Color Perception and Color Blindness. In normal light, the eyes differentiate many colors easily. This is believed to be accomplished through specific receptor areas in the retina, capable of differentiating the various colors from one another. However, we lose this ability in dim light, and at twilight all objects appear gray. The French have an apt expression for this: *"Dans la nuit, tous les chats sont noir"* (At night all cats are black).

The retinal receptors which are probably responsible for color perception are sensitive to the four basic colors—red, green, yellow and blue. Individuals who can't differentiate one or two of the basic colors are said to be *colorblind.*

About 10 out of 100 men and less than 1 of 100 women show some degree of color blindness. This is a hereditary condition, and is probably due to a congenital lack of the proper color receptors in the eye. It is usually passed from a colorblind grandfather through a normal mother to a colorblind grandson, and is therefore called a sex-linked characteristic.

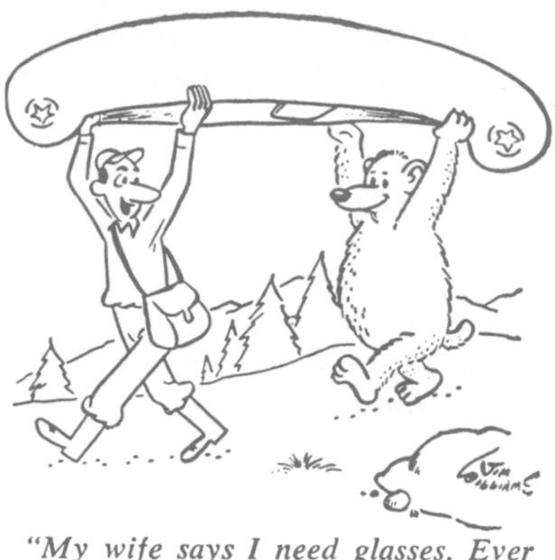

"My wife says I need glasses. Ever hear anything so silly, Ed?"

(From *Modern Medicine,* September 15, 1956.)

Common Visual Defects

As rays of light enter the lens, they are bent, or refracted, and brought to a focus on the proper part of the retina. Unfortunately, few eyes refract light rays perfectly, and even though they may be close to perfect at some stage of life, the aging process may alter the lens or muscle and cause visual defects.

The chief reason for this is that perfect focusing depends on a number of factors: the transparency and curvature of the lens, its thickness or thinness, and the ciliary muscles around the eyeball which support and modify its size.

We can see near and far objects clearly because our lenses have the capacity of *accommodation,* changing their shape to adjust to distances.

Myopia, or nearsightedness, literally means half-closing the eyes, or squinting, which is exactly what near-sighted people do to focus. Only objects held very close to the eye are clearly in focus, and everything else is blurred. In this condition the lens is thicker and more convex than normal, and the eyeball is too long. Entering light rays are bent so sharply that they come to a focus *before* they reach the retina. Glasses with concave lenses shift the point of sharp focus farther back so that it is on the retina. About 5 per cent of children are myopic.

Hyperopia, or farsightedness, means "beyond the eye" and is a common complaint of children, occurring in about six of ten. It is just the opposite of myopia. Objects far away are very clear, but those close at hand are blurred. The eyeball is too short in hyperopia, the lens is thinner than normal, and the light rays are brought to a focus *behind* the retina. Hyperopia is corrected by glasses with *convex* lenses which reduce the divergence of the light rays and bring them to a focus on the retina, instead of behind it.

Most young people with this condition can accommodate satisfactorily for close

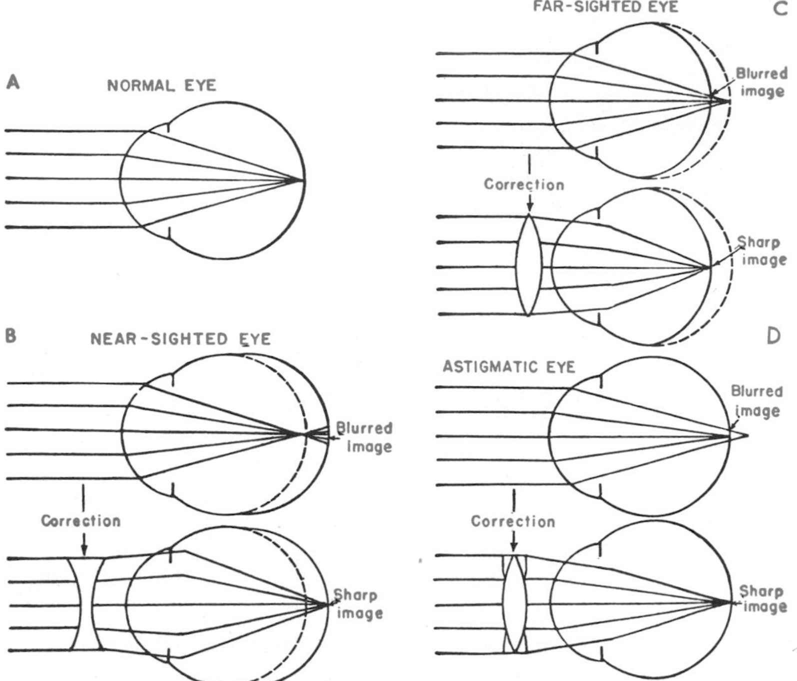

Figure 29–2. Diagram illustrating common abnormalities of the eye. **A,** Normal eye, in which parallel light rays coming from a point in space are focused as a point on the retina. **B,** Near-sighted eye, in which the eyeball is elongated so that parallel light rays are brought to a focus in front of the retina (on dotted line, which represents the position of the retina in the normal eye) and so form a blurred image on the retina. This situation is corrected by placing a concave lens in front of the eye. This diverges the light rays, making it possible for the eye to focus these rays on the retina. **C,** Far-sighted eye, in which the eyeball is shortened and light rays are focused behind the retina. A convex lens converges the light rays so that the eye focuses them on the retina. **D,** Astigmatic eye, in which light rays passing through one part of the eye are focused on the retina, while light rays passing through another area of the lens are not focused on the retina, owing to unequal curvature of the lens or cornea. A cylindrical lens can correct this by bending light rays going through only certain parts of the eye. (From Hunter and Hunter: *College Zoology*. Philadelphia, W. B. Saunders Co.)

work without glasses, although some experts believe that glasses are desirable in all cases, and will save the eyes from strain.

Presbyopia literally means "old eyes," and indicates that the elasticity of the lens and the power of accommodation are reduced. As the far-sighted person ages, distant vision often remains perfectly clear, but his lenses can no longer accommodate to close objects. The result is that he may hold a book at arm's length to bring the print into sharp focus. Corrective glasses are usually essential at this stage, and often *bifocals* are recommended. These contain a lens for distant objects in the upper part, and for close objects, in the lower.

Astigmatism means "without a point." Incoming light rays focus at different points, instead of a single one. This condition is due to uneven curvature of the lens, and both nearsighted and farsighted individuals may be astigmatic. Most people have a slight degree of astigmatism, which doesn't disturb their vision. However, severe astigmatism can be extremely annoying, causing fatigue, headaches and eyestrain unless it is corrected by specially ground lenses.

Strabismus or crossed eyes is fairly common in young children, but frequently outgrown. It usually results from eye muscle irregularities, making one eye more farsighted than the other. Because of this imbalance, the normal eye tends to be over-

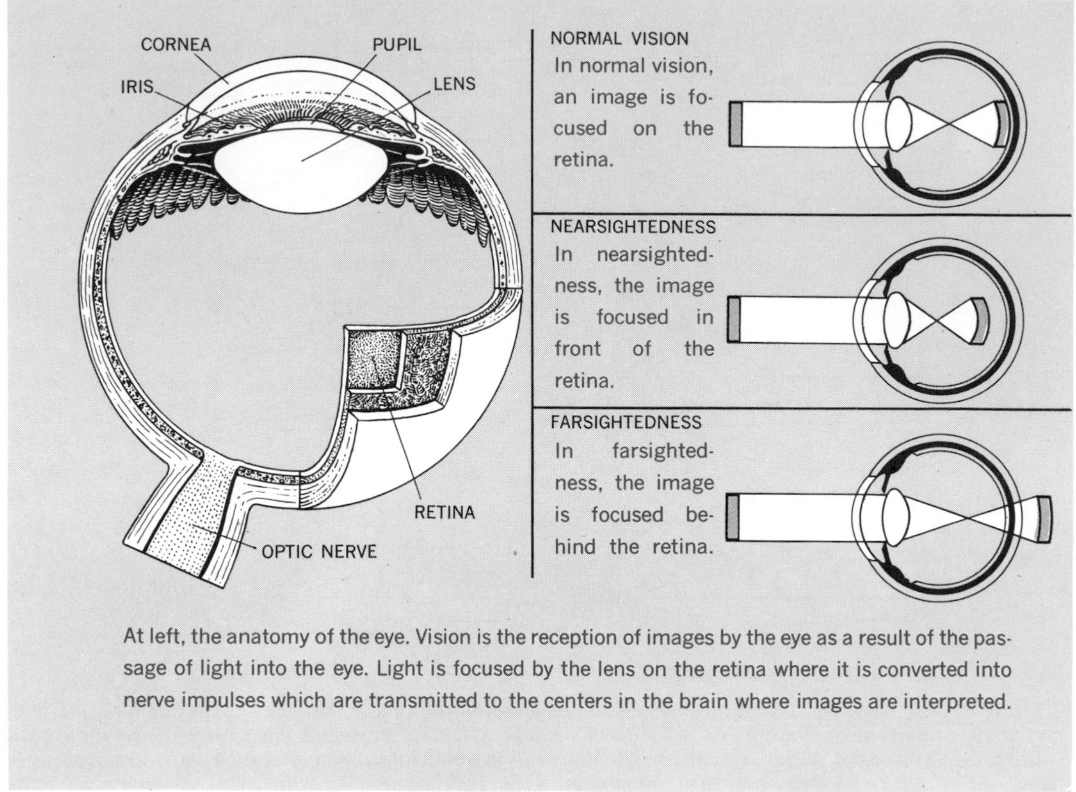

At left, the anatomy of the eye. Vision is the reception of images by the eye as a result of the passage of light into the eye. Light is focused by the lens on the retina where it is converted into nerve impulses which are transmitted to the centers in the brain where images are interpreted.

worked, and the muscles of the farsighted eye stop working entirely, fixating the eye in one position. Crossed eyes are the result.

Corrective glasses, exercises and covering the sound eye to force the other one to function may be adequate measures to resolve this difficulty. In extreme cases, surgery is necessary.

Eye Exercises and Eyestrain

Exercising the eyes can help certain conditions, and they rarely do any harm. But no eye exercises to correct eyestrain should be carried on as a substitute for wearing glasses unless specifically recommended by an expert in this field. This is an area where faddists should be particularly avoided. Eyesight is far too important to be jeopardized in any way.

The major causes of eyestrain are the eyes themselves. Near-sightedness, farsightedness, astigmatism and strabismus all introduce strain, and many of these conditions, if uncorrected, may cause severe headaches, fatigue and other symptoms such as nausea.

In addition, it is possible to strain the eyes by subjecting even well compensated eyes to unusual conditions for prolonged periods of time. Intense, unrelieved focusing on small objects may fatigue the eye muscles and cause temporary blurring of vision. This is readily relieved by rest. Movies can cause eyestrain if the lighting is poor, the film flickering, if you sit too far to one side, or watch too many movies. Television falls into pretty much the same category as movies. It won't hurt your eyes if you have a fairly large screen, unless you have the room totally dark, sit at too close an angle, or watch too steadily for a long time.

Eyewashes and Eyedrops

Unless these are recommended by a physician to relieve a specific condition, the routine use of eyedrops or eyewashes is not desirable. Nature provides adequately for this in the tear ducts.

Goggles and Sunglasses

Shatterproof goggles should be used in all industries where there are hazards to the eyes, for example, where lathes or grinding machines are used.

Good, optically ground sunglasses are also desirable protective devices. (Cheap ones, made from ordinary glass, may cause distortion and headaches.) If you already wear glasses, you can have sunglasses ground to your prescription, or can clip optically ground sunglasses to your regular glasses. However, no ordinary sunglass is sufficiently dense to permit looking directly at the sun without damage to the eyes.

Automobile drivers should not wear sunglasses or tinted lenses at dusk or at night. Even tinted windshields have been reported to reduce "visual distance" 10 to 30 per cent, and cause a corresponding increase in accident rates.

Illumination

Poor illumination for close work may also overwork the eye muscles and cause strain. Reading with a light which is either too dim or incorrectly placed is a common failing. The correct *intensity* of illumination will vary for different activities, much brighter light being required for severe visual tasks, such as reading fine print, drafting or working with very tiny objects of any kind. Lamps should be placed to throw the light over your left shoulder if you are right-handed, and over the right shoulder if you are left-handed.

The proper *distribution* of light is equally important. Glare, contrast, shadows and illumination of specific objects must be considered. Direct lighting may provide maximum utilization of the available light, but may be so bright that it causes undesirable shadows and glares. Eye fatigue and discomfort are greatest in the presence of glare, caused by unshaded light bulbs, or reflection from glossy surfaces such as certain papers, polished metals or glass desk tops. Diffused lighting provides even, general illumination and avoids shadows and glare. This can be achieved most easily by using indirect illumination—throwing the light toward ceiling or walls, from which it can be deflected to a room. Shielding light bulbs with diffusing plastics or similar materials is also helpful to the eyes.

Extreme contrasts in light and dark areas of a room or a work area should be avoided because this is a major cause of eyestrain. It is very fatiguing to the eyes to be forced to accommodate rapidly and repeatedly to extremes of light and darkness. To prevent this, illumination experts recommend that work areas such as desk tops and blotters should be light in color, beige or gray, so that the light falling on the white pages of a book or writing paper will not be in too marked contrast to its surroundings. This is also the reason behind keeping a lamp lighted in the room where you are watching television.

Importance of Color. The proper use of color has both physical and psychological significance. Certain colors or intensities of color produce specific reactions. Red, orange, and yellow are usually considered warm, and blues and greens, cool. However, the dark, heavy shades seem warmer whereas the pale, pastel shades appear cooler.

The amount of light reflected from various colors and woods varies tremendously, and should be considered in select-

Table 29–1. Reflection of paint, paper, and wood*

Color	*Per Cent Reflected*	*Color*	*Per Cent Reflected*
White	85		
Light		*Dark*	
Cream	75	Gray	30
Gray	75	Red	13
Yellow	75	Brown	10
Buff	70	Blue	8
Green	65	Green	7
Blue	55		
Medium		*Wood finish*	
Yellow	65	Maple	42
Buff	63	Satinwood	34
Gray	55	English oak	17
Green	52	Walnut	16
Blue	35	Mahogany	12

*From U.S. Navy Electronics Laboratory, as reproduced in *The Human Machine* by Shilling.

ing paints or papers for interior decoration, and for eye protection as well.

Green chalkboards are better than black ones. The Illuminating Engineering Society recommends backgrounds of soft gray, blue, green, and blue-green as easy on the eyes. These colors possess a good light reflectance without being too bright. An industrial color code has recently been incorporated into safety practices: certain parts of hazardous equipment are painted orange to warn of the danger of cutting, crushing, burns or shock. Red is used to mark fire protection devices, and green indicates first-aid equipment.

It is important to remember both in the choice of clothes and paints for exterior use that light colors reflect the sun's rays and therefore reflect heat, whereas dark colors absorb heat. For this reason, white and pastel colors have become popular in the tropics.

Contact Lenses Versus Glasses

Glasses have been made so attractive in colors and shapes of frames that the resistance many people feel about wearing them is rapidly diminishing. There seems little reason to deprive oneself of good vision because of vanity about wearing glasses.

For people who continue to be sensitive about wearing glasses—and this is apt to be particularly true for actresses and others whose beauty is their stock in trade—*contact lenses* have proved very helpful.

Although Leonardo da Vinci first conceived the idea of correcting faulty vision by placing a lens in direct contact with the eye, it took more than 400 years to perfect a tiny, comfortable, inconspicuous lens. The contact lenses used today fulfill all these specifications. Essentially the only deterrents to their widespread use are the rather high cost and the fear about placing anything in contact with the eye.

Contact lenses are now being made of an almost paper-thin plastic, 1/3 inch in diameter, or about as large as the tip of a cigarette. After the first week or two, most people find them so comfortable that they are hardly conscious of them. Plastic lenses can be used to correct most ordinary

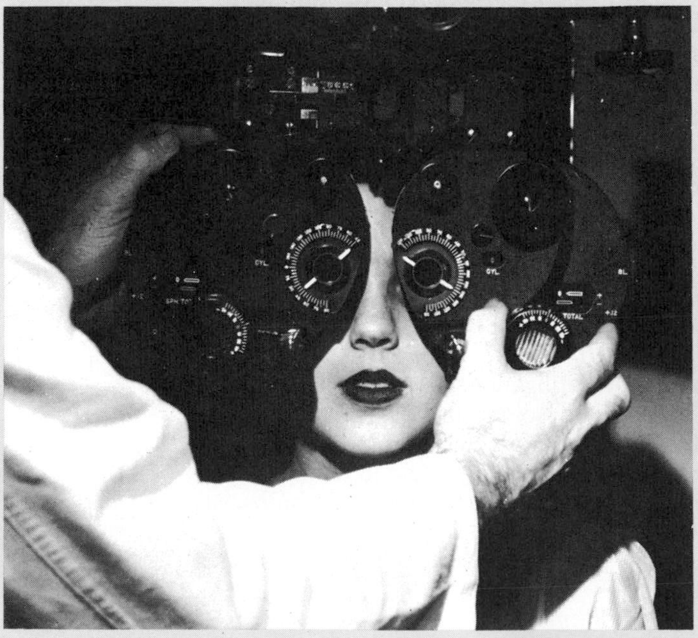

Regular eye examinations are recommended, especially for children and for people over 40. Both the ophthalmologist and the optometrist are qualified to examine eyes and prescribe glasses. In addition, the ophthalmologist is trained to treat eye diseases.

eye defects. In addition, they can be used to match normally mismatched iris colors (for example, one blue and one brown eye), they can be tinted for photophobia, and they are even available today as bifocal lenses.

Because plastic doesn't attract grease as easily as glass, contact lenses are easier to keep clean than glass. Also, they don't "steam up" as glass does. Someone has pointed out that plastic contact lenses "enable the nearsighted to shower and shave without losing the soap, and to swim without losing the family."

Eye Specialists

Several different groups of professional experts deal with the eye, and it is important to know who can do what. An *ophthalmologist* (oculist) is an eye specialist with

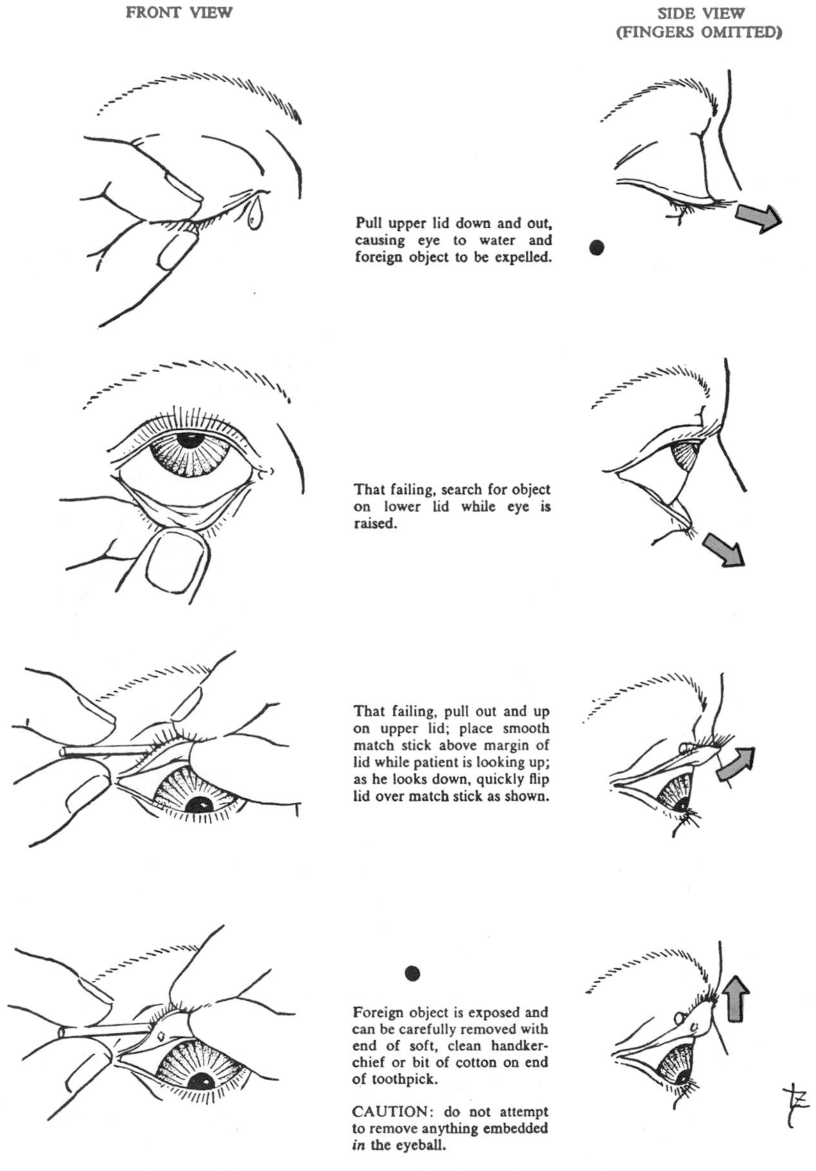

Figure 29–3. Removing a foreign object from the eye.

an M.D. degree, trained in surgery of the eye, as well as its diseases. An *optometrist* is not a medical doctor, but he has received the training necessary for examination of the eyes, in order to prescribe eyeglasses. An *optician* fills the prescriptions made by ophthalmologists or optometrists. He is the counterpart of the pharmacist who fills prescriptions for medicines. Neither the optometrist nor the optician can treat diseases of the eye or perform eye surgery.

Eye Surgery

A variety of eye afflictions may be helped considerably and sometimes completely relieved by surgery. These include strabismus or crossed eyes, opacity of the cornea, cataract of the lens, detached retina, and glaucoma.

Diseases (and Degeneration) of The Eyes

Reddening and inflammation of the eye may result from a minor irritation or infection of the conjunctiva or the iris, but it may also indicate a more serious illness. *No eye infection or chronic abnormality of vision should be neglected. It always calls for a visit to a physician.*

Conjunctivitis, usually called pink eye, is a very infectious, but generally minor, irritation of the conjunctiva. The eyes become red, the lids swell, and they may be stuck together in the mornings by a thick secretion. Fortunately, this condition usually yields quickly to the proper eyewashes or ophthalmic ointments.

Eye Injuries

"Black eyes" are really nothing more than a discoloration of the eyelid, due to a bruise or injury, and do not involve the actual eyeball at all. The black and blue features are due to changes in the blood pigment because of damage to blood vessels in that area. They clear up by themselves, and the traditional beefsteak method is useless. It would be better to eat the steak than to apply it to the eye.

A cinder, soot particle, or piece of dirt may lodge in the eye in such a way that the tears don't wash it away. Rubbing often aggravates the situation, and embeds the particle more deeply. If bathing the eye with a mild, sterile antiseptic solution like saturated boric acid doesn't remove the offending material, it is best to try to locate it by exposing the lids as shown in Figure 29–3.

Home and industrial accidents are responsible for a large number of eye injuries and total blindness. Eye injuries are among the costliest permanent disabilities, according to the National Safety Council, and in 1957 amounted to 60,000, or about 3 per cent of the total number of industrial accidents.

Any kind of eye injury, major or minor, should be seen by a qualified, experienced physician, to prevent infection or serious damage. (The major diseases of the eye, glaucoma and trachoma, as well as blindness, are described in Chapter 17, "The Disabling Diseases.")

THE EARS: HEARING AND EQUILIBRIUM

Next to sight, the sense of hearing is probably the most important both in the learning process and in the enjoyment of life. A deaf child learns to speak only with great difficulty, and even then will not talk normally.

Hearing protects us from impending dangers—an approaching car, falling rocks, ferocious animals.

People who have never heard or lose their hearing have described the terrible loneliness of a world in which communication with other human beings through the auditory sense is no longer possible. (Hearing impairment, which affects 18½ million Americans, is described in Chapter 17.)

How We Hear

The ear is made up of three parts, the *outer ear,* the *middle ear,* and the *inner ear.* The parts you see, the *lobe* and the *ear canal,* make up the outer ear. This canal leads to the *eardrum* and the middle ear in which lie the "bones of hearing," called the *hammer, anvil* and *stirrup* because of their resemblance to these objects. The middle ear is connected to the upper rear part of the throat by the *eustachian tube,* and with the *mastoid cells* inside the skullbone just behind the outer ear. The inner ear contains the *semicircular canals* (or *labyrinth*), which are essential to our sense of balance, and the *cochlea* in which nerves carry the sounds from the outer world to the brain.

The outer and middle ear are *conducting* mechanisms which convey sound waves to the cochlea. The cochlea of the inner ear, shaped like a shell, contains the nervous elements—the sound receptors.

Sound is the result of vibrations in the air, and it has *pitch, intensity,* and *timbre.*

The pitch refers to the number or frequency of vibrations per second and explains why all the notes on a piano sound different. The human ear discriminates frequencies as low as 20 and as high as 20,000, although some animals pick up much higher frequencies.

The intensity, or loudness of sound, is measured by an arbitrary unit, called a *decibel.* A whisper made 4 feet away corresponds to 20 decibels; normal conversation at 20 feet is rated at 50 decibels; a

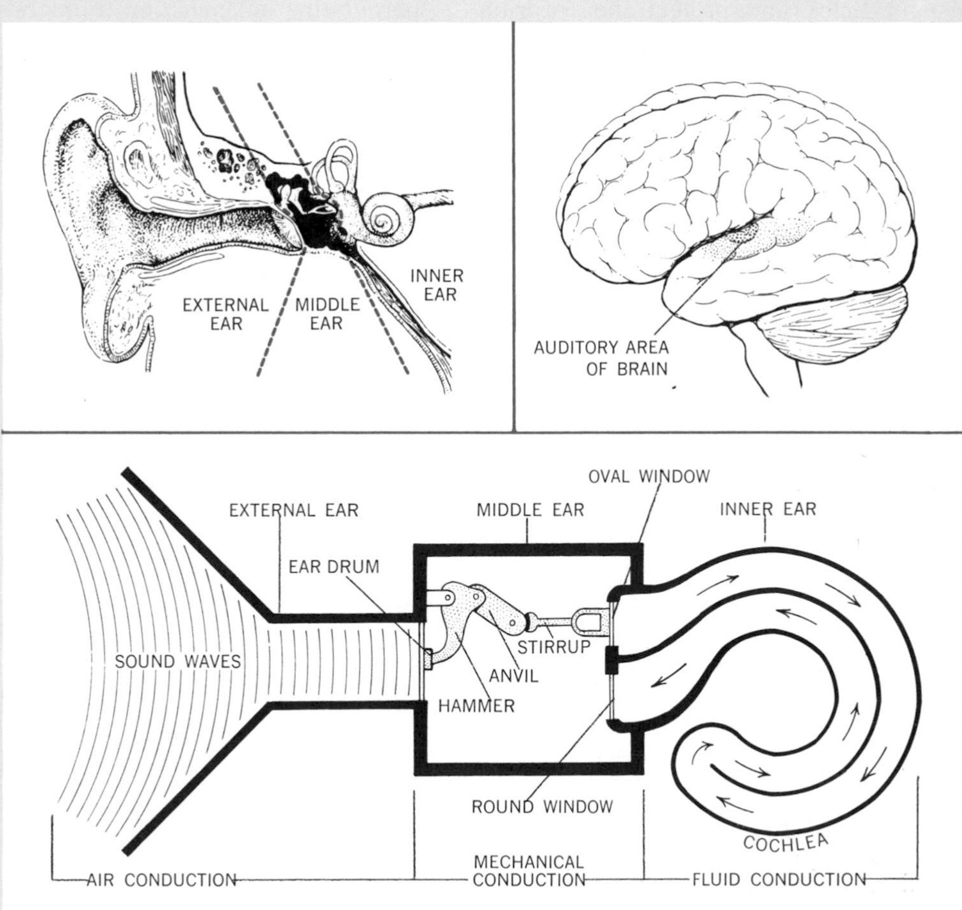

As sound is conducted from the external ear to the inner ear, the sound waves undergo considerable transformation. The eardrum, the ossicles, and the cochlea act as a mechanical transformer to concentrate the sound waves so that they can be picked up by nerve endings in the inner ear and transmitted to the brain.

pneumatic drill produces a sound intensity of about 120 decibels.

The timbre of sound refers to its quality and various overtones. Timbre explains why vibrating instruments, like the violin, piano, and accordion, as well as human voices, all sound different.

The outer ear is shaped to catch sound waves and direct them into the ear canal. This is why a dog cocks his ears. Many animals still possess the ability to turn the outer ear to the source of sound. But except for those distinguished individuals who can still wiggle their ears, we have lost this faculty. The muscles are still there, but they are rudimentary, evolutionary vestiges in most of us.

The skin lining of the ear canal is rather hairy. These hairs and the wax secreted into the ear are very important: they catch dust particles and protect the eardrum.

The ear canal directs the sound toward the eardrum, which is a thin, tough, slightly rounded membrane, separating the middle and the outer ear. Because it is thin and flexible, it vibrates with the sound waves, and can transmit these vibrations to the three small middle ear bones, the hammer, anvil and stirrup. (The scientific names for these bones are *malleus, incus,* and *stapes.*)

When these tiny bones are set into vibration, they can transmit the vibration to the inner ear. The stirrup, or stapes, which is attached to a membrane which covers and protects the fluid in the inner ear, is responsible for this task.

The stapes vibrates and sends the vibration across the membrane of the inner ear. It passes through the fluid there by waves, and then reaches special nerve endings. The impulses are finally conducted to the *auditory nerve* which carries them to the brain where the impulse is identified as sound.

The Eustachian Tube

The eustachian tube connects the middle ear cavity with the mouth, and its major function is to equalize the pressure on both sides of the eardrum. When a plane climbs, the atmospheric pressure decreases; as the pressure in the middle ear increases, the eustachian tube is forced open, to equalize the internal and external pressure on the eardrum. When the plane descends, the atmospheric pressure is increasing, and the pressure in the middle ear will now be too low, until the eustachian tube opens to equalize this differential and relieve the unpleasant symptoms which develop. If we swallow periodically as we descend from higher levels in a plane, this forces the eustachian tubes to open more rapidly.

If the eustachian tube is clear, opening occurs automatically. But if the tubes are blocked, and they often are if you have a cold, equalization becomes difficult, and the external pressure on the eardrum may be painful and sometimes even dangerous.

Blocking of the eustachian tube in severe inflammatory conditions is sometimes hazardous to the middle ear because it permits the inflammation to migrate to the inner ear. The earaches we occasionally experience during colds develop when the eustachian tube is clogged and can't open to relieve pressure on the eardrum.

Balance and Equilibrium

One natural force we are normally not aware of is the magnetic pull of the earth's

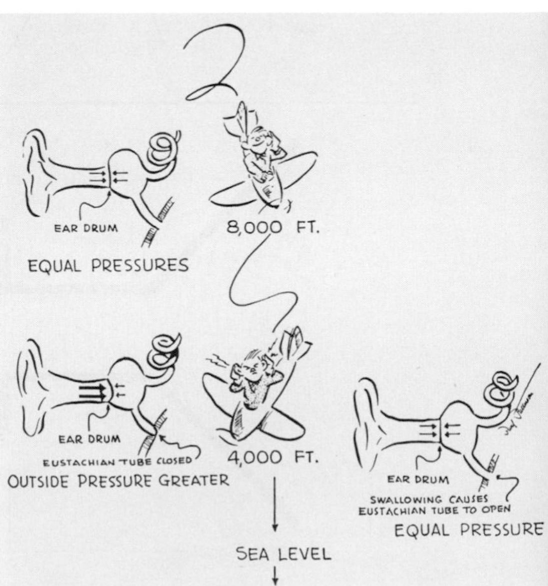

Figure 29–4. The function of the eustachian tube. (From Langley and Cheraskin: *The Physiology of Man.* New York, McGraw-Hill Book Co., Inc., 1954.)

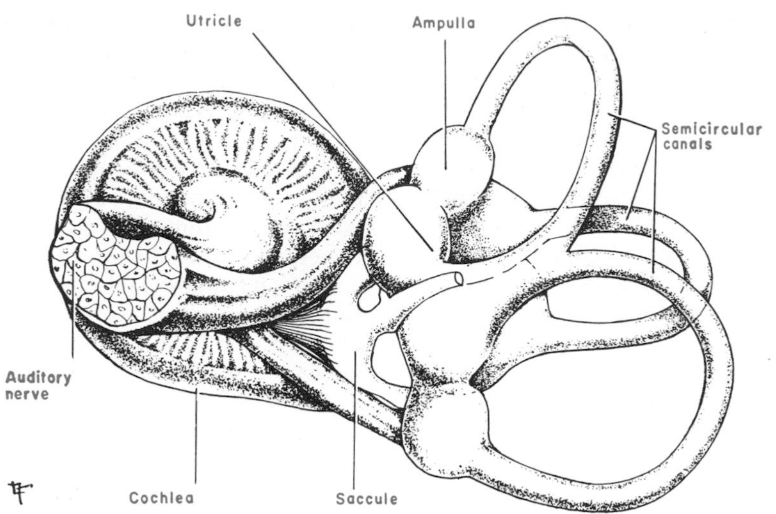

Figure 29–5. The nonacoustic labyrinths of the internal ear. Each of the semicircular canals lies in a plane perpendicular to the planes of each of the other two canals. (From Villee: *Biology*. 4th Ed., Philadelphia, W. B. Saunders Co., 1962.)

hard core. The only time we are conscious of it is when something goes wrong with the sensory organs which control our balance and equilibrium.

In addition to the cochlea, the inner ear contains several other structures–the *saccule, utricle,* and the *semicircular canals.* Together, these make up the *labyrinth* of the ear, so called because of its twisted shape. These structures connect via a nerve to the brain, and keep us upright against the pull of the earth's gravitational force; they also keep us in equilibrium when we are moving.

The saccule and utricle counteract the pull of gravity, and tell us which way is up or down. This may not always seem necessary, especially if you can see, but suppose you are swimming under water, or walking in complete darkness. Then you have to rely on these sensory organs of static equilibrium.

The working parts of the saccule and utricle are minute hair cells. Resting on top of these are the *ear stones,* or *otoliths,* which are actually concretions of calcium carbonate. These ear stones are extremely sensitive to gravitational pull, and act as a righting mechanism to keep us in the upright position.

The semicircular canals contain fluid and are arranged at right angles to one another–one in the horizontal plane, and the other two in the vertical plane, corresponding to the three planes in space. Whenever the head is tipped or rotated, the fluid moves and stimulates a nerve. This produces consciousness of the movement and reflex action to compensate for the rotation by moving the head in the opposite direction.

Under normal conditions, the fluid in the canals moves fast enough to maintain equilibrium. However, if there are rapid and continuous waves of motion, the canals may not be able to readjust rapidly enough. The result is motion sickness–and you can develop car sickness, air sickness, elevator sickness, sea sickness, train sickness, even swing sickness. Several good antimotion sickness medicines (such as Dramamine) are available today, but they must be taken well in advance.

How to Care for The Ears

Ear infections do not usually come from outside, but from the nose and throat via the eustachian tube. That is why inflamed tonsils and adenoids, a severe cold, sore throat or sinusitis are usually accompanied by a sense of pressure or pain in the ears.

Infection, especially in children, may spread up the eustachian tube into the middle ear.

If the middle ear becomes seriously infected, the hearing device may be destroyed. The infection may spread, causing rupture and destruction of the eardrum. It may continue into the mastoid cells, and unless checked there can enter the nearby brain and its covering. Children are very susceptible to middle ear infections. Before the development of sulfonamides and antibiotics, *mastoiditis* was a common and rightly dreaded disease, especially in children. Now these infections can be controlled successfully. Operations for infected middle ears and mastoids, so common until recent years, are seldom necessary today.

Infections which injure the hearing can also be caused by *foreign objects,* such as beads or pencil erasers, which very young children sometimes push into the ear canal. Adults can cause similar trouble by cleaning their ears with hairpins, match sticks or other long objects. Let a doctor clean wax out of your ears. There is a lot of sense in the old saying, "Never put anything smaller than your elbow into your ear."

Avoid violent nose-blowing. This sometimes leads to infection of the middle ear.

A *chronic running ear* is also an infected ear, and will respond to the proper therapy. If uncontrolled, it may lead eventually to deafness.

Swimming is rarely hazardous to the ears unless there is infection in the nose, sinuses or throat. Learning how to breathe in through the mouth and out through the nose when you are swimming will help prevent such infection. Occasionally the eardrum is perforated by the pressure of high diving. Although pain and bleeding sometimes result from this, a perforated eardrum does not necessarily cause permanent harm or hearing damage, if attended to.

Don't swim in stagnant waters and uninspected pools because infections can start from unclean water remaining in the ears.

Cosmetic Surgery of the Ears

Protruding or folded ears can be a source of great embarrassment, especially to young children, and should be corrected by plastic surgery. Children are born with ear deformities. They do not come about—as commonly believed—because an infant lies upon his ears and molds them.

The operative procedure is a very simple one: an elliptical section of skin and cartilage is removed from the angle between the ear and the skull.

For psychological reasons, the best time for such an operation is before the child starts school, where he would be subjected to the "big-ears" comments and jokes from his classmates. In terms of surgical efficiency, the optimum age for the operation is 13 or 14, when the ear has attained almost maximum size. However, this is a minor operation and can actually be done at any age—even on college students.

THE NOSE AND THROAT—SMELL AND TASTE

The nose, with its bones, cartilage, nerves, and mucous membranes (which contain glands secreting a watery fluid), is the organ of smell. Even more important, it is the means by which we take air into our bodies. We can (and some people do) get along by breathing through the mouth. Although this is not dangerous, the nose is a far better ventilator. It filters out dust, provides moisture, and acts as an air conditioner by warming the air before we take it into our lungs.

How We Smell and Taste

The sensations of smell and taste are very closely related. The *olfactory,* or smell, receptors, located in a crevice high up in the nasal cavity, are really an extension of the brain, much like the retina in vision.

One theory explains the sense of smell as a chemical process. We sniff in vapor-laden air, or it simply diffuses up into the nose, to reach the olfactory receptors. The vapors evolved from various substances are then thought to be dissolved in the fluid which bathes the olfactory membrane. Finally, the nerve endings in this

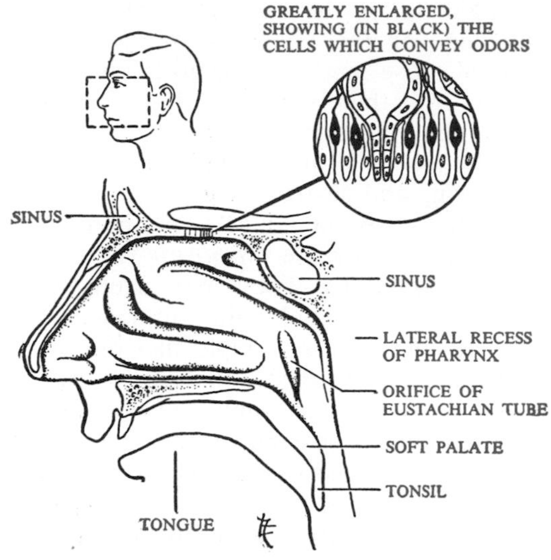

Figure 29–6. The nose.

membrane send a message to the brain which decides from experience what it is that we are smelling.

In animals, the sense of smell is very acute, far more highly developed than in man. It helps provide them with food and protection, and it is important in sexual activity, as well.

Even in man, smell is a highly developed sense. We learn to differentiate many different kinds of odors, and place most of them in one of the following classifications: fragrant (as in flowers), spicy (cinnamon), fruity or ethereal (oranges), resinous (pine or balsam), burnt (tar), and putrid (rotten eggs).

It is very unlikely that we have specific receptors for every odor we encounter, but the exact mechanism for differentiation of smells is poorly understood.

The threshold for smell varies with different materials and may be extremely low: we can smell 0.00000000004 ounce of vanilla vapor dispersed in a quart of air. Certain cheeses can be detected at almost as low a threshold.

Taste qualities are usually divided into four primary groups: bitter, sweet, sour and salt. However, many substances do not fall into any of these categories, and we can still taste them, and differentiate them from others, closely related. Try the blindfold test on pieces of raw potato and carrot.

The major receptors for taste sensations are the *gustatory neurons,* which end in specialized cells embedded in the taste buds of the tongue. However, taste buds are also found on the floor of the mouth, palate, pharynx, tonsils and the epiglottis. Here, again, as in smell, the taste bud is apparently excited and stimulated when it comes in direct contact with a *solution* of the material. We taste salt after it is *dissolved* in the mouth.

The sense of smell contributes strongly to taste sensations. This is why food loses so much of its flavor when we have a cold and our smell receptors are waterlogged and blocked. Hold your nose while you eat your next piece of Roquefort cheese. Most of the taste will be gone, and you will be left merely with a sensation of sharpness or tanginess.

It is possible to map the taste buds of the tongue fairly clearly. When we do this, we find that the tip is most sensitive to sweet substances, the sides to sour, the tip and sides to salt, and the back, to bitter. Perhaps this is why gourmets treat foods differently. They sip some foods slowly, hold some on the tip of the tongue and toss others to the back of the mouth. The brandy lover sniffs his brandy, then rolls it around his mouth.

To some extent, tastes depend on contrast. Milk and wine both taste a little acid if you drink them with a salad, because the salad dressing contains vinegar. The sweetness of foods is relative. Coffee tastes much more bitter if consumed with a very sweet dessert than when it is drunk with bland breakfast foods, like cold cereals.

Our threshold for tastes, as for smells, varies widely. Quinine is a very bitter medicine, and it tastes bitter even when diluted out to one part in a million. Sugar, on the other hand, is apparently much less sweet: at a dilution of 1 part in 200, it no longer imparts a sweet taste.

Although the tastes for most common foods are fairly universally experienced, the ability to taste certain chemicals varies among different individuals, and is inherited. This has led to the concept of a "tasting gene."

One substance widely studied from this point of view is the compound, phenylthiocarbamide, usually called PTC. A. L.

Fox reported that he once had occasion to prepare a fairly large quantity of this chemical. As he placed it in a bottle for storage, some of the fine particles were dispersed in the air as dust. One of his co-workers complained strongly of the bitter taste of the dust, which surprised Fox because he had inhaled a good deal of it and had not been conscious of a bitter taste. When Fox tested all the workers in his own and adjoining laboratories, he found a marked difference in their ability to taste PTC.[1]

This problem has interested geneticists, and extensive study of the taste of PTC by thousands of people suggests that it is related to heredity, as are many other biochemical reactions. Some people find it tasteless except in very high concentrations. A large number describe a very bitter taste, even in low concentrations.

Tonsils and Adenoids

The two tonsils are situated at the back of the throat, just above the level of the tongue. Normally, they are so small that they are barely visible, but when infected, they may swell until they almost fill the pharynx opening. Inflamed tonsils can cause sore throats and fevers, and may act as foci of infection which spreads to other tissues.

The *adenoids* may be considered to be small tonsils, located in the part of the throat behind the nasal passages. When they enlarge, they sometimes block the outlet from the nose so much that the affected person breathes chiefly through the mouth. Also, enlarged adenoids may block the eustachian tube which connects the middle part of the ear with the back of the throat. This condition may cause pain in the ears or a sense of pressure. It can also lead to infections in the middle ear, and, occasionally, interference with hearing.

In years past, tonsils and adenoids were removed almost routinely in all young children. However, in recent years, there has been a marked reversal in attitude toward this operation. It is *not* recommended unless the tonsils are chronically infected, or the adenoids interfere with normal nose and ear health. The chief reason for this is that both tonsils and adenoids are made up of *lymphoid tissue,* and lymph cells are actually beneficial in waylaying and destroying germs.

If the tonsils and adenoids are chronically infected, they are *harboring* instead of *destroying* germs. They may need to be removed. Fortunately, the surgical measures required are so simple that this is an extremely safe operation. Many physicians delay tonsillectomy and adenoidectomy as long as possible, however, because tonsil and adenoid tissue—like the thymus, another lymphoid tissue—usually shrinks spontaneously after about the tenth year of life.

The Sinuses

The *sinuses* are air spaces inside the bones of the face and skull, lined with mucous membrane, and communicating through tiny openings with the nasal cavity. The *frontal sinuses* are found in the bone above and behind the eyebrows; the *maxillary sinuses,* in the bones of the cheek beneath the eyes; the *ethmoid sinuses,* near the side of the nose and the inner portion of the eyes, and extending into the skull; and the *sphenoid sinus,* in the skull above the level of the throat.

The function of these hollow spaces is to lighten the weight of the head, and to increase the resonance of the voice.

Deviated or crooked septum refers to a deformity of the cartilagenous partition which separates the two sides of the nose. When the deviation interferes with breathing, or obstructs the openings into the sinuses, it has to be straightened out surgically.

Nasal polyps are grapelike growths within the nose which are thought to be allergic in origin. They are very common and nonmalignant, but they usually have to be removed if they obstruct breathing.

Care of the Nose and Throat

Perhaps the best possible advice about your nose and throat is not to do anything

[1]Fox, A. L.: *Proceedings National Academy Science, 18*:115, 1932.

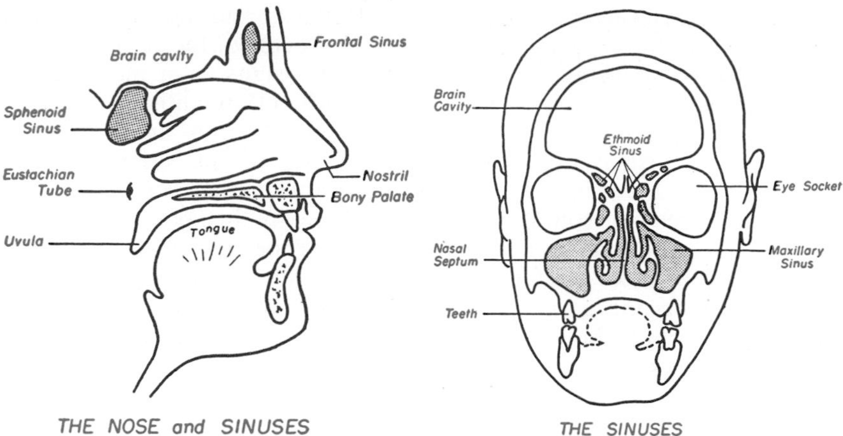

Figure 29–7. The nose and sinuses. (From Rothenberg, R. E.: *Understanding Surgery*. New York, Pocket Books, Inc., 1955.)

about it unless specifically directed by a doctor.

Don't use nose drops, sprays, gargles or inhalers, unless your doctor tells you to. They won't cure chronic sinusitis or postnasal drip or sore throats, and their continued use can cause irritation of the delicate mucous membranes. Gargles containing a mild analgesic agent (a painkiller) like aspirin are safe to use and may soothe a sore throat, but they won't cure it.

Blowing the nose, and blowing it hard, has been a time-honored remedy for colds, but it is very much overdone. Unfortunately, blowing hard is a very common cause of ear infections. If you try to clear a stuffed nose by blasting air through the nostrils, you increase the pressure in the back of your throat. This may open up the eustachian tubes connecting to the middle ear, and force mucus or pus into the middle ears, where bacteria can multiply and lead to middle ear infections. It is especially dangerous to blow the nose by closing one nostril, and blasting through the other one, or blocking both nostrils momentarily to build up an explosive force. The safest procedure is probably to wipe away the secretions which appear at the nostrils and not to blow at all.

Nosebleed

How to stop a *nosebleed* is an essential part of the first-aid information everyone should have. It may simply mean that a small blood vessel in the nose needs to be cauterized or packed. Your doctor can do this in a few minutes. On the other hand, nosebleeds in children are sometimes a sign of rheumatic fever. They may also herald the onset of typhoid fever. Contrary to popular notions, they are rarely caused by high blood pressure. If your nose bleeds frequently without any obvious cause, it requires your doctor's attention. A simple nosebleed may respond to the following measures: gently press the nostril closed; sit with head tilted forward, and apply an ice pack to the back of the neck and to the bridge of the nose.

Nose-picking may aggravate a weakened blood vessel and initiate bleeding.

Common Diseases of the Nose and Throat

Many diseases to which we are subject probably gain entry through the nose: influenza, tonsillitis, poliomyelitis, pneumonia, scarlet fever, and many others. A good deal of disease is transmitted through the air because people sneeze and spray out the organisms with which they are infected. Covering your nose and mouth during a sneeze is a kindness to your neighbor. You can reduce some infections which gain entry through the nose simply by observing ordinary hygienic measures such as frequent washing of the hands.

Various conditions can cause congestion of the nose, such as the *common cold,*[2] *hay fever* and *similar allergies, sinusitis, nasal polyps, chronic infections,* and a *deviated* or *crooked septum.*

Sore throats are almost as common as colds, for a certain amount of inflammation in the throat usually results from the cold itself. They may even be due to irritation caused by excessive smoking. If cutting down on your smoking and gargling with aspirin every two to three hours doesn't bring relief in a few days, visit your doctor or a hospital clinic.

Any *acutely sore throat* accompanied by fever may mean trouble. It may indicate the early stages of diphtheria, scarlet fever, a septic sore throat (an acute streptococcus infection), or a serious infection of the tonsils (tonsillitis). If these conditions are treated promptly, they can usually be cured just as quickly. You may wonder why your doctor gives you an injection or pills to swallow instead of applying something directly to the infected throat area. He does this because local applications do not reach the bacteria (they are below the surface), whereas medication taken internally attacks them through the blood stream. *Penicillin* works wonders in most throat infections. Be careful to avoid getting fatigued or chilled while you are recovering from a sore throat. These simple precautions may help prevent a serious illness, such as pneumonia or Bright's disease (a kidney disease), from developing.

Sinusitis develops when there is an inflammation of the mucous membrane lining the sinuses. It is usually caused by infections in the nasal cavity such as colds, but can also follow infections in the upper jaw, swimming or diving, injury to the bones containing the sinuses, or anatomical blocking of the sinuses. Sinus infections can be extremely painful, with unusual tenderness, severe headaches and sometimes fever.

Pus dripping from the back of the nose into the throat is responsible for the unpleasant condition called *postnasal drip.*

[2]Because the common cold is the commonest disease which afflicts mankind, it is discussed as a major nuisance ailment on page 187.

Redness and swelling of the inner parts of the eyelids, the portions near the nose, may be signs of a more serious form of sinusitis (ethmoiditis).

Sinus infections are usually diagnosed on the basis of the symptoms, by x-ray, or by transillumination of the sinuses. This is done by inspecting the sinuses with a very strong light in a dark room; if a particular sinus shows cloudiness and fails to light up, it means that an inflammation is present. It is usually treated by medicines which shrink the mucous membranes and by antibiotics. In extreme and chronic cases of sinusitis, surgical measures may be necessary.

Hoarseness is a sign that something may be wrong with your *larynx.* The larynx, which projects itself on the outside of the body as the Adam's apple, is part of the breathing apparatus. Its main function, however, is to act as a voice box in producing sounds. If you have been shouting and cheering at a football game the day before, the reason for the hoarseness is obvious. But if hoarseness or a change in your voice comes on without apparent cause, and lasts longer than a few days, it may indicate some potentially serious condition of the larynx.

You are probably familiar with a fairly common condition of the neck called *swollen glands.* This is an enlargement of the *lymph nodes,* usually called the lymph glands. If these glands are painful, it means that there is an infection somewhere in the head. It may be due to sore throat, tonsillitis, sinusitis or other types of infection, or stem from a cut or sore on the scalp. Relatively painless swollen glands may be caused by potentially serious illness, such as tuberculosis and Hodgkin's disease.

Plastic Surgery of the Nose

Tremendous progress has been made in the field of plastic surgery. For this we have evil to thank for good, because wars and accidents have accelerated the advance of plastic surgery.

Our modern concept of beauty focuses attention on the nose—its size, its shape and precise location in the middle of the face. Undoubtedly much of this emphasis is unwarranted, and a man or woman who is homely according to popular standards, whether because of nose, ears, mouth or eyes, can actually be vivacious, charming and very attractive. Yet certain individuals are born with, or develop through accidents, noses which are so disproportionately large or crooked that their whole lives are colored and shadowed by them. They feel they are ugly and unattractive, become shy and self-conscious as a result, and are often deeply unhappy. Sometimes the unhappiness is projected on society, and criminal or delinquent behavior results, largely because of these malformed features.

Plastic surgery can be very helpful in such situations—although it is not a cure-all for neuroses. It can be performed under local anesthesia, causes relatively little pain, and, if properly done, does not leave a visible scar.

THE SKIN AND ITS SENSATIONS[3]

The skin is the largest organ of the body—19 square feet in size and weighing about seven pounds. It has a variety of important functions. The first and most obvious of these is to serve as an envelope, a *protection* against germs and cold and the drying out of the body's vital fluids. The skin is resilient and tough enough to protect the soft underlying tissues from bruises and other mechanical injuries. In addition, it helps *regulate* the body's temperature by the evaporation of perspiration and by contracting or relaxing superficial blood vessels. It acts as a *sensory organ* because of its many nerve endings. It can *absorb* certain substances, and it also plays a part in the process of elimination.

Skin is made up of two layers, the outer (called the *epidermis* or *cuticle*) and the inner (the *dermis, corium,* or *true skin*). The amount of pigment in the inner layer determines whether skin will be black or yellow, brunette or blond. *Hairs* are epidermal growths, and *nails* are a modification of the epidermal cells. The *sebaceous glands,* which open into the *follicles* from which the hairs emerge, produce lubricating and protecting oils. The *sweat glands* lie coiled about in the dermis with ducts leading to the surface.

The skin has a tremendous power of rejuvenation, and is constantly being shed, little by little, and replaced. Also, it reflects the state of the body, as well as the state of the mind. You can plainly see when someone is blushing from embarrassment, or pale with fear, or showing the pallor of illness.

Skin Sensations and Receptors

The skin is an important sensory organ. Through it, we receive a great deal

[3]Care of the skin and skin diseases is discussed in Chapter 27.

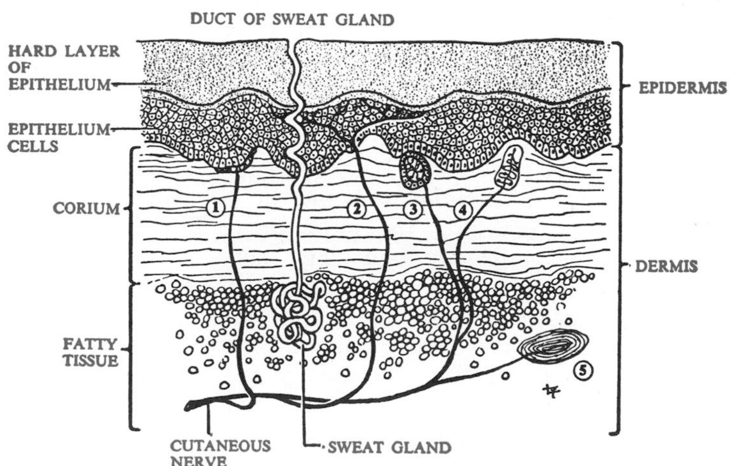

Figure 29–8. Structure of the skin. The numbers indicate the sensory nerve endings: **1,** warmth; **2,** pain; **3,** cold; **4,** touch; and **5,** deep pressure.

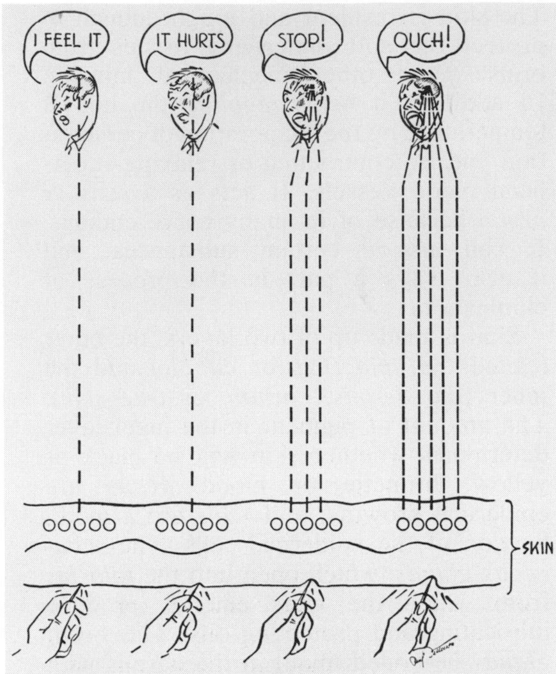

Figure 29–9. The mechanism by which change in intensity of stimulation is perceived. As the intensity of stimulation increases, more receptors become active and each receptor fires more rapidly. (From Langley and Cheraskin: *The Physiology of Man.* New York, McGraw-Hill Book Co., Inc., 1954.)

of information about our immediate surroundings. Our perception of warmth, cold, pain, touch, and pressure depends on intact, properly functioning sensory pathways in the skin.

Both skin layers contain nerve endings which respond to specific stimuli, such as cold, heat, and pain, The nerves involved are eventually bundled together and communicate with the spinal cord.

If your finger touches a hot stove, the sensitive nerve endings in the skin communicate to the spinal cord and then to the brain, which sends down the warning message: TAKE AWAY THE FINGER! The greater the stimulus, whether it is heat, cold or pressure, the more nerve endings are activated, and the more active your response. Also, some areas of the body are much more richly endowed with nerve endings than others. For example, the finger tips and the lips are far more sensitive to pressure and pain than the skin on the midarm and the back, or the ear lobe.

Nature's generosity in providing so many reactive nerve endings in the skin has a double purpose. It assures maximum protection against painful stimuli. Also, it makes us exceedingly sensitive to objects we touch. Think of the assurance a blind individual can gain by developing his sense of touch more highly. Without it, he could not even read Braille. The remarkable sculpture, fine sewing and other very delicate handwork made by sightless people all depend on delicate *kinesthetic* perception.

INTERNAL PAIN AND PRESSURE

Sensations of pain and pressure from the interior of the body are very common. For example, we can experience pain in the stomach, colon, bile duct or ureter; we are conscious of sensations in the muscles and joints, of hunger and thirst, of fullness in the bladder and rectum. However, these pain and pressure feelings differ somewhat from what you experience on the skin. You are apt to feel a dull ache rather than a sharp, highly localized pain. Internal pain is much less definitely localized, and there are probably fewer pain fibers. Also, internal pain nerves apparently respond to stimuli in a different way from the skin. It is possible to cut, tear, pinch, and even burn the meaty substance of almost any internal organs without producing pain.

It is interesting that the brain substance itself, generally thought to be so sensitive and so highly reactive, can be cut, pushed and stimulated in a variety of ways without any sensation of pain. During brain surgery, the coverings of the brain have to be desensitized with a local anesthetic because *they* are sensitive, but the brain substance itself can be operated upon *without any anesthetic.*

REFERRED PAIN

Sometimes a pain which originates in one area is felt in a completely different, perfectly healthy part of the body. This is called *referred pain.* For example, some visceral pain is felt on the skin. Heart pain can radiate into the arm or the shoulder or can mimic the pain of an intestinal upset. Patients with sinus infection sometimes get severe aching in the teeth because of referred pain; on the other hand, a toothache may cause a headache or a pain in the neck.

The reason for these referred pains from internal organs or tissues is not too clear. The most likely explanation is that the pain sensations from one area spread into the neurons that normally conduct pain sensations from another area, and we end up by being confused about the original source of the pain.

LOSS OF SENSORY RESPONSES

In certain diseases, there is a partial or complete loss of sensitivity to stimuli like pressure, pinprick, heat and cold, which are ordinarily very painful. This occurs in the condition called *syringomyelia,* because there is destruction of the nerve fibers in the spinal cord. Similar sensory losses can also be a symptom of neuritis, tumors of the spinal cord, multiple sclerosis and some severe emotional disturbances and hysterias.

Questions

1. "Keep your senses about you" is no idle command. What is the importance of our senses to normal behavior? to the learning process?
2. Describe how the eye and the ear function.
3. In animals, certain senses are more heightened than in humans, but humans too can increase the sensitivity of hearing if they are deprived of sight. How do you think this occurs?
4. What is "color-blindness," and how is it related to the sex of the individual?
5. Differentiate *myopia, hyperopia, astigmatism* and *strabismus.*
6. What is the best illumination for close work to prevent eyestrain? Why is it hard on the eyes to watch television in a completely darkened room?
7. Why does blocking of the eustachian tube cause a temporary deafness?
8. Do you think you could taste a completely insoluble substance?
9. What is the function of tonsils, adenoids and other types of lymphoid tissue?
10. Why do we have sinuses, and what causes sinusitis?
11. Name four functions of the skin.
12. How does the skin control some protective voluntary movements?
13. What is the difference between *sebaceous* and *sweat* glands?
14. What does *referred pain* mean?

Topics for Discussion

Reactions of the senses to space travel.
Eye versus camera.
Contact lenses.
Hearing aids.

Reading Suggestions

The Sense of Smell, Roy Bedichek. Doubleday, New York, 1960. A brillant discussion of olfaction in humans and lower animals. Very comprehensive and very readable.

The Truth About Your Eyes, Derrick Vail. Collier Books, New York, 1962 (paperback). A detailed description of your eyes and how to care for them. Written by a physician for laymen.

The Senses, Wolfgang Von Buddenbrock. University of Michigan Press, Ann Arbor, 1965. A well written paperback describing the senses and their combined action.

You and Your Brain, Judith Groch. Harper & Row, New York, 1963. A simplified but accurate description of the human brain. Especially good for the nonscience student.

Structure and Function in Man, Stanley W. Jacob and Clarice A. Francone. W. B. Saunders, Philadelphia, 1965. A basic textbook in integrated anatomy and physiology. It contains a very up-to-date discussion of the senses. Well illustrated.

Perceiving the World Around You, In *The Wonderful Human Body,* The American Medical Association, 1961. A very readable discussion of the senses. Well illustrated.

Function of the Human Body, Arthur C. Guyton. W. B. Saunders, Philadelphia, 1964. A very readable college level physiology book. Good description of the physiology of the senses.

Common Diseases of the Ear, Nose and Throat, Phillip Reading. 3rd Ed., Little, Brown & Co., Boston, 1961. A well written synopsis of some diseases that all laymen should be acquainted with.

SECTION NINE

SPECIAL CONSIDERATIONS

30

HANDLING EMERGENCIES THAT THREATEN LIFE

Any of us, at any time, can be confronted with a situation in which the application of first-aid principles may save our own life or some other person's. The five major emergencies in which first aid can be life-saving are *severe bleeding, suffocation, heart stop* (cardiac arrest), *poisoning, and shock.*

Two basic rules apply in all serious emergencies: (1) Never lose your head. This is a time for quick, clear thinking and decisive action. If the sight of severe bleeding makes you so shaky that you forget what to do, sit down for a minute with your head between your legs until you can recover enough to carry out the necessary measures. (2) Summon help. Call a doctor, the police, or the nearest hospital as soon as possible after first aid has been given. Better still, try to get someone else to call while you are treating the injured.

BLEEDING AND HEMORRHAGE

The danger from a severe cut or wound arises from the possibility of fatal blood loss. The simplest and most effective way to stop bleeding is direct pressure on the wound with a gauze pad, or better still, a thick compress of gauze. In an emergency, any clean cloth will do, and if bleeding is serious, you may have to use your bare hands. Direct pressure on the wound (or in the wound if it is very wide) will stop nine of ten cases of bleeding. Hold the dressing firmly in place for a few minutes. If no blood soaks through, bind the gauze or cloth with tape or strips of cloth.

If the bleeding is in an arm or leg, it helps to raise the limb higher than the body, because there is less blood in an elevated limb.

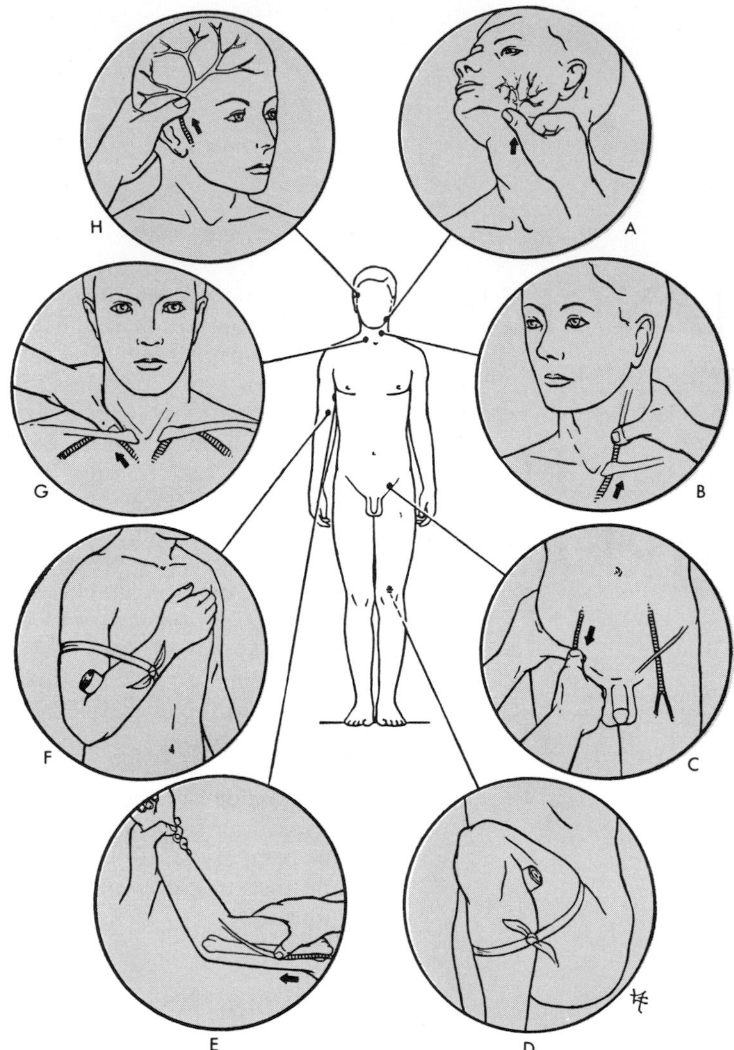

Figure 30–1. Pressure points on arteries. The arrows show the direction in which the blood flows through the arteries. Pressure points are located between the wound and the heart. **A,** For bleeding from face. **B,** For bleeding from head and face. **C,** For bleeding from leg (the inguinal ligament is shown as it passes over the artery). **D,** For bleeding from below knee. **E,** For bleeding from arm. **F,** For bleeding from below elbow. **G,** For bleeding from shoulder and entire arm. **H,** For bleeding from scalp and upper part of head.

Bleeding is different in arteries and veins. Blood from a *vein* flows steadily; it is dark in color, almost a bluish-red. *Arterial* blood is bright red and comes out in spurts, caused by the heartbeat. Venous bleeding can always be stopped by direct pressure on the wound, and although this does not staunch arterial bleeding in every case, it should be tried first. If it fails, press your finger or hand over the nearest pressure point shown in Figure 30–1.

Warning Against Use of Tourniquet

The authors mention the tourniquet primarily to discourage its use. It is only in very rare cases that its application is ever justified. It is dangerous to apply, causes tissue damage and gangrene if left on, and may cause shock if it is removed. Remember, evenly applied direct pressure is all that is needed to control most bleeding cases. However, if all else fails, you may have to use a tourniquet. The material selected for a tourniquet should have a flat surface and be an inch or more in breadth. Apply it above the site of the injury within half an inch of the wound. Tighten the tourniquet until blood flow stops, and leave it in place until medical assistance arrives. Never cover a tourniquet with bandages or blankets. Leave it in the open, where it can be seen by the doctor and where you can get to it.

A tourniquet is indicated in any case in which the accident causes loss of a limb. In such cases, the amputated part of the body should be sent to the hospital with the victim.

ASPHYXIA (SUFFOCATION) AND CARDIAC ARREST (HEART STOP)

Sudden cessation of breathing or of the circulation of the blood constitutes an emergency of the very highest order. Fortunately, it is now possible for anyone with a little training to institute artificial respiration or artificial circulation. In fact, it is possible to carry out both these life saving procedures at once if the circumstances demand it.

Asphyxia. Asphyxia is due to shortage of oxygen, and the sensations are those of choking or suffocation. Breathing is difficult, and sometimes the asphyxiated person is not breathing at all. However, even if breathing stops, the heart continues to beat for a few minutes. If you can apply artificial respiration successfully you may save a life in cases of electric shock, drowning, or any other accident in which breathing stops.

To combat asphyxia, you should begin artificial respiration at once. This is accomplished by forcing air from your own lungs into the victim's mouth, allowing him to exhale naturally. The following steps should be taken:

1. *Place the victim on his back and pull his jaw up and back.* The front of the neck should be stretched and the head tilted definitely backward to open the airway. This procedure alone will allow some victims to breathe if the mouth is open.

2. *Insert your thumb between the victim's teeth and open the mouth, but not wide.* You must be able to cover it completely with your own mouth. Clear the mouth and throat of any obstructions.

3. *Pinch shut the victim's nose and place your mouth tightly over his mouth.* If the victim is a child, you may place your mouth over both his mouth and nose. Blow forcefully into the victim's mouth—more gently if it is a very young child. During the first minute, blow quite rapidly, then slow down to 20 times a minute for young children. With older children and adults, blow air in only 12 times a minute.

4. *As soon as you see the chest expand, remove your mouth so that the unconscious victim can exhale passively;* then repeat the cycle of breathing. In young children, it may be necessary to press the abdomen gently to prevent too much air from accumulating.

5. *When the victim begins to breathe by himself, continue to assist him by blowing in as he inhales.*

6. *Don't give up too soon.* Fortunately, this technique can be kept up for many hours, because it takes very little energy.

Cardiac Arrest. This term means that the heart has stopped beating. Artificial respiration is of no value in this instance, because the blood cannot deliver oxygen to the tissue. The blood must be circulated by artificial means.

Artificial circulation is based on the principle of squeezing the heart between the rib cage and the spine. The following steps should be taken:

1. *Place the victim on his back and kneel on one side of him.*

2. *Place the heel of one hand directly over the victim's breastbone* (sternum) in the center of his chest. Now place the heel of your other hand on top of the first hand. The fingers do not touch the chest wall; all the pressure is transmitted through the heels of the two hands.

3. *To start circulation, push the breastbone toward the spine for a distance of about 1½ to 2 inches;* then release. Repeat this procedure at a rate of 60 times a minute.

If two people are available and if the

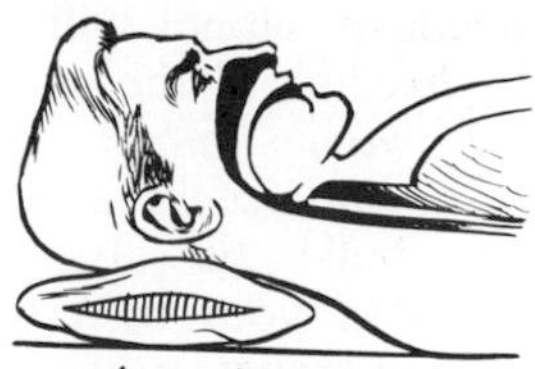

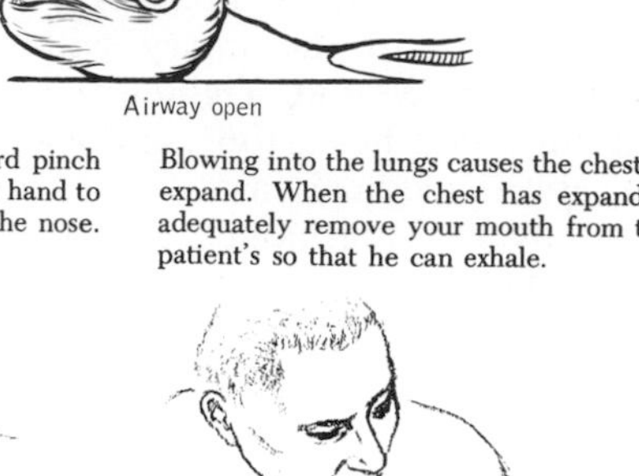

Place one hand under the patient's chin and the other on top of his head. Lift up on the chin and push down on the top of the head to tilt the head backwards.

Put the thumb of the hand under the jaw into the patient's mouth; grasp the jaw and pull it forward.

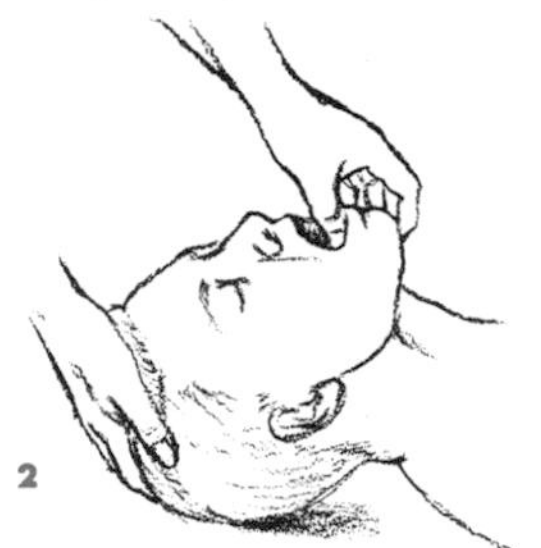

While holding the jaw forward pinch the nostrils closed with the other hand to prevent leakage of air through the nose.

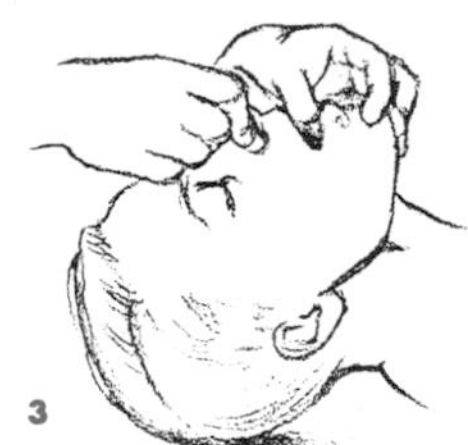

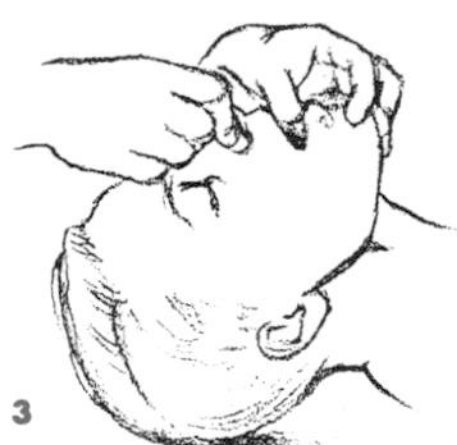

Take a deep breath; place your mouth tightly over the patient's and blow forcefully into his lungs.

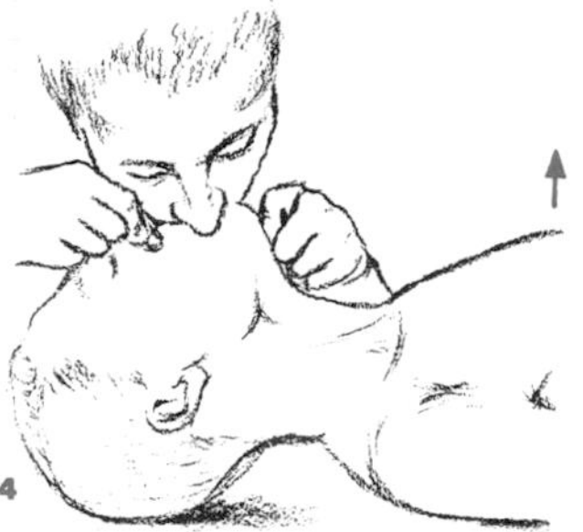

Blowing into the lungs causes the chest to expand. When the chest has expanded adequately remove your mouth from the patient's so that he can exhale.

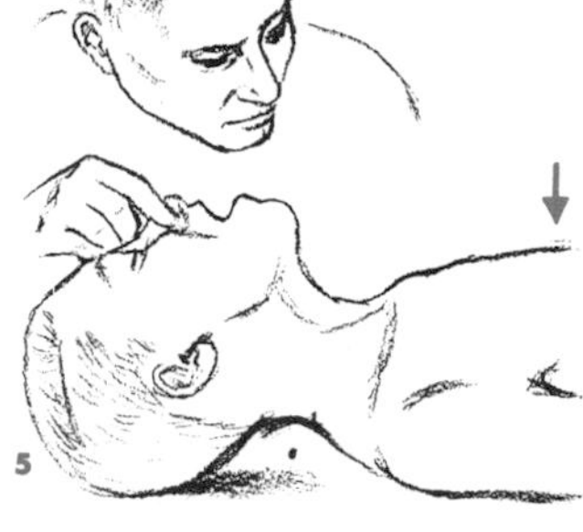

Repeat this sequence of maneuvers every 3 to 4 seconds until other means of ventilation are available.

If you cannot open his mouth blow through his nose. In infants cover both mouth and nose with your mouth. Blow gently into a child's mouth, and in infants use only small puffs from your cheeks.

TECHNIQUE OF ARTIFICIAL RESPIRATION BY MOUTH-TO-MOUTH METHOD

(Nealon)

Figure 30–2.

conditions warrant it, one should instigate artificial circulation and the other artificial respiration. When your efforts are effective:

1. The pupils of his eyes will constrict.
2. The victim's bluish color will change to his normal color.
3. A carotid pulse wave (on the side of the neck) must occur with each compression of the heart.
4. The victim may move or start to breathe.

In the event that you find yourself alone with a victim who has no circulation or respiration, it will be necessary to compromise the procedures just outlined:

1. *Quickly ventilate the lungs three times.*
2. *Apply manual heart compression 15 times.*
3. *Ventilate the lungs two times.*
4. *Compress the heart 15 times.*
5. *Repeat this cycle continuously.*

If you find it necessary to administer either artificial circulation or respiration, be sure that you remain with the victim until a doctor arrives or until the victim reaches a hospital. This is necessary because respiration or circulation may stop again.

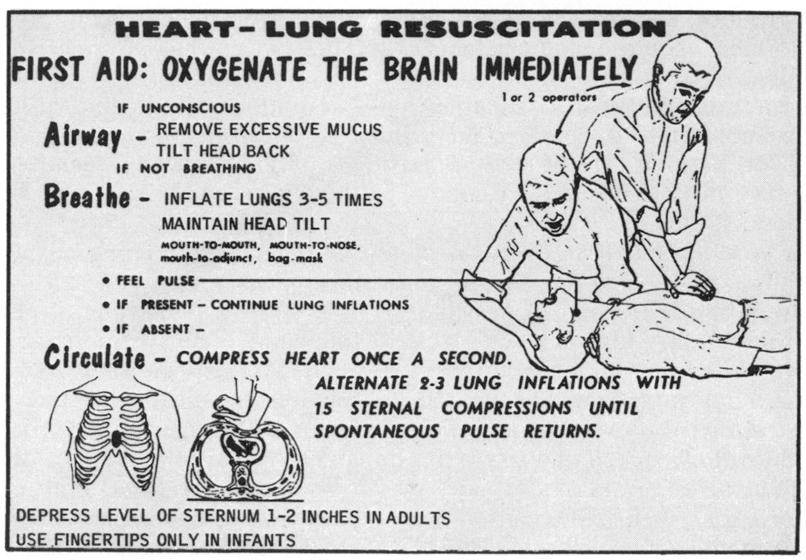

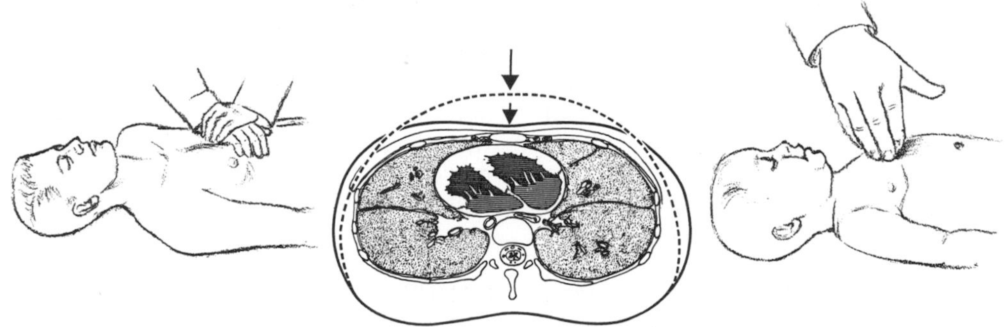

TECHNIQUE OF RESUSCITATION BY CLOSED CHEST CARDIAC MASSAGE
(Kouwenhoven, Jude, and Knickerbocker. J.A.M.A. 173:1064, 1960.)

Figure 30–2. (Cont'd)

POISONING

Three essential procedures in poisoning are:

1. *Always save the container and any remaining poison.* Take both to the doctor or the hospital in case it is necessary to identify the poison before specific treatment can be started.

2. If someone has taken a poison that is an acid or alkali (this includes lye), *he should be forced to drink as much water as possible* to dilute it before it can corrode tissue. The water should be followed by milk, olive oil, or egg white. Do not induce vomiting because heaving may rupture an already weakened esophagus. This is also the treatment for persons who have swallowed kerosene and gasoline. These products are not very dangerous if they are merely swallowed and retained in the stomach. The danger arises if they are drawn into the lungs, and this may easily occur during vomiting.

3. For almost all other types of poisons, you should try to *induce vomiting as soon as possible* by placing your finger down the victim's throat. If this isn't successful, dissolve two tablespoons of salt in a glass of warm water and force this salty water

down to produce nausea and vomiting. Keep forcing liquids and inducing vomiting for half an hour to wash out the stomach, and continue this treatment even while the victim is being taken to the doctor or hospital. If the poison is unknown, save the vomitus. Call a doctor *after* you have started first aid.

Someone who has taken an overdose of sleeping pills should also be forced to drink water and made to vomit, if possible. If he is conscious, give him as much black coffee as he will drink; if he is drowsy, walk him around until he wakes up. *He needs immediate medical attention and preferably hospital care if he is unconscious and cannot be aroused.*

Food poisoning is usually caused by bacterial contamination, but toadstools or poisonous mushrooms, certain berries, and shellfish and other foods which have "spoiled" or have been improperly canned can also be highly toxic.

The symptoms are usually acute and come on soon after eating the contaminated food. They may include pain or tenderness in the abdomen, nausea, vomiting, diarrhea, weakness, and in mushroom poisoning, dimness of vision and behavior resembling alcohol intoxication.

The stomach should be washed out with large quantities of water as in other types of poisoning. However, excessive vomiting should be avoided because it is so exhausting. Keep the patient warm and give him strong coffee or tea as a stimulant. Find a doctor as soon as possible, especially if toadstools, poisonous berries, or tainted shellfish have been eaten. Poisoning due to improperly canned food *(botulism)* is less apt to be fatal, but medical treatment is still necessary.

SHOCK

Shock may follow any accident, especially one that is extremely painful or involves a considerable loss of blood. An individual in shock becomes very pale, and his skin feels cold and clammy. He breathes rapidly and his pulse beat is faster than normal, but faint. Partial or complete unconsciousness may develop, and severe shock can result in death. These symptoms are not usually seen in a person who has merely fainted.

To prevent shock and speed up recovery:

1. *Keep the victim lying quietly with his feet higher than his head* (except where there is a head injury), and cover him with warm blankets.
2. *If he is fully conscious, give him warm drinks.*
3. *Stop any bleeding,* if possible. Shock following major hemorrhage, automobile accidents or gunshot wounds usually requires medical aid and blood transfusions. However, if you can reduce blood loss, you may prevent a fatal outcome.
4. *Try to relieve the pain.* Fracture pains can be agonizing. If no pain-stopping medicine is available, talk reassuringly to the patient, and hold his hand. This may rally his vital forces enough to delay the onset of acute shock. Unless it is an absolutely critical situation and no help can be brought to the scene of the accident, *don't move a patient with a severe fracture* without expert help. If you find you must move him, try to construct a splint such as that shown in Figure 30–3.

OTHER EMERGENCIES THAT THREATEN LIFE

Flaming Clothes or Hair

Pour water on the victim if it is readily available, but don't go for water if it is not handy. Take a rug, coat, or blanket and smother the flames. If you try to beat out the flames with your hands, you may injure the burned person, as well as yourself.

Contact with Live Electric Wire

The key safety theme in this accident is *dryness.* Never pull the victim off without precautions, because you may be electrocuted, too. You must provide perfect insulation before you attempt to remove anyone connected to a high voltage wire, because electricity passes rapidly through

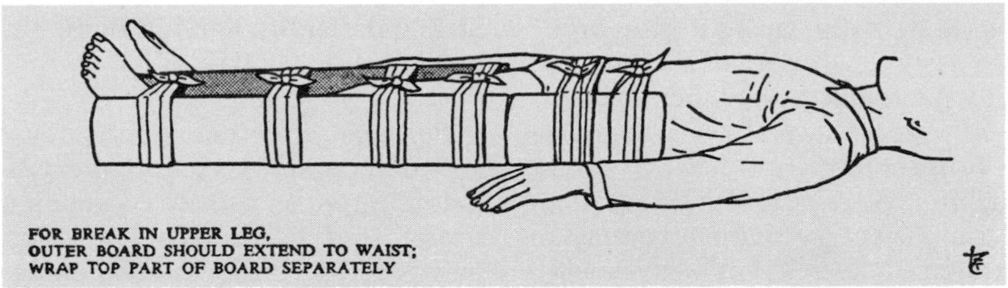

Figure 30–3. Splinting the leg.

water or moist articles. Stand on something dry, and use perfectly dry sticks, newspapers, or gloves over your hands.

Sunstroke or Heatstroke

High fever, dizziness, headache, dry, hot skin, red face, and rapid pulse are the usual symptoms, but unconsciousness may develop in severe sunstroke or heatstroke.

The first thing to do is to *call a doctor.* Then put the victim in a cool place, and loosen his clothing. Apply cold water over the body quickly and in large quantities to reduce the fever; use a garden hose (gentle stream, not full force) or place him in a bathtub of very cold water.

Snake Bite

Poisonous snakes native to the United States include the rattlesnake, the copperhead, the cottonmouth moccasin, and the coral snake. Of these, the coral snake causes the least trouble. It seldom attacks

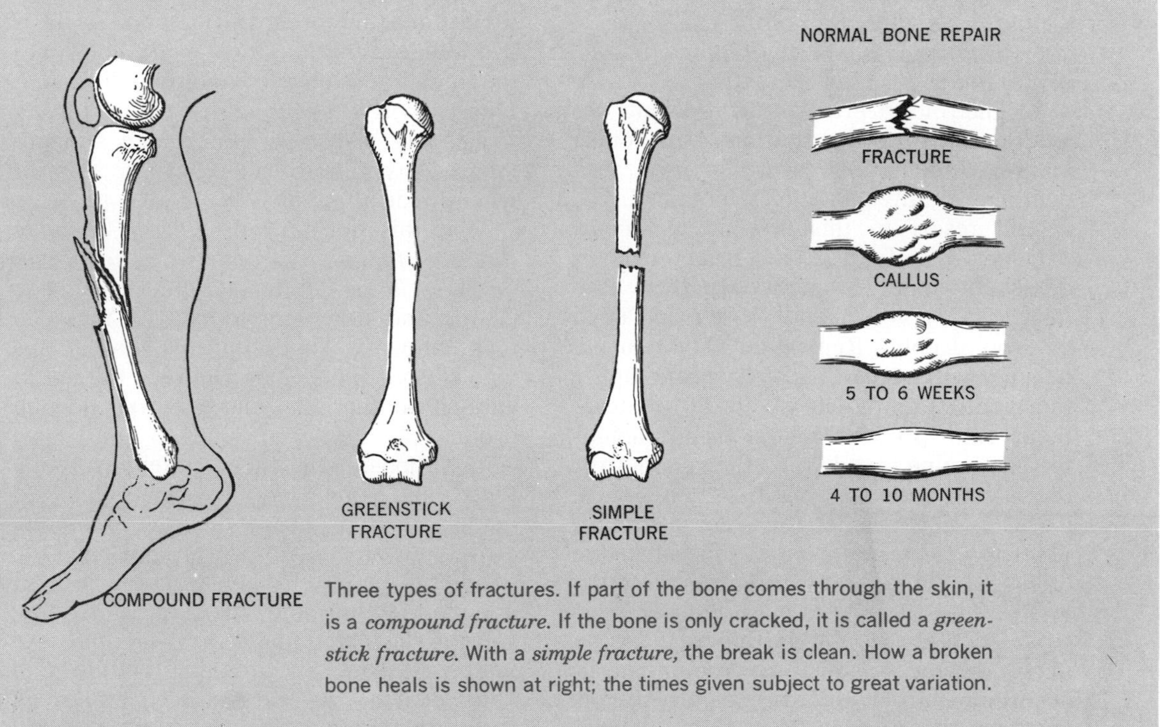

Three types of fractures. If part of the bone comes through the skin, it is a *compound fracture.* If the bone is only cracked, it is called a *greenstick fracture.* With a *simple fracture,* the break is clean. How a broken bone heals is shown at right; the times given subject to great variation.

unless provoked; even then, it can only hold on to a very small part of the human body such as the toe. But the other snakes, which are pit vipers, may attack when not provoked. Fortunately, however, a polyvalent antivenin is available against the poisons of these vipers. Anyone planning a trip into a snake-infested country should take antivenin with them and learn how to inject it. It is reassuring to know, however, that only 10 per cent of the persons bitten by pit vipers die even when not treated.

In case of poisonous snake bite (if the bite is poisonous there will be immediate pain and swelling, and the skin will turn purple):

1. *Stop activity at once.*
2. *Apply a constriction bandage above the bite.* This should be applied only tightly enough to impede venous and lymphatic drainage. It is not a tourniquet and should not occlude the arterial blood supply. It should be released 1 minute of every 30 minutes until antivenin can be administered. The compression should be reapplied further from the wound if swelling progresses.
3. *Ice should be applied directly to the wound to localize the venom.*
4. *Antivenin should be obtained as soon as possible.*
5. The older practice of opening the wound and applying suction is no longer employed by doctors. However, if neither a doctor nor antivenin can be obtained, you should resort to this first-aid technique.

Using a knife or razor blade, make a cross cut about 1/4 inch deep over each fang mark. Avoid blood vessels and don't cut too deeply. Remember that you are dealing with venom in body tissue, not in the blood stream. The object of this technique is to prevent venom from reaching the circulating blood. Suck the venom from the wound with a first-aid suction device; if this is unavailable, use your mouth. If you use your mouth, spit out the sucked-in fluid frequently. The venom is harmless if swallowed unless you have cuts or open sores in your mouth. If this is the case, avoid sucking, because the venom can be absorbed into your own blood stream. Keep up the suction for at least an hour.

Strangulation by Foreign Body in Throat or Glottis

Perhaps no other emergency calls for so much coolness and judgment as strangulation. Suppose you are eating dinner with a friend, and he swallows a large piece of meat the "wrong way," catching it in the glottis, the upper part of the windpipe. If he is lucky, nature will bring it up in a violent fit of coughing. But sometimes even coughing doesn't dislodge it, and he begins to choke. If no doctor or hospital is near enough at hand, what should you do?

1. While you are trying to remove the meat, have someone *call the police and explain the emergency.* If the glottis is completely obstructed, you have very little time because the human body can tolerate oxygen deprivation for only about 15 minutes, at most.
2. *If you can see the tip of the obstructing object* (with the help of a flashlight or lamp, if necessary), *try to grasp it* with your fingers, or crook your little finger around it. Then *pull.* Don't *push,* because this will only make the situation worse. If this doesn't work, try the nearest substitute for forceps—tweezers, a beer can opener, anything that might hook into the meat and enable you to pull it out. Don't worry about cutting the throat. Your only task is to relieve the strangulation. Any minor bleeding can be stopped when medical aid arrives.
3. If this doesn't work, *try to dislodge the obstruction by combined gravity-pull and coughing.* Put the victim nearly upside down, and urge him to cough. You can help him by squeezing his lower ribs vigorously. This may loosen the meat enough so that you can grasp it and pull it out.
4. Suppose all these attempts have failed, and your friend is turning blue. No medical help is heard on your doorstep. Now you must say a prayer, and open the windpipe below the obstruction. Forget about infection and bleeding. *Take the sharpest steel implement you have*—a knife, scissors, or anything with a real cutting edge—*and get to work.* If possible, have someone pull the head back to stretch

the neck. Your target is the hard "pipe" you feel below the Adam's apple. Cut horizontally if you can find the open space between the rings of cartilage. If not, just make an opening in any way you can. When you have succeeded, you will hear air being sucked in. Make the opening sufficiently large so that air comes in freely enough to restore the person's normal color.

Never attempt this drastic procedure unless you are sure that (a) the person has really inhaled a foreign body, (b) it cannot be dislodged, (c) no medical help can be obtained immediately, and (d) the air stoppage is so complete that the person is suffocating.

Questions

1. Why does blood spurt from a cut artery? Contrast the color of arterial and venous blood.
2. When should you apply a tourniquet?
3. Describe at least four major emergencies in which first aid can save a life.
4. Name some causes of food poisoning.
5. Describe the mouth-to-mouth technique for artificial respiration.
6. How do you remove a person from contact with a live wire?
7. What is the difference between heat *stroke* and heat *exhaustion?*
8. What is the recent change in thinking about treatment of snakebite?
9. How and when should you administer artificial circulation?

Topics for Discussion

First aid in burns.
First aid in animal and insect bites.
First aid for frostbite.

Reading Suggestions

Textbook in First Aid, American Red Cross. Doubleday & Co., Garden City, N. Y., 1957.

Family Guide to Emergency Health Care, U. S. Department of Defense and U. S. Department of Health, Education and Welfare, 1963. U. S. Government Printing Office, Washington, D. C. An up-to-date publication on family emergency care.

A New Fight Against Sudden Death, Ann Cutler. Look, Dec. 1, 1964, p. 44. An account of recent advances in resuscitation including artificial respiration and artificial circulation.

Home Health Emergencies, Equitable Life Assurance Society of the United States, New York. A guide to home nursing and first aid in family health emergencies.

First Aid Diagnosis and Management, W. H. Warren, *et al.* Appleton-Century-Crofts, New York, 1960. An informative guide to first aid.

Emergency Medical Guide, John Henderson. Blakiston, McGraw-Hill, New York, 1963.

First Aid Training, M. Fishbein and L. W. Irwin. Lyons & Carnahan, Chicago, 1961.

31

COMMUNITY HEALTH

Public health philosophy embraces human life from the preconception period until death; it considers the total environment of land, water and air; it includes all ways of life–urban, suburban and rural; it ignores no disease or condition antithetical to human welfare, and its area of concern includes the whole world. Space medicine promises soon to knock down even that boundary line.

HERMAN HILLEBOE

Because maintaining a healthy mind and body is so largely a personal responsibility, much of the emphasis in previous chapters has been on what each of us can and should do for his own sake. However, just as our world has grown larger, more complex, and more interdependent, so have the problems of health and the dangers to the individual grown beyond the ability of any one person, or even any small group, to control them. So individuals work together and communities develop services and safeguards for the sake of every individual.

Dramatic episodes fill the pages of medical history. A life saved by a new surgical technique, a baby given a chance to live by replacement of his blood, a piece of plastic inserted in place of a defective heart valve–impressive as such incidents are, even more significant are the activities of the many public health agencies and services, which may develop methods that help entire communities or nations avoid disease or disaster. On a personal basis, the special knowledge and skills of community health representatives many times have saved one man's life; in doing so, a community health agency has protected many more men, women, and children from a potentially serious health menace.

In this chapter, some health services are reviewed. Their scale of operation ranges from the international to the community, and their organization is official, professional, or voluntary. Their goal is the same in each instance–the protection of the individual and the attainment of the highest possible standard of health for everyone.

SAFEGUARDS TO OUR HEALTH

If there were not adequate control and purification of drinking water, we might

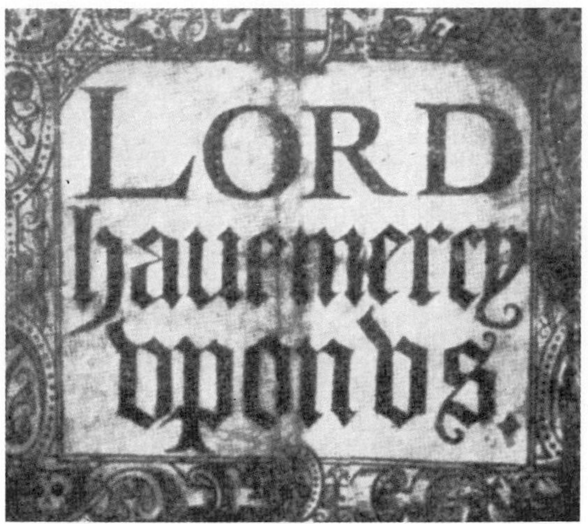

Figure 31–1. 16th century wood block used to mark houses stricken by plague.

soon return to the horror of seventeenth century London, so ravaged by polluted water that the death rate exceeded the birth rate. (In the United States today, the birth rate is nearly *two and one half times* the death rate.) Or we might suffer the fate of 6 million American Indians, half the total Indian population, who fell victims to smallpox in 1841 before the rigid enforcement of smallpox vaccination by public health officials. Even today smallpox persists in many areas of Africa, Asia, and South America—a day's journey to the United States by jet plane—but we are protected because public health laws stipulate that no one can enter the United States without a vaccination certificate.

Sometimes it is difficult to comprehend how many safeguards are provided for our health. You awaken in the morning when the alarm clock goes off, and walk to the bathroom still in the throes of sleep. But groggy or not, you have no fear about drinking a glass of water or brushing your teeth with it. In fact, you are so completely confident of its purity that you never even give it any thought, thanks to your municipal water purification plant. When you brush your teeth with a standard brand of toothpaste, you aren't worried about swallowing some potentially poisonous chemical because you know it has been certified as safe by the Food and Drug Administration of the Federal Government.

The oranges you eat for breakfast have undoubtedly been sprayed and perhaps even dyed to give them a more attractive color, but neither the spray nor the dye would be permitted by health authorities if it had toxic properties. The milk you drink is free of dangerous microorganisms because pasteurization is required by law in most communities, and the ham you enjoy with your eggs comes from inspected pigs. If you are having breakfast in a restaurant or college dormitory, the kitchens have undoubtedly been inspected by the municipal Board of Health and must therefore adhere to certain rules of cleanliness; if you live in a state with high health standards, the food-handlers, too, have taken periodic health tests to guarantee that they are free from tuberculosis and communicable diseases like typhoid.

On your way to class, you might pass the science building where radioactive isotopes are being used in research. It may never occur to you that this is potentially a very hazardous area, but there is no danger to you because rigid regulations control the disposal of all radioactive wastes.

Perhaps you need to consult a doctor because you've sprained your ankle in a tennis game, or visit your dentist for an aching tooth, and one of them writes a prescription which a pharmacist must fill. Whether you realize it or not, you're in good hands, because all these professional people must have demonstrated a desirable level of training and skill in order to be licensed to practice.

These are but a few examples of the efficient, seemingly automatic controls which make so many aspects of our lives in the twentieth century healthy and safe. The credit must go to the remarkably well organized health agencies throughout the nation and the world.

Three types of organizations carry on these activities—the *official* public health departments, which are supported through taxation and organized on an international, federal, state, or local basis; the *voluntary* agencies, maintained through fund-raising appeals or similar charitable sources, and controlled by groups of interested citizens, with the necessary full-time professional

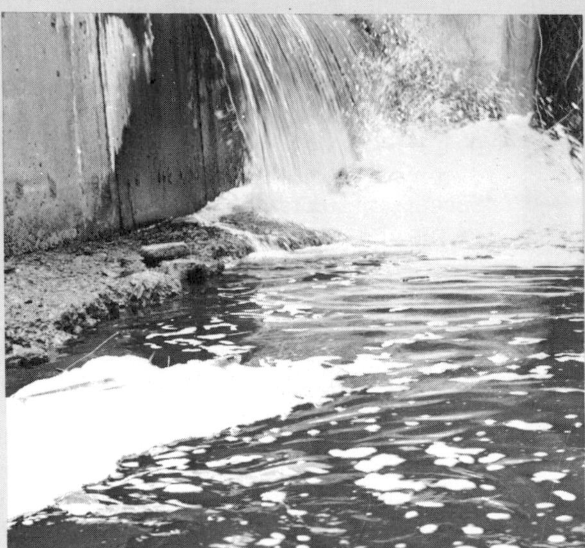

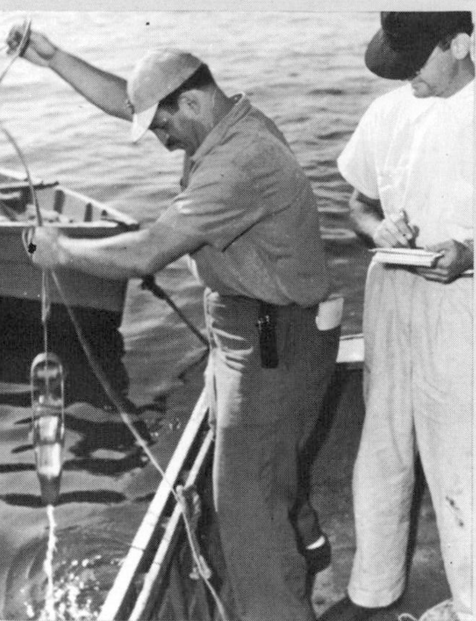

Foam floating on a small stream, left, is from household detergents, the chemicals of which are an increasing source of water pollution. At right, health experts take samples of water for laboratory testing, to determine the level of pollution in a public water supply.

personnel; and the *professional societies* in medicine and allied fields.

OFFICIAL HEALTH AGENCIES

World Health Organization

In a report made when he was a U. S. Senator, Hubert Humphrey praised the work of the World Health Organization and the valuable contribution the United States has made to it:

> In recent years, it has for the first time in the history of man become technically possible to obliterate, or hold under control, many of the historic scourges. The World Health Organization has played an invaluable role in this process. Despite limited financial resources . . . (it) has helped spearhead innumerable advances in health among nations. No country has done more for the health of the human family than the United States of America.[1]

Disease knows no boundary lines, national, racial, or religious, and the extraordinary importance of this in these days of high speed travel has finally been fully recognized in the establishment of the WHO. Even as early as 1831, the need for international cooperation in solving world health problems was the impetus for organizing the Egyptian Quarantine Board to prevent the spread of plague diseases through mercantile contacts between nations. The League of Nations Health Commission was founded in 1923, and despite a very small staff and minimal financial support, it succeeded in conducting excellent epidemiological surveys on disease and assisting in the health services of backward nations.

WHO was founded in 1948 as an outgrowth of the United Nations, and its constitution stresses these inspiring objectives:

Health is a state of complete physical, mental and social well-being, and not merely the absence of disease or infirmity.

The enjoyment of the highest attainable standard of health is one of the fundamental rights of every human being without distinction of race, religion, political belief, economic or social condition.

[1] *United States and the World Health Organization: Teamwork for Mankind's Well-Being,* U.S. Govt. Printing Office, Washington, 1959.

The health of all peoples is fundamental to the attainment of peace and security, and is dependent upon the fullest cooperation of individuals and States.

The achievement of any State in the promotion and protection of health is of value to all.

The membership and responsibilities of WHO have grown as the size of the United Nations itself has increased. At the end of 1963, WHO had 120 nation-members, and its budget for 1964, $34 million, was the largest in its history. WHO works from its international headquarters at the Palais des Nations in Geneva, Switzerland, through six regional offices—Brazzaville, Congo Republic, for Africa; Washington, D. C., for North and South America; New Delhi, India, for Southeast Asia; Copenhagen, Denmark, for Europe; Alexandria, United Arab Republic, for the Eastern Mediterranean, and Manila, the Philippines, for the Western Pacific.

WHO's efforts, valiant and effective as they are, cannot nearly meet the worldwide need. Nearly half the 3.3 billion people in the world are afflicted with preventable or curable chronic diseases, and millions die needlessly simply because the existing knowledge and techniques of modern medicine are not available to them. WHO operates to fill these needs and in fact works very efficiently with its modest allotment of funds. Its mission is formidable for many reasons, one of the most pertinent being the shortage of physicians and other trained medical personnel in much of the world. In the United States, we have one physician for about every 800 persons; in some areas of the world, the ratio is one physician for every 50,000 men, women, and children.

Specifically, the major aims of WHO are:

1. To strengthen the health services of member nations, improving the teaching standards in medicine and allied professions, and advising and helping generally in the field of health.

2. To promote better standards for nutrition, housing, sanitation, recreation, economic and working conditions.

3. To improve maternal and child health and welfare.

4. To advance progress in the field of mental health.

5. To encourage and conduct research on problems of public health.

When WHO was established, it assigned priority to the major killing and disabling diseases of member nations, working on an emergency basis, for two reasons. First, World War II left great areas devastated or at least deprived of adequate public health facilities and personnel. Second, the organization's funds were too limited for any but the most immediate needs. Now, however, WHO has moved from the emergency tasks of the immediate postwar period to long-range programs. Such programs are essential if the newly developing countries are to enjoy the benefits of new knowledge acquired during recent years, especially in more effective control over communicable diseases.

Some of the diseases on which WHO concentrates are little known to young Americans today. Others still are a health problem in the United States but much less so than they were a generation ago. WHO, for example, works to combat the following diseases:

Malaria. This is still a devastating disease, affecting 150 million persons every year and killing as many as 1½ million. WHO has made substantial progress in fighting malaria. In 1963 alone, this organization protected 44 per cent of the population in Southeast Asia previously exposed to malaria.

Communicable Diseases. Smallpox, typhus, yellow fever, leprosy, influenza, yaws, and tuberculosis are serious problems in many places. WHO has reduced the incidence of many of these diseases. The mortality from tuberculosis, for example, has been declining sharply in recent years, both as a result of advances in detection and treatment and through the work of WHO (see Table 31–1).

Water-borne Diseases. Cholera and typhoid fever, for example, are caused by inadequate sanitation measures and the resulting contamination of drinking water.

Diseases Resulting from Malnutrition. WHO extends its work to environmental health. In 1963, it helped 57 countries establish clean drinking water supplies. The health organization has recently established a new Expert Advisory Panel to combat the growing problem of air pollution, and it is studying and advising its members on new problems—such as the unexpected development of strains of pests that resist insecticides.

In many other fields, WHO is moving against dangers to human health and safety—planning, developing, and operating public health services; developing protection against the hazards of radiation; studying problems of human genetics; and establishing services to rehabilitate the sick and the crippled.

Finally, WHO is organized to work in emergency situations. In 1963 alone, staff members were on the scene to help after tornadoes struck Cuba and Haiti; after an earthquake hit Yugoslavia; after cholera broke out in Korea, Malaya, and Burma; and after an epidemic of typhus broke out among the people of Yemen. Some years earlier, in 1957, WHO headquarters in Geneva learned that Singapore was in the midst of an influenza epidemic, and a short time later, that the disease had broken out in China and spread to Hong Kong. Samples of the influenza virus responsible for this virulent epidemic were quickly flown to the World Influenza Center in London, and identified as a new strain of the virus. Public health, research and pharmaceutical laboratories were mobilized, and a successful vaccine was soon produced. Within five months the epidemic had spread over five continents, and in the fall and winter of 1957–1958, nearly half the people in the United States were affected by respiratory ailments serious enough to keep them out of school or work for at least one day. Undoubtedly, a significant portion of these infections was due to the so-called Asian flu, but the American people didn't panic, despite vivid memories of the devastating influenza epidemic of 1917–1918. They realized that public health officials had the situation well under control and that effective vaccines were reaching many Americans in ample time to prevent serious respiratory illnesses from developing. Without the vigilance of WHO and other health agencies, the flu epidemic would probably have been much more severe.

Table 31–1. Mortality from tuberculosis of all forms* per 100,000 population (1959)

Country	*Death Rate*
Chile	54.6
Singapore	39.7
Japan	35.5
Puerto Rico	29.2
Finland	28.6
Colombia	27.8
UAR	23.8
France	23.2
Ireland	18.2
Italy	18.2
Belgium	17.0
Switzerland	15.8
England and Wales	8.5
Sweden	7.2
United States	6.5
Israel	6.1
Norway	6.1
Australia	5.5
Canada	5.5
New Zealand	4.5
Denmark	4.0
Netherlands	3.6

*From the World Health Organization Epidemiological and Vital Statistics Reports, 1959, published 1962.

WHO also plays a vital role as a clearing-house for all types of global health and disease information, in promoting uniform quarantine standards throughout the world, and in setting up international standards for the manufacture of vaccines, antibiotics and similar medications. It protects us against importation of disease, and also guards the health of U. S. citizens travelling abroad. In its 120 member countries, WHO staff personnel are plotting the paths of disease and studying the health patterns of nations. And its teams of physicians, nurses, sanitary engineers, and other health experts are travelling through deserts, jungles and mountains, by foot, by camel and by plane, to carry medicines and medical equipment, as well as modern skills and knowledge to impoverished peoples throughout the world.

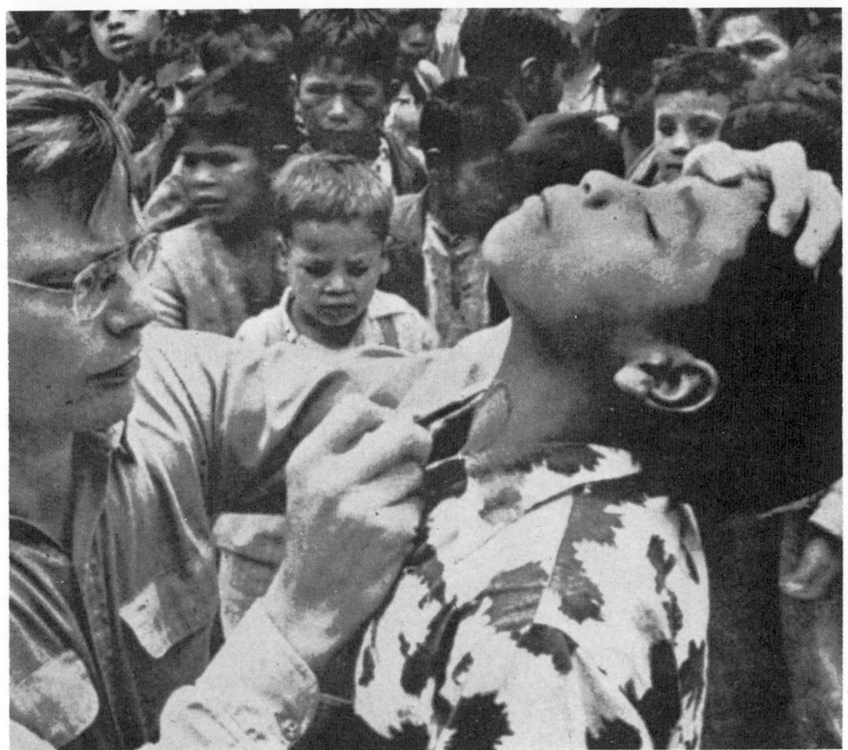

Figure 31–2. Examination of Guatemalan school children for goiter by WHO physicians.

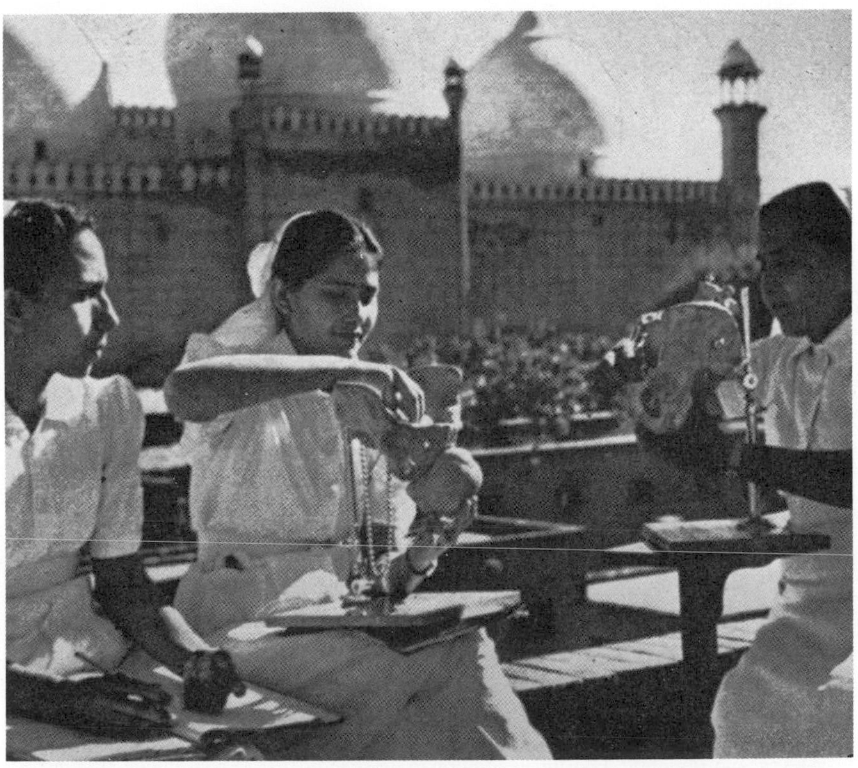

Figure 31–3. Class for midwives in India organized by WHO maternal and child health team.

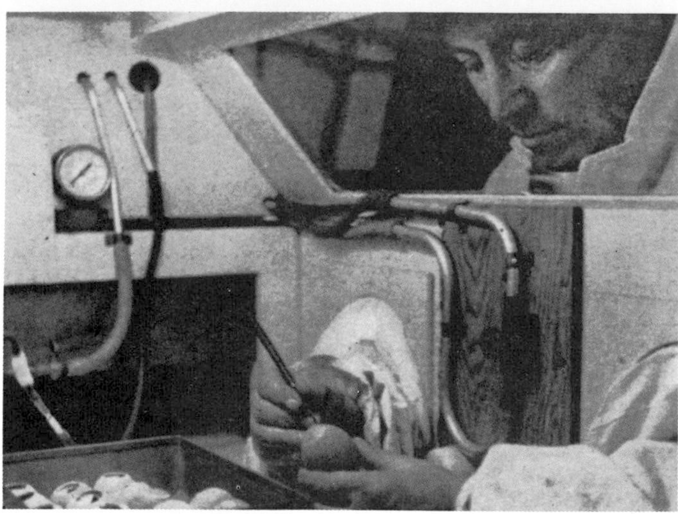

Figure 31–4. WHO technicians prepare Asian flu vaccine at World Influenza Center in London.

Federal Public Health Activities

The United States Public Health Service, which today is an enormous structure with a wide variety of important activities, was started in 1798, almost with the birth of the nation. The 13 struggling colonies had to depend on the seas both for protection and trade. To encourage enlistment and expansion of the small merchant marine, the government established a Marine Hospital Service to provide medical care for seamen when they were ashore. The first hospital was established on

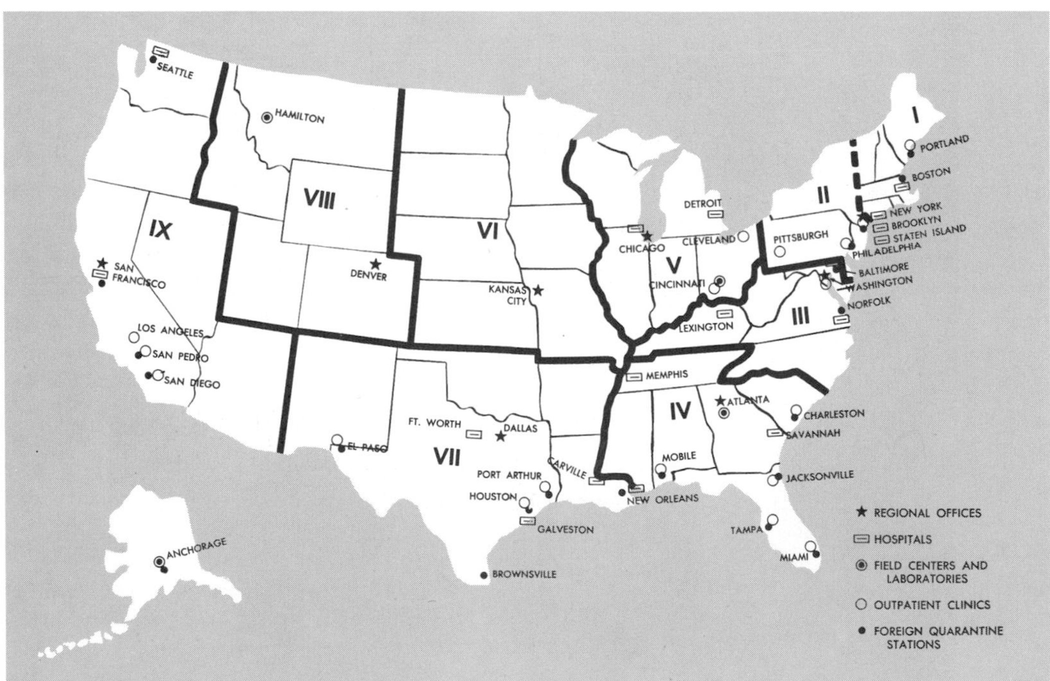

Figure 31–5. Public Health Service offices in the United States. Regional offices have now been established in Anchorage, Alaska, and Honolulu, Hawaii, in addition to those indicated. (From *Public Health Service Today,* U. S. Govt. Printing Office, Washington, D. C.)

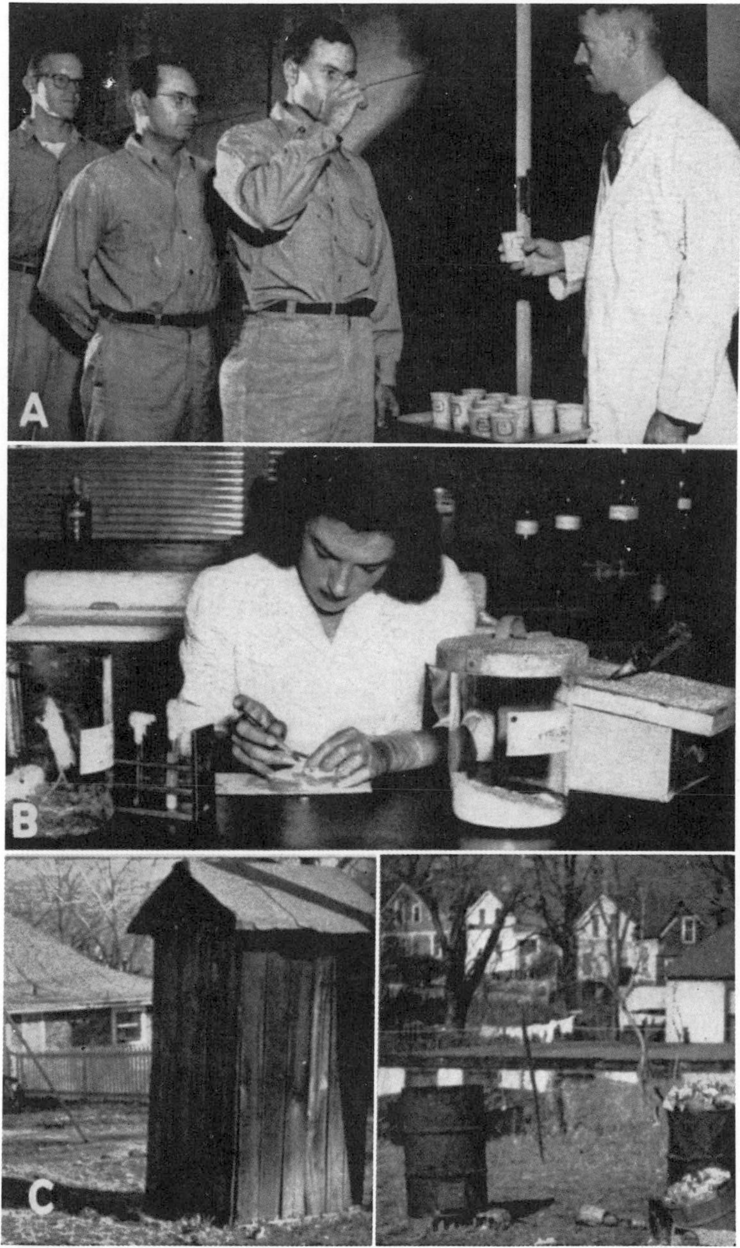

Figure 31–6. Some activities of the Communicable Disease Center. **A,** During studies to determine the possible toxicity of DDT residues in foods, volunteers have taken for several months without detectable injury over 100 times the amount a person might inadvertently consume. **B,** Rabies investigations at the Center have shown the mouse inoculation test is the most accurate laboratory method for diagnosing rabies. **C,** Eliminating privies and unsanitary refuse disposal. (From Public Health Service Publication No. 491, Communicable Disease Center, Atlanta, Ga.)

Castle Island in Boston Harbor, and each seaman contributed 20 cents from his monthly pay to help support it. As we pushed our frontiers westward, hospitals were established at Mobile, Paducah, New Orleans, Natchez and other places on major waterways, and by 1853 the Marine Service had reached the West Coast and had set up a hospital in San Francisco.

New problems soon developed, requiring greater extension of public health services. The major ones were widespread epidemics of yellow fever, smallpox, and cholera. The evolution of the nation from a rural to an urban civilization brought with it the accompanying problems of sanitation, hygiene and water pollution. It became apparent that some public health organization must take the responsibility for studying and regulating the relationship of people to *their total environment*—where they live and work, their water, sanitary facilities, food, and air.

In 1912, the Marine Hospital Service was disbanded, and the U. S. Public Health Service established; it is interesting that this branch of the government fulfills its historic function and still controls the marine hospitals for the benefit of members of the merchant marine. Today, the U. S. Public Health Service represents an extremely important section of the Department of Health, Education and Welfare. This was established in 1953, and is organized as follows:

1. *Public Health Service*
   - Office of the Surgeon General
   - National Institutes of Health
   - Bureau of State Services
   - Bureau of Medical Services
2. *Office of Education*
3. *Social Security Administration*
   - Office of the Commissioner
   - Bureau of Federal Credit Unions
   - Bureau of Old Age and Survivors' Assistance
   - Children's Bureau
4. *Office of Vocational Rehabilitation*
5. *Food and Drug Administration*
6. *St. Elizabeth's Hospital* (for the mentally ill)
7. *Welfare Administration*

The 34,000 employees of the Public Health Service, representing more than 300 occupations, participate in functions that increase in variety and in scope almost yearly. In its *medical and hospital services,* PHS operated, in 1963, a total of 65 hospitals, 25 outpatient clinics, and 42 Indian and Alaskan native health centers. In its *community health* program, PHS helps the states and communities develop preventive, curative, and restorative services for the general public. *Environmental health* activities include research and assistance to state and local agencies in air and water pollution, radiological hazards, occupational hazards, and sanitation problems. Through the National Institutes of Health, the government supplies funds for about 40 per cent of all *research and training* programs in the nation. *Health information resources* include the National Library of Medicine and the National Center for Health Statistics, and as a contribution to *international health,* PHS works with WHO, the Pan American Health Organization, and many universities.

The *National Institutes of Health* carry on extensive laboratory research and clinical investigations, and also make research, teaching, and training grants to scientists in other institutions through eight National Research Institutes. Another of its sections, the Division of Biologic Standards, sets up standards for the safety, purity and potency of vaccines, toxins and antitoxins, serums, and related biological products.

The *Bureau of State Services* provides assistance to the state and local community health programs, both financial and technical, in addition to many other activities. Funds are apportioned according to state needs, with the larger amounts going to the poorer states to raise their health levels. They cover general health, control of venereal disease, tuberculosis, heart disease and cancer, mental health activities, construction of hospitals and sewage disposal plants, and water pollution control. The National Office of Vital Statistics is also part of this bureau and is responsible for valuable records on the health of the nation, births, deaths, marriages and divorce, and the incidence of communicable diseases.

Public health education, occupational

health, radiological hazards, accident prevention and poison control centers are also under the jurisdiction of this branch. Air pollution studies, as well as water pollution and milk and food sanitation, are an important part of the work of State Services, which also includes the Communicable Disease Center. This center gives aid in threatened epidemics—as in the Asian flu outbreak of 1957-1958—and in disasters, such as hurricanes.

Some important activities of the *Bureau of Medical Services* are the operation of hospitals and out-patient clinics for merchant seamen, as well as for officers and enlisted men in the Coast Guard and Public Health Service, and civil service employees; enforcement of foreign quarantine regulations for air, land, and sea traffic and medical examination of immigrants and ship or plane crew members arriving in this country. This division is also responsible for hospitals and health services for the American Indians and Alaskan natives; design and construction of hospitals and other health facilities; and provision of medical care to prisoners in the 30 institutions under the federal prison system.

Federal institutions have become an extremely important adjunct in medical research in recent years, and we owe much of the development of effective anti-malarial agents to the cooperation of prisoners who volunteered to serve as guinea pigs in these experiments even though it meant contracting malaria. Urgent research problems during World War II gave a tremendous impetus to the use of prison inmates as experimental subjects, but actually as far back as 1915, they were part of a critical study on the vitamin deficiency disease, pellagra, conducted by Joseph Goldberger of the U. S. Public Health Service. As a result of these experiments, Goldberger clearly established that injecting blood from a pellagra patient into a normal volunteer did not produce pellagra, and that it was therefore not an infectious disease. He proved that it was a condition of dietary origin which could be induced by feeding a limited diet of grits, rice, and potatoes, and that it could be cured by adding milk, eggs, lean meat, and vegetables to the diet.

Prisoners have also been used in investigations leading to vaccines for infectious hepatitis and syphilis; the effect of DDT

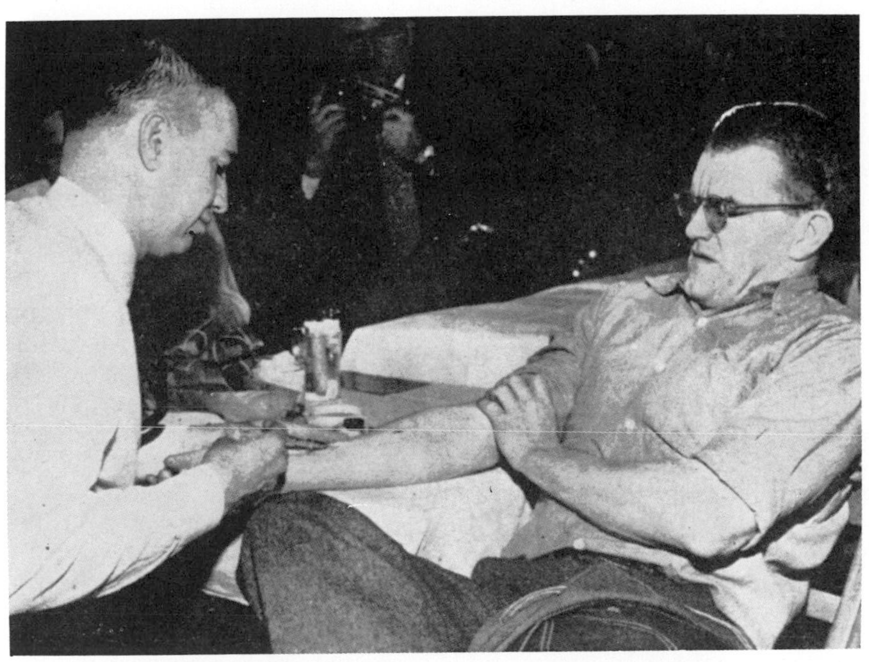

Figure 31–7. Injection of cancer cells in prison experiment.

contamination in foods; the occupational hazards of noise; and studies on mental illness and cancer. All experiments conducted in prisons must conform to rules laid down by the American Medical Association, and all subjects are fully informed about any hazards before they are permitted to volunteer. The calls for volunteers are usually so popular that they are often oversubscribed several times. One man with a life sentence who volunteered for cancer studies apparently expressed the sentiments of many other prisoners when he said, "All my life I've been a stinker. This is the first worthwhile thing I've ever done."

Children's Bureau

In addition to the Public Health Service, many other divisions of the Department of Health, Education and Welfare contribute to our well-being. The Children's Bureau, which has been operating since 1912, assists the states in extending and improving maternal and child health and welfare, and in making provisions for crippled children. Long-term chronic illnesses, congenital malformations of various kinds, blindness, deafness, and mental retardation are now, rightly, regarded as crippling conditions. This bureau has always been an outstanding and forward-looking government agency and is now studying and attempting to correct situations leading to our increasing juvenile delinquency as well as problems of migratory workers' children.

Food and Drug Administration (FDA)

The responsibility of protecting the health and well-being of consumers of foods, drugs (medicines), and cosmetics against contamination, deterioration, toxicity or quackery is under the control of this division. In typical actions of the FDA, various lots of fresh and canned produce were condemned because of too high an insecticide content; distributors of a chili powder were forced to recall it because it contained dangerous amounts of broken glass; numerous criminal prosecution suits were instituted against wholesalers who were shipping filthy or partially decomposed foods; defective or misbranded medicines were recalled by pharmaceutical houses; quack medicines and devices were seized and their promoters prosecuted. The vigilance of this department has ensured high standards in a great many products essential to our continued good health.

Office of Vocational Rehabilitation

Another important health program of the federal government, extremely meaningful both economically and emotionally to its recipients, is the rehabilitation of handicapped persons. In 1964 nearly 115,000 such individuals were restored to useful activity through the work of the Office of Vocational Rehabilitation, mostly people with amputations and other crippling conditions, but also patients suffering from emotional problems or recovering from mental illness, epileptics and many cerebral palsied, and blind persons. In addition, this agency prepares demonstration projects on disabling conditions and rehabilitation for the states, and provides them with funds and other types of assistance.

Other Government Agencies Advancing Health

There are many other government agencies which contribute significantly to our health and well-being. The Department of Health, Education and Welfare, for example, supports the American Printing House for the Blind in Louisville, Kentucky, and the world's only college for the deaf, Gallaudet College in Washington, D.C., a fully accredited school. The American Printing House for the Blind prints the official schoolbooks for the blind and also maintains large catalogs of Braille books, Talking Books (phonograph records), recorded tapes, and Braille music publications, providing a rich collection of educational material from kindergarten through the high school grades.

The Social Security Administration as

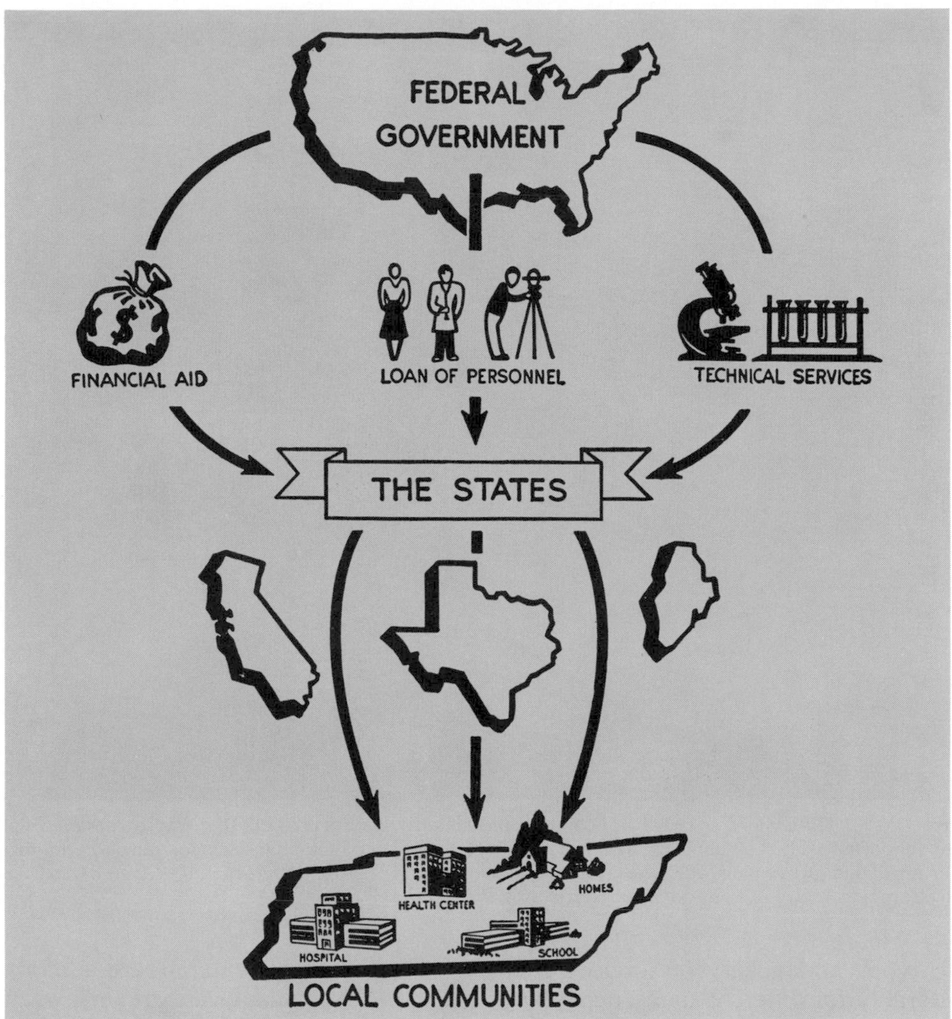

Figure 31–8. Federal health aid to states and local communities. (From *Guide to Health Organization in the United States*. U.S. Government Printing Office, 1953.)

of 1963–64 reported that it was protecting 92.1 million persons through the old-age, survivors, and disability programs. Those Americans now making regular contributions to this agency with funds matched by their employers are thus guaranteed some measure of economic security for themselves and their families, a protection against loss of income from retirement, disablement, or death. In addition, several million more received federal support on state or local welfare or assistance lists, or through unemployment compensation while they were searching for new jobs.

In addition to these and other agencies of the Department of Health, Education and Welfare that contribute to better health, the United States Army, Navy, and Air Force have excellent medical care programs for servicemen, officers, and their families; and the hospitals of the Veterans Administration provide good facilities for the exservicemen in our nation.

Health Control at the State and Territorial Level

All the states and the territorial possessions of Puerto Rico, the Virgin Islands, and Guam have health departments to administer state health programs and assist local municipalities.

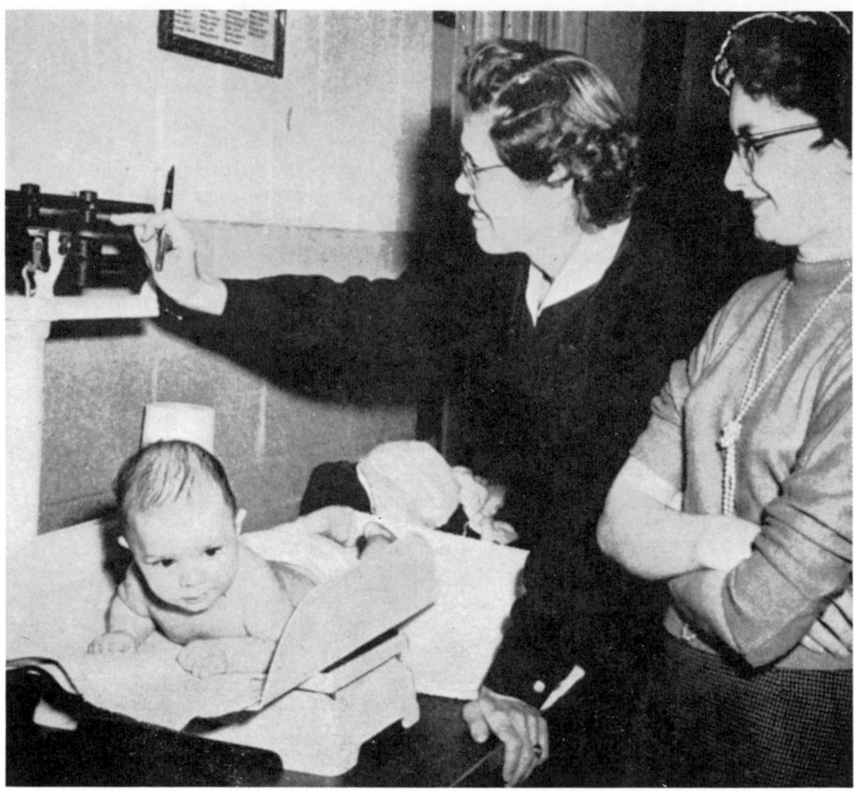

Figure 31–9. Division of maternal and child health. Healthy infants are kept that way by periodic checkups at state-supported well-baby clinics. Emphasis on complete health of the baby includes nutrition, mother-child relationships, and prevention of disease through immunization. (From *1957 Annual Report*. Department of Health, Commonwealth of Pennsylvania, Harrisburg, Pa.)

The types and quality of services vary considerably for different states, depending largely on their wealth and the progressiveness of their administration, but usually include the following: *communicable disease control, maternal and child health, public health nursing, public health laboratories, environmental sanitation, vital statistics,* and *health education.* The Department of Health of the Commonwealth of Pennsylvania exemplifies a thorough coverage of health problems.

This Department, created in 1905, was reorganized in 1962 to meet contemporary public health problems more effectively and efficiently. For the fiscal 1965, the Department's budget was nearly $14.5 million, and another $9.5 million was spent in aid to hospitals throughout Pennsylvania. In almost every sector of life where health is at stake, the Department of Health has a role. Here are some examples:

The Sanitary Water Board administered the Pennsylvania clean stream laws, halted industrial and civic water pollution, and controlled the installation and use of disposal systems.

Nearly 2000 alcoholics received advice and assistance, and a small number was admitted to a commonwealth rehabilitation center for treatment.

Nursing service was made available throughout Pennsylvania in about one-third of whose counties no other free nursing care was available.

The Air Pollution Commission and its seven regional control centers undertook an intensified program to control existing atmospheric contaminants and to try to prevent further pollution.

Patients suffering from tuberculosis and from mental illnesses were treated in Pennsylvania hospitals.

In addition, Pennsylvania protected its citizens by issuing licenses only to qualified physicians, pharmacists, nurses, dentists, and others who work in the medical and allied professions. The operation of laboratories, supervision of drug and cosmetic products, and surveying and licensing of restaurants, institutions, industries, and clubs that served food and beverages rounded out the public health service functions of the commonwealth.

Local Health Departments

National and state public health services operate for the benefit of everyone, yet immediate responsibility for meeting health problems closest to home often rests with the health departments of cities, towns, and counties. To a large degree, they may parallel the work of state and national agencies, but they may also offer services and assistance not otherwise easily available to the community. Local boards of health also carry out many routine but important licensing services, to ensure that food-handlers, barbers, and others who work with or for people in ways that could affect health are themselves in good health.

The Department of Public Health of Philadelphia is representative in size, financing, and scope of local health organizations in other large American cities. In Philadelphia, a community of over 2 million, the 1965 operating budget for health purposes was $7.5 million. In addition, the Department operates Philadelphia General Hospital for the needy, for city employees, and for research and training at a cost of another $15 million annually.

A range of services from prenatal care to programs for the elderly is offered through the city's ten community health centers. Philadelphia maintains a public health nursing service and, since 1954, has offered the community a mental health center. This center serves more than 5000

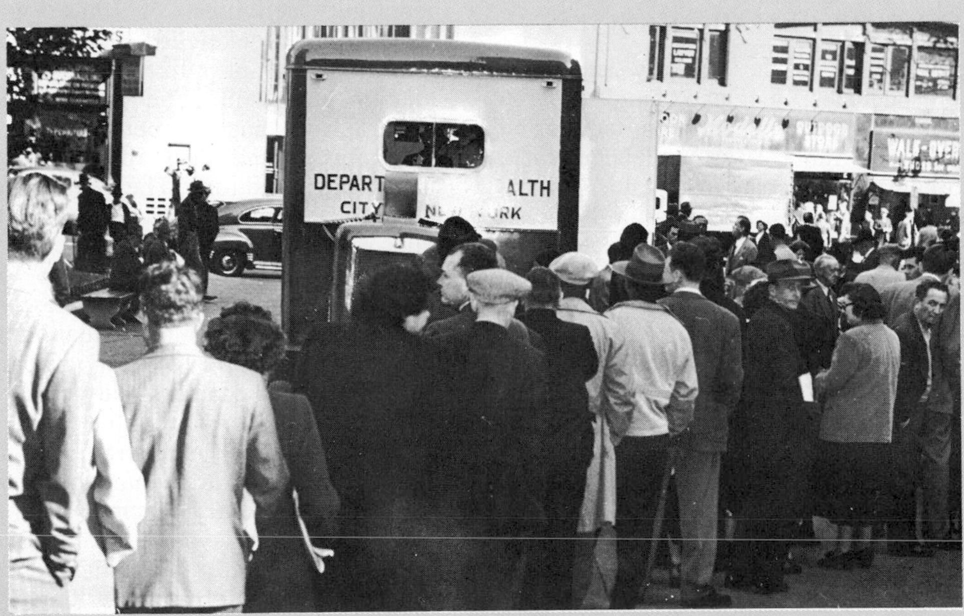

This crowd is in line at a New York City Health Department mobile chest X-ray unit which conveniently provides X-rays free of charge. Like other cities that provide similar public health services, New York uses units such as this in its campaign to control tuberculosis and other chest diseases.

patients annually through diagnosis and, when necessary, placement in mental hospitals. Another 2500 persons are treated on an outpatient basis. Air pollution, mosquito and rodent control, radiation hazard control, and a dental health program are among the other services that the city offers.

This public health staff has been industrious in bringing the advantages of new advances in medicine to public attention. Polio immunization programs were undertaken in the early 1960's when the Salk vaccine was made available, and in 1963 and 1964 the Sabin preparation was distributed (see p. 460). An extensive publicity campaign brought tens of thousands of families to neighborhood schools for the Sabin immunization series.

Most of the work of the Department of Public Health is done without fanfare, however. As in most other communities, the staff usually works without the awareness of most of the residents, but its role is vital to all those who live in the complicated and crowded surroundings of this large American city.

VOLUNTARY HEALTH AGENCIES

In addition to the publicly supported health agencies, we also have a large number of voluntary groups, supported by gifts and fund drives, which may also be organized at a national, state, or local level. Some of these, such as the National Tuberculosis Association which was started in 1892, pioneered in giving medical care to the tuberculous poor before public funds became available.

In certain communities, these voluntary agencies supply services which are not otherwise available—such as home nursing visits—or they complement community activities. The American Cancer Society, the American Heart Association, the National Foundation, and many others have been helpful in providing medical care and treatment in expensive chronic illnesses, and also in health education and the support of medical research.

There are over 100,000 national, regional, and local voluntary health and welfare agencies soliciting contributions from the general public, which gives over $1.5 billion every year. This has stirred up some criticism and resentment because the public is being asked to contribute to many individual health drives, as well as support activities in their own community through their Community Chest or its equivalent. Much of the success of these voluntary organizations and the valuable contributions they have made depend on the public's sympathy and kindness. An appeal for funds for a specific disease, such as polio or cancer, evokes a much greater pull at the heart strings—and a corresponding loosening of the purse strings—than a request for funds for unspecified or general health needs. Nevertheless, because the number of voluntary agencies has increased so rapidly in recent years, it may soon become necessary to combine all the individual appeals into a single drive for medical and health support, or the voluntary agencies may "kill the goose that has been laying the golden egg."

In fact, concern over the proliferation of fund-raising agencies and over the increasing number of questions by the public about the great number and increasing activities of these groups moved the Rockefeller Foundation to invite a group of citizens to study the situation in detail. The group included industrialists, businessmen, college and university executives, union officials, and magazine editors. They examined the problem in great detail and made three major recommendations:

1. A National Commission on Voluntary Health and Welfare Agencies should be formed to study the situation on a continuing basis, to develop criteria for appraising the agencies, and to act as a court of appeals.

2. Every agency supported by public contributions should account to the public for its programs and financing.

3. A uniform system of accounting should be adopted, to be developed by the American Institute of Certified Public Accountants.

The special committee's work was published in *Voluntary Health and Welfare Agencies in the United States,* published by The Schoolmasters' Press in 1961. The committee members listed a

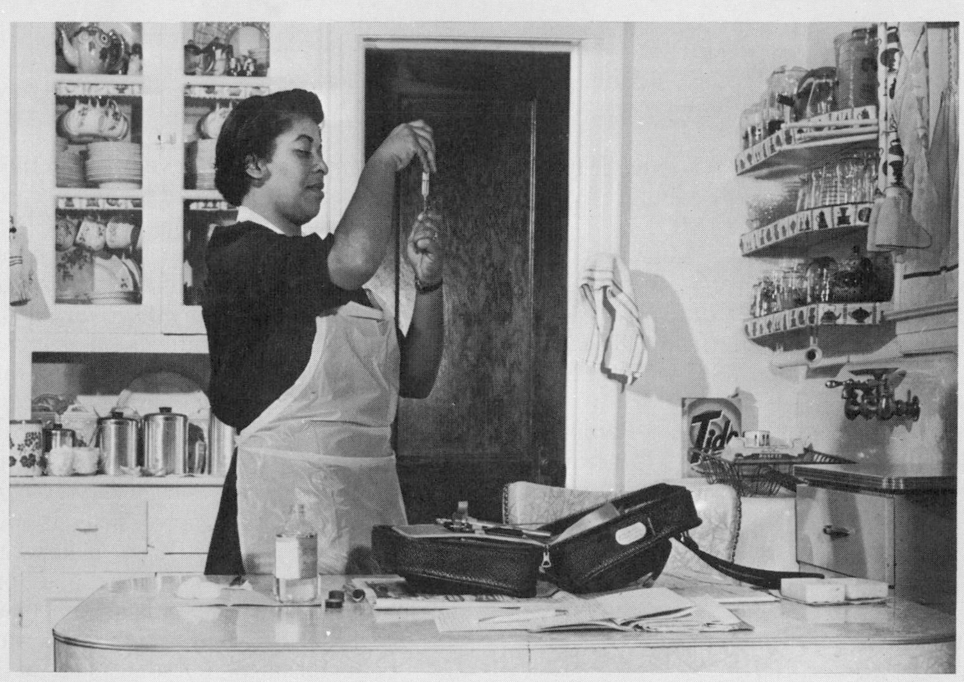

Visiting nurse prepares to give an injection to a patient at home. Her visits are a public health service of the New York City Health Department. This type of assistance for people who are unable to leave their homes is available from public and private health agencies in various parts of the country.

detailed account of public contributions, extrapolating them to 1970. They pointed out significantly:

> It is true, of course, that the multitude of services and the competition for ideas and methods provided by these voluntary agencies have produced progress which otherwise might not have been possible. For democracy, though, we always pay a price. That we expect. But we need to be sure that the price is a necessary concomitant of democracy and that the product is worth the price.

Some of the important nationally organized voluntary health agencies which provide information and, in many cases, treatment as well for specific diseases are:

Accident Prevention: National Safety Council, 425 North Michigan Avenue, Chicago, Ill. 60611.

Alcoholism: Alcoholics Anonymous (National), Box 459, Grand Central Annex, New York, N. Y. 10017.

Blindness: National Society for the Prevention of Blindness, Inc., 16 E. 40th Street, New York, N. Y. 10016.

Cancer: American Cancer Society, Inc., 218 E. 42nd Street, New York, N. Y. 10017.

Cerebral Palsy: United Cerebral Palsy Associations, Inc., 321 W. 44th Street, New York, N. Y. 10036.

Diabetes: American Diabetes Association, Inc., 1 East 45th Street, New York, N. Y. 10017.

Drug addiction: Addicts Anonymous, Box 2000, Lexington, Kentucky.

Epilepsy: National Epilepsy League, Inc., 203 North Wabash Avenue, Chicago, Ill. 60601.

Hearing Defects: American Hearing Society, 919 Eighteenth Street, N.W., Washington, D.C. 20006.

Heart Disease: American Heart Association, 44 East 23rd Street, New York, N. Y. 10010.

Infantile Paralysis and Other Crippling Diseases: The National Foundation, 800 Second Avenue, New York, N. Y. 10017.

Mentally Ill or Retarded: National Association for Mental Health, Inc., 10 Columbus Circle, New York, N. Y. 10019.

Multiple Sclerosis: National Multiple Sclerosis Society, 257 Park Avenue South, New York, N. Y. 10017.

Muscular Dystrophy: Muscular Dystrophy Associations of America, Inc., 1790 Broadway, New York, N. Y. 10019.

Rehabilitation: American Rehabilitation Committee, Inc., 28 East 21st Street, New York, N. Y. 10010.

Sterility: The Planned Parenthood Federation of America, 515 Madison Avenue, New York, N. Y. 10022.

Tuberculosis: National Tuberculosis Association, 1790 Broadway, New York, N. Y. 10019.

Venereal Disease: American Social Health Association, 1790 Broadway, New York, N. Y. 10019.

PROFESSIONAL SOCIETIES

Physicians, public health workers, dentists, and professional workers in allied fields all have their own professional societies, such as the American Medical Association, the American Public Health Association, the American Dental Association, and the national nursing organizations. These do not provide health services in the direct sense, but, indirectly they are important in the health field. All of them, for example, set the standards for professional and medical education and thereby determine the caliber of personnel employed in health and medical activities. The *Joint Committee on Hospital Accreditation* is concerned with improving hospital standards so that patients will get the best possible service and treatment. Before a physician can become a specialist in any area, he must be accredited by the *specialty licensure board* in his particular area of interest, certifying that he has the necessary training and attainments. Many of the professional societies also carry on educational programs in the field of health or accident prevention, and some are actively involved in surveys of important diseases.

MEDICAL RESEARCH

The remarkable achievements in modern medicine and public health must be credited to the inspiration of a long line of dedicated scientists, going back several hundred years in many cases. No one man or group can be acclaimed for any discovery. When a research team announces a successful vaccine for diphtheria, polio, or rabies, the isolation of a penicillin, the synthesis of a hormone, the slowing down of a cancerous process by medicines, or the technique for lifesaving surgery, you can be certain that the triumphal peak is merely the top of a pyramid. Below it lies a body of data, collected patiently and painstakingly by many scientists, unacclaimed in most cases, and often unrewarded except in terms of personal satisfactions. "One researcher takes up where another leaves off. Each new bit of information helps to narrow down the area of search until the scent is unmistakable and science can close in for the kill.[2]

This is vividly illustrated by the history of the development of the Salk vaccine for polio, which signalized the beginning of the end of this much-feared, crippling disease. Merely the highlights of this climax cover many centuries and many nations:

Anton van Leeuwenhoek, a Dutch investigator known as the "Father of Bacteriology," first revealed the world of microorganisms with his minute but powerful lenses in 1676.

Edward Jenner, the English physician, successfully vaccinated against smallpox in 1796 by inducing the milder cowpox.

Louis Pasteur (1822–1895), described as the greatest French scientist of all time, demonstrated that bacteria could be killed by heat, the process we call pasteurization. His vaccines for anthrax and rabies, developed about 1885, can be considered the first true vaccines, and represent the beginning of modern immunology.

Eli Metchnikoff, a Russian scientist, performed

---

[2]*Medical Advance,* Vol. III, No. 3, Fall, 1955, National Fund for Medical Education, New York.

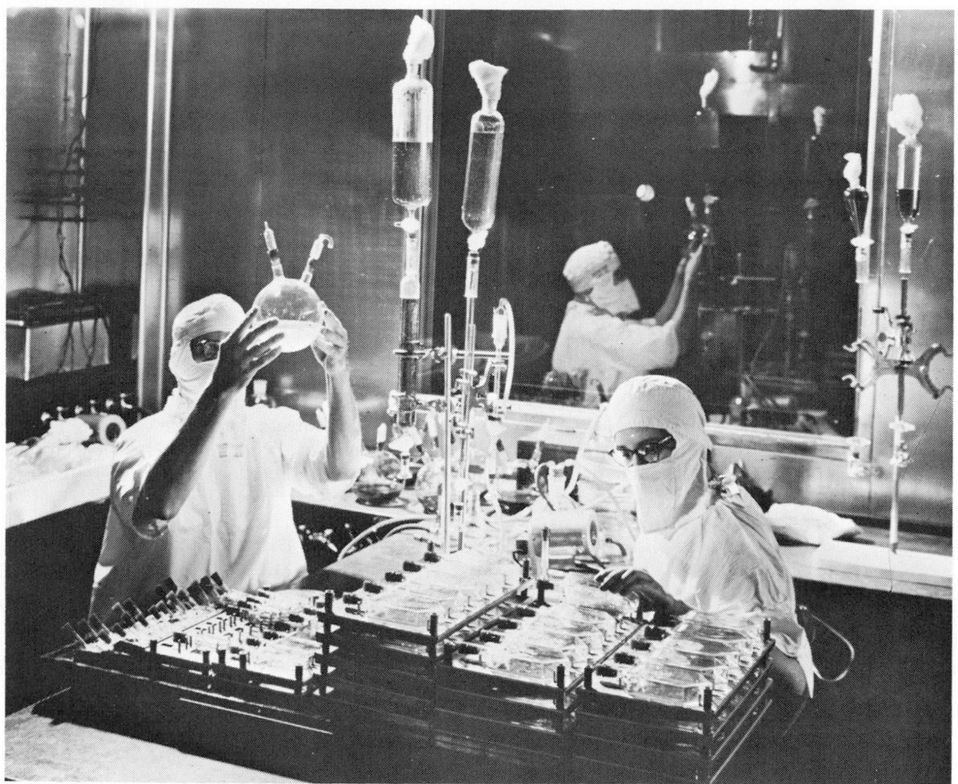

Figure 31–10. Cancer research. Living cells are handled by workers wearing sterile masks at the National Cancer Institute in Bethesda, Maryland, where cells are raised in cultures and then studied to determine how they grow, multiply, and sometimes become cancerous. (From Changing Patterns of a Nation's Health, *Life Magazine,* Feb. 17, 1958. Copr. 1958, Time, Inc.)

experiments in 1882 which advanced the science of immunology.

Dmitri Iwanowski, also a Russian, helped in our understanding of the viruses by his studies in 1892 of the *tobacco mosaic virus,* which causes a disease of tobacco leaves.

Karl Landsteiner, a Viennese scientist, who later came to the famous Rockefeller Institute for Medical Research in New York, showed in 1909 that polio was caused by a virus, an organism smaller than a bacterium, and that it could be transmitted to monkeys.

Simon Flexner, an American investigator (and first director of the Rockefeller Institute) proved that polio could be passed from humans to monkeys and from monkey to monkey (1909). He also demonstrated that serum from monkeys who recovered from polio carried antibodies against the disease which could protect healthy monkeys.

John A. Kolmer of Temple University School of Medicine and Maurice Brodie and William Park in New York City tried to prepare vaccines against polio in the early 1930's. These sometimes worked but at other times failed to have any effect. (As more knowledge of polio accumulated, it was shown that there were several polio viruses, not just one, and the early vaccines were not effective against them all.)

William McD. Hammon of the University of Pittsburgh School of Medicine showed that polio antibodies remained in the blood of human beings who had recovered from the disease. Subsequently, other scientists demonstrated that pooled serum from adults (most of whom could be presumed to have had genuine or abortive polio at some time in their lives) conferred a short-lived immunity against polio.

In the early 1950's, three research scientists at Harvard Medical School—John F. Enders, Thomas H. Weller and Frederick C. Robbins—broke through the impasse in the preparation of effective polio vaccine: a method of growing polio virus outside an animal's body. Until that time, the only source of the virus for vaccine preparation was the brain and spinal cord of infected monkeys or mice. Enders and his team found a way of culturing polio virus on monkey kidney cells, kept alive in test tubes with a special nutrient fluid developed at the Connaught Medical Research Laboratories in Toronto, Canada. This was a critical step forward in the preparation of an effective vaccine, and led to the Nobel prize for these investigators.

Meanwhile, Jerome T. Syverton and his associates at the University of Minnesota Medical School developed speedier methods for establishing a diagnosis of polio and the demonstration of immunity. Until their work, the only way to do this was to inject material into a monkey and wait to see if polio developed. Syverton's method for rapid diagnosis was to add fecal matter or other preparations suspected of containing polio virus to a test-tube culture of a special strain of cancer cells, called "HeLa cells." If the cancer cells died, it indicated that polio virus was present. He was able to demonstrate antibodies to polio in blood samples by adding a known culture of polio virus *plus the blood* to HeLa cells. If they survived despite the presence of polio virus, it proved that the blood contained antibodies, and the blood donor was immune.

Dorothy M. Horstmann at Yale University School of Medicine and David Bodian of Johns Hopkins University School of Hygiene and Public Health showed independently about 1952 that polio virus circulates for brief periods in the blood of experimental chimpanzees. Subsequent work indicated that the virus might be present in the blood of human beings before the illness began.

Howard A. Howe and Isabel Morgan of Johns Hopkins Medical School found that they could rob the virus of its ability to cause disease by treating it with certain chemicals. But with their technique, *the virus still retained the power to stimulate immune antibodies and act as a true vaccine.*

The virus responsible for infantile paralysis was now trapped, and teams of researchers concentrated on methods of preparing safe and effective polio vaccine for large scale use. Dr. Jonas E. Salk and his co-workers at the University of Pittsburgh School of Medicine were among the first to be successful, and in field trials conducted on human subjects in 1954, the Salk vaccine proved 60 to 70 per cent effective against type I polio and 90 per cent effective against types II and III. We now possess a successful preventive measure for another human scourge.

Even more recent than the Salk vaccine are the oral vaccines – particularly the one developed by Dr. Albert B. Sabin. The Sabin vaccine contains harmless weakened strains of polio virus disguised in a pleasant-tasting liquid. It is usually taken in three doses about six weeks apart.

Although there is obviously great virtue in a polio vaccine that can be taken by mouth, the Sabin vaccine has not superseded the Salk vaccine but so far has merely supplemented it. Both vaccines have proved safe and effective. Which one to be used in a given case is a question to be answered by the individual physician and the public health officials.

Proof for the enthusiasm most Americans feel about medical research is found in their generous support of both voluntary fund drives and increased government spending for better health and more and happier years of life.

The major support for research in medicine today comes from six sources: the *federal government,* now the leading donor; *voluntary health drives,* like those of the

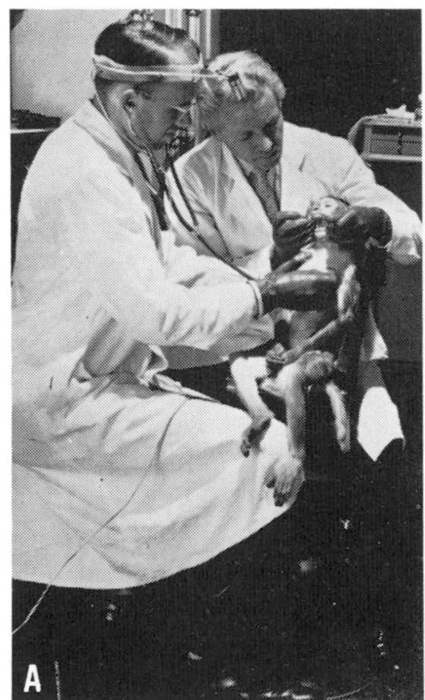

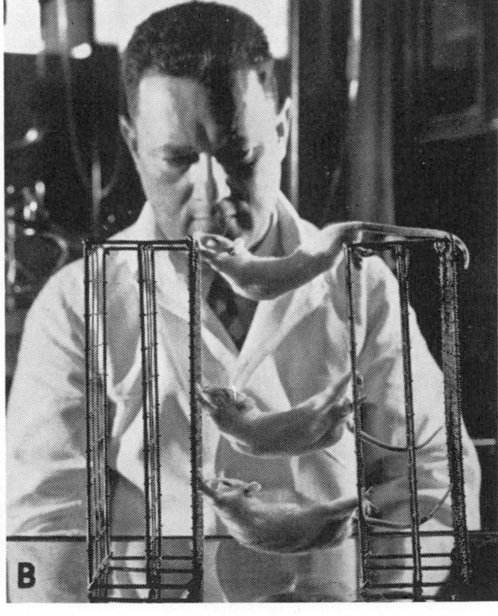

Figure 31–11. Medical research. **A,** Studies on tooth decay at Harvard Dental School. Monkey's teeth have mineral content removed with acid to see whether chemicals in saliva can rebuild teeth. **B,** Drugged rats grip racks and hang in dazed rigidity akin to catatonic state of mental patients, in schizophrenia study at the New England Institute for Medical Research in Boston. (From Changing Patterns of a Nation's Health, *Life Magazine,* Feb. 17, 1958, Copr. Time, Inc.)

American Cancer Society and the American Heart Association; *privately endowed foundations,* such as the Rockefeller, the Commonwealth, the Josiah Macy, the Hartford and the Markle Foundations; *privately endowed institutions,* outstanding among which are the Rockefeller Institute for Medical Research in New York, the Henry Phipps Institute for research in tuberculosis in Philadelphia, and the Carnegie Institution of Washington. *Pharmaceutical companies* also make sizable research grants, and many *medical schools* have large endowments to support research in medicine, which they supplement with additional funds from the above sources.

The Federal Government actually entered the medical research scene quite early, when part of the appropriation to the Army and Navy for the health of military personnel was diverted to original studies after 1875. But the big push for greater government support resulted from the shrinking of private endowment funds because of the depression of 1929. In 1937, Congress authorized an initial appropriation of $750,000 for the buildings and facilities of the National Cancer Institute and an additional $700,000 to aid and support cancer research.

Just before World War II, the total national expenditure for medical research was $45 million, but because of the many urgent medical problems during the war years and the increased public interest and willingness to support medical research, this amount quickly increased. By 1964, public and private expenditures for research related to medicine and health totaled nearly $1.7 billion, 65 per cent of which came from the Federal Government. The government's role alone has grown from a budget allotment of $27 million in 1947 to $1.2 billion in 1964. By 1964, Federal funds for medical and health-related activities accounted for about 15 per cent of all government research and development money. Of the $1.2 billion budgeted in 1964, 90 per cent went for research activities and the balance for new facilities. The accompanying charts show how Federal support for these activities has increased and how it compares to non-Federal and private support.

Today the Department of Health, Education and Welfare, the Department of Defense, Atomic Energy Foundation, Veterans Administration, the Department of Agriculture, the Armed Forces, and the National Science Foundation all contribute to basic and applied research problems in the field of medicine, and to the training of research scientists through pre- and postdoctorate fellowships. A new and very

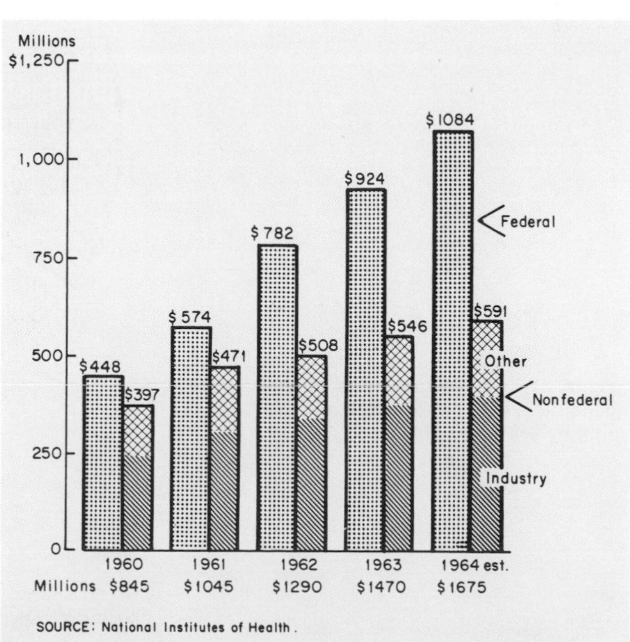

Figure 31–12. Recent trends in sources of support for performance of health-related research, 1960–64.

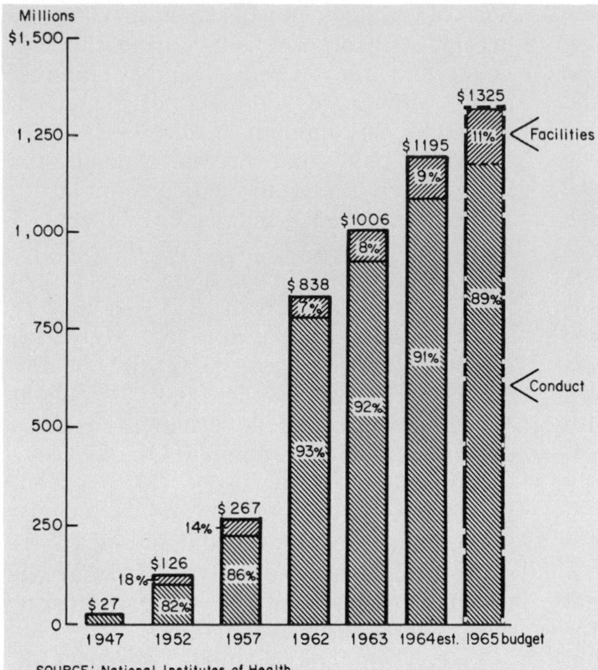

Figure 31–13. Federal support for health-related research, 1947–65.

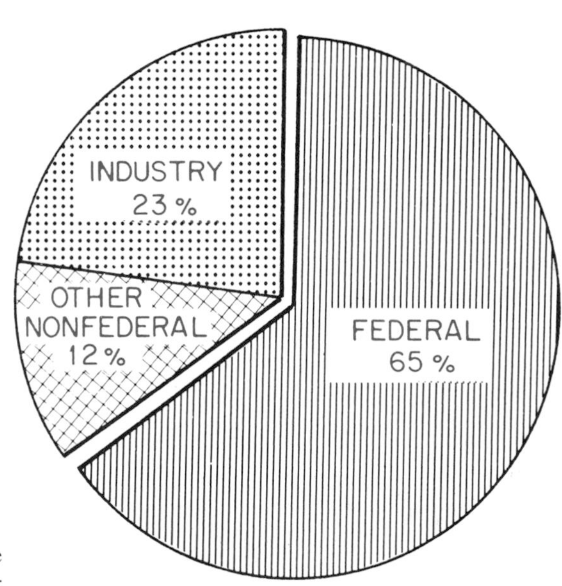

Figure 31–14. National total of public and private expenditures for performance of health-related research by source of support, 1964.

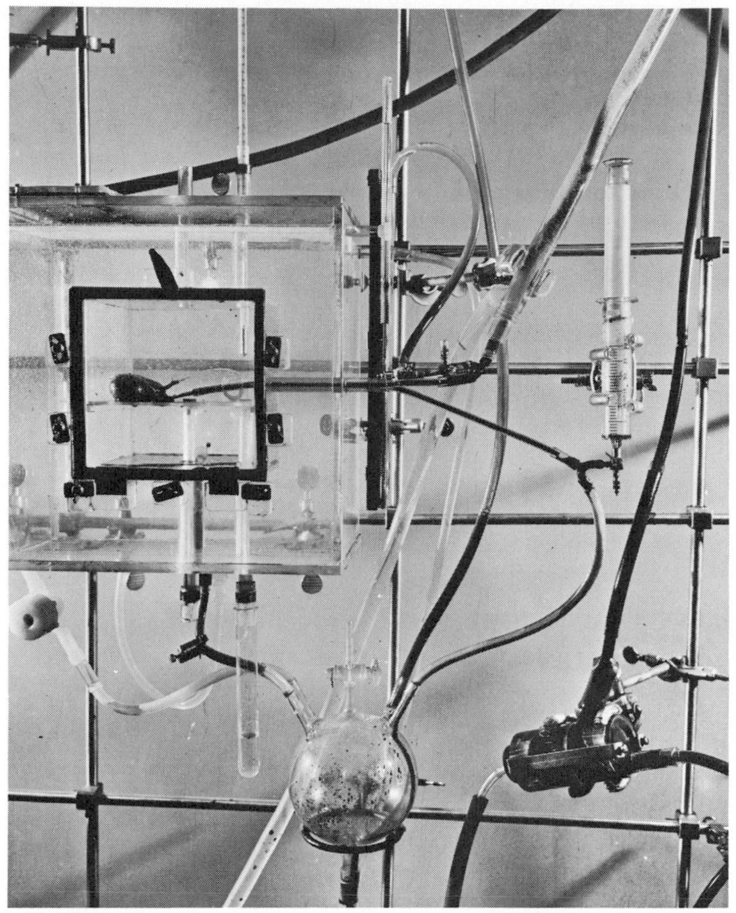

Figure 31–15. Isolated kidney, taken from a dog, continues functioning in a square plastic cage at the Harvard Medical School. Via a pump *(lower right)* the kidney is given whole blood to determine how an organ can be kept alive outside the body. (From Changing Patterns of a Nation's Health, *Life Magazine,* Feb. 17, 1958. Copr. 1958, Time, Inc.)

significant development, sparked by the voluntary health agencies, is to grant so-called "career investigatorships" to a small number of scientists who have distinguished themselves in their chosen area of research. These fellowships guarantee *lifetime support,* and certainly indicate that the research scientist is finally beginning to receive the recognition and credit he deserves.

American medical research today is of the highest order, and our Government is now actively assisting scientists in other countries by encouraging interchange of ideas, exchange programs for training in research, and by actual research grants to other nations. The budget approved for medical research through the Department of Health, Education and Welfare alone amounted to $800 million for fiscal 1965. Yet a group of consultants, headed by Stanhope Bayne-Jones, formerly dean of the Yale University School of Medicine and now Technical Director of Research, Office of the Army Surgeon General, has recommended that this is still far too low, and that the United States should raise its expenditures for medical research to *one billion dollars* a year by 1970.

The 1965 appropriation of $800 million is expended through the eight National Institutes of Health in Bethesda, Md., as follows:[3]

National Institute of Allergy and Infectious Diseases: $68,445,000.

National Institute of Arthritis and Metabolic Diseases: $113,176,000.

National Cancer Institute: $140,926,000.

National Institute of Dental Research: $20,135,000.

National Heart Institute: $125,398,000.

[3]Budget of the United States Government, 1965.

National Institute of Mental Health: $188,917,000.

National Institute of Neurological Diseases and Blindness: $88,428,000.

National Institute of Child Health and Human Development: $43,169,000.

These Institutes and the Clinical Center, opened in 1953 to permit them to round out medical research programs by adding clinical studies to laboratory research, constitute probably the largest and one of the most outstanding research centers in the world. Here scientists of every discipline are seeking better methods for preventing, diagnosing and treating the major diseases of man, studying everything from the most minute structures of the cell, visible only in the electron microscope, to the patient as a whole.

OVERPOPULATION: A HEALTH MENACE

No one is comfortable in an overcrowded room. Some people have to stand, the air may be smoky and unpleasant, and the pleasures of social contact turn into the displeasures of unsociable crowding. However, the scope and complexity of a world that is becoming overcrowded (some areas of our planet already are saturated) far exceed the little problems of a stuffy room, from which, after all, one can escape. "Population explosion" is not a tired phrase but a threat to the health of all of us. The concept of too many people is more than a subjective fear; overpopulation, in the context of lagging food production, insufficient health services, too few doctors and nurses, and inadequate housing, constitutes a health menace. It is the analog of a disease.

The world's population is now about 3.3 billion. Given the current net increase of 2 persons per second, the population of the earth will double approximately each 40 years. At this rate, by the end of the twenty-seventh century, each unfortunate human being will have about one square foot of ground to squirm around on. Such a situation surely will not occur, of course, for if war or disease—the classic controllers of population—do not intervene, mankind will have been forced long before 2700 A.D. to take firm and drastic steps to control his numbers.

In some countries—India, Egypt, and many new nations of sub-Sahara Africa—an ironic situation is developing. All the hard work, the funds, and the great hopes being invested in projects designed to raise the living standard, very likely will be negated by the flood of humans certain to pour over the land if present birth rates (and declining death rates) continue. On this subject, Dr. John Rock, world-renowned gynecologist and a pioneer in the development of the oral contraceptive, has written in his book, *The Time Has Come:*

> Early in the 1950's . . . the prospect of the Aswan High Dam became symbolic of the fellaheens' great expectations for a better life. Designed to provide electric power for industry and irrigate two million acres of farmland, Aswan was Egypt's banner hope for combating hunger and idleness.
>
> Now, even as the massive ramparts of the dam only begin to rise above the Nile Valley, Egypt's leaders are concerned that the project's goal of substantially raising living standards for the populace may not be met. The dam is scheduled to be fully operative by 1972. By then, there will be some thirteen million more Egyptians than when the Nasser regime began in 1952, an increase of almost 60 per cent. It is therefore highly questionable whether Aswan's hydroelectric capacity can do more than ensure the nation's current subsistence level.

In the United States, the standard of living is high (although millions of families, struggling on marginal incomes, have not noticed this fact), and an increase in numbers does not appear to be an obvious threat. Nevertheless, overcrowded schools, the increasing difficulty in entering colleges and universities, jammed highways, cluttered suburbs, the encroachment of communities on parks and other open spaces—all these are visible evidence that the United States is no longer an open land, ready to welcome and accommodate anyone willing to come and to work. Dr. Donald Bogue, Associate Director of the Population Research and Training Center, University of Chicago, has warned:

> We possibly are facing a sudden spurt in population growth that could make the baby boom of 1946 look small . . . . It is difficult to escape the conclusion that voluntary family limitation, with each couple utilizing means that it finds acceptable on religious, esthetic, and physical grounds, is the alternative to some much more radical choices only a few years from now.

The size of the future population of the United States is pointed up in Table 31-2.

Table 31–2. Increase in population according to age group*

	Persons up to 19 Years of Age
1963	74,145,000
1950	51,343,000
	22,802,000 increase, or 45 per cent
	Persons 20 to 44 Years of Age
1963	58,962,000
1950	56,962,000
	2,000,000 increase, or 3.5 per cent
	Persons 45 Years of Age and Older
1963	55,423,000
1950	43,019,000
	12,404,000 increase, or 27.9 per cent

*From *Statistical Abstract of the United States,* 1964.

The overall population of the United States grew from 151,324,000 in 1950, to 188,530,000 in 1963—or 24.5 per cent. But clearly, if the youngsters, whose category has grown almost twice as fast as the population at large, reproduce at the same accelerated pace as their parents, the meaning of "population explosion" will be much more frightening to Americans of 1980 than to those of our own day, who are less than worried about Egypt or India.

Dr. Frederick E. Flynn, of the Catholic College of St. Thomas, related the problem neatly to health when he remarked, "And if reason and medicine bid us take off excess weight, surely reason and humanity bid us reduce overpopulation."

OCCUPATIONAL HEALTH PROBLEMS

Because nearly half the adult population is employed in some industrial activity, occupational hazards and accidents assume great importance in the health of the nation. Certain industries and types of work are more dangerous than others, with mining and quarrying leading the list, and the comparatively low accident rate in many potentially hazardous occupations is due primarily to their excellent safety programs. Recognition of the part that fatigue and human factors play—as well as the "accident-proneness" of certain individuals—has also been very important. In addition, industrial physicians must be watchful that diseases of nonoccupational origin are not aggravated by the job itself. For example, a worker with anemia will develop an even more severe anemia if he is exposed to certain chemicals.

The chief occupational hazards are usually classified as *chemical, physical,* or *infectious* agents.

Chemical Agents

Chemicals which may be dangerous do their damage either as dusts, vapors or contact agents, and the greatest number of

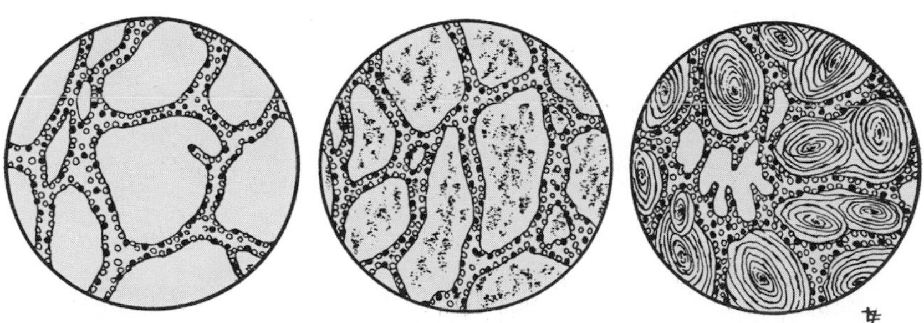

Figure 31–16. Foreign elements in the lungs. **Left,** Microscopic section of a normal lung. **Center,** Similar section showing the presence of ordinary dust particles. **Right,** Section showing changes due to silica dust.

Table 31–3. Workmen's compensation payments in the United States.*

Year	Payments
1940 –	$ 255,653,000
1945 –	408,374,000
1950 –	614,702,000
1955 –	915,665,000
1960 –	1,288,167,000
1962 –	1,465,200,000

*Payments include cash and medical benefits. From Statistical Abstract of the United States, 1964.

claims for workman's compensation in New York State in recent years, for example, was due to lung disease (*pneumoconiosis)* from inhalation of toxic dusts.

Dust may come from ginding, cutting, crushing, or drilling lead and other metals, or from organic substances of plant or animal origin, such as coal, flour, sugar, feathers, and leather. If the dust particles are above a certain size, they will settle rapidly and present no hazard, but smaller particles remain suspended in air for a long time, and may be inhaled to do lung damage. The most dangerous inorganic dust is silica, which can increase the severity of tuberculosis or cause the disease called *silicosis,* characterized by fibrous nodules throughout the lung. Asbestos workers sometimes develop a similar, but less severe, lung inflammation, *asbestosis,* and hard and soft coal miners are subject to a disabling shortness of breath because of the effects of coal dust on lung tissue. Most organic dusts are less harmful because the particles are bigger, but they are often responsible for allergies, skin irritations, and even asthma. A tremendous reduction in medical conditions due

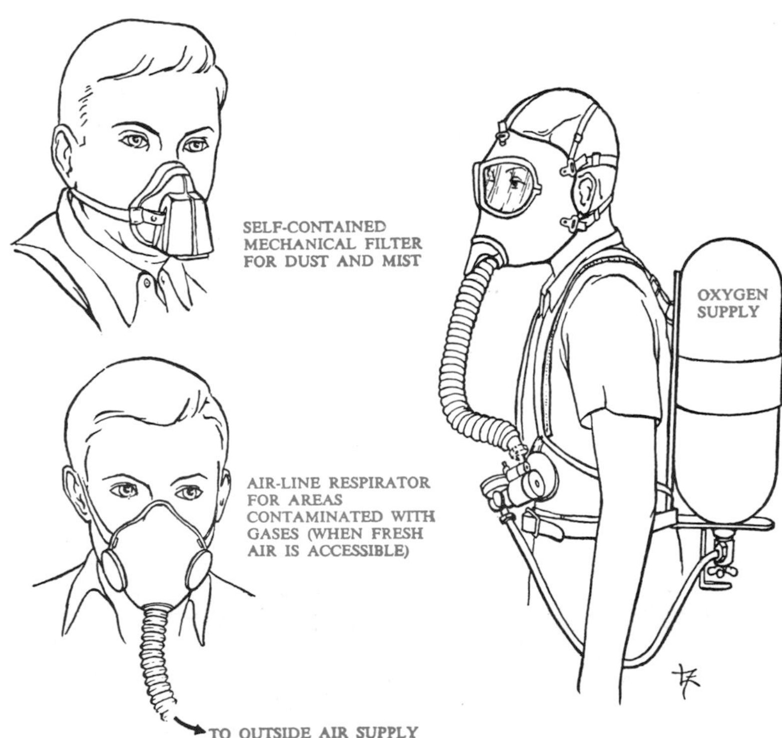

Figure 31–17. Types of protectors for respiration.

to inhalation of dust can be achieved by adequate protective devices – good ventilation and exhaust systems, or helmets and respirator masks.

Dangerous *gases* and *vapors* include carbon monoxide, ammonia, hydrogen sulfide, and sulfur dioxide; solvent vapors such as gasoline, benzol or carbon tetrachloride; and fumes from lead, zinc, and other toxic elements.

The chief hazards from chemical agents are asphyxiation, by interfering with the cells' oxygen supply; irritation of the eyes and the upper respiratory tract; systemic poisoning by such chemicals as lead, benzol, and carbon tetrachloride; lung damage by dusts; contact dermatitis; and even cancer in rare instances from asbestos and certain chemical compounds.

Physical Agents or Conditions

Pressure abnormalities. Men working in occupations where the atmospheric pressure is very high (compressed-air workers or divers) are subject to the "bends," or caisson disease. This problem is encountered in boring subway tunnels under rivers. The opposite condition, high altitude, can produce symptoms of oxygen deprivation, air embolism, and blockage of the middle ear via the eustachian tubes.

Radiation. The hazards from radiation stem from radium, high voltage x-rays or the newer radioactive elements, and can produce blood changes and even cancer (see Chapter 32). Welders are exposed to a high intensity of *ultraviolet* rays, and need special masks or goggles to prevent eye damage; also the *infrared rays* which are commonly used commercially in drying operations may cause eye or skin inflammations.

Abnormally high temperatures. Dehydration results, and is often responsible for muscle cramps and even heat exhaustion. Addition of extra salt to drinking water will prevent these conditions.

Dampness. This is a problem of coal miners, tankmen, and vatmen, and may lead to frequent colds, coughs, and rheumatic diseases. Water-proof clothing, rubber boots and gloves, and drain channels to carry off excess water are valuable protective devices.

Noise. Nerve deafness is not uncommon after exposure to excessive noise.

Infectious Agents

Infectious agents are a smaller problem in the United States than in less industrialized and less sanitary nations. However, bacterial, fungal, and parasitic diseases of occupational origin still occur. For example, workers who handle cattle are subject to *undulant fever* (brucellosis), and leather workers sometimes contract *anthrax* from the bacilli on the hides. Slaughterhouse workers must be on guard against tetanus and brucellosis.

Prevention of nonoccupational diseases is also of great importance to industry, because these are responsible for absenteeism due to sickness as well as for decreased productivity. This is one of the reasons for the increased medical care programs in many industries.

Recent years have brought about tremendous improvements in working conditions and a corresponding reduction in occupational hazards, largely because of excellent industrial health legislation, services provided by government and nongovernmental organizations, trade unions and voluntary control measures instituted by the industries themselves. The first of such laws was passed in 1842, the Child Labor Law in Massachusetts. Until that time it was not uncommon for children as young as seven or eight to spend 10 hours a day in factories.

Another major step was the passage of the first Workmen's Compensation Law in 1913 in New York State, governing the liability of the employer in accidents – or even death – of his workers. Both of these laws began to humanize conditions for working men, women, and children who were unfortunately regarded by many employers as little more than beasts of burden. By 1925, practically every state had some form of workman's compensation legislation, and subsequent measures extended the control of working conditions and the responsibility of employers. Today, the U.S. Public Health Service, the U.S.

Bureau of Mines, the U.S. Department of Labor, the Armed Services, state and local health agencies, and even nongovernmental agencies, such as industrial hygiene associations, medical societies, labor organizations, and various health and welfare organizations, are directly or indirectly concerned with the promotion of industrial health.

These comments by Dr. Hugh Garland epitomize in simple terms industrial medical problems.[4]

"It has already been stated that there is no field of medicine which offers greater scope for prevention than the industrial medical field . . . . The late Sir Thomas Legge . . . after much practical experience in the field of prevention enumerated the following now famous axioms:

> Unless and until the employer has done everything—and everything means a good deal—the workman can do next to nothing to protect himself, although he is naturally willing enough to do his share.
>
> If you can bring an influence to bear external to the workman (i.e., one over which he can exercise no control), you will be successful; and if you cannot or do not, you will never be wholly successful.
>
> All workmen should be told something of the danger of the material with which they come into contact, and not be left to find it out for themselves—sometimes at the cost of their lives.

[4]Garland, H.: *Medicine,* St. Martin's Press, Inc., New York; and The Macmillan Co., of Canada, Ltd., 1953.

ATMOSPHERIC POLLUTION

Atmospheric pollution is becoming an increasingly greater hazard in major cities of the world, and unless drastic measures are taken to curtail it, it will become worse instead of better because of steadily expanding mechanization. *Smog* is the heavy, low-lying layer of air, compounded of smoke plus fog, and containing all the other air pollutants which rise from an urbanized center. According to experts analyzing our air, metropolitan inhabitants are daily breathing in an unsavory and distinctly unhealthy mixture of such things as soot, tiny cinders, ground-up paper, wood slivers and cloth fibers, lime, paint specks, cement,

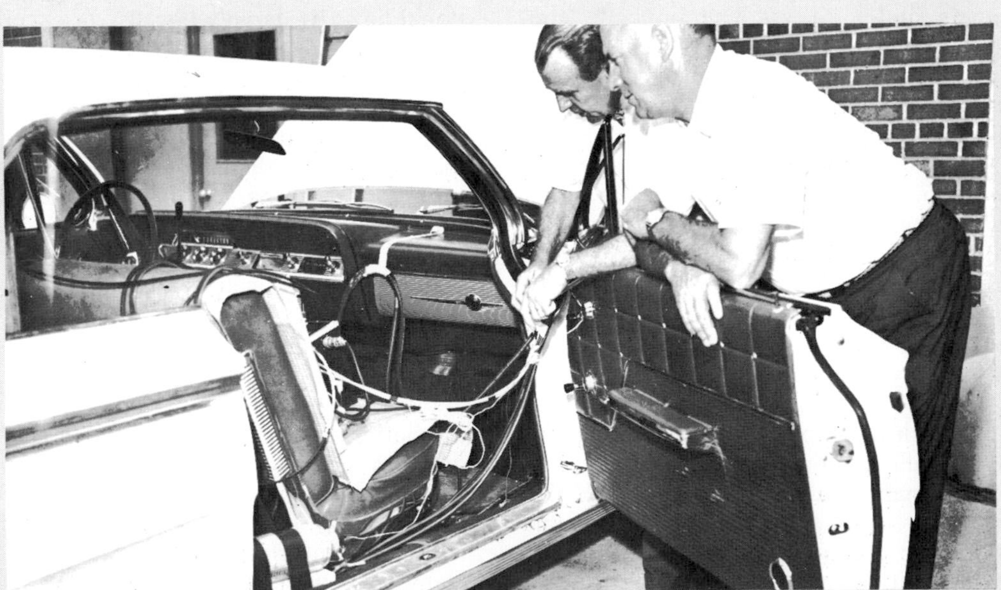

An increasingly important part of sanitary engineering is the control of air pollution, especially in large cities where there are many automobiles and industries. This automobile, at a United States Public Health Service Sanitary Engineering Center, is being used in a study of the causes and prevention of smog. It has special instruments that collect exhaust fumes for scientific study.

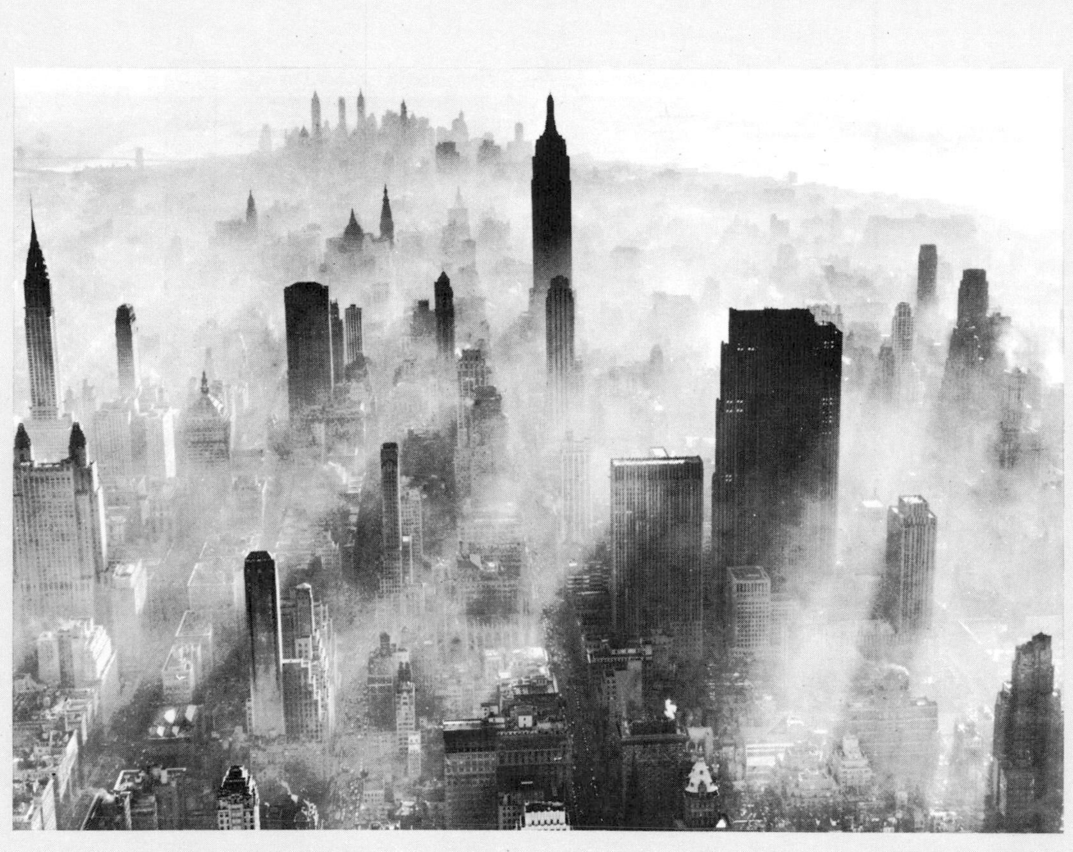

Air pollution in Manhattan, New York City, on an otherwise clear day. Most urban air pollution comes from automobiles, buses and trucks, heating furnaces, and factories.

and a variety of gaseous and finely suspended solid chemicals. Automobile exhaust, smoke from homes and industries, fires from burning leaves, and erosion of all types are contributory factors. Weather conditions also profoundly influence the layering of this dirty air over cities.

Even on foggy days, enough sunlight penetrates the smog to convert some of the floating gases into quite toxic substances, and authorities in this field are agreed that peroxides and ozone derivatives produced in this way are a very serious source of danger.

When the concentration of ozone in the air reaches 0.1 parts per million (ppm) there is an adverse effect on growing green plants, and at 0.2 parts per million, the damage becomes severe. Ozone levels of 0.1 ppm are not uncommon in Los Angeles, which has been especially troubled by the smog problem in recent years. The first "smog alert" there is called at 0.5 ppm, and this requires that all but the most essential traffic be halted. It is reached several times a year but, fortunately, rarely lasts more than a few hours. According to Clarence A. Mills, exposure to 0.5 ppm for less than four hours is harmless, but when the level exceeds 1 ppm for this period of time, it is probably hazardous.[5]

[5]Mills, C. A.: Respiratory and cardiac deaths in Los Angeles smogs, *American Journal of Medical Science, 233*:379, 1957.

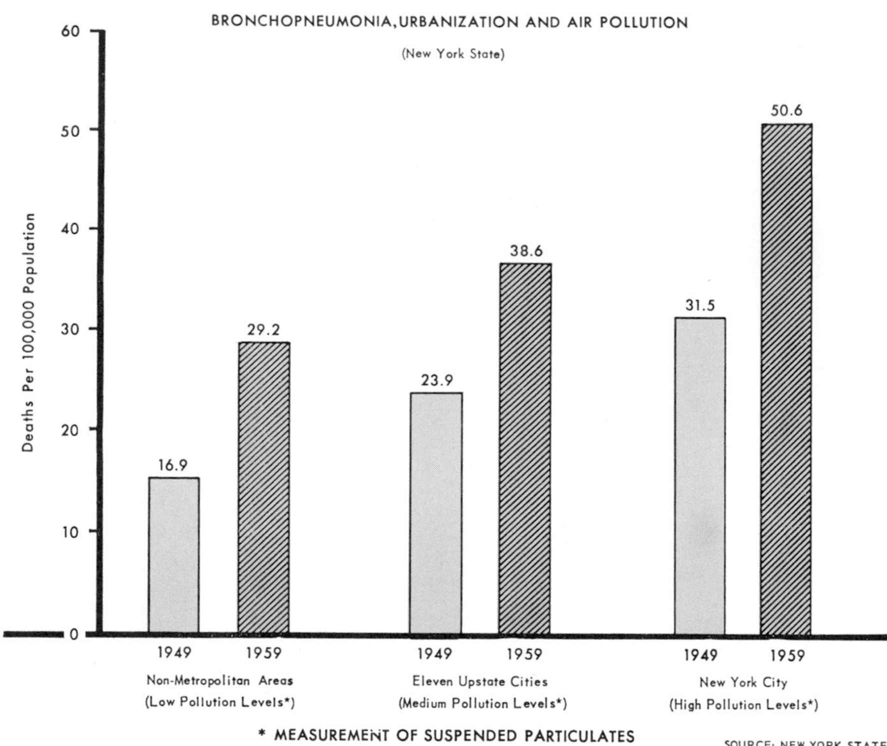

Figure 31–18. Rising bronchopneumonia death rates are associated with an urban factor, of which air pollution is probably a part. (From Hilleboe and Larimore: *Preventive Medicine.* 2nd Ed., Philadelphia, W. B. Saunders Co., 1965.)

The economic losses from atmospheric pollution—fuel waste, paint and cement damage, increased bills for cleaning and structural maintenance, and erosion of all types by corrosive chemicals in the air—are tremendous. Crop damage in the United States is in the millions: $5 million in the Los Angeles area alone and at least $1 million in San Francisco. However, the danger to human health is of even greater concern. Physicians close to this problem feel that smog is responsible for, or even aggravates, eye and respiratory tract irritations, asthma, chest pain, coughs, and shortness of breath. Older people are especially sensitive.

Although this has not been proved in humans, smog has also been implicated in cancer; experimental animals develop skin and lung cancer when exposed to, or injected with, atmospheric pollutants.

The cumulative effects of smog on man are unknown. But it might be relevant to consider that it wasn't until the growth rate of seedlings in the Los Angeles area was *reduced one-half* that anyone took notice of smogs there and realized that air pollution was responsible.[6]

Physicians in areas with only one major industry have commented that when the plant was on strike there was a marked drop in the number of respiratory complaints. As soon as work—and atmospheric pollution—resumed, the colds, coughs, and bronchitis returned.

If the problem involved nothing more serious than minor respiratory disturbances, we would not be so concerned about atmospheric soiling as a major public health problem; however, it is infinitely more dangerous. In the latter part of October 1948, the steel town of Donora, Pennsylvania, scarcely noticed the heavy haze which settled over the area because dirt and smoke were commonplace there.

[6]Went, F. W.: Air pollution, *Scientific American,* *63*:192, 1955.

But as the days went by, the haze thickened because warm air over the bowl-like valley prevented the smoke from rising upward, and instead it rolled along the ground, blending with particles of moisture in the foggy air. By the time the wind finally blew the smoke out of the valley, 20 people had died of serious respiratory illnesses and thousands more were ill.

The tragedy that hit London in December, 1952, was far worse. An extremely heavy, low-lying fog mixed with smoke to make a smog that transformed day into night, seeped into homes, and filled the hospitals of London with its choking, coughing victims. The smog hung over the city for a week, and when it finally dissipated, an estimated 4000 people were dead.

In most cases, such serious situations as those in Donora and London are due to unusual atmospheric conditions which trap the smoke and fog, and make a blanket of dirty air called an "inversion" layer settle over the city. According to H. A. Leedy, president of the Midwestern Air Pollution Prevention Association of Chicago:

> Contrary to popular belief, the largest contributor to air pollution is not industry. It is the individual who complains the most—the resident . . . . The thousands of homes and small apartment furnaces, and the millions of automobiles, trucks and buses produce far more pollution than does industry.

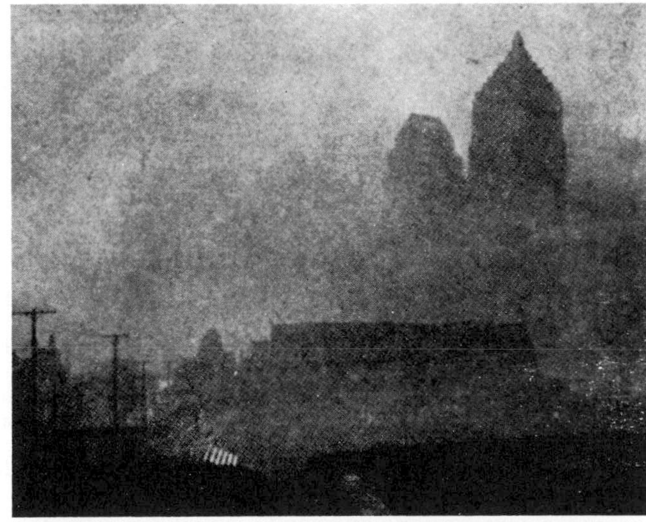

Pittsburgh in winter of 1946. Laws regulated industrial smoke, but home owners continued to burn soft, smokey coal.

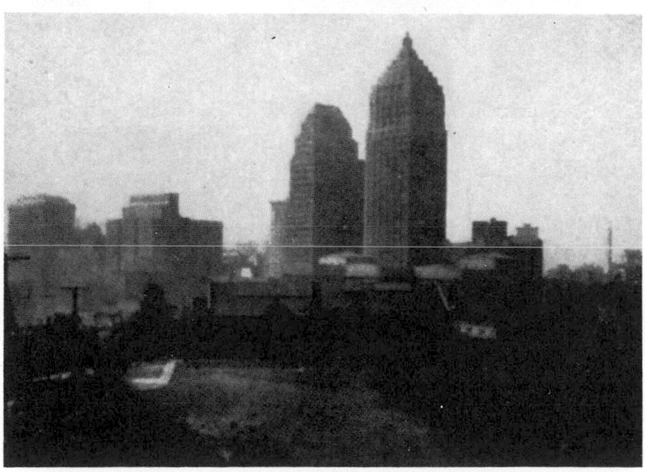

Pittsburgh, 1947. Same view shows how tighter antismoke law banning all use of soft coal cleared up city's smog. (Courtesy of Wide World Photos, Inc.)

Figure 31–19. Smoke reduction in Pittsburgh, Pennsylvania.

Fortunately, most major cities have become aware of the serious health menace of smog, and some are taking strong steps to correct it. The success of united community action in solving this problem is dramatically illustrated by what has happened in Pittsburgh, notoriously the "smoky city" ever since it became highly industrialized and a major consumer of soft coal. A comprehensive control program, started in 1941 and interrupted by the war, was resumed in 1946, under the guidance of the United Smoke Council. All consumers were required to employ either smokeless fuel or stokers which prevented smoke production. By the winter of 1947 the typical day-long smogs of Pittsburgh winters were eliminated, and a slow but steady diminution continued over the years. Today Pittsburgh is an outstanding example of what united community activity and pressure can achieve in preventing atmospheric pollution. It has become remarkably clean for a highly industrialized metropolis, and has achieved a dramatic diminution in soot and dustfall. The economic and health benefits are incalculable, and Pittsburgh residents can now justly boast of their city's striking beauty. Pittsburgh's fuel bill increased somewhat when control measures were instituted, but an estimated $25 million in annual cleaning bills alone was saved.

Cities must have clean air to survive. Stringent air-control regulations have become almost as important to our health as water commissions and sanitation laws.

Following the lead of the cities and states that recognized the dangers of air pollution and took action, the Federal Government began to move. In the Clean Air Act of 1963, new Federal responsibilities were recognized in controlling and combating the contamination of the atmosphere. (In the same year, incidentally, there was a new emphasis on the control of water pollution, including new research grants and funds for the construction of eight new water pollution laboratories.) The effects of air pollution have long been noted, and the relationship between a contaminated atmosphere and poor health has been extensively studied recently. The unlikelihood of escape from this condition, by means other than control at the source, is pointed up in a recent book, *Preventive Medicine,* by Dr. Herman E. Hilleboe and Dr. Granville W. Larimore:

> The air over many cities of the world fosters growing intra-urban deserts where human habitation is undesirable, vegetation is sparse and scrubby, and property is in a state of deterioration. The bulging suburbs provide no escape. The ex-urbanite's automobile, his leaf and trash burning, the nearby smoking dump, and the bus- and truck-choked arterial roads that keep his community alive are creating serious problems in the most countrified developments.

Questions

1. Describe how public health activities help protect your health during the course of a day.
2. What are some of the aims of the World Health Organization?
3. Do you think that, given truly adequate financial support, the World Health Organization could eradicate almost all widespread infectious diseases in the backward countries?
4. What are some of the health areas covered by the Department of Health, Education and Welfare?
5. What are the responsibilities of the National Institutes of Health?
6. Describe some of the activities of the health department in your own city or county.
7. Was the Salk vaccine a completely original discovery, or did it depend on earlier scientific work?
8. Define "smog" and describe its dangers to health.
9. What shifts in emphasis can you see in the work of the Public Health Service?
10. What professions, besides medicine, contribute to the health of the public? In what ways?
11. Do some services offered by the federal, state, and community governments overlap? Is this a wasteful duplication of effort?
12. What health services does your own community provide? What others do you think it should provide? Do you think your fellow citizens would be willing to pay for additional public health facilities and personnel?
13. From your own observation, what are some of the problem areas in which the Food and Drug Administration works?
14. Can you trace the development of some other vaccine, as the development of the Salk and Sabin vaccines was traced in the text?
15. List the sources of funds for medical research in the United States today and the approximate percentages of the total contributed by each.
16. What are the three most dangerous areas of work, in terms of accidental deaths and disabling injuries?
17. What are some of the substances that pollute the atmosphere?

Topics for Discussion

Investigate activities of at least one of the voluntary health agencies mentioned in this chapter.

Contributions of unionism to healthful working conditions.

Contributions of pharmaceutical houses to medical research.

Activities of professional medical societies.

The fairness of asking prisoners to volunteer for hazardous experiments in medical research.

Influence of WHO on international cooperation in other areas.

Areas of public health that you think demand more attention and funds.

Strictness or laxity of state licensing practices.

Increase in fund-raising agencies and public reaction.

Desirability of a central fund-raising administration.

Desirability of federal control of *all* medical research.

Contributions of nonphysicians to advances in medical knowledge and public health protection.

Adequacy of workmen's compensation laws.

New hazards in industry resulting from new technology.

Problems associated with rising population.

Reading Suggestions

Preventive Medicine, H. E. Hilleboe and G. W. Larimore. W. B. Saunders Co., Philadelphia, 1965. A useful reference book.

Eleven Blue Men, Berton Roueche. Berkley Publishing Co., New York (paperback), 1965. This is an absorbing, humorous, informative account of true medical mysteries many of which were solved by public health experts. The title derives from the account of eleven men in various parts of New York City who developed poisoning of their red cell hemoglobin after eating contaminated food in the same restaurant.

Voluntary Health and Welfare Agencies in the United States, Robert H. Hamlin. Schoolmasters' Press, 1961. A study of philanthropy in America, as expressed through the voluntary health and welfare organizations.

Better Communications for Better Health, Helen Neal (ed.). Columbia University Press, New York, 1962. A discussion of problems and aspects of communications in the overall field of health.

An Introduction to Public Health, H. S. Mustard and E. L. Stebbins. Macmillan, New York, 1959.

Control of Communicable Disease in Man: An Official Report, 9th Ed., The American Public Health Association, 1960.

Communicable Disease Control, Gaylord W. Anderson, Margaret G. Arnstein, and Mary R. Lester. Macmillan, New York, 1962.

Our Synthetic Environment, Lewis Herber. Knopf, New York, 1962. Advances in science also have brought new dangers, and some of them affect us with every breath. The author describes and discusses some menaces of a synthetic world.

Administration of Community Health Services, Eugene A. Confrey (ed.). International City Managers' Association, Chicago, 1961.

The World Health Organization: Its Global Battle against Disease, Albert Deutsch. Public Health Affairs Pamphlet, 1958.

Civilization and Disease, Henry E. Sigerist. University of Chicago Press, 1961. A detailed account of the influence of disease on various aspects of civilization.

Silent Spring, Rachel Carson. Houghton Mifflin, Boston, 1962. By now, a classic account of the dangers of the indiscriminate use of insecticides to wildlife and to ourselves.

The United States and the World Health Organization: Teamwork for Mankind's Well-being. Senate Subcommittee on Reorganization and International Organizations, April 1961. An excellent summary of health problems in many countries and of the work of WHO and the United States in trying to resolve them.

The Public Health Service—Background Material Concerning the Mission and Organization of the Public Health Service, 1963. A survey of the programs, activities, and organization of the United States Public Health Service, prepared for the Interstate and Foreign Commerce Committee of the House of Representatives.

Health Care for the Community, John B. Grant. Johns Hopkins Press, Baltimore, 1963.

The Family: A Focal Point in Health Education, Iago Galdston, International Universities Press, New York, 1961. The relationship of health education to the activities of the family in many of its aspects.

Regionalization and Rural Health Care, Walter J. McNerney and Donald C. Rudel. University of Michigan Press, Ann Arbor, 1962. A detailed account of an unusual experiment, in which three health centers and two hospitals in a rural area worked under a regional agreement.

Radiological Health Practices, American Public Health Association, 1959.

Airborne Infections. Richard L. Riley and Francis O'Grady, Macmillan, New York, 1961.

Let's Clear the Air, National Conference on Air Pollution. U.S. Public Health Service, 1962.

The Poisons in Your Food, William Longgood. Simon & Schuster, New York, 1960.

The Function of Food Additives, J. F. Mahoney. American Journal of Public Health, *51*:1101, 1961.

Radiation: What It Is and How It Affects You, Jack Schubert and Ralph E. Lapp. Viking Press, New York, 1957.

Motor Vehicles, Air Pollution and Health, a Report of the Surgeon General, U.S. Department of Health, Education and Welfare, Washington, 1962.

Air Pollution and Medical Research, J. R. Goldsmith. Science, *141*:832, 1963.

The Troubled Air, U.S. Public Health Service Publication 977, December 1962.

Fish and River Pollution, J. R. Erichsen Jones. Butterworth & Co., London, 1964.

The Breath of Life, Donald E. Carr. Norton, New York, 1965. Discusses the problem of polluted air, which the author considers as serious as nuclear fallout.

Does Overpopulation Mean Poverty? Joseph M. Jones. Center for International Economic Growth,

Washington, 1962. An authoritative presentation of facts about population growth and economic development.

The Time Has Come, John Rock. Knopf, New York, 1963. A distinguished physician, who happens to be Catholic, discusses some means of ending the battle over birth control.

People—Challenge to Survival, William Vogt. William Sloane Associates, New York, 1960.

On Population, essays by Thomas Malthus, Julian Huxley and Frederick Osborn. New American Library of World Literature, New York, 1960. Malthus' classic essay (1830) is included with essays by two contemporary authors.

The Population Ahead, Roy G. Francis, ed. University of Minnesota Press, Minneapolis, 1958. The population growth and the problems it presents are examined by nine scholars in this field.

Population, Evolution, Birth Control: A Collage of Controversial Readings, Garrett Hardin. San Francisco. Freeman. A representative selection of short articles from the literature on population, with teaching notes.

Catholics and Birth Control: Contemporary Views on Doctrine, Dorothy Dunbar Bromley. Devin-Adair, New York. The author, not a Catholic, presents a carefully documented survey of the published views on the birth control controversy.

What Are the Facts about the Population Crisis? National Health Education Committee, New York (paperback). Single copies free on request.

Health in Industry, Donald Hunter. Penguin Books, Baltimore, 1959.

Accident Facts, National Safety Council, Chicago, 1964.

The Health of People Who Work, A. Q. Maisel. National Health Council, New York, 1959.

Accident Prevention, by the Program Area Committee on Accident Prevention. McGraw-Hill, New York, 1961.

32

RADIATION: BENEFITS AND HAZARDS

Radioactive compounds have been known for about 60 years, and their use in medicine for both diagnosis and treatment has been of immeasurable value. The nuclear era, which started when we first learned how to split the atom and release its energy and radioactivity, is much more recent. Yet in a short period of time we have made tremendous advances in understanding both the beneficial and harmful aspects of atomic energy.

From the time man first made fire, he had to learn to master every new source of energy in order to take the greatest advantage of it, and, at the same time, protect himself from its hazards. This is also true for atomic power.

There has been so much publicity in the past few years about the dangers of x-rays and other sources of radiation, that many people have become very anxious and actually refuse to submit to *necessary* x-rays that their doctors recommend. As R. H. Chamberlain, Professor of Radiology at the University of Pennsylvania, has pointed out:

> This attention is worthwhile . . . for there are hazards . . . that need careful control. It is equally important that no misconceptions or exaggerations . . . prevent any patient from receiving the great benefits in modern medical care that derive from . . . x-rays and other ionizing radiations.[1]

Radioisotopes are made in the nuclear reactor (or pile) by splitting uranium-235 and other atoms. With this technique, scientists have already made about 900 radioisotopes of the elements which are found in nature. The most important in medical diagnosis and therapy are radio-

[1]*Medical Use of Ionizing Radiations,* Modern Medicine, Sept. 1, 1958.

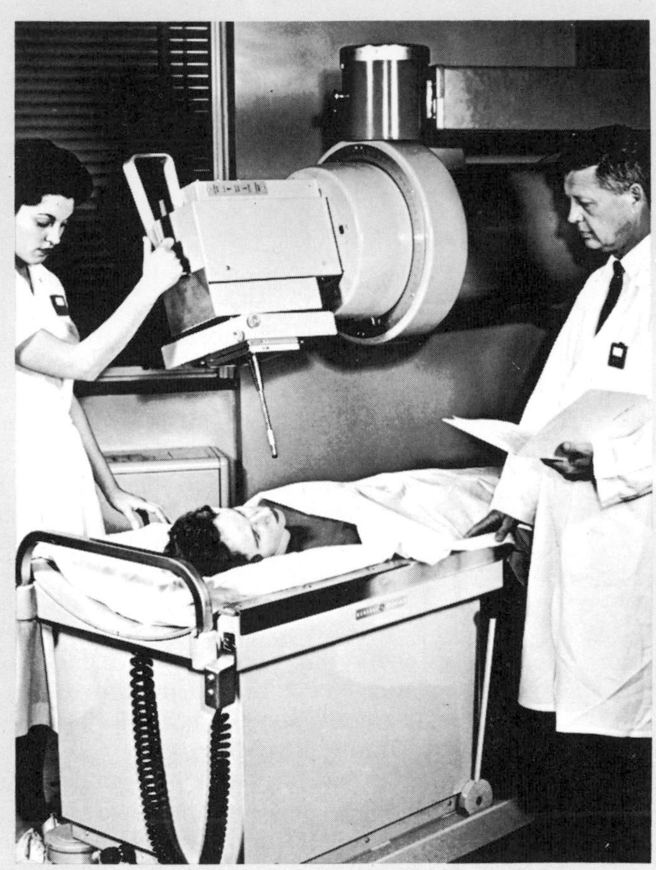

A cancer patient is about to receive radiation therapy from a medium-sized X-ray machine. This form of treatment has been of help to a great many people with various types of cancer.

active *cobalt* (cobalt-60), which is used to destroy cancer cells, and *iodine-131*, employed chiefly for the diagnosis of thyroid disease, and the treatment of cancer of the thyroid and overactive thyroid gland. *Phosphorus-32* has proved to be valuable in localizing brain tumors and in the therapy of chronic leukemia, and *gold-198*, in cancer of the prostate gland.

Radioactive cobalt has been called "the poor man's radium": a rod of cobalt-60 half the size of a cigarette costs $21,600 and its radioactivity is equivalent to 4 pounds of radium, which sells for *36 million dollars*. This isotope has made it possible for hospitals with only moderate means to use intense radiation therapy against cancer. With cobalt-60, a beam of very high energy, equivalent to a three million volt x-ray machine, can be focused directly on the tissue to be irradiated.

RADIOACTIVE SCANNING

One of the most dramatic diagnostic tools available to medical science today is the photoscanner. This instrument makes it possible to take a picture of the radiation distribution in various organs of the body. From this picture, your doctor can determine how well your various organs are functioning. For example, if a certain radioactive chemical does not reach a part of your lung, it may indicate a pulmonary embolism; if gold-198 fails to accumulate

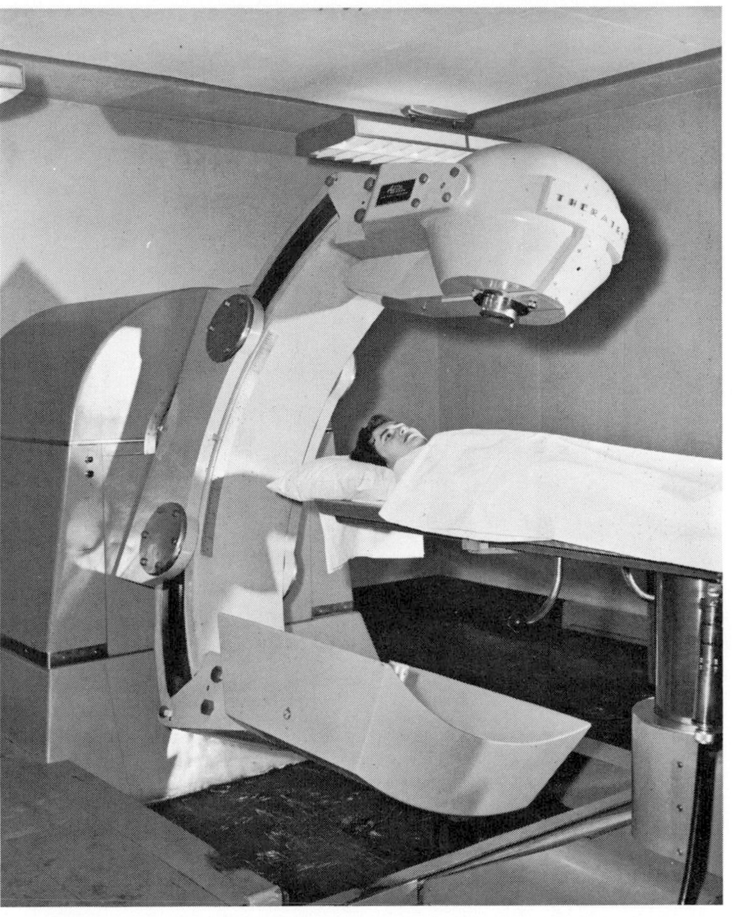

Figure 32–1. Cobalt irradiator. The cobalt element is housed in a lead cylinder in the head of the unit. The C shaped unit rotates a full 360 degrees around the patient, who lies flat. (Courtesy of the American Cancer Society.)

in a spot in your liver, a tumor may be suspected; or if a certain chemical concentrates in a specific area of the brain, it may indicate a tumor in that area. Currently, the photoscanner is used to scan the brain, thyroid, parathyroid, lungs, heart, liver, spleen, kidneys, and bones.

HOW MUCH RADIATION ARE WE EXPOSED TO?

One of the unfortunate features of radioactive emanations is that their effect is cumulative and adds up over the years. It stays with us—like poisoning by lead. Scientists have calculated that over a 30 year period—say from infancy to age 30—we absorb on the average 4.3 R from the natural background, 3 R from diagnostic x-rays and fluoroscopy, and at present, 0.1 R from weapons-testing.[2] However, if nuclear tests continue, the latter effect would be multiplied 25 times, and amount to about 2.5 R. In radiation for therapeutic purposes, the situation is quite different, of course; as much as 6000 R may be used on *very limited* areas of the body, but only the area irradiated is damaged.

HAZARDS OF RADIATION

According to a nationwide survey of public health officers conducted by the American Public Health Association, "Radiological health is the most important newly emerging public health problem."

[2]The roentgen (R) is a measure of the effect of radiation; it is the amount of radiation that produces 1.6×10^{12} ion pairs per gram of air.

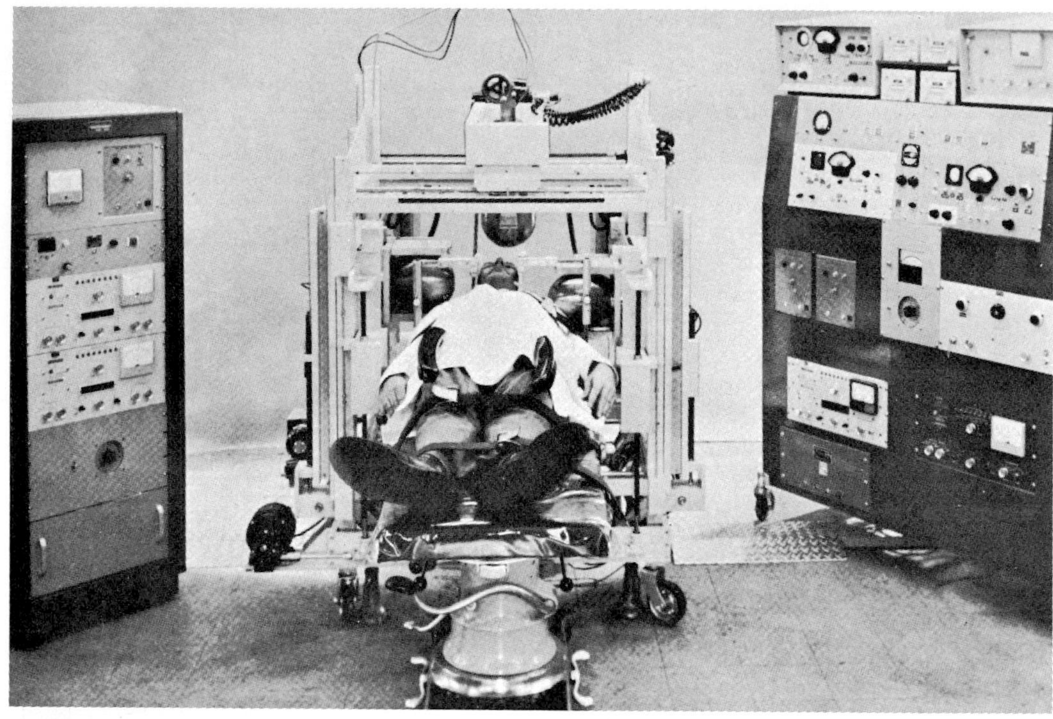

Figure 32–2. The Tetrascanner–a unique device in use at National Institutes of Health–scans four areas of brain simultaneously to detect tumors. Greater quantities of radioactive material (radioiodinated human serum abumin) are absorbed by tumorous tissue, making this a valuable diagnostic aid. The most important advantage of this device is that it is much faster than conventional scanners. (From Tressel, G. W.: *Today's Health,* May, 1965.)

It is estimated that by 1970 at least 1200 radiological health experts and 4000 radiological technicians will be needed in the United States.

Established facts are that exposure of the entire body to 800 R causes certain death, and 400 to 600 R carries with it a 50/50 chance of dying. Lower levels, 30 to 80 R, produce *genetic damage* and double the number of defective children, causing mental deficiency, epilepsy, vision and hearing defects, and malformations of various kinds–skeletal, neuromuscular, skin, blood, and endocrine organs. Other hazards are the *shortening of the life span* and *malignancies.*

Genetic Damage

Numerous studies on experimental animals–from fruit flies to the higher mammals–have shown that radiation damages the genes, and this damage is then transmitted from generation to generation. We now have ample evidence that human beings are at least as sensitive as lower animals: a study of 98 pregnant women living within a 2000 meter radius (about a mile) of the center of the Hiroshima and Nagasaki atomic explosions, showed that less than one-fourth of their infants were born alive and normal; miscarriages and stillbirths occurred in 23 per cent; one-fourth of the infants who survived the neonatal period had congenital abnormalities, including mental retardation.

Because of the disturbing information which has accumulated, the Committee on Genetic Effects of the National Academy of Sciences has recommended that during the first 30 years of life, reproductive tissue–the gonads–should not receive more than 10 R of man-made radiation plus the 4.3 from natural background

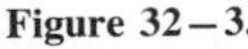

Figure 32–3.

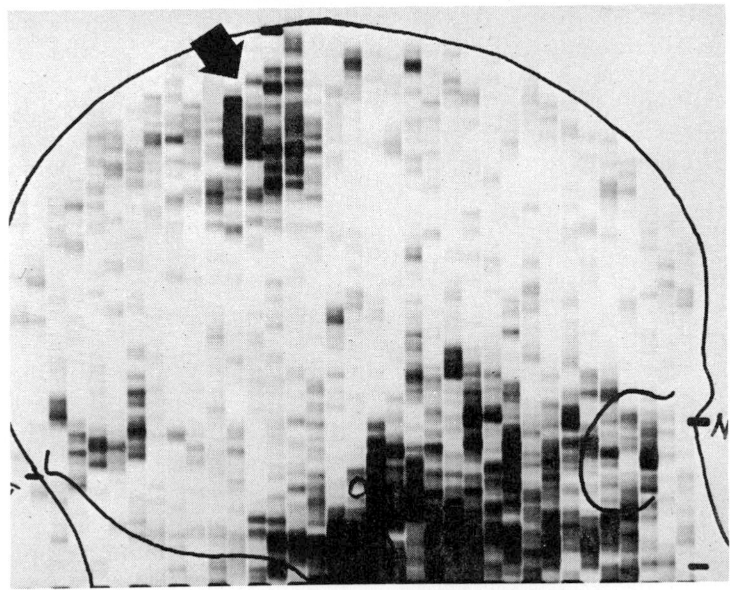

Figure 32–3. Film recordings made by brain scanner. In a patient with choriocarcinoma, the tumor is detected *(arrow)* 24 hours after injection of the isotope. Other dark areas are normal patterns. (From Tressel, G.W.: *Today's Health,* May, 1965.)

Figure 32–4.

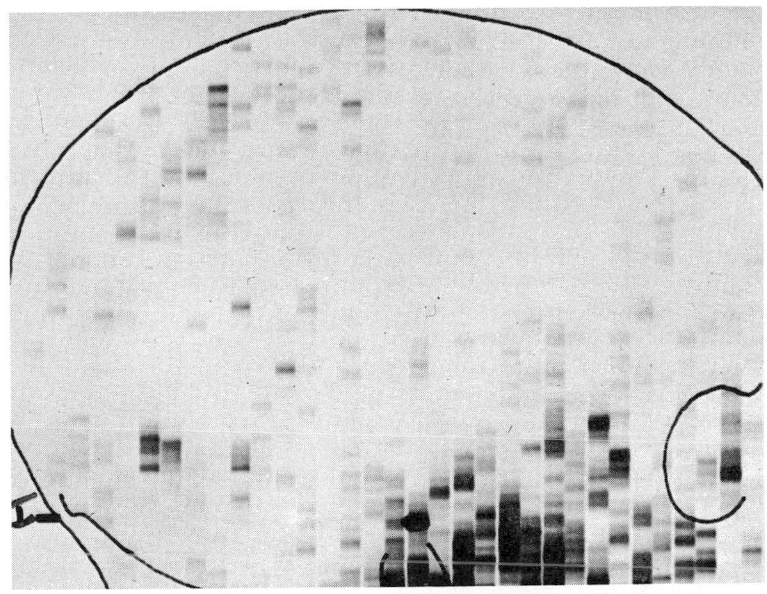

Figure 32–4. Same patient after chemotherapy. (From Tressel, G.W.: *Today's Health,* May, 1965.)

sources.[3] However, according to experiments conducted by Michael A. Bender, of Johns Hopkins University, even 10 R may be too high.

Bender studied the amount of damage sustained by pure cultures of human cells after exposure to only 25 and 50 R and found many changes in the chromosomes. He concluded from his experiments that the danger to human genes is "much higher than that which has been generally assumed to occur for such low doses. In fact, the present experiments . . . lend great weight to the belief . . . that there is no 'safe' dose of radiation."[4]

Unfortunately, as Wendell G. Scott, Professor of Clinical Radiology at Washington University School of Medicine has pointed out:

> In genetic damage to the reproductive cells, the hereditary defect will be present in every cell of the offspring to whom it is transmitted via (either the) egg or sperm, and no tissue can escape the consequences of the defect. The sole safeguard in each of such cases is the general probability that the set of genes inherited from the other parent will not carry the same defective gene.[5]

Effect on Life Span

Douglas Grahn, an Atomic Energy Commission scientist, has calculated that every roentgen of radioactivity absorbed from fallout in testing will shorten the average length of life as much as 12 days. From the fallout which has already been deposited in soil and water, the average person will absorb approximately 1 R, which represents a few days to two weeks off his life. However, if nuclear testing should continue, this could reach a level as high as 8 R, which means one to three months off his life. Most of this so-called somatic damage (which means effect on the whole cell rather than the chromosomes) is attributed to strontium-90, the long-lived isotope which gets into food and ultimately reaches the bones, where it is stored for a long time.

[3]*Biological Effects of Atomic Radiation.* Report to the Public. National Academy of Science-National Research Council, *Science, 124*:60, 1956.

[4]Medical Science, September 15, 1957.

[5]Radiation Hazards, *Journal of the American Medical Association,* May 23, 1959.

In 1959 the little island of Saltholm in Denmark—which fortunately, has only 22 inhabitants—suffered a minor tragedy because of radioactive fallout. The inhabitants were ordered by the government to stop drinking rainwater, their only source of fresh water, because it had reached a level four times greater than was considered the danger point. This increase resulted from Soviet and American weapons testing in distant areas.

Malignancies

For reasons unknown, there has been an increase in the incidence of leukemia in the past 20 years, and many experts suspect that part of this may be related to the expansion of diagnostic radiology and radiation treatments for various diseases. It has been well known for a long time that in experimental animals irradiation in sufficiently high amounts will lead to leukemia. U.S. radiologists, who are using radiation techniques constantly, reportedly die ten times as often from leukemia as do other groups of physicians.[6] In addition, physicians have reported that many more than the expected number of leukemia cases developed in patients who had received radiation for ankylosing spondylitis (a form of arthritis), and in infants and children who were irradiated to reduce enlarged thymus glands.[7, 8]

Another disturbing report is that children born to mothers who received radiation exposure to the abdomen for diagnostic reasons during pregnancy developed twice as many cases of leukemia as did the controls.[9] There is also evidence that cancer of the thyroid increases markedly in patients who received thymus irradiation

[6]March, H. C.: Leukemia in radiologists, *Radiology, 43*:275, 1944.

[7]Court-Brown, W. M., and Doll, R.: Hazards to man of nuclear and applied radiations, Medical Research Council, London, 1956.

[8]Simpson, C. L., Hemplemann, L. H., and Fuller, L. M.: Neoplasia in Children Treated with X-rays for Thymic Enlargement, *Radiology, 64*:840, 1955.

[9]Stewart, A., Webb, J., Giles, D., and Hewitt, D.: Malignant Disease in Childhood and Diagnostic Irradiation in Utero, *Lancet, 2*:447, 1956.

as infants and children, or x-ray treatment for other benign conditions of the head and neck.[10]

How to Reduce Hazards from Radiation

In the United States alone, 38 million x-rays are made every year for diagnostic purposes, and for the most part, they are indispensable for better understanding of how to treat the disease. There are no indications, in general, that when x-rays are taken by experts and with all precautions, the patient receives excessive amounts of radiation. However, now that scientists are stressing the fact that there may be *no such thing as a completely harmless dose of radiation,* radiologists are becoming even more cautious. In a sense, as Walter D. Claus of the Atomic Energy Commission has stated, the *maximum permissible dose* is a philosophical concept, and represents an estimate of what people can afford to pay, in terms of potential personal damage, for the benefits of x-rays and other types of radiation.

We should certainly *not* refuse to be x-rayed when such tests are needed in treating and curing disease. However, as the Genetics Panel of the National Academy of Sciences pointed out in their report, "Medical authorities of this country should initiate a vigorous movement to reduce the radiation exposure from x-rays to the lowest limit consistent with medical necessity; and in particular that they take steps to assure that proper safeguards always be taken to minimize the radiation dose to the reproductive cells." Most x-ray specialists are in full agreement with these warnings, and the following program has been urged to reduce hazards in this area:

1. Use common sense and *never* pressure your doctor into taking x-rays. He knows when they are necessary.
2. Tuberculin testing, instead of repeated x-rays, should be used to detect tuberculosis, especially in young people under 20. X-rays are recommended only when the tuberculin test is positive, to determine whether the disease is active.
3. Fluoroscopy should be employed only when it is definitely required for diagnosis.
4. X-rays are *not* necessary to measure the pelvis of a pregnant mother, in order to determine the ease of delivery. There are other methods available, which do not subject the gonads of the fetus as well as of the pregnant woman to radiation hazards.
5. Dental x-rays should be taken only when necessary, and not routinely. The new type of panoramic dental x-ray machine developed at the National Bureau of Standards, which photographs the entire mouth on a single film, reduces exposure to x-ray tremendously.
6. Fluoroscopic machines should *not* be used to fit shoes. In 1957, more than 10,000 such shoe-fitting machines were used by 40,000 shoe salesmen with no professional experience in the administration of radiation. In some surveys, as many as 85 per cent of these machines were defective, and some of them were found to be operating at *three times* the radiation level recommended as safe by the National Academy of Science. Their use has been banned in the State of Pennsylvania, and perhaps other states will soon recognize this danger, too.
7. X-ray should be employed for therapy (different from *diagnosis,* because much larger amounts of radiation are necessary) only when the disease is more serious than the potential hazard of the x-ray. For example, it should not be used to reduce the size of the thymus gland in children.
8. Many luminous watch dials deliver far more radiation than is consistent with safety, because the luminous paint is radioactive. Unless you are assured that there is no significant radiation hazard in such a watch, you might be better off buying another type.

Questions

1. Contrast the beneficial effects of medical x-rays with some of the dangers.
2. How are radioisotopes employed in medicine?
3. How can excessive isotopic and x-ray radiation affect future generations?

[10]C. L. Simpson, L. H. Hemplemann and L. M. Fuller, *op. cit.,* p. 840.

Topics for Discussion

Radioactive isotopes of medical importance.

Radium dial painters (as discussed in *From Hiroshima to the Moon,* by Daniel Lang, Simon & Schuster, New York, 1959).

Training and duties of radiologist.

Hiroshima today.

Reading Suggestions

A Report of Fallout in Your Food, Roy Hoopes. The New American Library of World Literature, New York, 1962. The effect of fallout on the world's food supply is discussed in an easy-to-understand fashion.

Nuclear Energy As a Medical Tool, George W. Tressel. Today's Health, May 1965, p. 50. An excellent article with good illustrations.

Fallout, Food and Man; Report of Symposium at Meeting of Federation of American Societies for Experimental Biology. Science, June 21, 1963.

Genetics in the Atomic Age, Charlotte Auerbach. Essential Books, Fair Lawn, N.J., 1956. A very readable short volume reviewing essential concepts of genetics and the effect of radiation on hereditary characteristics.

Radiation: What It Is and How It Affects You, Jack Schubert and Ralph E. Lapp. Viking Press, New York, 1957. A sound, thoughtful presentation of the problem by two experts.

Film

Diagnosis and Therapy With Radiation. This film deals in a semitechnical manner with all aspects of atoms-for-peace research. It is available without charge from 10 AEC film libraries.

PROMISES OF HEALTH FOR THE FUTURE

Medicine has certainly kept pace with advances in other sciences, and we can anticipate that the future will bring even greater improvements in our health and longevity than have the past 50 years. Perhaps eventually, with all nations working together through the World Health Organization, all communicable diseases will be eradicated. Certainly the day isn't too far distant when practically all infectious disease will be under control. The marvellous bonus to this is that preventing the after-effects of disease—rheumatic heart disease, Bright's disease and the like—would reduce tremendously the number of serious chronic ailments which now bedevil mankind. And when these chronic diseases do develop, despite our best efforts to prevent them, the use of treatments now available, and perhaps even better treatments in the future, will quickly return patients to a normal life.

Inflammatory conditions such as appendicitis will in most cases probably be controllable by medicines, and no longer require surgical intervention. We have already seen this happen with mastoid infections.

Many of the problems attending embryonic development will be solved in coming years. We have learned that radiation, nutritional deficiencies, certain infectious diseases and chemical agents are responsible for some developmental defects, and, knowing this, we can already prevent some of these hazards. Exposure of girls to German measles before they reach the childbearing age eliminates the dangers from this disease. Perhaps we will find other hazardous viruses against which we can vaccinate and halt any deleterious effect to the developing baby.

Infant and maternal mortality have dropped steadily through the past five decades, and there is no reason to anticipate that this decline will not continue. Understanding the reasons for premature births and making it possible for all mothers to carry their babies to term will sharply reduce neonatal deaths.

We can look forward to some reduction in hereditary diseases by greater acceptance of the science of eugenics and its aids to marriage counseling. Some, like hemophilia, we can already control even when they do develop. We will lose much of our fear of gene-linked diseases when we realize that they are often no worse than, and sometimes no different from, diseases which are acquired after birth, and can be controlled just as well. The future will undoubtedly bring techniques for supplementing and correcting defective enzyme systems in genes.

Despite a tremendous research push, we do not yet possess a truly curative agent for cancer, but we can already save or prolong many lives by the medicines, surgical techniques, and radiation therapy we now have available. It is extremely likely that more effective medicines will be developed, and it is even conceivable that entirely new treatments for cancer will emerge from present-day research. For example, if viruses prove to be responsible for some human malignancies, it may be possible to immunize against them as has been done so successfully with polio.

We know today that certain forms of mental disease or the predisposition to them are of genetic origin, and that others appear to result from emotional stresses during early childhood. We have also learned that some drugs and medicines can induce mental aberrations under special conditions, emphasizing the possibility that mental disease may result from a change in body chemistry or metabolism. If this proves true, we may before too long learn what these defects are and correct them with the proper supplements or medicines. We also have a tremendous body of knowledge relating to the emotional environment which shapes our children into stable, resourceful adults. When all this knowledge is generally applied, mental illness will show a sharp decline.

The time may come when we will be able to replace hopelessly diseased organs by normal, functioning ones. Already we can successfully transplant parathyroid glands, arteries, corneas, bones and teeth. In a number of instances, one of a pair of identical twins suffering from advanced and incurable kidney disease has been saved from certain death by successful implantation of a normal kidney from the other identical twin. If we succeed in solving some basic problems in the field of tissue transplantation, the way will be clear for a complete set of spare parts—including the heart, lung, kidneys, and other organs and tissues!

In medical research laboratories, new ideas are being born which will some day shape into realities beneficial to all mankind. They will materialize even more quickly if we provide all possible support for research into the cause and cure of disease, and for implementation and use of the knowledge attained.

FILM SOURCES

FILM SOURCES

Because teaching films become obsolete rapidly and new ones are being added constantly, we present the following list of *sources* for films to supplement a college course in health.

The Educational Film Guide, published by H. W. Wilson Co., 950 University Avenue, New York 52, N.Y., includes a listing of health films, published annually and kept up-to-date with monthly supplements. Information on each film includes type and length, synopsis of content and general evaluation.

Blue Book of Non-Theatrical Films, published periodically by Educational Screen and Audio-Visual Guide, 2000 Lincoln Park West Building, Chicago 14, Ill.

Educators' Guide to Free Films, published by Educators' Progress Service, Randolph, Wis.

Health Education Series, Text-Film Department, McGraw-Hill Book Co., Inc., New York 36, N.Y.

A List of Sources of Films on the Subject of Health is available from the Council on Scientific Assembly, Motion Pictures and Medical Television, American Medical Association, 535 N. Dearborn Street, Chicago, Ill.

INDEX

Page numbers in **bold face** indicate illustrations. Page numbers followed by the letter "t" indicate tabular information.